Histopathological Atlas of the Inner Ear

Dalian Ding · Peng Li · Weidong Qi ·
Jianhui Zhang · Haiyan Jiang · Liling Li

Histopathological Atlas of the Inner Ear

WORLD PUBLISHING CORPORATION

Springer

Dalian Ding
Balance and Auditory Research Center
Department of Otolaryngology-Head and Neck Surgery
University of Mississippi Medical Center
Jackson, MS, USA

Weidong Qi
Department of Otolaryngology Head & Neck Surgery
Huashan Hospital Fudan University
Shanghai, Shanghai, China

Haiyan Jiang
Balance and Auditory Research Center
Department of Otolaryngology-Head and Neck Surgery
University of Mississippi Medical Center
Jackson, MS, USA

Peng Li
Department of Otolaryngology Head & Neck Surgery
The Third Affiliated Hospital of Sun Yat-Sen University
Guangzhou, Guangdong, China

Jianhui Zhang
Department of Otolaryngology and Head and Neck Surgery
The Third People's Hospital of Chengdu
Chengdu, Sichuan, China

Liling Li
Department of Otolaryngology Head & Neck Surgery
The Third Affiliated Hospital of Sun Yat-Sen University
Guangzhou, Guangdong, China

ISBN 978-981-95-6337-1   ISBN 978-981-95-6338-8 (eBook)
https://doi.org/10.1007/978-981-95-6338-8

Jointly published with World Publishing Shanghai Co., Ltd
The print edition is not for sale in China (Mainland). Customers from China (Mainland) please order the print book from: World Publishing Shanghai Co., Ltd.

This Springer imprint is published by the registered company Springer Nature Singapore Pte Ltd.
The registered company address is: 152 Beach Road, #21-01/04 Gateway East, Singapore 189721, Singapore

Foreword

It is an honor for me to join Professor Ding Dalian's team in the creation of this work, which has been yet another invaluable learning opportunity for me. Earlier this month, while organizing my emails, I discovered that Professor Ding and I have exchanged nearly 400 letters since 2013. As this manuscript nears completion, I would like to express my deepest admiration and gratitude toward him, though my words may fall short of capturing the full extent of my respect.

My initial impression of Professor Ding came from his published articles, monographs, and the training courses he conducted. At that time, my understanding of him was vague, yet I was deeply struck by his rigorous pursuit of truth and his unwavering dedication to otological research. It was not until I entered his laboratory that I truly came to know him. In late February 2014, my flight to Buffalo was delayed due to weather, and by the time I landed, it was already 10 p.m. As I stepped out of the airport, I saw Professor Ding waiting at the arrival gate from afar, and my anxiety from the long journey instantly melted away. In a foreign land, amidst Buffalo's icy winter, his quiet presence was profoundly comforting. From that moment on, a profound mentor–student bond and an unforgettable friendship began—one that has deeply shaped my academic and personal journey.

With a distinguished career spanning over five decades, Professor Ding has made seminal contributions to otological research, authoring more than 420 scientific publications and 240 conference abstracts presented both domestically and internationally. His work has profoundly influenced multiple generations of researchers, and his lifelong dedication has been instrumental in advancing China's morphological studies of the inner ear. Professor Ding belongs to the youngest cohort of the "Laosanjie" (1968 junior high school graduates). Although technically a junior high school graduate, his formal education was abruptly interrupted in 1966 due to the socio-political upheavals of the time, leaving him with only an elementary-level education when he was sent to the countryside as an "educated youth." Professor Ding's remarkable path has seen him assume diverse roles—farmer, sanitation worker, nurse, laboratory technician, and chief technologist—each undertaken with unwavering determination despite formidable challenges. Undeterred by adversity, he then embarked on a decade-long intellectual odyssey, devoting all his evenings and weekends to relentless self-improvement. Through night schools, he systematically completed secondary education curricula that historical circumstances had denied him in youth. His perseverance culminated in admission to the Department of Biological Engineering at Fudan University, where he earned his degree in genetics with an outstanding academic record (average score: 92/100). This achievement not only redeemed lost educational opportunities but also laid the foundation for his subsequent scientific contributions.

At the age of 60, through 4 years of persistent dedication, Professor Ding attained his PhD in biochemistry from the University of Tokyo—a testament to lifelong learning. On his return to Buffalo following the successful dissertation defense, I had the privilege of meeting him at the airport. During our ride back, he recounted his examination experience with uncharacteristic animation; his every gesture radiated a childlike delight that I found profoundly moving. This academic achievement held particular significance: for an established doctoral advisor like Professor Ding, pursuing this degree represented not a professional necessity but rather the realization of a deeply personal aspiration.

Professor Ding exemplifies scholarly dedication through his meticulous work ethic. Weekends invariably find him in the laboratory, where he methodically analyzes experimental results, composes research articles, and rigorously reviews manuscripts for both domestic and international journals. His hands-on involvement in every experimental procedure sets an uncompromising standard that inspires equal diligence among his students. Characterized by intellectual vitality and independence from conventional wisdom, Professor Ding demonstrates remarkable energy and decisive execution in research. He continuously refines experimental protocols during implementation, consistently yielding robust and reproducible findings. With characteristic humility, he often quips, "Smooth experiments sometimes require a bit of luck—perhaps I'm just frequently favored by fortune." Yet in truth, his apparent "luck" represents nothing less than five decades of accumulated expertise and tireless dedication—each success meticulously built upon profound scientific mastery and exhaustive effort.

Before leaving Buffalo, I meticulously compiled all of Professor Ding's publications into a personal digital library. I also prepared PowerPoint tutorials on confocal microscopy operation protocols and quantitative cellular damage curve analysis. Together with Gao Kelei and Jiang Haiyan, we recorded instructional videos documenting Professor Ding's specialized techniques in inner ear dissection and organ culture. These carefully prepared materials were presented to him as a farewell gift the day before my return to China, with the hope that they would both alleviate some of his teaching responsibilities and serve as valuable learning resources for future visiting scholars.

After returning home, Professor Ding and I maintained occasional contact through WeChat, yet for 10 years, we have preserved our tradition of email correspondence. I have kept every single letter we exchanged—each message vividly conveys his thoughtful guidance and unwavering support as a mentor, as well as the steadfast assistance and implicit trust of a true friend. As this manuscript approaches completion, I wish to express my deepest gratitude to Professor Ding, who has been both my teacher and friend, commanding both my respect and affection. I am certain that this rare and precious bond we share will endure forever.

Guangzhou, China
June 2022

Li Peng

Preface

Histopathological Atlas of the Inner Ear is a new work following our previous publications: Handbook of Anatomy and Inspection of the Inner Ear in Guinea Pigs, Morphology of the Inner Ear, and Science of the Inner Ear.

This unique atlas compiles approximately 800 high-quality images of the inner ear labyrinth, comprehensively showcasing the gross anatomy of the bony and membranous labyrinth of the inner ear as well as the microstructure under the light microscope and the ultrastructure under the electron microscope. Although many previous books have covered inner ear anatomy and pathology, this atlas provides more detailed physical images of these structures. In addition to exhibiting the standard images of the anatomical structure and histomorphological characteristics of the cochlea and vestibular sensory organs, this atlas also shows the evidence of a series of primary and secondary pathological changes in the sensory hair cells and the peripheral neurons. These changes were induced by various damaging factors. This atlas will illustrate some new scientific discoveries and academic views with the help of images and image captions. As pathology serves as an authoritative diagnostic tool in medical research, the pathological images and their image captions contained in this atlas are based on facts, clarifying the etiology, pathological process, pathological mechanisms, and lesion outcomes of damage to the inner ear. Thus, previously hidden and unique inner ear lesions are clearly revealed to readers.

This atlas is designed to bridge the gap between past findings and future advancements in inner ear research; enables researchers to better understand the underlying mechanisms and progression of inner ear disorders; and supports the diagnosis, treatment, and prevention of inner ear diseases with essential theoretical insights.

Jackson, MS, USA — Dalian Ding

Contents

About the Authors

Prof. Dalian, Ding, Ph.D., previously served successively in the Department of Otorhinolaryngology at Wuhan Union Hospital for 8 years, in the Otology Research Laboratory at Shanghai Second Medical University for 17 years, and at the Center for Hearing and Deafness at the State University of New York at Buffalo for 30 years. He is currently working at the Balance and Auditory Research Center in the Department of Otolaryngology–Head and Neck Surgery at the University of Mississippi Medical Center. Dr Ding graduated from Fudan University and the University of Tokyo. He has published more than 430 scientific articles and more than 200 international conference abstracts. The series of techniques for inner ear pathological research that he established or improved have been recognized and widely used by peers. He is praised by many peers as the man who drills into the inner ear.

Peng, Li MD, Ph.D., is a professor and chief physician serving as deputy director of the Department of Otorhinolaryngology and director of Otologic Surgery at the Third Affiliated Hospital of Sun Yat-sen University. He was a visiting scholar at the Center for Hearing and Deafness, University at Buffalo, State University of New York. Dr. Li specializes in otologic microsurgery and research on auditory and speech disorders, with extensive expertise in diagnosing and treating ear diseases, as well as performing microsurgical procedures for conditions such as otitis media and otosclerosis. He currently holds editorial board membership at the Chinese Journal of Otology and serves as the cochlear implant program director at his hospital. In addition, he holds several key positions in otological academic societies in Guangdong province. Dr. Li has led 10 national and provincial-level research projects and has published over 60 papers in SCI-indexed and core Chinese journals.

Prof. Weidong Qi, MD, is an otolaryngologist who has a special interest in ear and skull base disorders. He is the deputy director of the Department of Otorhinolaryngology (ENT)—Head and Neck Surgery at Huashan Hospital affiliated to Fudan University. He was a visiting scholar and postdoctoral fellow at the State University of New York at Buffalo (USA). His main research focus includes auditory neuropathy, drug ototoxicity and protection, and gene therapy for deafness. He is proficient in inner ear anatomy and inner ear morphology, as well as auditory electrophysiological techniques. He has published over 40 papers and edited two books.

Jianhui Zhang MD, Ph.D., director and chief physician of the Department of Otorhinolaryngology Head and Neck Surgery at Chengdu Third People's Hospital, Sichuan, China. Dr. Zhang received his medical degree from North Sichuan Medical College in 2002, followed by a master's degree in clinical medicine from the same institution in 2010. He completed his PhD in Otorhinolaryngology Head and Neck Surgery from Xiangya School of Medicine, Central South University, in 2018.

Dr. Zhang holds 12 academic appointments, including graduate supervisor at Southwest Jiaotong University, North Sichuan Medical College, and Southwest Medical University; chair of the Otolaryngology Head and Neck Disease Prevention Committee, Sichuan Preventive Medicine Association; standing committee member of the Otorhinolaryngology Head and Neck Surgery Society, Sichuan Medical Association; vice chair of the Otorhinolaryngology Committee, Sichuan Association of Integrative Medicine; and member of the National Clinical Research Center for Otorhinolaryngology Diseases (Minimally Invasive Head and Neck Surgery Group).

His research elucidates hearing loss and allergic rhinitis mechanisms, with parallel clinical excellence in cochlear implantation and ENT disorder management. A prolific scholar, he has published research in ten SCI journals and five leading field journals, in addition to contributing to Atlas of Inner Ear Histopathology (ISBN: 978-7-5232-1012-3, 2024). Dr. Zhang has performed Sichuan's first endoscopic transoral-nasal combined approach odontoidectomy (now established as a standard procedure). He also received the 2023 Sichuan Science and Technology Award (Third Prize) for his research on ototoxic deafness. As an active research supervisor, he currently mentors six postgraduate students, with two graduates already trained. He currently leads five government-funded research projects (provincial/municipal) as PI. Recognized as a leading authority in his field, Dr. Zhang continues to advance both clinical practice and research in otorhinolaryngology.

Haiyan Jiang has served as a technician, assistant laboratory technician, and experimenter in the Alpine Respiratory Physiology Laboratory and the Hypoxia Laboratory at the Shanghai Institute of Physiology from 1977 to 1997. Haiyan Jiang continued to work as a research technician in the Center for Hearing and Deafness Research at the University at Buffalo, State University of New York, from 1997 to 2021. After years of part-time study, Haiyan Jiang graduated from the Department of Bioengineering of Fudan University in 1989. Haiyan Jiang is proficient in a variety of inner ear science techniques, including laboratory animal auditory function testing, inner ear pathology examination, inner ear organ culture, and molecular biology testing of inner ear samples. To date, she has published 108 papers in domestic and international journals and 72 international conference abstracts. She has also been invited to participate in numerous international otology conferences in the USA and European countries.

Liling Li female, is a doctoral student in the Otorhinolaryngology program at Sun Yat-sen University, enrolling in 2024. Her research focuses on presbycusis, heavy metal ototoxicity, and drug-induced ototoxicity.

1 Anatomy of the Vestibular System

Prior to introducing the anatomical structure of the vestibular sensory organs, we begin with an overview of the general structure of the inner ear via a schematic diagram (Fig. 1.1). The color-coded schematic identifies key structural components: red denotes sensory hair cell regions, yellow indicates endolymph-containing spaces within the membranous labyrinth, light blue shows perilymph-filled areas between the bony and membranous labyrinths, and orange marks peripheral neuronal elements.

The membranous labyrinth resides within the bony labyrinth cavities of the petrous temporal bone, comprising the cochlear duct, vestibular organs (utricle and saccule), and semicircular canals [1–5]. The peripheral vestibular system specifically includes the saccule, utricle, and three semicircular canals, excluding the cochlear structures. Due to its deep encapsulation within the temporal bone, direct visualization of inner ear anatomy proves challenging. However, carefully grinding of the surrounding bone to fully expose the bony labyrinth reveals clear anatomical relationships and landmarks [2, 4, 6, 7] (Fig. 1.2). Micro-CT imaging provides additional three-dimensional visualization of both surface topography and internal cavities of the vestibular labyrinth (Fig. 1.3). In addition, when we further peel off the shell of the bone labyrinth, the entire membranous labyrinth will be fully exposed (Fig. 1.4).

1.1 Bony Vestibular Labyrinth

The vestibular cistern is the place where all the vestibular receptors gather. It is an irregular, hollow bony cavity that connects anteriorly with the cochlear scala vestibuli and posteriorly with the semicircular canals. The lateral bony wall of the vestibular cistern participates in forming part of the inner bony wall of the tympanic cavity. In the center of the lateral wall of the vestibular cistern, there is an oval-shaped opening called the oval window. The oval window was covered by the plate of stapes and sealed by surrounding annular ligament [1–5] (Fig. 1.5). On the medial wall of bony promontory of middle ear cavity in rats and mice, there is a stapedial artery passing between the anterior crus and posterior crus of the stapes. The round window niche is located behind the stapes artery [8] (Fig. 1.6). However, larger mammals such as chinchillas, guinea pigs, rabbits, and monkeys do not have this stapedial artery. The superior bony wall of the vestibular cistern participates in the formation of the bony wall at the bottom of the superior tympanum (Fig. 1.7). The inferior bony wall of the vestibular cistern participates in the formation of the skull base of the petrous part of the temporal bone. On the outside of the lower part of the vestibular cistern, an ampulla of the posterior semicircular canal and a single non-ampullary end of the lateral semicircular canal enter the vestibular cistern in turn from front to back. The medial bony wall of the vestibular cistern participates in the formation of part of bony wall of the internal auditory canal, and also partly participates in the separation of the vestibular cistern and the posterior cranial fossa.

In the center of the medial wall of the vestibular cistern, there is a vestibular crest that runs diagonally from the upper part of the front to the lower part of the back. A prominent vestibular crest traverses this medial surface obliquely from anterosuperior to posteroinferior, dividing two key recesses—the spherical recess (housing the saccule) anteriorly and the elliptical recess (containing the utricle) posteriorly. In the lower portion of the medial bony wall of the vestibular cistern, there is a secret opening called the vestibular aqueduct, which communicates with the endolymphatic sac via the endolymphatic duct in the bony slit behind the petrous portion of the temporal bone. The posterior opening of the bony slit in the petrous portion of the temporal bone containing the endolymph sac is tightly covered by the sigmoid sinus. The posterior bony wall of the vestibular cistern separates the vestibular cistern from the subarcuate fossa.

At the position where the posterior bony wall of the vestibular cistern forms an angle with the superior bony wall, the ampulla of the superior semicircular canal and the ampulla of

D. Ding et al., *Histopathological Atlas of the Inner Ear*,
https://doi.org/10.1007/978-981-95-6338-8_1

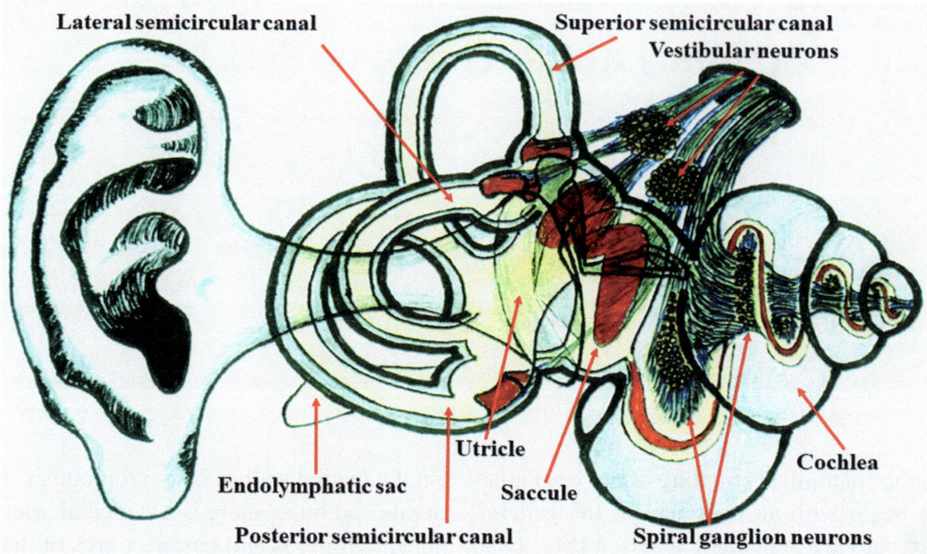

Fig. 1.1 Diagram of the anatomical structure of the ear. This diagram illustrates anatomical relationships from the external auditory structures to the internal auditory canal. The central region demonstrates four functionally distinct compartments of the inner ear: the red zone designates the sensory epithelia of both cochlear and vestibular end organs; yellow delineates the endolymphatic spaces of the membranous labyrinth; light blue identifies the perilymphatic compartment surrounding the membranous labyrinth; while orange marks the neural elements, including cochlear spiral ganglion neurons and vestibular ganglion cells

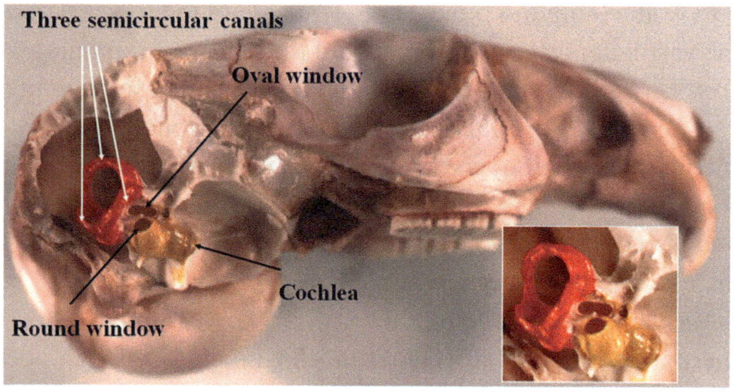

Fig. 1.2 Photo of the bony labyrinth in chinchilla. An electric drill is used to grind away the surrounding osseous tissue of the temporal bone of the chinchilla to fully expose the bony labyrinth. Labels indicate the three semicircular canals, oval window, round window, and cochlea. An inset provides a close-up view of these components, with the semicircular canals in red and the cochlea in yellow

the lateral semicircular canal enter the vestibular cistern from the top and the lateral, respectively. At the medial side of the lower part of the posterior bony wall of the vestibular cistern, the common crus formed by the confluence of the superior semicircular canal and the posterior semicircular canal enters the vestibular cistern[1–5, 9–14] (Fig. 1.8).

The three bony semicircular canals are located behind the vestibular cistern, forming three perpendicular hollow bony canals bent into two-thirds. Taking the chinchilla as an example, the lateral semicircular canal forms an angle of about 30°, the superior semicircular canal forms an angle of about 90°, and the posterior semicircular canal is roughly parallel to the horizontal plane.

In summary, the ampulla ends of the bony lateral semicircular canal and the bony superior semicircular canal enter the vestibular cistern at the upper part of the vestibular cistern, and the ampulla end of the bony posterior semicircular canal enters the vestibular cistern at the lower part of the vestibular cistern. The vestibular cistern has a total of seven openings, three of which are communicated with the ampullas of the three semicircular canals, one of which is communicated with a single nonampullated end of lateral semicircular canal, and another one is formed by the union of the nonampullated ends of superior and posterior canals and is termed the common crus. In addition, the largest opening facing the front of the vestibular cistern is communicated with the scala vestibuli of the cochlea, and the smallest opening at the lower portion of the medial wall of the vestibular cistern leads to the endolymph sac through the endolymphatic duct [1–5, 15].

1.2 Membranous Vestibular Labyrinth

The vestibular membranous labyrinth is a system of interconnected sacs and ducts within the vestibular bony labyrinth, which precisely matches the shape of the vestibular bony labyrinth. The vestibular membranous labyrinth is filled with endolymph, and the space between the vestibular membranous labyrinth and the vestibular bony labyrinth is filled with perilymph.

The vestibular sensory hair cell regions are distributed in five different locations within the vestibular membranous

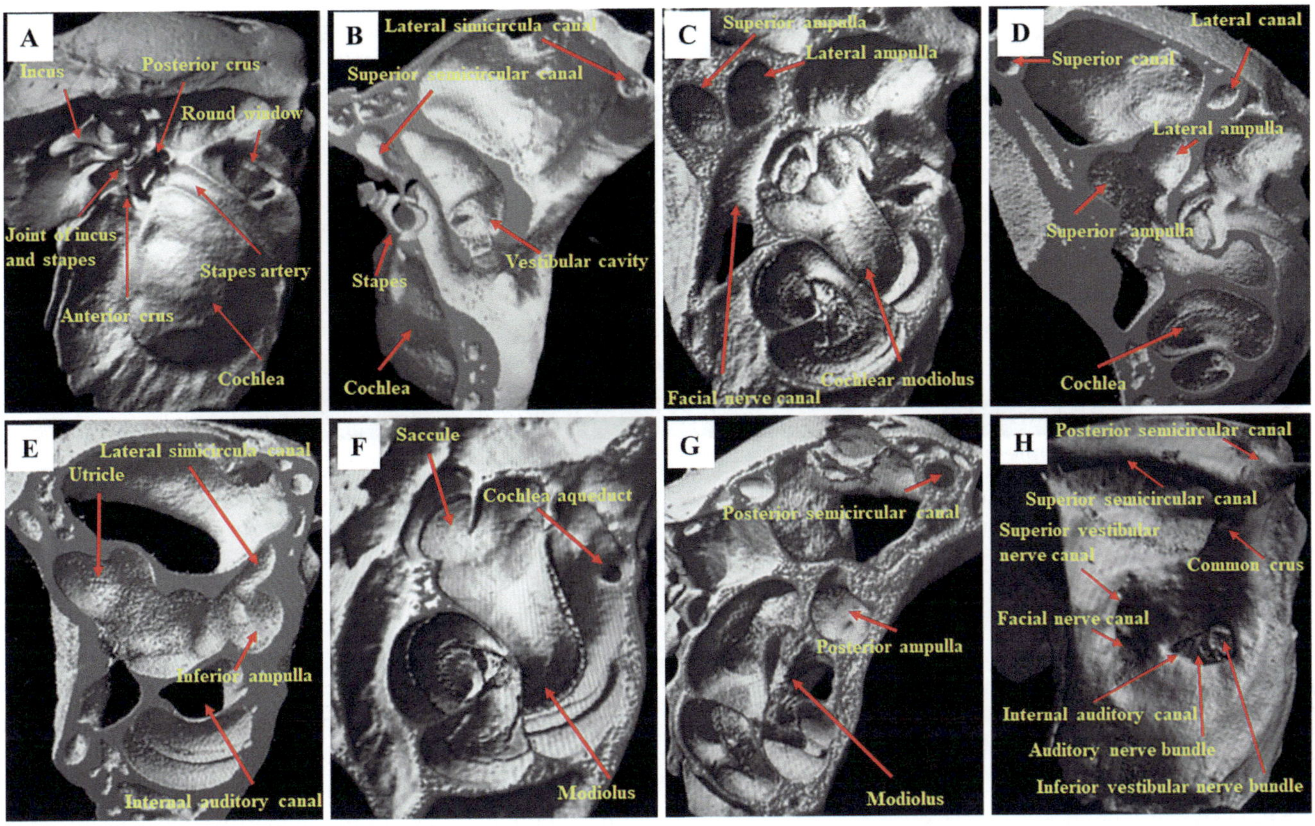

Fig. 1.3 An X-ray scanned 3D image of the mouse's inner ear cavity. The bony structure of the inner ear cavity in mice is displayed layer by layer in the horizontal or sagittal plane using X-ray scanning and 3D imaging technology of Micro CT. (**A**) A sagittal view of the medial wall of the tympanic cavity reveals the surface structure of the promontory. (**B**) A horizontal cross-sectional view at the top portion of the vestibule cavity reveals the structural spaces entering the superior aspect of the vestibule. (**C**) A sagittal section of the temporal bone reveals the structures of the ampullae of the superior and lateral semicircular canals, as well as the modiolus of the cochlea. (**D-H**) Sagittal sections of the temporal bone reveal at various levels, demenstrate the luminal structures of the cochlea and vestibule

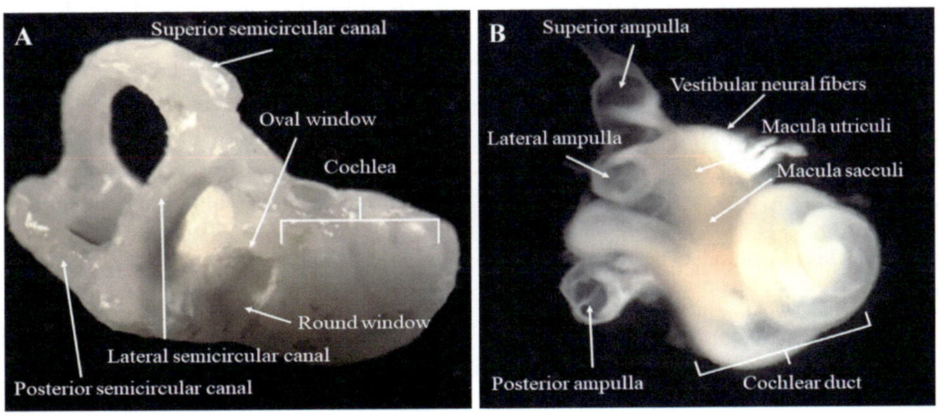

Fig. 1.4 Exposure of the entire bony labyrinth and the membranous labyrinth of the rat. (**A**) The entire bony labyrinth of the rat was exposed by grinding away the bone tissue surrounding the temporal bone with an electric drill. (**B**) The bony wall of the bony labyrinth was removed to expose the entire membranous labyrinth inside

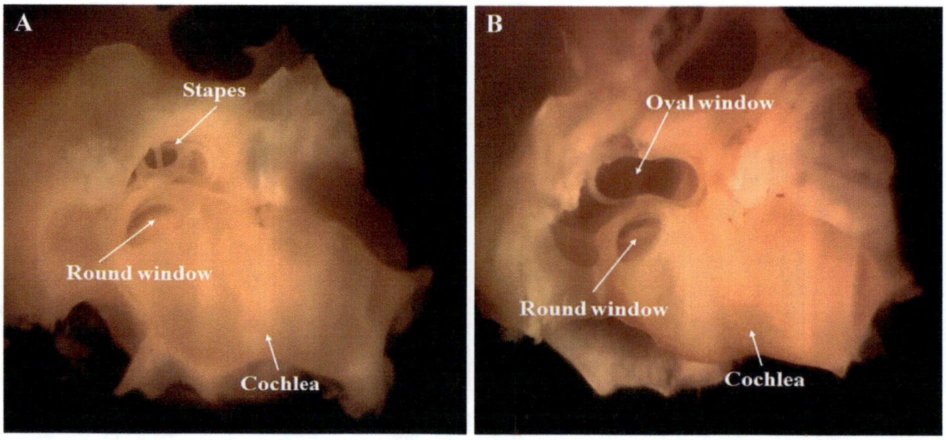

Fig. 1.5 Surgical exposure of the internal wall of the tympanic cavity in chinchilla. (**A**) The round window membrane seals the round window niche, while the stapes footplate occupies the oval window. A bony columella traverses between the anterior and posterior arches of the stapes, potentially serving to restrict stapes mobility and maintain its anatomical position. (**B**) After stapes removal, the saccular and utricular maculae become partially visible through the oval window opening

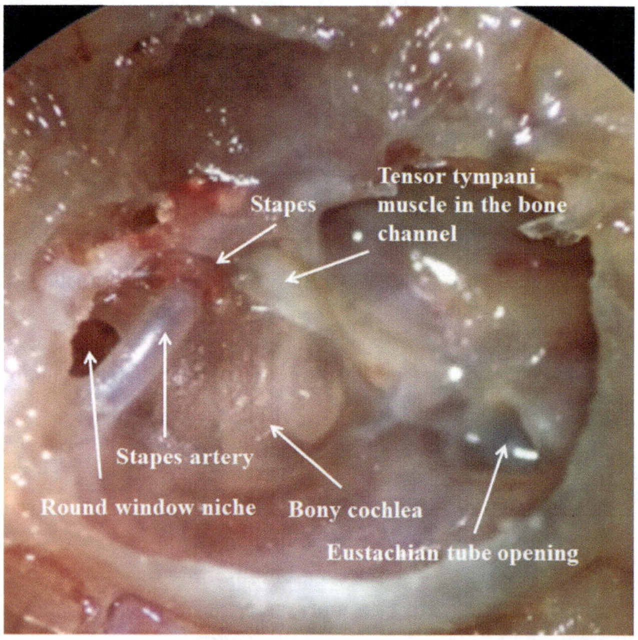

Fig. 1.6 Surface morphology of the medial wall of the tympanic cavity in the mouse. The stapedial artery passes between the anterior and posterior crus of the stapes, and the round window niche is partially covered by the stapedial artery. (Courtesy of Li et al. [8])

labyrinth, namely the saccular macula in the saccule, the utricular macula in the utricle, the crista within the ampulla of lateral semicircular canal, the crista within the ampulla of the superior semicircular canal, and the crista within the ampulla of posterior semicircular canal.

The vestibular sensory epithelium is composed of two layers of cells. The hair cells are located on the surface of vestibular end-organs, and the supporting cells are located at the bottom of the hair cells. The cuticular plate of the supporting cells is connected to each other to form a reticular membrane on the surface. The cuticular plate of each hair cell is embedded in a mesh of the reticular membrane, and its cuticular plate is flush with the cuticular plate of the supporting cells. There is one kinocilium and dozens of stereocilia in the ciliary bundle on the surface of the cuticular plate of each vestibular hair cell. The kinocilia are arranged at one end of the cuticular plate of vestibular hair cell. The stereocilia bundles are closely attached to the kinocilia and are located in the center of the cuticular plate. The consistent arrangement of kinocilia and stereocilia arrays determines the morphological polarization axis of vestibular hair cells, a critical determinant of its electromechanical transduction property [1–4, 16] (Fig. 1.9).

There is an arc-shaped area in the middle of the macula of saccule and the macula of utricle, respectively, termed the striola zone. The kinocilia of hair cells in the striola area are not arranged in a uniform direction, but on both sides of the striola region of macula of saccule and utricle, the location of kinocilia on hair cells is toward a different direction. The kinocilia on the hair cells in the marginal region of the macula of saccule face away from the striola, while the kinocilia on the hair cells in the marginal region of the macula of utricle face the striola [1–4, 16].

The kinocilia and stereocilia of vestibular sensory hair cells are firmly anchored into the otolithic membrane on the macula of saccule and utricle or inserted into the gelatinous cupula on the crista ampullae of semicircular canals. When a displacement of the otolith membrane or cupula occurs due to motion, head movement, or temperature-induced inertial flow, ciliary deflection causes depolarization (stereocilia bending toward kinocilia) or hyperpolarization (stereocilia bending away from kinocilia) of membrane potential of hair cells leading to release

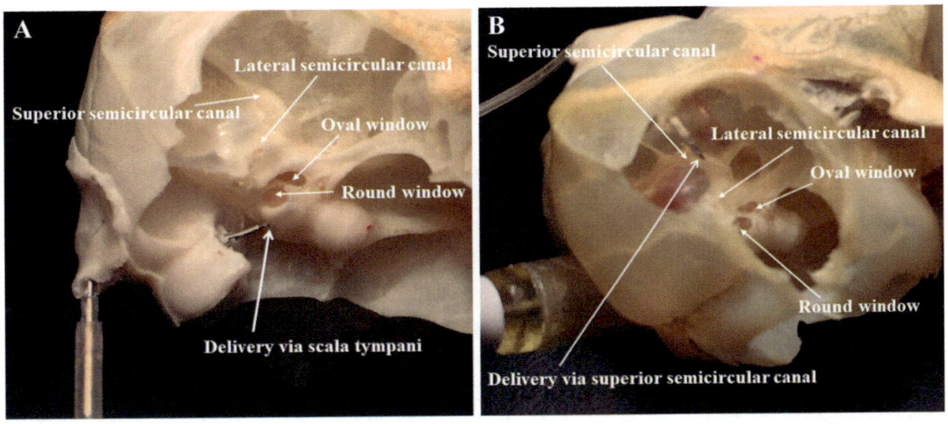

Fig. 1.7 Micro-osmotic pump implantation from the chinchilla tympanic cavity. (**A**) The pump catheter is inserted into the tympanic cavity through a surgical opening below the posterior tympanic cavity, and then inserted into the scala tympani of the cochlea through a small hole on the tympanic bony wall below the round window niche, enabling controlled chemical delivery for cochlear drug/gene therapy. (**B**) Alternatively, the pump catheter is inserted into the superior tympanic cavity through a surgical opening, and then advanced into the superior semicircular canal lumen or lateral semicircular canal lumen for targeted drug/gene delivery of vestibular therapy

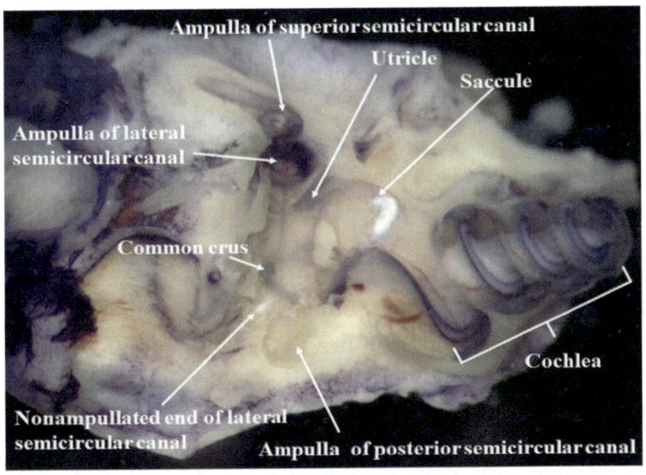

Fig. 1.8 The vestibular sensory epithelial areas and the cochlear membrane labyrinth were exposed by opening the bony lateral wall of the inner ear cavity in the guinea pig. (Courtesy of Ding et al. [14])

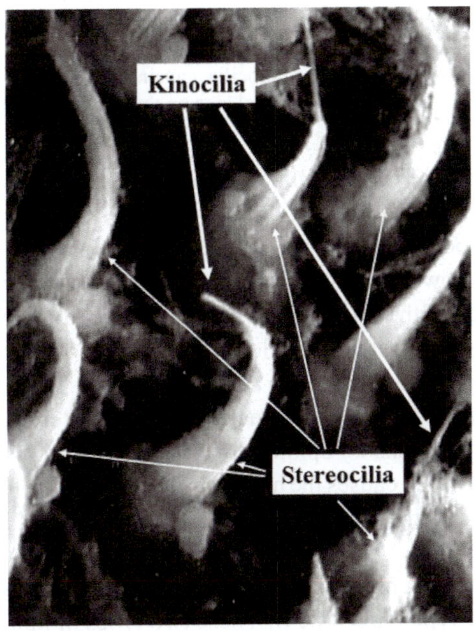

Fig. 1.9 Scanning electron micrograph of the cilia bundle of vestibular hair cells. The cilia bundle of vestibular hair cells consists of a single kinocilium (the tallest cilium) accompanied by multiple stereocilia of graded heights

of neurotransmitters and resulting in excitation or inhibition of vestibular ganglion neurons. When linear acceleration is perpendicular to the striola zone of the macula of saccule or utricle, the hair cells in the marginal areas at both sides of the striola will show completely opposite reactions: the hair cells located in the marginal zone on one side of the striola, their stereocilia bending toward the kinocilia will cause depolarization of the hair cells; while the hair cells located in the marginal zone on the other side of the striola, their stereocilia bending away from the kinocilia will cause hyperpolarization. This push-pull mechanism generates asymmetric neural firing patterns that propagate through vestibular pathways, enabling the central nervous system to precisely decode head position and movement [1, 4, 16, 17] (Fig. 1.10).

In the crista of the lateral semicircular canal, the kinocilia of all hair cells are toward the utricle, while the location of kinocilia on all hair cells in the cristae of the superior and posterior semicircular canals is toward the semicircular canal. Although the polarization of kinocilia of hair cells on each crista of ampulla is toward the same direction, since the shape of the crista is a horizontal saddle-shaped bulge in the ampullary cavity, when the overlying cupula is swinging with the flow of endolymph, the bundle of cilia inserted into cupula

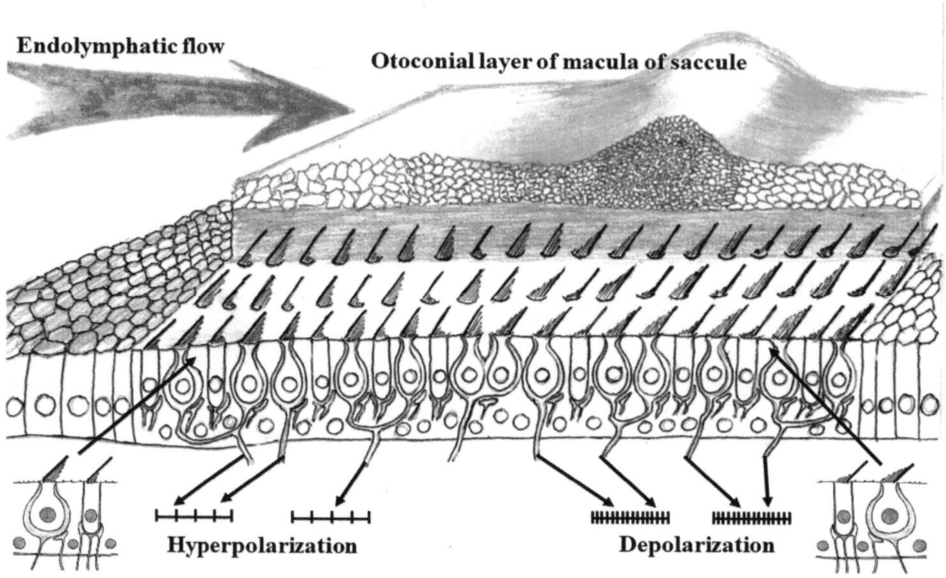

Fig. 1.10 Bidirectional mechanotransduction stimulation in the linear acceleration perpendicular to the striola zone of the saccule causes the hair cells in the marginal areas at both sides of the striola to produce opposite reactions. Taking the macula of saccule as an example, in the marginal area facing the acceleration source, the stereocilia of the hair cells deflected away from the kinocilia, causing the hair cells to hyperpolarize and inhibit. In the marginal area on the other side of the striola, the stereocilia deflection was toward the kinocilia, causing the hair cells to depolarize and excite. This asymmetric stimulation, occurring simultaneously in the same vestibular sensory organ, causes half of the hair cells to produce an inhibitory response and the other half to produce an excitatory response, allowing the body to accurately detect linear movements of the head. (Courtesy of Ding et al. [16])

on one side of crista will be deflected in the same direction of cupula. In contrast, the cilia of hair cells on the other side of crista occur in the opposite direction of bending due to a swirling flow towards the crista. Therefore, the hair cells on both sides of the crista of ampulla are in a completely opposite unbalanced state in which the hair cells on one side are excited and on the other side are inhibited. This means that the same direction of acceleration may produce different stimulus signals to the sensory epithelium on both sides of the crista of ampulla, which causes the hair cells on either side of the crista to emit diametrically opposite neural input signals [16] (Figs. 1.11 and 1.12).

Vestibular sensory hair cells can be divided into two different types, type I and type II. These two types of hair cells are different from the morphology of the cilia bundle, the shape of the hair cell body, and the synaptic connection of the afferent nerve and the efferent nerve [16, 18] (Fig. 1.13). While both type I and type II vestibular hair cells possess round cuticular plates bearing ciliary bundles, their stereociliary architectures differ significantly. Type I hair cells exhibit lusheng-shaped stereociliary arrays (resembling the Chinese reed instrument) with gradually decreased height from the kinocilia outwards (Fig. 1.13A). Conversely, type II hair cells display compact clusters of uniformly short stereocilia (Fig. 1.13B). These two distinct stereocilia morphologies are one of the reliable features for distinguishing hair cell subtypes [16] (Fig. 1.13C). The shapes of the soma of vestibular type I hair cells and type II hair cells are also completely different. The cell body of the type I hair cells is flask-shaped, while the cell body of the type II hair cells is cylindrical. Therefore, two different types of vestibular hair cells can be distinguished based on their body shape in vestibular sections [19–21]. In addition to the different morphologies of the cilia bundles and the shape of the cell soma, the afferent and efferent nerve connections to the type I and type II vestibular hair cells are also different. In the vestibular afferent system, the vestibular type I hair cells are located within unique wine glass-shaped afferent terminals from medium-to-large vestibular nerve fibers. The upper edge of the wine cup-shaped type I afferent nerve terminal is precisely aligned with the constriction neck of the type I hair cell, so that entire cell body of the type I hair cell, except its cuticular plate of the type I hair cell, is enclosed by the type I afferent nerve cup. In contrast, the type II afferent nerve terminals from the vestibular thin nerve fibers establish direct synaptic connections at the base of the type II hair cells. In the vestibular efferent system, the vestibular efferent nerve terminals below the type I hair cells only establish synaptic connections with the afferent nerve fibers below the type I afferent nerve cup, but do not contact directly with the vestibular efferent nerves connected to type II vestibular hair cells establish direct synaptic connections at the base of type II hair cells. These distinct innervation patterns provide additional criteria for differentiating hair cell subtypes [1–4, 16] (Figs. 1.13C and 1.14).

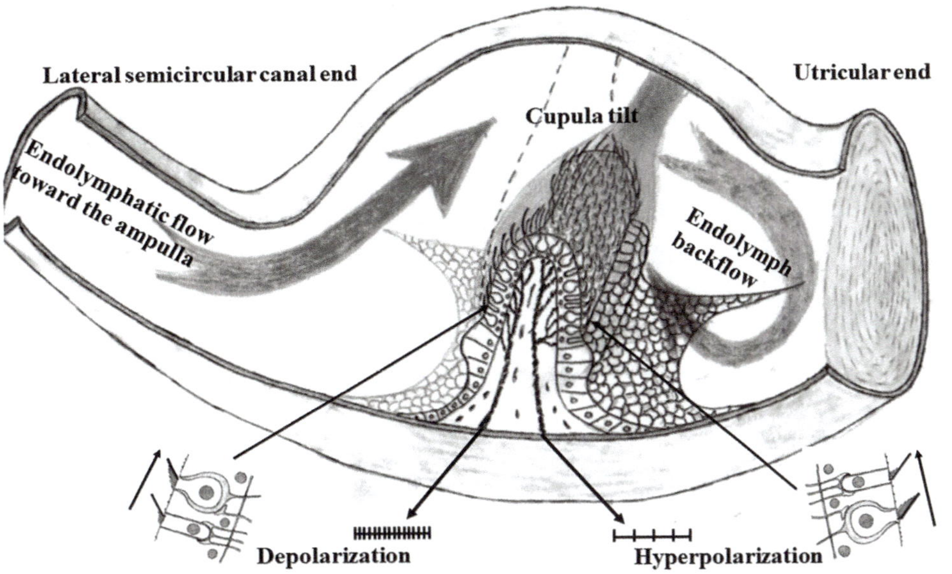

Fig. 1.11 Endolymph flow in the same direction causes the hair cells on both sides of the ampullary crista to produce opposite afferent nerve output signals. Using the lateral ampullary crista as an example, although the kinocilia of all hair cells on this crista are uniformly oriented toward the utricle, when the endolymph flows toward the crista and pushes the cupula in the direction of utricle, the dam-shaped crista and the above cupula block the endolymph fluid from flowing into the utricle. This causes the stereocilia of the hair cells facing the semicircular canals to be deflected toward the crista as the endolymph flows toward the crista. On the contrary, due to the vortex formed by the obstruction of the ampullary crista and cupula, the stereocilia of the hair cells on the other side of the ampullary crista facing the utricle will also be deflected toward the crista along with the vortex, causing the hair cells on both sides of the ampullary crista to synchronously release hyperpolarized and depolarized afferent nerve output signals respectively. This demonstrates that although the kinocilia of hair cells on both sides of the crista are arranged to the same direction, the saddle-shaped structure of the ampullary crista and the sealed swing of the cupula cause the fluid on both sides of the crista to flow to opposite directions, thereby causing the hair cells on one side of the crista producing excitatory stimulation signals, while the hair cells on the other side of the crista produce inhibitory stimulation signals. (Courtesy of Ding et al. [16])

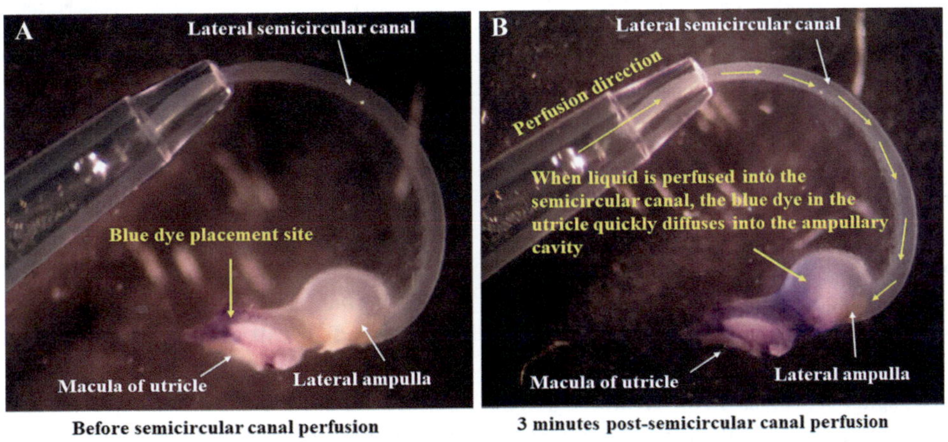

Fig. 1.12 Demonstration of fluid flow within the lateral semicircular canal. (**A**) The blue dye was placed in the utricle. (**B**) Three minutes after the colorless liquid was injected into the ampulla through the semicircular canal, the blue dye preplaced in the utricle quickly diffused from the utricle to the surface of the ampullary crista facing the utricle, suggesting that perfusion from the semicircular canal to the ampullary cavity can cause the fluid in both sides of the ampullary crista to flow toward this crista. (Courtesy of Ding et al. [16])

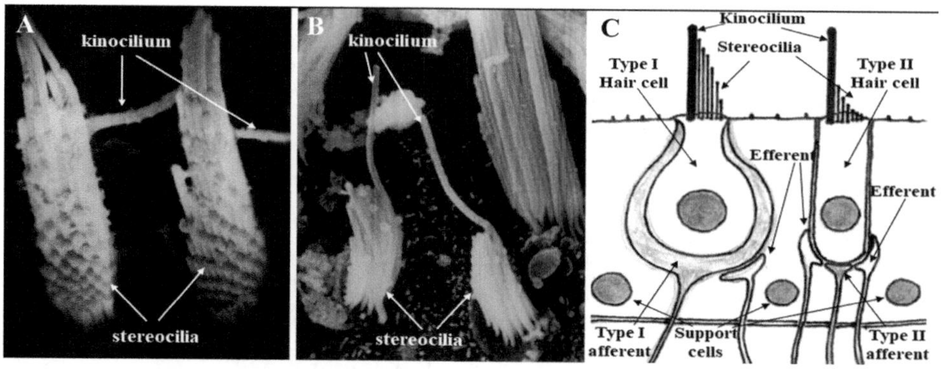

Fig. 1.13 Morphological differences between vestibular type I and type II hair cells. (**A**) Type I hair cells have kinocilia located on one side of the cuticular plate, with the length of the stereocilia decreasing in a stepwise pattern. (**B**) Type II hair cells also have kinocilia located on one side of the cuticular plate, but the stereocilia are only a short tuft. (**C**) Schematic comparison, highlighting key differential features: stereociliary structures, the soma morphology (flask-shaped vs. cylindrical), and the different afferent/efferent innervation patterns. (Courtesy of Ding et al. [16])

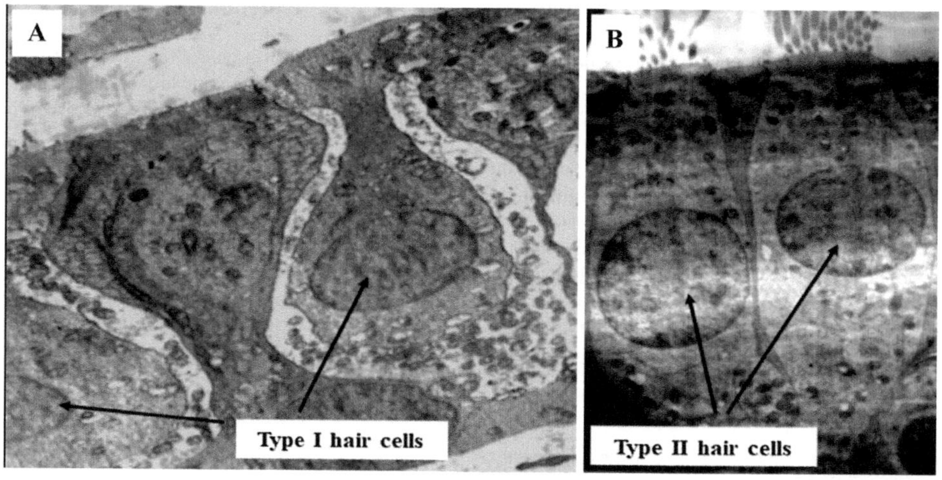

Fig. 1.14 Ultrastructural comparison of vestibular hair cell subtypes. (**A**) Type I hair cell exhibiting characteristic amphora-like morphology (bulbous base, constricted neck, and expanded apex), completely enveloped by a calyceal afferent terminal from a large-diameter vestibular nerve fiber. (**B**) Type II hair cell demonstrating cylindrical morphology with bouton-type afferent synapses, lacking calyceal encapsulation

1.2.1 Saccule

The saccule is shaped like an inverted stomach-like cystic membranous structure, which is located in the spherical recess on the medial wall of vestibular cistern at the anterior and inferior of the vestibular crest. The medial wall of the saccule is tightly attached to the osseous spherical recess. In the central region of the medial wall of the saccule, there is a thickened hook-shaped area that lies in a predominantly vertical position and is covered by the otolithic membrane, termed the macula of saccule. Since the location of macula of saccule is exactly facing the oval window on the lateral wall of the vestibular cistern, once the stapes is removed or the lateral wall of the vestibular cistern is opened, the white otolith membrane in a hook shape covering the macula of saccule will be clearly visible. The saccule has two openings, one opening is the ductus reuniens on the lateral side of the lower end that communicates with the cochlear duct, and the other is the saccular duct at the back of the lower end of saccule, which leads to the endolymphatic sac through the endolymphatic duct [1–4] (Fig. 1.15).

The medial wall of the saccule is tightly anchored to the bony medial wall of the vestibular cistern. Afferent and efferent nerve fibers and blood vessels from most of the macula of the saccule pass through the small holes in the middle sieve spot zone, where afferent nerve fibers pass through the middle sieve spot zone to connect with the inferior vestibular ganglion neurons at the bottom of the cochlear neuroforamen [1–4].

The macula of saccule is bisected by a narrow curvilinear zone traversing through its central region, termed striola. On both sides of the striola zone are marginal areas. The surface of the macula is covered with an otolith membrane with double-layer structures. One structure layer is a basal gelatinous

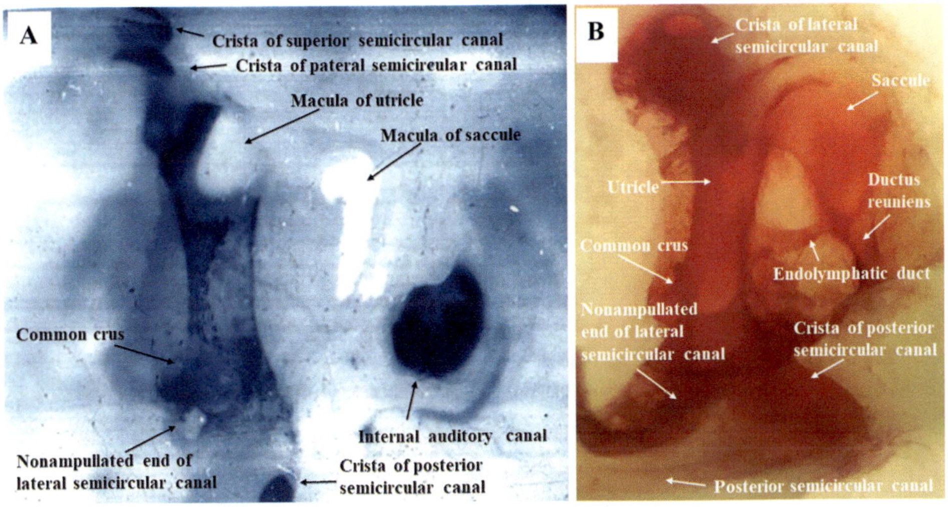

Fig. 1.15 Exposure of the vestibular membranous labyrinth within the vestibular cistern. (**A**) The lateral wall of the vestibular cistern was opened surgically and the modiolus of the cochlea was removed to fully expose the saccule and utricle. White otolithic membranes were seen covering the surface of the macula of the saccule and utricle. (**B**) The membranous structures of the saccule in the vestibular cistern show that the ductus reuniens leads to the scala media of cochlear basal turn at the lower lateral portion of the saccule, and the endolymphatic duct leads to the endolymphatic sac posteriorly at the lower and medial portion of the saccule. The membrane structure of the utricle in the vestibular cistern is dumbbell-shaped, thin in the middle, and bulging at the upper and lower ends. The ampulla and non-ampulla ends of the three membranous semicircular canals communicate with the utricle from the upper and lower ends of the utricle, respectively

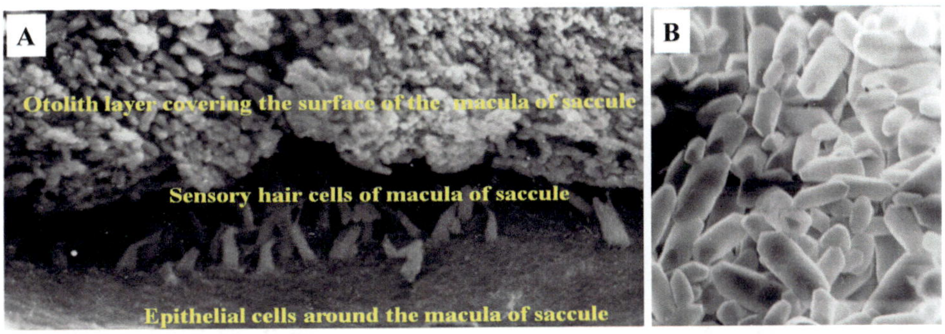

Fig. 1.16 Micrographs of scanning electron microscopy reveal the surface structure of the otolith membrane on the macula of saccule. (**A**) Lateral view of the otoconial layer overlying hair cells. (**B**) A high-magnification micrograph reveals the characteristic calcite crystalline architecture of otoconia

layer adjacent to hair cells; the ciliary bundles of the hair cells are inserted into the substantia jelly of the otolith membrane, so the ciliary bundles of the hair cells can be deflected by the displacement of the otolith membrane caused by changes in gravity or inertia. Another structure layer is the superficial otolith particles composed of calcite crystalline calcium carbonate (Fig. 1.16). The otolith membrane covering the surface of the saccule maculae is thicker above the striola zone and thinner at the edges of marginal area, so it looks like a highland with a hillside terrain. In addition, the size of otolith particles varies vertically within the layer, with smaller crystals superficially and larger particles near the gelatinous interface where they interact with cilia bundles of hair cell cilia [1, 2, 4].

Under a dissecting microscope, the white otolith membrane covering the surface of the macula of saccule clearly marks its exact location (Fig. 1.17A). After removing the otolith membrane, specific staining can clearly show all the sensory hair cells in the entire macula of saccule (Fig. 1.17B). The striola zone predominantly contains type I hair cells, while the marginal region shows equal distribution of type I and type II cells. This regional specialization may correlate with innervation patterns, where the larger calyceal afferents enveloping type I hair cells (occasionally encompassing two to three type I hair cells per calyx in the striola) occupy more space than the bouton-type synapses of type II hair cells, resulting in slightly lower hair cell density within the striola zone compared to the marginal region[14, 19] (Fig. 1.18).

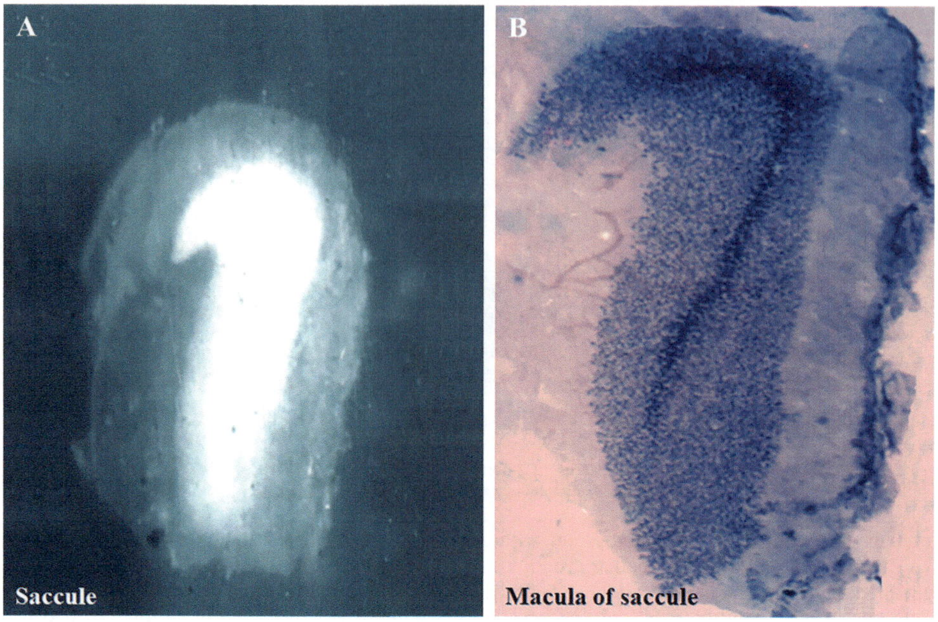

Fig. 1.17 Micro-dissection of entire saccule and the surface preparation of macula of saccule. (**A**) The white otolith membrane covering the saccular macula marks its precise location. (**B**) Succinate dehydrogenase staining labels all hair cells blue in the surface preparation of entire macula of saccule

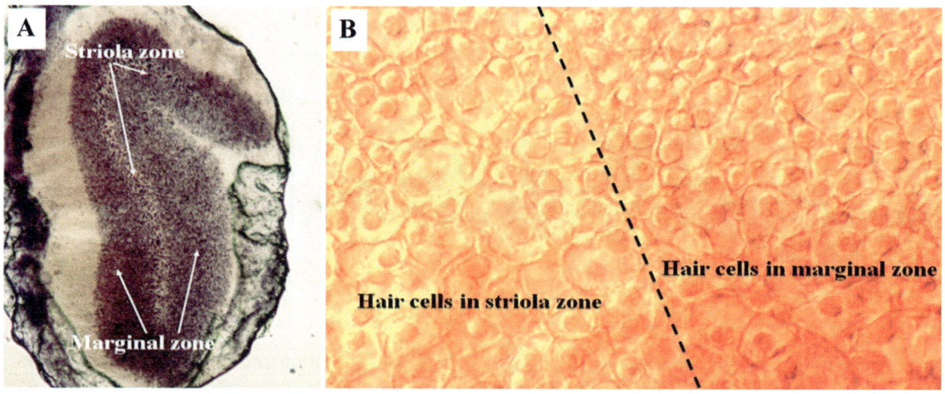

Fig. 1.18 Regional division in macula of saccule. (**A**) Surface preparation of macula of saccule demonstrates lower hair cell density in the striola zone compared to marginal regions. (**B**) High-magnification view reveals that the striola zone mainly contains type I hair cells, typically with two to three type I hair cells clustered per calyceal afferent terminal. In contrast, marginal region shows equal distribution of type I and type II hair cells, and there is usually only one type I hair cell located within one calyx of type I afferent nerve terminal. The difference in density of vestibular hair cells in the striola and marginal zones may be due to the difference in the number of type I hair cells in these two areas and the fact that the expansive calyceal afferent terminals in striola occupy more space

The cells surrounding the macula of saccule are a uniform single layer of squamous epithelial cells without dark cells. Therefore, the saccule can neither produce endolymph nor absorb endolymph. This means that the endolymph in the saccule can only be derived from the secretion by the epithelium and dark cells in the stria vascularis on the cochlear lateral wall and enters the saccule through the ductus reuniens. Since the saccule lacks dark cells, the endolymphatic fluid that enters the saccule cannot be absorbed. The only way to solve the absorption of endolymphatic fluid in the saccule is to be transported to the endolymphatic sac through the endolymphatic duct and then absorbed by the epithelial cells in endolymphatic sac, thus realizing the longitudinal flow circulation pattern of endolymphatic fluid from the cochlear duct through the saccule to the endolymphatic sac. Furthermore, since there are no dark cells in the saccule, the degenerated otoliths that fall off from the otolith membrane of the saccule can only be transported to the endolymphatic sac through the endolymphatic duct, which means that the otoliths that fall off from the otolith membrane of the saccule can only be phagocytosed and degraded by the epithelial cells in the endolymphatic sac [1–4, 11].

1.2.2 Utricle

The utricle, located in the oval depression on the medial wall of the vestibular cistern, behind and adjacent to the saccule, is a dumbbell-shaped cystic membranous tube with bulging upper and lower ends (Figs. 1.15A and 1.19A). The utricle has a total of six openings. At the back upper portion of the utricle, there is an opening to communicate with the ampulla of superior semicircular canal. At the lateral side of the opening of the ampulla of the superior semicircular canal, there is an opening to communicate with the ampulla of the lateral semicircular canal. In the front of the lateral portion at the lower end of the utricle, there is an opening that communicates with the ampulla of the posterior semicircular canal. Behind the opening of the ampulla of the posterior semicircular canal, there is the opening to connect the single non-ampullated end of lateral semicircular canal. Underneath the medial wall of the utricle, there is an opening to communicate with the common crus, which is formed by the confluence of the superior semicircular canal and the non-ampullary end of the posterior semicircular canal. In addition, there is a cleft-shaped opening at the anterior of inferior portion of the utricle communicating the endolymphatic duct. This opening has a valve that opens unidirectionally toward the endolymphatic duct. Therefore, the endolymph can only flow from the utricle to the endolymphatic sac, but not from the endolymphatic duct to the utricle [1–4, 11].

The macula of utricle is in the coronal position at the enlarged upper portion of the utricle. The layer of surface of the sensory hair cells on macula of utricle is facing the back, while the nerve fibers and capillaries are on the dorsal side of macula of utricle leading to the small holes at superior sieve spot on the medial bony wall. The shape of the macula of utricle is a fan-shaped plate. The otolith membrane clearly marks the position of the surface of the macula of utricle (Fig. 1.19A). The macula of utricle is divided into two areas by a narrow curvilinear zone which extends through the middle. Like the macula of saccule, this zone is also termed the striola (Fig. 1.19B). Most of the hair cells in the striola area are type I hair cells. In the marginal area on both sides of the striola, type I hair cells and type II hair cells are evenly distributed. In the marginal regions on both sides of the striola, the kinocilia of all hair cells are arranged on the side facing the striola zone [16]. Therefore, when the body produces an accelerated movement along the plane perpendicular to the striola of utricle, the hair cells in one side of the marginal area of utricle will be depolarized to be excited, while the hair cells in the other side of marginal area of utricle will be hyperpolarized to be inhibited. This may indicate that one stimulus in the same direction produces a reversed stimulation pattern to the hair cells in the marginal areas on both sides of the striola of utricle.

Around the macula of utricle is a transitional zone covered by transitional epithelium. The periphery of the transitional epithelial zone is covered with a large number of dark cells (Fig. 1.20). Since dark cells have dual functions of secreting and absorbing endolymph, endolymph in the utricle can be secreted and absorbed by local dark cells. Therefore, the endolymph in the utricle shows a circulatory pattern of radiation flow. Perhaps only when the endolymph in the utricle is

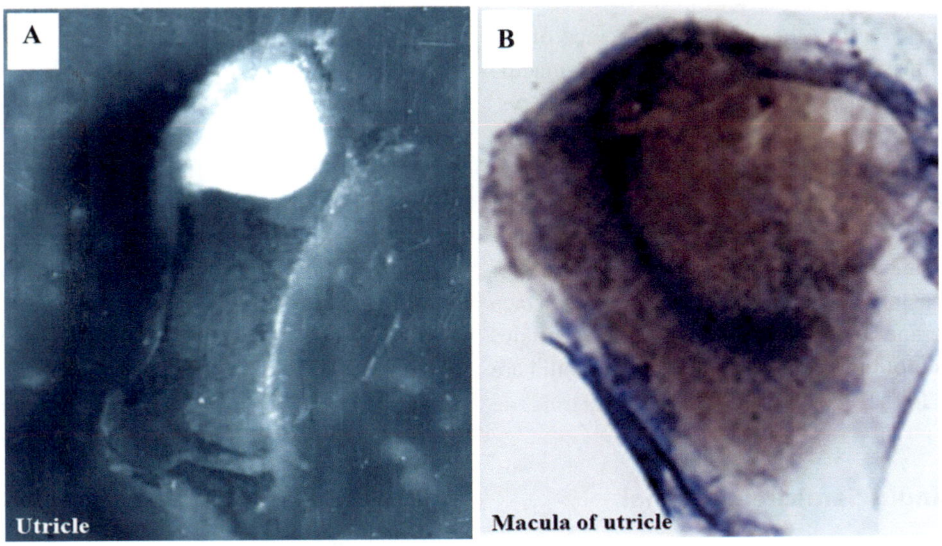

Fig. 1.19 Micro-dissection of entire utricle and the surface preparation of macula of utricle. (**A**) The white otolith membrane covering the macula of utricle marks its precise location. (**B**) After removing the otolith membrane, the macula of utricle was laid flat on the glass slide to expose the underlying sensory epithelial cells for microscopic examination

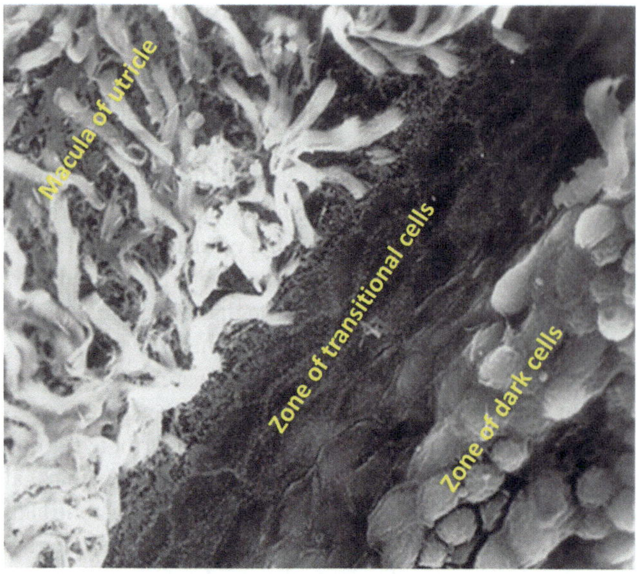

Fig. 1.20 Scanning electron microscopy shows the transitional epithelial border and dark cell zone outside the transitional epithelium at the periphery of the macula of utricle in guinea pig

excessively secreted, the endolymph will be discharged through the thickened cleft-shaped opening to the endolymph sac. In addition, the degenerated otoliths that fall off from the otolith membrane of the macula of utricle may also be phagocytosed and degraded by the dark cells in the utricle. The degenerative otoliths may also fall into the posterior ampulla cavity or the single non-ampullated end of lateral semicircular canal or the common crus of the superior or posterior semicircular canals. Once the otolith particles fall on the cupula on the top of the ampullary crest, they may induce the symptoms of benign paroxysmal positional vertigo [1, 2, 4, 22].

The otolith layer covering the gelatinous surface of the macula of utricle is the same as the otolith layer on the macula of saccule, composed of calcium carbonate with a calcite crystal structure with a specific gravity of 2.71. However, unlike the otolith membrane covering the surface of the macula of the saccule, the otolith layer on the striola zone of macula of utricle is thinner, but thicker on its marginal area. This makes the otolith membrane covering the surface of the macula of utricle look like a basin. The otolith particles near the surface of the otolith membrane are smaller, while the otolith particles near the gelatinous otolithic membrane and hair cell cilia are larger [1, 2, 4].

1.2.3 Membranous Semicircular Canal

The three membranous semicircular canals are in close contact with the osseous wall at the convex side of their ampullary ends, while the rest portion of the semicircular canals is suspended in the perilymph with the help of connective tissue trabeculae. The membranous semicircular canals are filled with endolymph, but the space between the membranous semicircular canals and the bony semicircular canals is filled with perilymph. The crista of ampulla is located within the ampulla cavity equivalent to the position at the junction of the convex edge of the semicircular canal and the bone wall. The shape of crista of ampulla is a horizontal saddle-shaped bulge, and its direction is perpendicular to the bending direction of the semicircular canal. In guinea pigs and larger mammals, the structure of the three ampullary crestae is basically the same with a saddle-shaped crista across the bottom of the ampullae. The direction of saddle-shaped ampullary cresta is perpendicular to the bending direction of the semicircular canal. The surface of the ampullary crest is covered with a gelatinous cupula, and the cilia of hair cells are inserted into the gelatinous cupula on the top of crista (Fig. 1.21). Avian species demonstrate divergent crista architecture with a central non-sensory epithelial ridge bifurcating the sensory epithelium into dual regions, creating a characteristic cruciform morphology (Fig. 1.22). In rodents smaller than guinea pigs, such as mouse and rat, the ampullary crista of lateral semicircular canal mirrors the mammalian saddle-shaped pattern, while the superior and posterior cristae resemble the crista structure of avian organization with the central division of sensory areas. This raises unanswered questions about the mechanisms underlying the functional differentiation of the different stimulation patterns between the horizontal and vertical semicircular canals in mice and rats (Fig. 1.23) [1–4].

The basal region of ampullary crista anchors to the osseous wall via connective tissue, with both neural fibers and vascular channels traversing the perforated bony interface to establish connections with vestibular ganglion neurons and vasculature respectively; specifically, the afferent nerve fibers from the superior vestibular ganglion neurons and vestibular efferent fibers cross the superior cribriform area and establish synaptic connections with the sensory hair cells on lateral and superior crests. whereas the afferent fibers from the inferior vestibular ganglion neurons and efferent fibers course through inferior cribriform pathway to connect the sensory hair cells on the posterior crista [1–4].

The hair cells on the crista of ampulla, like those in the macula of saccule and utricle, are classified into type I and type II variants. The location of the kinocilia on all hair cells in each individual ampullary crista exhibits uniformly oriented kinocilia, and the kinocilia of hair cells on ampullary crista of the lateral semicircular canal are facing the utricle, while the kinocilia on hair cells in crista of superior and posterior semicircular canals are toward their respective semicircular canals [1, 2, 4, 16].

The surface of the ampullary crista is surmounted by a sail-shaped gelatinous cupula that extends to the opposite wall of the ampullary cavity. The cupula extends from the top of the

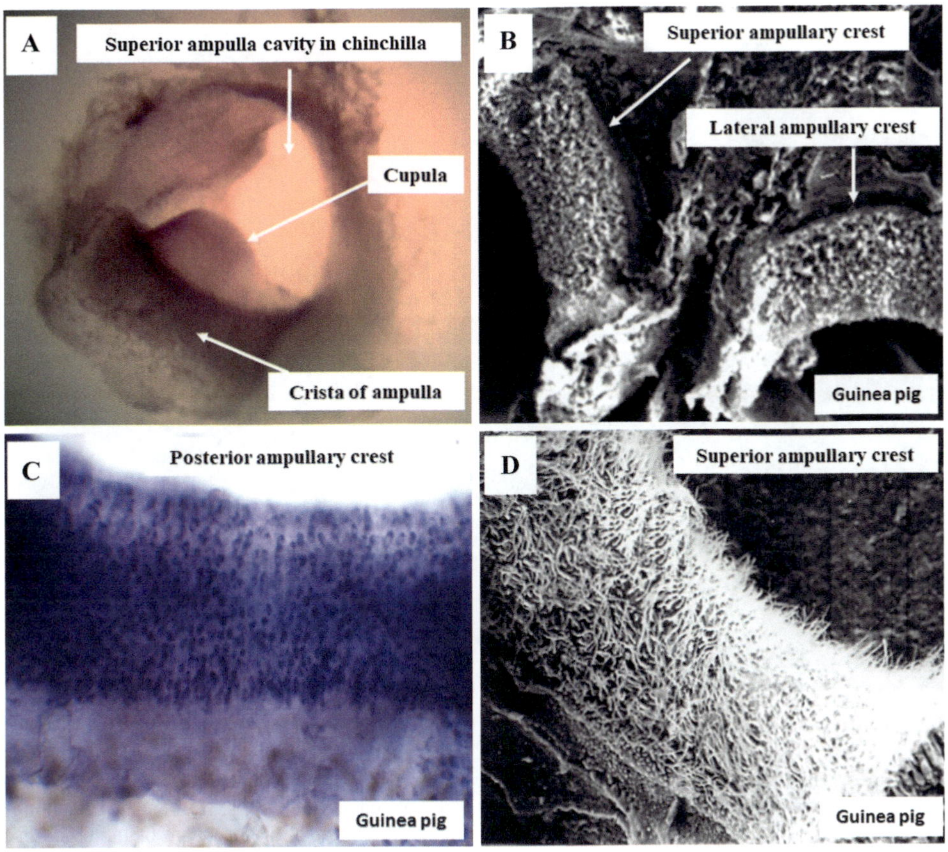

Fig. 1.21 View of the crista of ampullae under light microscope or scanning electron microscope. (**A**) Macroscopic view of the cupula positioned on the saddle-shaped ampullary crista in superior ampullary cavity in chinchilla under dissecting microscopy. (**B**) Scanning electron micrograph showing the saddle-shaped cristae in both superior and lateral ampullae of guinea pig. (**C**) The surface preparation of ampullary crista with succinate dehydrogenase staining shows the saddle-shaped crista in the posterior ampulla of chinchilla under a light microscope. (**D**) Ciliary bundles on the surface of hair cells on the superior ampullary crista of guinea pig were observed under a scanning electron microscope

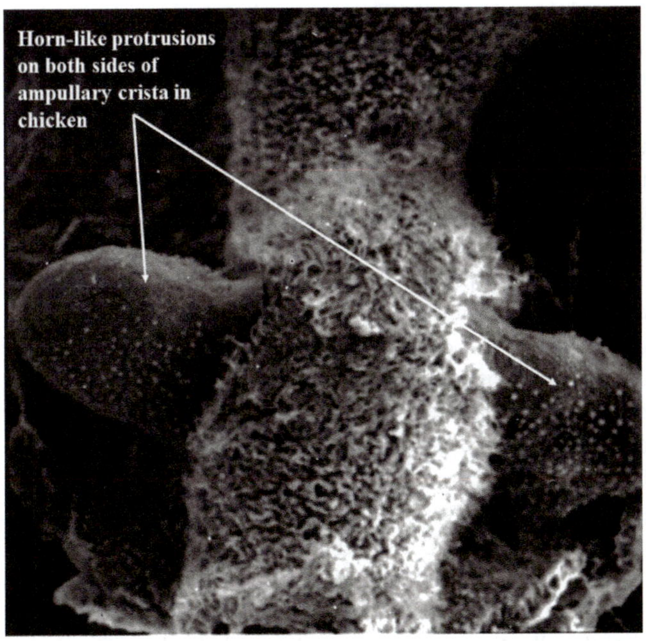

Fig. 1.22 A scanning electron micrograph shows the unique cruciform morphology of avian ampullary cristae. This photomicrograph shows the horn-like processes extending symmetrically from the middle of the crista ampullae of birds, with their surfaces covered by columnar epithelial cells

ampullary cristae to the entire opposite wall of the ampullary cavity, which means that the endolymph in the semicircular canals can only communicate with the endolymph in the utricle through the opening at the non-ampullary end of semicircular canals, but the endolymph cannot enter the utricle through the ampulla cavity. The ciliary bundles of sensory hair cells on the crista are embedded in the gelatinous matrix covering their tops.

Take the lateral semicircular canal as an example, when the overlying gelatinous cupula is swinging with the flow of endolymph toward the ampullary crista, the ciliary of hair cells on the side of crista facing the semicircular canal will be tilted in the same direction of gelatinous cupula bends toward the crista. However, the cilia of hair cells on the other side of ampullary crista facing the utricle will also be tilted to the ampullary crista due to a swirling flow towards the crista from utricle. The hair cells on both sides of the crista of lateral ampulla will therefore be in an unbalanced state, where they are excited at one side of the crista but are inhibited at the other side, resulting in precisely balanced bidirectional signaling [1, 2, 4, 16].

There are two transitional epithelium zones on both sides of ampullary crista. The lateral area of transitional zone is a crescent-shaped area of dark cell aggregation. In pigmented guinea pigs and C57BL/6J mice, these melanin-rich dark cells

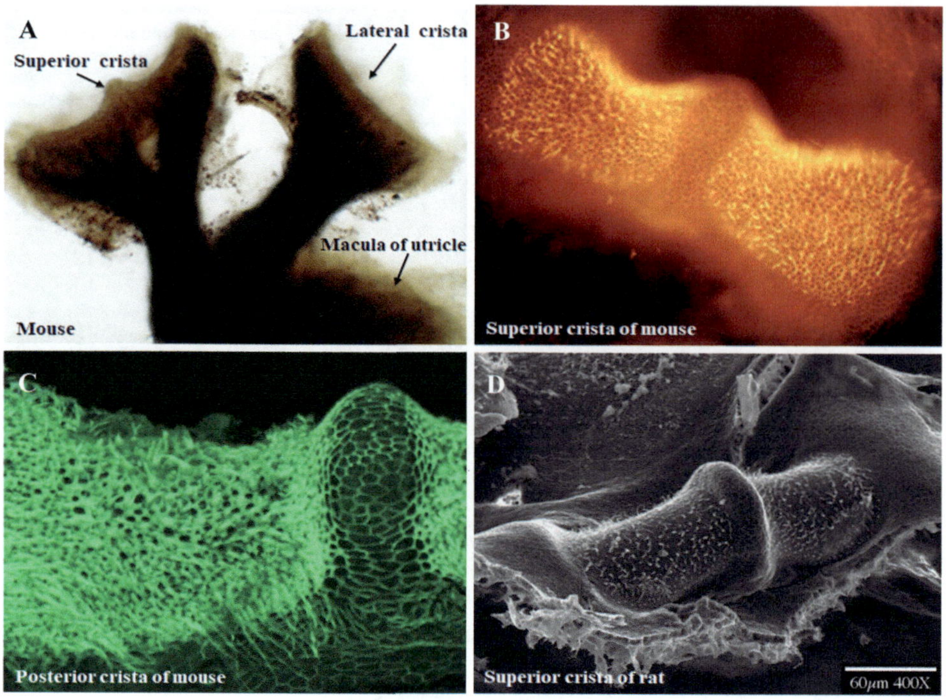

Fig. 1.23 Shape of the ampullary cristae of the vertical semicircular canals in mouse and rat. (**A**) Under a dissecting microscope, the lateral crista in mouse is saddle-shaped, while the superior crista has a central ridge. Note that the nerve fibers at the base of the superior crista bifurcate to both sides of the midline and project to the hair cell zones on both sides of the crista. (**B**) Phalloidin staining shows that the superior crista develops a distinctive central bulge partitioning the sensory epithelium into two areas in mouse. (**C**) Phalloidin staining shows that the cells in the central bulge of the posterior crista of mice do not have ciliary bundles. Therefore, it can be judged that the epithelial cells on the midline bulge of the crista ampullae in the vertical semicircular canals are not sensory hair cells. (**D**) Under a scanning electron microscope, the epithelial cells on the bulge of the crista in superior semicircular canal of the rat divide the sensory hair cells into two areas. This raised non-sensory epithelium ring at the middle of the crista looks like a "life buoy"

form two towards the opposite crescent-shaped domains (Fig. 1.24). The melanin-containing dark cells are also scattered throughout the membrane of the semicircular canals. This phenomenon of dark cells distribution on the membranous semicircular canals and in the crescent-shaped areas in the ampullary cavity suggested that dark cells not only maintain local endolymph homeostasis by secreting and absorbing the endolymph, but also participate in the phagocytosis and clearance of otolith fragments shed from the macula of utricle into the ampullary cavity and semicircular canals [1, 23].

1.2.4 Endolymphatic Duct and Endolymphatic Sac

The saccule duct arising from the dorsal side of the lower portion of the saccule joins with the utriculosaccule duct to form a small epithelial-lined channel in the bony labyrinth of the petrous temporal bone, termed endolymphatic duct. This endolymphatic duct then courses backward in the petrous portion of the temporal bone (Fig. 1.25). As it reaches the location beneath the common crus, the upper and lower gaps of the bony tube begin to widen. Consequently, the membranous endolymphatic duct gradually expands upward and downward to form the endolymphatic sac. The rearward opening of the bony slit where the endolymphatic sac is situated is tightly covered by the sigmoid sinus in the sulcus of the sigmoid sinus [1, 24, 25].

The endolymphatic duct resides within a bony canal known as the vestibular aqueduct. The inner surface of the endolymphatic duct is lined with squamous epithelium or cuboidal epithelial cells. The enlarged portion of the endolymphatic duct extending backward forms the endolymphatic sac.

The anterior part of the endolymphatic sac is situated in a niche on the posterior surface of the petrous bone, while its posterior part is located within the layers of the dura mater of the posterior fossa. The endolymphatic sac can be divided into three parts: the proximal part lies within the bony niche; the anterior portion of the intermediate part is also located in the bony niche, whereas the posterior portion of the intermediate part is situated between the layers of the dura mater; the distal part is located within the layers of the dura mater overlying the transverse sinus [1, 11, 24, 25]. The epithelial cells on the inner surface of the proximal portion of the endolymphatic sac are slightly taller than those in the endolymphatic duct. The surface

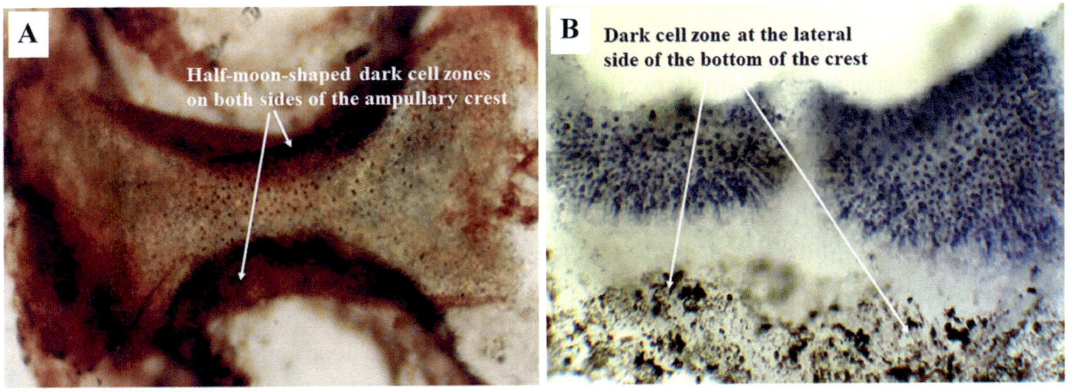

Fig. 1.24 Superior and side views of the ampullary crista of pigmented rodents. (**A**) Superior view reveals paired melanin-rich dark cell regions forming two crescent-shaped areas in both sides of crista in the guinea pig. (**B**) Side view shows pigment-containing dark cells concentrated in the basal meniscal zones in the C57BL/6J mouse

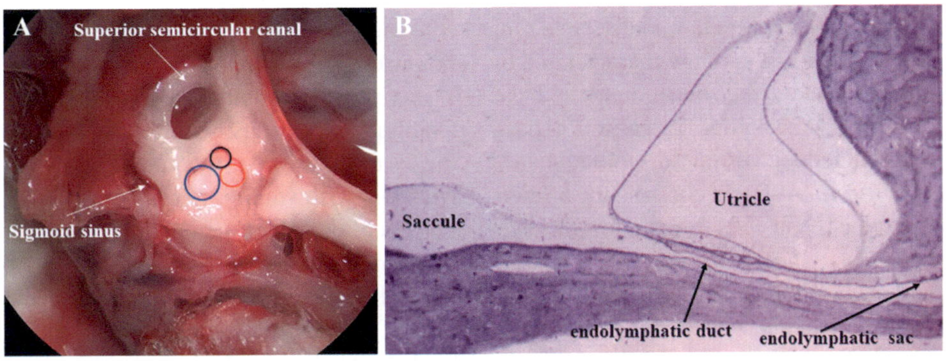

Fig. 1.25 Anatomical landmarks of the lateral bony wall of the posterior cranial fossa. (**A**) The lateral osseous wall of the posterior cranial fossa sequentially reveals the superior semicircular canal, superior vestibular canal, facial nerve canal, and auditory canal from superior to inferior orientations. The sigmoid sinus is embedded in the S-shaped groove under the dura mater at the junction of the temporal bone and occipital bone, covering the bony fissure of the endolymphatic sac. (**B**) Horizontal section of a guinea pig temporal bone parallel to the endolymphatic duct and endolymphatic sac, showing the pathway from the sac to the endolymphatic duct and then to the endolymphatic sac. (Courtesy of Ding et al. [16])

cells in the intermediate portion of the endolymphatic sac are uneven and covered with irregularly arranged tall columnar cells. These cells can be divided into two categories: one is the light cells with clear cytoplasm, more pinocytic vesicles and microvilli; the other is the dark cells with dense cytoplasm, fewer pinocytic vesicles and microvilli. The inner surface of the distal endolymphatic sac is lined with cuboidal light cells and dark cells, with the number of light cells outnumbering the dark cells [1].

Cell fragments and degenerated otoliths can be found in the endolymphatic sac cavity. Suspended leukocytes with obvious pinocytosis can also be visible, particularly macrophages. In this way, the endolymphatic sac is not only regarded as the absorption site of endolymph, but also as the "graveyard" for phagocytosis and decomposition of otoliths that fall off the otolith membrane of the saccule. This means that the endolymphatic sac can be an immune organ of the inner ear [4, 26–28].

1.3 Vestibular Nervous System

The area with small holes on the medial bony wall behind the elliptical recess of the vestibular cistern is termed the superior sieve spot zone. The superior vestibular nerve fibers and blood vessels pass through this superior sieve spot zone leading to the macula of utricle, the superior portion of the macula of saccule, and the ampullary cristae of the lateral and superior semicircular canals. The area of small holes on the medial bony wall just in front of the spherical recess of vestibular cistern is called the middle sieve spot zone. The blood vessels and one of the inferior vestibular nerve bundles pass through this middle sieve spot zone leading to the main portion of macula of saccule, except the anterosuperior portion of the macula of saccule. The area of small holes at the medial bony wall under the front of spherical recess of vestibular cistern is called the inferior sieve spot zone. Another nerve fiber bundle of the inferior vestibular nerve and capillaries pass through this inferior sieve spot zone leading to the ampullary crista of posterior semicircular canal [1–4].

The inferior vestibular nerve fibers beneath the supporting cell layer of the macula of the saccule are arranged horizontally (Fig. 1.26A), while the superior vestibular nerve fibers beneath the supporting cell layer of the macula of the utricle are arranged in a fan shape (Fig. 1.26B). The vestibular nerve fibers are arranged in a vertical and horizontal crisscross pattern beneath the supporting cell layer of the ampullary crista (Fig. 1.26C).

1.3.1 Vestibular Afferent Nervous System

As mentioned earlier, the vestibular sensory epithelium contains two different types of hair cells with distinct patterns of afferent nerve connections. The afferent terminals connecting to type I hair cells have chalice-like endings characterized by a wider opening, a thinner neck, and a round, enlarged base, resembling an ancient Greek wine bottle. The entire cell body of the type I hair cell is embedded within this goblet-shaped afferent nerve ending (Fig. 1.27A–D). In contrast, the afferent terminals connecting to type II hair cells form button-like synaptic connections at the base of the type II hair cells, following a typical synaptic pattern (Fig. 1.27A, C).

The vestibular afferent nerve fibers connecting to the macula of utricle, superior portion of macula of the saccule, the ampullary cristae of the lateral and superior semicircular canals all enter the superior vestibular neuroforamen through small holes in the bone wall of the superior sieve spot zone. The superior vestibular ganglion neurons are located in the superior vestibular neuroforamen (Fig. 1.28A). The nerve fibers of the inferior vestibular ganglion neurons respectively pass through the middle and inferior sieve spot zones on the medial bony wall of the vestibular cistern to establish synaptic connections with the hair cells in most areas of the macula of saccule and the hair cells on the ampullary crista of the posterior semicircular canal. The soma of the inferior vestibular neurons is distributed at the bottom of the cochlear neuroforamen (Fig. 1.28B). Vestibular afferent neurons are bipolar neurons (Fig. 1.29A). The superior and inferior vestibular ganglion neurons extend in the rostral-caudal direction through the superior vestibular canal and cochlear neuroforamen, respectively. The nerve fibers of the peripheral end pass through the small holes on the bony wall of the sieve spot zone to enter the vestibular cistern, and then establish synaptic connections with the sensory hair cells on each vestibular end-organ. The axons of central end of the vestibular neurons converge into nerve bundles in the superior vestibular canal and cochlear neuroforamen, respectively, and then merge to form the vestibular nerve tract after entering the intracranial to lead to the vestibular nucleus in the brainstem [1–3, 20, 21].

Peripheral vestibular neurons are divided into two types. One type of neurons, with thicker nerve fibers, is located in the rostral portion of the ganglion region. The other type of neurons, with smaller nerve fibers, is located in the caudal portion of the ganglion region. The large nerve fibers primarily terminate at the goblet-shaped endings of type I hair cells, while the small nerve fibers terminate at the base of type II hair cells. These two types of neurons and their nerve fibers can be distinguished by double labeling using antibodies against Peripherin and Tubulin [1–4, 29] (Fig. 1.29B).

The central axons of the superior and inferior vestibular ganglion neurons merge together after entering the intracranial space and cross from the posterior aspect of the cochlear nucleus to the vestibular nuclei in the brainstem. Afferent nerve

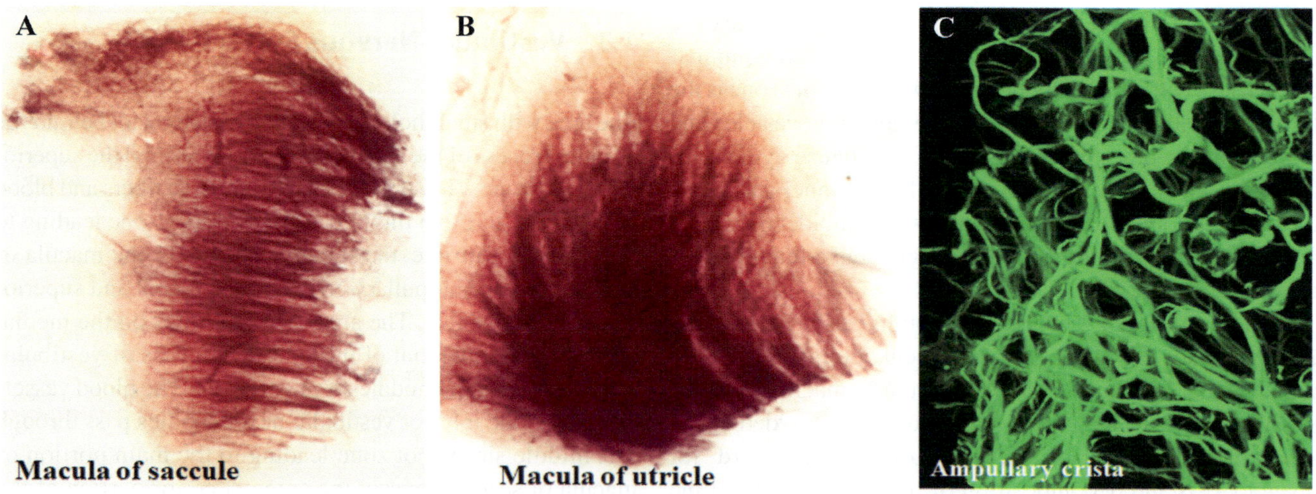

Fig. 1.26 Arrangement of nerve fibers at the base of vestibular end-organs. (**A**) The nerve fibers under the supporting cells of the macula of saccule are arranged horizontally. (**B**) The nerve fibers under the supporting cells of the macula of utricle are arranged in a fan-shaped pattern. (**C**) The nerve fibers beneath the supporting cells of the ampullary crista are arranged in a pattern of vertical and horizontal

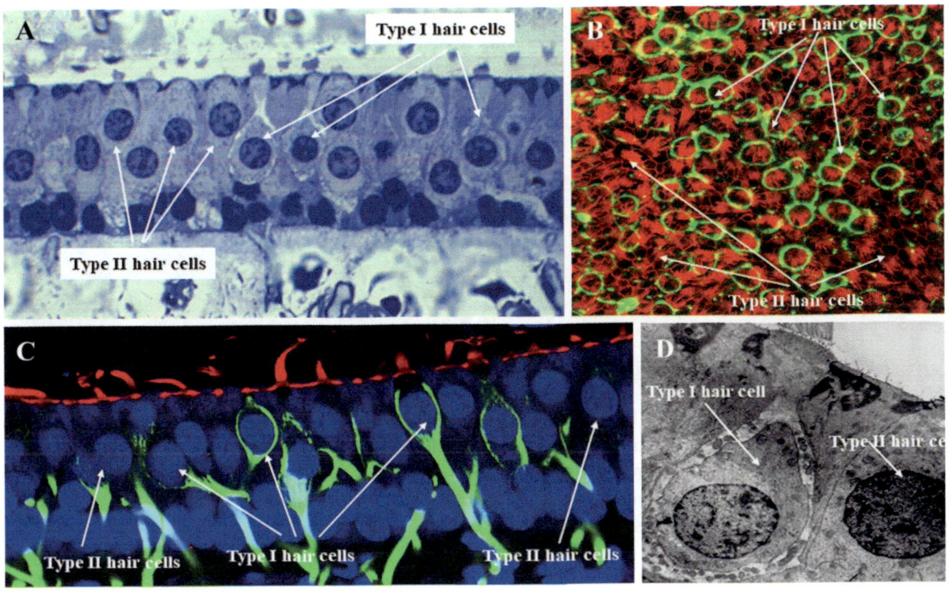

Fig. 1.27 Two different types of hair cells in the vestibular organ are shown from two different viewing angles: sectioning and spreading. (**A**) Cross-sectional section of the macula of utricle showing flask-shaped type I hair cells and columnar-shaped type II hair cells. (**B**) Surface preparation of macula of utricle with neurofilament staining shows the nucleus of a type I hair cell surrounded by a ring of type I afferent nerve endings (green fluorescence), while the type II hair cells do not have such a ring of afferent nerve terminals surrounding their nuclei. (**C**) Cross-sectional image of the utricle macula showing flask-shaped type I afferent nerve endings surrounding the soma of type I hair cells and button-shaped afferent nerve synapses at the base of type II hair cells. (**D**) A view under the transmission electron microscope reveals the different morphologies of type I and type II hair cells

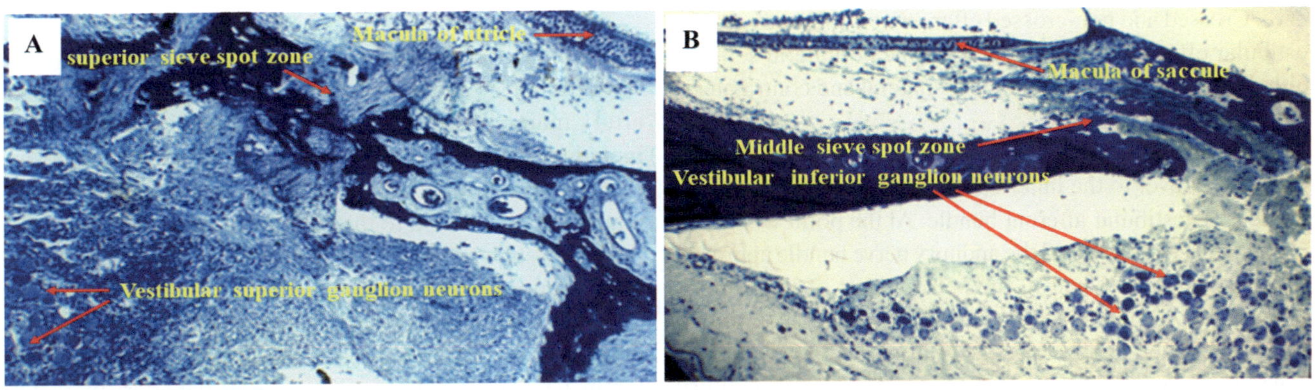

Fig. 1.28 Cross-sectional sections of the superior and middle sieve spot zone showing the vestibular sensory epithelium on the macula of saccule or utricle, and the superior vestibular ganglia or inferior vestibular ganglia and their nerve fibers on both sides of the ethmoid plaque, respectively. (**A**) A cross-sectional slice of the superior sieve spot zone shows the hair cells on the macula of utricle and the soma of the superior vestibular ganglion neurons in the superior vestibular canal and their superior vestibular nerve fibers passing through the superior sieve spot zone. (**B**) A cross-sectional slice of the middle sieve spot zone shows the hair cells on the macula of saccule and the soma of the inferior vestibular ganglion neurons in the cochlear neuroforamen and their inferior vestibular nerve fibers passing through the middle sieve spot zone

fibers from the macula of the utricle and the superior portion of the macula of saccule primarily terminate in the lateral vestibular nucleus. Afferent fibers from most area of the macula of saccule terminate in the inferior vestibular nucleus, while afferents from the cristae of three ampullae mainly terminate in the superior vestibular nucleus and the medial vestibular nucleus [1, 12].

1.3.2 Vestibular Efferent Nervous System

The efferent circuit in the nervous system transmits nerve impulses from the central nervous system to the sensory end organs. Studies have shown that the vestibular descending efferent nerve pathway and its ascending afferent nerve pathway remain parallel, connecting the vestibular center with the

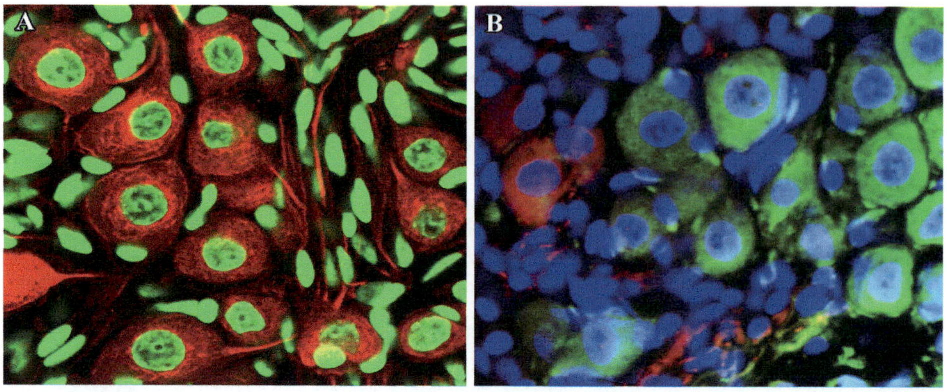

Fig. 1.29 The vestibular ganglion neurons consist of bipolar neurons oriented in a rostral-caudal direction. (**A**) Double staining of the cell bodies of superior vestibular neurons. The neurons were labeled in red using an anti-Tubulin antibody, and the nuclei were stained in green with ToPro-3. (**B**) Triple staining of vestibular neurons. Vestibular neurons connecting to type I hair cells are labeled in green with an anti-Tubulin antibody, vestibular neurons connecting to type II hair cells are labeled in red with an anti-Peripherin antibody, and nuclei are stained in blue with ToPro-3

peripheral vestibular end organs. The vestibular efferent nerve originates from the brainstem and terminates at the hair cells or primary afferent nerve fibers in the cristae of the ampullae and the maculae of the saccule and utricle. Approximately 200–300 efferent neurons innervate each terminal of the vestibular end organs. The cell bodies of the vestibular efferent neurons are located in the brainstem, roughly in the region between the abducens nerve and the superior vestibular nucleus, as well as in the dorsal portion of the descending branch of the facial nerve. Crossed and non-crossed efferent nerve fibers from the vestibular efferent neurons project to the peripheral sensory epithelium of the vestibule on the ipsilateral and contralateral sides, respectively [1, 30].

The vestibular efferent nerve fiber and the cochlear efferent nerve fiber travel to the inner ear along the auditory afferent bundle and vestibular afferent bundle. At the point where the vestibular nerve bundle and the auditory nerve bundle approach the auditory nerve canal in the petrous part of the temporal bone, the vestibular efferent nerve bundle splits into two branches. One branch follows the inferior vestibular afferent nerve bundle and cochlear efferent bundle into the auditory nerve canal, then enters the vestibular cistern through the small holes in the bony wall at the middle and inferior sieve spot zones to innervate most of the hair cells in the macula of the saccule and all hair cells on the posterior crista of the ampulla. The other branch of the vestibular efferent nerve bundle accompanies the superior vestibular afferent nerve bundle through the vestibular nerve canal, entering the vestibular cistern via the small hole in the bony wall of the superior sieve spot zone to innervate all hair cells on the macula of the utricle, the hair cells on the upper portion of the macula of the saccule, and all hair cells on the superior and lateral cristae [1, 30].

The efferent nerve connections to the two types of hair cells in the vestibular sensory epithelium differ. The efferent nerve endings that innervate type I hair cells in the vestibular receptors are located beneath the "goblet"-shaped vestibular afferent terminals, establishing synaptic connections with the afferent nerve fibers but not directly connecting to the cell body of the type I hair cells. In contrast, the efferent terminals that innervate type II hair cells in the vestibular receptors form direct synaptic connections with the type II hair cells at the base of these cells (Fig. 1.30).

1.4 The Vascular System of the Vestibule

The intracranial blood supply primarily originates from the vertebral artery and the internal carotid artery. The vertebral artery mainly supplies blood to the posterior brain tissues, including the cerebellum, brainstem, and occipital lobe, and forms the posterior circulation. The internal carotid artery primarily supplies blood to the anterior brain tissues, including branches such as the ophthalmic artery, anterior choroidal artery, anterior cerebral artery, middle cerebral artery, and posterior communicating artery, forming the anterior circulation. The vertebral arteries enter the cranial cavity through the foramen magnum and join to form the basilar artery (part of the vertebrobasilar system), which then connects with the posterior communicating artery and anterior communicating artery from the internal carotid artery to form the cerebral arterial circle (Circle of Willis). It is important to note that the labyrinthine artery, which supplies the inner ear, originates solely from a branch of the basilar artery. Blood from the internal carotid artery cannot flow retrogradely into the basilar artery system. Thus, the labyrinthine artery branch of the vertebral artery is the exclusive source of blood supply to the inner ear [1, 31, 32].

1.4.1 Vestibular Artery Supply

The anterior inferior cerebellar artery arising from the vertebral artery gives off the labyrinthine artery. Near the cochlear

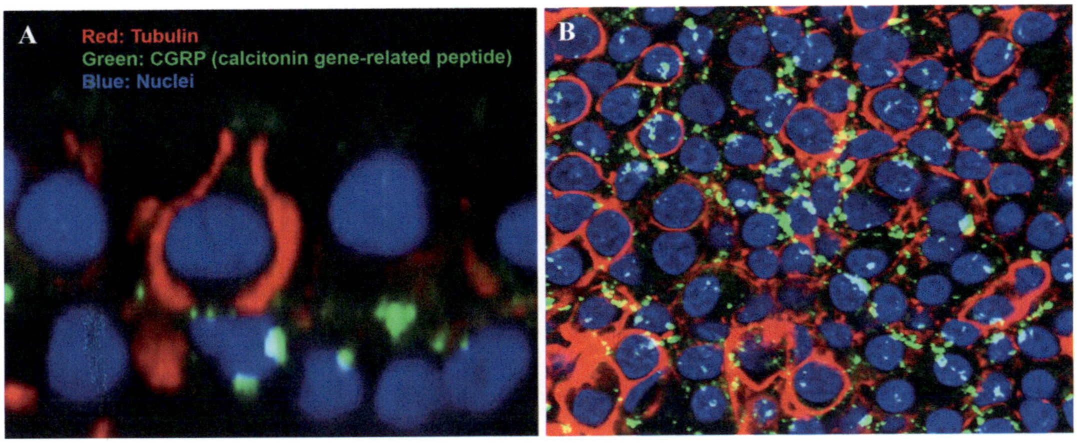

Fig. 1.30 Distribution of vestibular afferent and efferent nerve terminals. (**A**) Triple labeling of vestibular end-organs is shown from the viewing angle of the cross-section. The chalice-shaped type I afferent nerve terminal is labeled in red with anti-Tubulin antibody, the vestibular efferent nerve synapse is labeled in green with anti-CGRP antibody, and the nuclei of cells are stained in blue with ToPro-3. (**B**) From the viewing angle of the surface preparation of the macula, the ring-shaped red fluorescent signals surrounding the nuclei of type I hair cells represent type I afferent nerve terminals, the punctate green fluorescent signals indicate vestibular efferent terminals, and the blue fluorescent signals stain the nuclei of hair cells

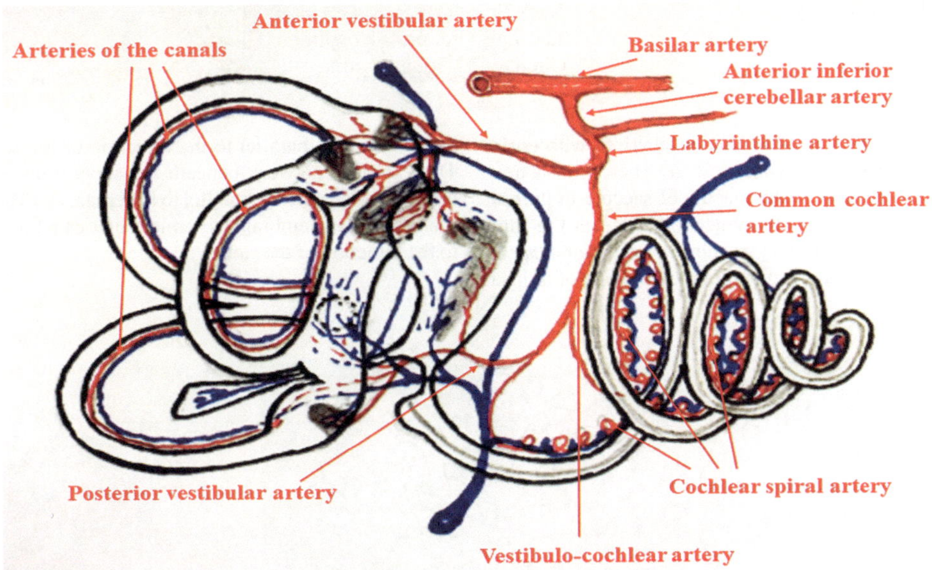

Fig. 1.31 Schematic diagram of the arterial supply in the membranous labyrinth in mammals

neuroforamen and vestibular neuroforamen, the labyrinthine artery branches into the common cochlear artery and the vestibular artery, which enter the cochlear neuroforamen and the vestibular neuroforamen, respectively. The vestibular artery enters the vestibular cistern from the vestibular neuroforamen and mainly supplies the upper portion of the utricle and the ampullae of the lateral and superior semicircular canals. Within the cochlear neuroforamen, the common cochlear artery further divides into the main cochlear branch and the vestibulocochlear branch. The main cochlear branch courses through the cochlear modiolus, forming a spiral artery that extends from the base of modiolus to the apex of the cochlea. The vestibulocochlear artery supplies the basal turn of the cochlea and enters the vestibular cistern through small foramina in the bony wall at the middle and inferior sieve spot zones, providing blood supply to the lower and inner portions of the saccule and utricle, as well as the posterior semicircular canal and the common crus (Fig. 1.31). In summary, three arteries supply the inner ear: 1. The anterior vestibular artery enters the superior vestibular neuroforamen from the labyrinthine artery to supply the superior portion of utricle and ampullas of lateral and superior semicircular canals. 2. The common cochlear artery enters the cochlear neuroforamen to provide blood supply to the cochlear basal turn and the main portion of the macula of saccule and the lower and medial portions of the saccule and utricle, as well as the ampulla of posterior semicircular canal and the common crus. 3. The posterior vestibular artery, another branch of the common cochlear artery, supplies the lower portion of the vestibular cavity. supplies the lower portion of the vestibular cavity. It is worth noting that the blood supply areas of these three arteries are different and there is no overlap in blood supply, which indicates that the occlusion of one artery will cause ischemia and hypoxia in its specific area without affecting the blood supply areas of the other two arteries [1, 31, 32].

1.4.2 Vestibular Capillaries

The dense capillary network supplying the vestibular sensory epithelium is located beneath the supporting cell layer of each vestibular end-organ. In mammals, the capillaries beneath the supporting cells of the macula of the saccule are arranged horizontally (Figs. 1.32A and 1.33A). In contrast, the capillaries

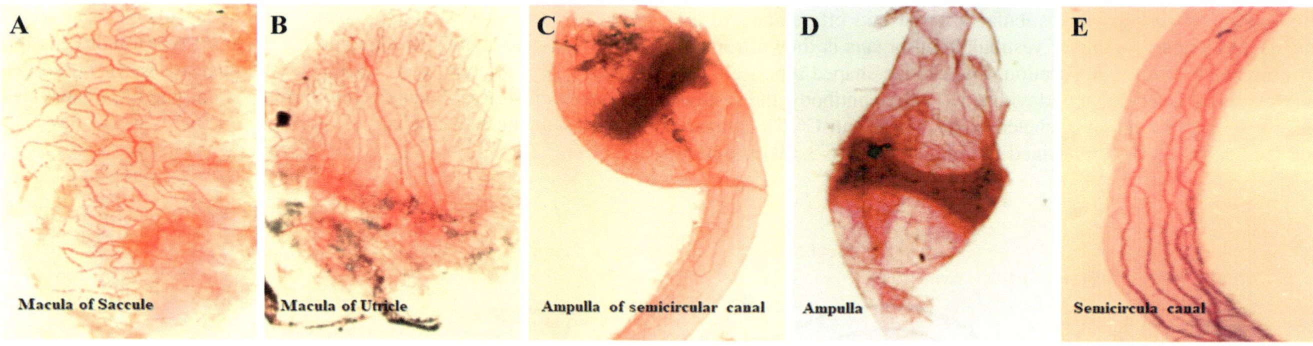

Fig. 1.32 The surface preparations of vestibular labyrinth with eosin staining show the erythrocytes in the capillaries. (**A**) The capillary network beneath the supporting cells of the macula of saccule in guinea pigs is arranged laterally. (**B**) The capillary network beneath the supporting cells of the macula of the utricle in guinea pigs is fan-shaped. (**C**) The dense capillary network in the membranous ampulla of guinea pig is basically parallel to the direction of the semicircular canal. (**D**) The capillary network beneath the supporting cells of the ampullary crista in guinea pigs is parallel to the crista. (**E**) The arrangement of capillaries on the membranous semicircular canal in guinea pigs is parallel to the direction of the canal

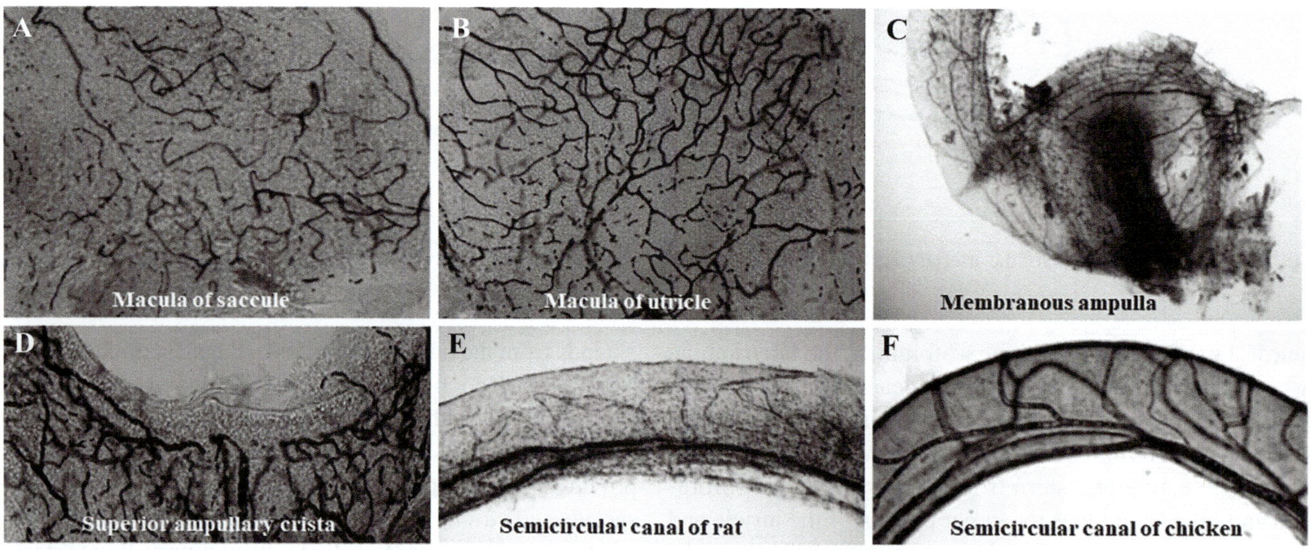

Fig. 1.33 The surface preparations of vestibular labyrinth with 3,3′-Diaminobenzidine staining shows erythrocytes within the capillaries. (**A**) The capillary network beneath the supporting cells of the macula of the saccule in rats is oriented perpendicular to the striola zone. (**B**) The capillary network beneath the supporting cells of the macula of the utricle in rats is criss-crossed. (**C**) The capillary network on the membranous ampulla of rats runs parallel to the semicircular canals. (**D**) The capillary network beneath the supporting cells of the rat ampullary crista is essentially parallel to the ampullary crista. (**E**) The arrangement of capillaries on the membranous semicircular canal of rat is essentially parallel to the semicircular canals. (**F**) The arrangement of capillary network on the membranous semicircular canal in chicken is like rings around the semicircular canal

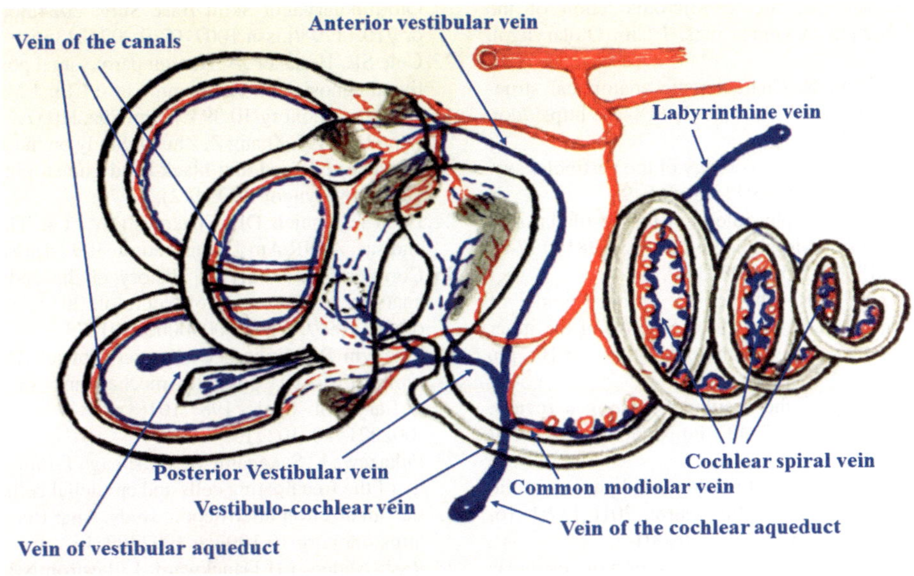

Fig. 1.34 Schematic diagram of the venous return of the membrane labyrinth in mammals

beneath the supporting cells of the macula of the utricle are arranged in a fan shape (Figs. 1.32B and 1.33B). On the membranous ampulla, the capillaries are oriented perpendicularly to the ampullary crista, but parallel to the semicircular canal (Figs. 1.32D and 1.33D). The capillaries beneath the supporting cell layer of the ampullary cristae are either parallel to the crista or arranged in a crisscross pattern (Figs. 1.32D and 1.33D). The capillary network on the membranous wall of the maculae is relatively sparse. The capillaries on the membranous wall of the semicircular canal in mammals are oriented parallel to the direction of the semicircular canal, with those near the membranous ampulla being slightly thinner in diameter than those farther from the ampullary end (Figs. 1.32E and 1.33E). If these capillaries represent the terminal ends of arteries, it suggests that arterial blood flow in mammals travels from the semicircular canal toward the ampulla. Conversely, if these capillaries mark the beginning of venous return, it indicates that venous blood flow in the semicircular canals of mammals travels from the ampullary end toward the semicircular canal (Figs. 1.32E and 1.33E). In contrast, the capillaries on the membranous wall of the semicircular canal in birds are arranged in a circular pattern around the semicircular canal, starting from the concave side edge of the canal [2, 4, 33, 34] (Fig. 1.33F).

1.4.3 Vestibular Venous Return

There are three approaches for the venous return of the inner ear, which are the labyrinthine venous route, the cochlear aqueduct venous route, and the vestibular aqueduct venous route. The venous blood from the middle turn and apical turn of the cochlea flows through the spiral veins in the cochlear modiolus to the labyrinth veins, which drain into the superior petrosal sinus. However, this pathway is not related to the vestibular venous return. In contrast, the cochlear aqueduct venous circuit and the vestibular aqueduct venous circuit are two critical pathways for vestibular venous drainage. The anterior vestibular vein drains blood from the utricle and the ampullae of the superior and lateral semicircular canals, while the posterior vestibular vein drains blood from the saccule and the ampulla of the posterior semicircular canal. The anterior vestibular vein forms the vestibular aqueduct vein at the vestibular aqueduct and follows the endolymphatic duct to the lateral sinus of the superior petrosal sinus. The posterior vestibular vein forms the cochlear aqueduct vein near the round window and follows the cochlear aqueduct to the lateral sinus of the inferior petrosal sinus (Fig. 1.34). Ultimately, these three venous pathways from the inner ear converge into the internal jugular vein [1, 33].

References

1. Schuknecht H. 2. Anatomy. In: Schuknecht H, editor. Pathology of the ear. 1st ed. Cambridge: Harvard University Press; 1974. pp. 40–96.
2. Ding D, Jiang S. Chapter 4: Inner ear anatomy and structure. In: Ding D, editor. Manual of anatomical examination of the inner ear of the guinea pig. Shanghai: Xuelin Publishing House; 1989. pp. 24–35.
3. Ding D, Li M, Jiang C, Salvi R. Chapter 3: Anatomy of temporal bone and inner ear. In: Ding D, editor. Morphology of the inner ear. Harbin: Heilongjiang Science and Technology Press; 2001. pp. 10–17.
4. Ding D, Qi W, Qu Y, Salvi R. Chapter 1: Anatomy of the inner ear. In: Ding D, editor. Science of the inner ear. Beijing: China Science and Technology Press; 2010. pp. 1–8.
5. Hayes SH, Ding D, Salvi R, Allman BL. Anatomy and physiology of the external, middle and inner ear. In: Celesia GG, editor. Eds. Disorders of peripheral and central auditory processing. Handbook of clinical neurophysiology. Vol. 10. New York: Elsevier; 2013. pp. 3–23.
6. Ding D, Luo S, Jin X. Microdissection of the vestibular end-organs in guinea pigs. Shanghai Med J. 1986;9(3):153–4.

7. Ding D, Zhao J, Huangfu M, Jin X. Microdissection of the whole membranous labyrinth in guinea pigs. J Clin Otolaryngol. 1987;1(1):9–11.
8. Li P, Gao K, Ding D, Salvi R. Characteristic anatomical structures of rat temporal bone. J Otol. 2015;10(3):118–24. https://doi.org/10.1016/j.joto.2015.11.002.
9. Guyot JP. [Review of anatomy and physiology of the vestibular system]. Rev Med Suisse Romande. 1993;113(8):665–9.
10. Sakka L, Vitte E. [Anatomy and physiology of the vestibular system: review of the literature]. Morphologie. 2004;88(281):117–6. https://doi.org/10.1016/s1286-0115(04)98134-9.
11. Ding D, Qi W, Qu Y, Salvi R. Chapter 15: Animal model of intra-labyrinthal hydrops. In: Ding D, editor. Science of the inner ear. Beijing: China Science and Technology Press; 2010. pp. 183–188.
12. Khan S, Chang R. Anatomy of the vestibular system: a review. Neurorehabilitation. 2013;32(3):437–43. https://doi.org/10.3233/NRE-130866.
13. Kingma H, van de Berg R. Anatomy, physiology, and physics of the peripheral vestibular system. Handb Clin Neurol. 2016;137:1–16. https://doi.org/10.1016/B978-0-444-63437-5.00001-7.
14. Ding D, Li P, Qi W, Zhang J. Quantitative observation of vestibular sensory hair cells in experimental animals. Chin J Otorhinolaryngol Skull Base Surg. 2022;28(1):11–18. https://doi.org/10.11798/j.issn.1007-1520.202290001.
15. Engstrom H. Microscopic anatomy of the inner ear. Acta Otol. 1951;40(1–2):5–22. https://doi.org/10.3109/00016485109138903.
16. Ding D, Qi W, Salvi R. Antiphase stimulation model of vestibular hair cells. Chinese J Otol. 2017;15(6):715–20.
17. Engstrom H, Bergstrom B, Rosenhall U. Vestibular sensory epithelia. Arch Otol. 1974;100(5):411–18. https://doi.org/10.1001/archotol.1974.00780040425002.
18. Merchant SN, Velazquez-Villasenor L, Tsuji K, et al. Temporal bone studies of the human peripheral vestibular system. Normative vestibular hair cell data. Ann Otol Rhinol Laryngol. 2000;181:3–13. https://doi.org/10.1177/00034894001090s502.
19. Ding D, Wang J, Salvi RJ. Early damage in the chinchilla vestibular sensory epithelium from carboplatin. Audiol Neurotol. 1997;2(3):155–67. https://doi.org/10.1159/000259238.
20. Ding D, Shi L, Xing Y, et al. Sagittal sectioning of temporal bones and quantitative measurement of neural densities in the inner ear in normal mice. Chin J Otorhinolaryngol Skull Base Surg. 2024;30(2):69–75. https://doi.org/10.11798/j.issn.1007-1520.202424331.
21. Ding D, Shi L, Xing Y, et al. Secondary neural damage in the inner ear induced by intratympanic gentamicin injection. Chin J Otorhinolaryngol Skull Base Surg. 2024;30(1):11–19. https://doi.org/10.11798/j.issn.1007-1520.202424356.
22. Cole SR, Honaker JA. Benign paroxysmal positional vertigo: effective diagnosis and treatment. Cleve Clin J Med. 2022;89(11):653–62. https://doi.org/10.3949/ccjm.89a.21057.
23. Ding D, Jin X, Zhang Z, Zhu Q. Study on the different susceptibility between red-eyed and black-eyed guinea pigs to gentamicin. Acta Otorhinolaryngol. 1995;9(2):70–74.
24. Lo WW, Daniels DL, Chakeres DW, et al. The endolymphatic duct and sac. AJNR Am J Neuroradiol. 1997;18(5):881–7.
25. Corrales CE, Mudry A. History of the endolymphatic sac: from anatomy to surgery. Otol Neurotol. 2017;38(1):152–6. https://doi.org/10.1097/MAO.0000000000001273.
26. Wackym PA, Friberg U, Bagger-Sjoback D, et al. Human endolymphatic sac: possible mechanisms of pressure regulation. J Laryngol Otol. 1987;101(8):768–79. https://doi.org/10.1017/s0022215100102713.
27. Fukazawa K, Sakagami M, Matsunaga T, Fujita H. Endocytotic activity of the free floating cells and epithelial cells in the endolymphatic sac: an electron microscopic study. Anat Rec. 1991;230(3):425–33. https://doi.org/10.1002/ar.1092300315.
28. Rask-Andersen H, Danckwardt-Lilliestrom N, Linthicum FH Jr, House WF. Ultrastructural evidence of a merocrine secretion in the human endolymphatic sac. Ann Otol Rhinol Laryngol. 1991;100(2):148–56. https://doi.org/10.1177/000348949110000211.
29. Gao K, Ding D, Sun H, Roth J, Salvi R. Kanamycin damages early postnatal, but not adult spiral ganglion neurons. Neurotoxic Res. 2017;32(4):603–13. https://doi.org/10.1007/s12640-017-9773-2.
30. Mathews MA, Camp AJ, Murray AJ. Reviewing the role of the efferent vestibular system in motor and vestibular circuits. Front Physiol. 2017;8:552 https://doi.org/10.3389/fphys.2017.00552.
31. Sugita M, Masutani H, Moriguchi M, Matsunaga K, Nakai Y. Distribution of arteries from brain stem to inner ear around the internal auditory canal. Acta Otolaryngol Suppl. 1991;486:45–52. https://doi.org/10.3109/00016489109134981.
32. Salgado-Lopez L, Leonel LCP, Aydin SO, Peris-Celda M. Surgical anatomy of the labyrinthine and subarcuate arteries and clinical implications. World Neurosurg. 2020;141:e880–7. https://doi.org/10.1016/j.wneu.2020.06.083.
33. Hansen JM, Qvortrup K, Friis M. Vestibular tributaries to the vein of the vestibular aqueduct. Acta Oto-Laryngol. 2011;131(1):9–13. https://doi.org/10.3109/00016489.2010.511260.
34. Ding D, Liu H, Qi W, et al. Ototoxic effects and mechanisms of loop diuretics. J Otol. 2016;11(4):145–56. https://doi.org/10.1016/j.joto.2016.10.001.

2 Sectioning Techniques of Vestibular Tissue

Pathology is a pivotal discipline in medical diagnosis and research, focusing on the etiology, pathogenesis, developmental patterns, morphological and metabolic alterations during disease or injury progression, as well as disease outcomes. The historical development of pathology can be traced back to the mid-eighteenth century. With advancements in optical microscopy and electron microscopy, coupled with innovations of the techniques in tissue preparations and the refinement of biological staining and labeling methods, pathology has evolved into a crucial "bridging discipline" connecting basic and clinical medicine. Within this context, vestibular pathology has emerged as a specialized field in scientific research of the inner ear, paralleling the progress in pathological techniques.

Tissue sectioning represents a fundamental sample preparation methodology in pathological studies, encompassing various techniques such as freehand sectioning, paraffin embedding sectioning, collodion embedding sectioning, gelatin-embedding frozen sectioning, and plastic resin embedding sectioning. In vestibular pathology research, collodion-embedding sections, gelatin-embedding frozen sections, and plastic resin-embedding sections have been extensively utilized due to their specific advantages.

The preparation of vestibular tissue sections follows a standardized protocol similar to that of other tissue samples, involving sequential procedures including tissue harvesting, fixation, decalcification, dehydration, penetration, clearing, embedding, sectioning, and staining. However, the specific protocols for vestibular organ sectioning may vary depending on the observation parameters, staining techniques, and embedding materials employed. To illustrate the general workflow of vestibular sectioning, we briefly describe below several conventional sectioning methods with temporal bone sections and single vestibular end-organ sections as representative examples.

2.1 Continuous Sectioning of the Whole Temporal Bone

Although temporal bone sectioning techniques may have been developed as early as the 1930s or before, the first comprehensive description of this methodology is widely attributed to Schuknecht's seminal work, *Pathology of the Ear*, published in 1974 [1].

2.1.1 Fixation of the Temporal Bone

The inner ear is deeply buried within the petrous portion of the temporal bone and contains highly hypoxia-sensitive sensory hair cells. Even brief hypoxia can induce significant pathological alterations in these cells, potentially mimicking tissue autolysis artifacts. Consequently, immersion fixation alone is insufficient, as delayed fixation may introduce experimental artifacts due to postmortem changes in the inner ear sensory epithelium. To avoid these issues, effective and rapid fixation must be achieved before the onset of postmortem degeneration. Cardiac perfusion under deep anesthesia, ensuring systemic circulation of the fixative, is widely recognized as one of the most reliable methods for optimal temporal bone fixation.

The perfusion fixation procedure is performed as follows: Under deep anesthesia, a midline cervical incision is made to expose the internal jugular vein, which is then occluded using a vascular clamp. Following thoracotomy to expose the cardiac chamber, a perfusion needle is inserted into the left ventricular cavity. Preheated (38°C) saline is perfused through the left ventricle into the aortic arch and into the arteries flowing throughout the body using a perfusion pump, while simultaneously making an incision in the clamped jugular vein to permit blood drainage. The transition to fixative perfusion (either 10% phosphate-buffered formalin or 2.5% phosphate-buffered glutaraldehyde) is initiated

D. Ding et al., *Histopathological Atlas of the Inner Ear*,
https://doi.org/10.1007/978-981-95-6338-8_2

when the venous effluent becomes clear, indicating adequate blood clearance. The perfusion is maintained for a minimum of 20 min to ensure complete systemic distribution of the fixative through the circulatory system. After the perfusion fixation is completed, the temporal bone is immediately separated, and then the stapes is removed to open the oval window. The fixative is then perfused directly into the vestibular cistern to ensure optimal preservation of the delicate inner ear structures. Finally, the specimen is immersed in fixative solution overnight to complete the fixation process. This rigorous protocol ensures rapid and effective preservation of the inner ear sensory epithelium in a near-physiological state, minimizing postmortem artifacts [1–5].

2.1.2 Temporal Bone Decalcification Techniques

After fixation, specimens intended for temporal bone sectioning require decalcification for routine inner ear pathology examination. The standard decalcification protocol typically employs either 5% nitric acid or 5% hydrochloric acid solution, with the decalcifying agent requiring daily replacement with fresh solution. For guinea pig temporal bones, calcium removal can typically be assessed after 3 days of treatment. The chemical verification method involves sampling the decalcification solution and adding saturated ammonium oxalate followed by ammonia—absence of white precipitate indicates complete decalcification, while its presence necessitates continued treatment [6, 7]. Alternatively, radiographic assessment may be employed to confirm calcium removal. It should be noted that these acidic decalcification methods are suitable only for conventional staining in routine pathological examinations and are incompatible with enzymatic histochemical metal labeling or immunohistochemical techniques. For specimens intended for immunohistochemical labeling, 10% disodium ethylenediamine tetraacetate (EDTA) solution is the preferred decalcifying agent, requiring daily solution replacement and a prolonged decalcification period of 5–7 days to ensure that the tissue is preserved in the best condition for subsequent histochemical staining and observations [4, 8, 9].

2.1.3 Temporal Bone Staining Techniques

There are certain technical difficulties in histologically processing temporal bone sections using conventional methods. Serial sectioning of collodion-embedded temporal bone requires sequential staining of individual sections in exact slicing order, resulting in low work efficiency and time-consuming and labor-intensive process. Similarly, gelatin or OCT embedding frozen sections of the entire temporal bone are also difficult to stain each single section effectively due to the contamination of the stain and the section rupture caused by the dissolution of embedding agent. Therefore, traditional hematoxylin-eosin staining is nearly impossible to perform slice-by-slice on temporal bone frozen sections. In view of the application limitations of the above-mentioned traditional temporal bone section staining method, we proposed an optimized scheme for overall staining of the entire temporal bone before sectioning [6, 10].

Following complete decalcification in hydrochloric acid, the temporal bones are flushed under running water for at least 3 h, and then rinsed thoroughly with distilled water to remove residual acid. The temporal bone is then immersed in the dilute solution of Ehrlich hematoxylin and placed in a 37°C incubator for 3 days. Post-staining treatment includes an extensive 24-h running water rinse to achieve uniform nuclear staining throughout the osseous and soft tissue components. This innovative pre-embedding staining methodology yields significant advantages, as all subsequently sectioned slices maintain complete histological staining prior to tissue processing, enabling immediate mounting and microscopic examination without requiring additional staining procedures [6, 7, 10].

The stock solutions of Ehrlich hematoxylin are separately prepared, including a 5% aluminum ammonium sulfate aqueous solution, a 2% hematoxylin solution in 95% ethanol, and a 10% glacial acetic acid solution in glycerin. These components form the basis for preparing Ehrlich's hematoxylin staining solution. To prepare stock solutions of Ehrlich hematoxylin, combine 100 mL of the 2% hematoxylin solution with 100 mL of 5% aluminum ammonium sulfate solution by dropwise addition while stirring continuously. After allowing the mixture to stand at room temperature for several days, add 100 mL of the 10% glacial acetic acid-glycerin solution with thorough mixing. The solution is then transferred to a cotton-plugged glass bottle and exposed to natural light for 2 months to facilitate oxidation. The mature stain, characterized by its deep purple coloration indicating complete oxidation, serves as the mixed stock solution for whole tissue staining applications [6, 7, 10]. Before staining the entire temporal bone, prepare the Ehrlich hematoxylin dilute solution according to the following recipe. The preparation method of Ehrlich hematoxylin dilute solution is to mix 6 mL Ehrlich hematoxylin stock solution with 5 mL glacial acetic acid and 66 mL 50% alcohol solution. The temporal bone is immersed in this solution at 37°C for 3 days to achieve the ideal overall staining effect.

2.1.4 Embedding of the Temporal Bone

The embedding method for temporal bones is selected based on the desired sectioning technique. For collodion-embedded continuous sections, specimens undergo complete dehydration followed by sequential infiltration with increasing concentrations of collodion prior to final embedding. When preparing paraffin-embedded serial sections, standard dehydration protocols are followed by paraffin infiltration and embedding.

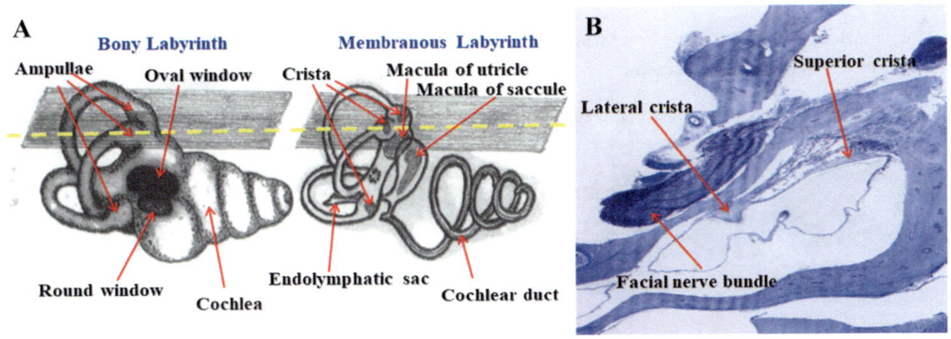

Fig. 2.1 Standardized transverse section of temporal bone at the vestibular cavity roof level. (**A**) Schematic diagrams of the guinea pig bony labyrinth and membranous labyrinth are shown from left to right. The yellow dashed line marks the slice plane at the top of the vestibular cistern. (**B**) Histological cross-section demonstrates orthogonal orientation of semicircular canal cristae: the superior ampullary crista appears in longitudinal profile while the lateral ampullary crista is sectioned transversely within the same plane. (Reproduced with permission from Ding et al. [14])

Frozen section preparation employs an alternative approach where specimens are directly embedded using a two-step gelatin gradient (10% followed by 25%) incubated at 37°C, eliminating the need for dehydration. During cryosectioning, the polymerized gelatin matrix provides critical structural support, maintaining the anatomical relationships between the inner ear cavities and membranous labyrinth while ensuring section integrity, as validated in previous research [6, 7, 11–13].

2.1.5 Slice of the Temporal Bone

The three-dimensional architecture of the vestibular system necessitates multiplanar sectioning for comprehensive structural analysis. Horizontal sections provide superior-inferior separation, sagittal sections divide left-right components, and coronal sections delineate anterior-posterior relationships. Among these orientations, cross-sectional temporal bone slices have become the gold standard due to their diagnostic utility and anatomical relevance.

Continuous sectioning along the horizontal plane enables complete reconstruction of the membranous labyrinth when required by specific experimental protocols. However, for routine histomorphological evaluation of vestibular end-organs, five strategically selected representative levels typically suffice to demonstrate essential pathological or developmental changes. This standardized approach balances thorough anatomical assessment with practical laboratory efficiency [14].

In rat temporal bone models, horizontal sectioning begins at the superior tympanum base. Initial cuts expose the ampullary cavities of superior and lateral semicircular canals by opening their bony walls, yielding sections of their cristae ampullares. Due to their orthogonal anatomical relationship, these cristae appear in perpendicular orientations on sections, with one crista displayed longitudinally and the other transversely (Fig. 2.1). The second standardized level parallels the stapes plane, intersecting the vestibular cistern to reveal utricular and saccular maculae cross-sections within the superior sieve region. This plane simultaneously demonstrates superior vestibular ganglion neurons and their nerve fibers, along with habenula perforata in the cochlear basal turn osseous spiral lamina. The nerve fiber density at these perforations serves as a reliable indicator of spiral ganglion neuron-hair cell connectivity integrity in the cochlea [3, 14] (Fig. 2.2).

The third critical sectioning plane traverses the cochlear modiolus, enabling concurrent evaluation of the organ of Corti on the cochlear basilar membrane, the spiral ganglion neurons in Rosenthal's canal, and the sensory hair cells on the macula of saccule. This comprehensive view facilitates correlative analysis between the hair cells on the macula of saccule, the posterior ampullary crista, and their shared inferior vestibular neuron projections (Fig. 2.3). The fourth optional plane is parallel to the endolymphatic duct and endolymphatic sac, which is mainly suitable for observing and studying the pathological changes of the endolymphatic duct and endolymphatic sac (Fig. 2.4). The fifth layer of the temporal bone cross section is the horizontal section of the ampullary crista of posterior semicircular canal. This section is equivalent to the slice at the bottom plane of the vestibular cistern and the cross-section of the habenular nucleus in the bony spiral plate can be collected again. Therefore, in addition to the pathological evaluation of the lesions of the posterior semicircular canal ampulla crest hair cells, the degree of damage to the cochlear spiral ganglion neurons and the surrounding auditory nerve fibers can also be evaluated [8, 9, 14–20] (Fig. 2.5).

The five standardized temporal bone section planes provide comprehensive evaluation of vestibular and auditory structures: The first plane assesses hair cell pathology in the superior and lateral semicircular canal cristae; the second plane simultaneously evaluates utricular macula hair cell integrity and superior vestibular ganglion neuron status (Fig. 2.6), while also serving as the optimal plane for stapes and annular ligament observation (Fig. 2.7); the third plane reveals saccular macula hair cell

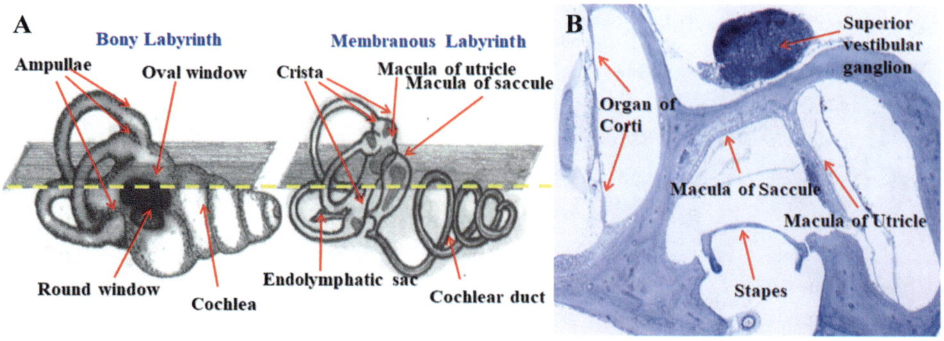

Fig. 2.2 Standardized transverse section of temporal bone at the stapes plane level. (**A**) Schematic representation of guinea pig osseous and membranous labyrinth anatomy (left to right). The yellow dashed line indicates the section plane corresponding to the oval window orientation. (**B**) In horizontal section parallel to the stapes, the saccular macula in transverse section is located on the medial wall of the vestibular cistern facing the footplate of the stapes, and the transverse section of the utricle macula posterior to the saccular macula can be seen. In the medial cranial bony wall separated from the macula of utricle, neurons in the superior vestibular tract can be observed at the same section. The portion of the cochlear basilar membrane located in front of the vestibular cistern and the peripheral auditory nerve fibers in the habenula perforata can also be observed. (Reproduced with permission from Ding et al. [14])

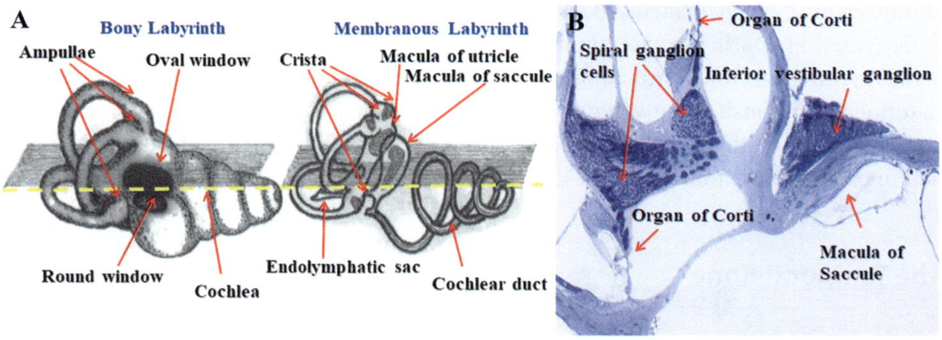

Fig. 2.3 Standardized transverse section through the cochlear modiolus plane. (**A**) Schematic representation of guinea pig labyrinthine anatomy (left to right) with the yellow dashed line indicating the section plane parallel to the modiolar axis. (**B**) In horizontal section parallel to the modiolus, the inferior saccular macula in transverse section on the medial wall of the vestibular cistern and the inferior vestibular ganglion neurons at the bottom of the cochlear modiolus can be observed. From this cochlear modiolus section plane, the section of the organ of Corti on the cochlear basilar membrane and the spiral ganglion neurons in Rosenthal's canal in the modiolus can also be observed. (Reproduced with permission from Ding et al. [14])

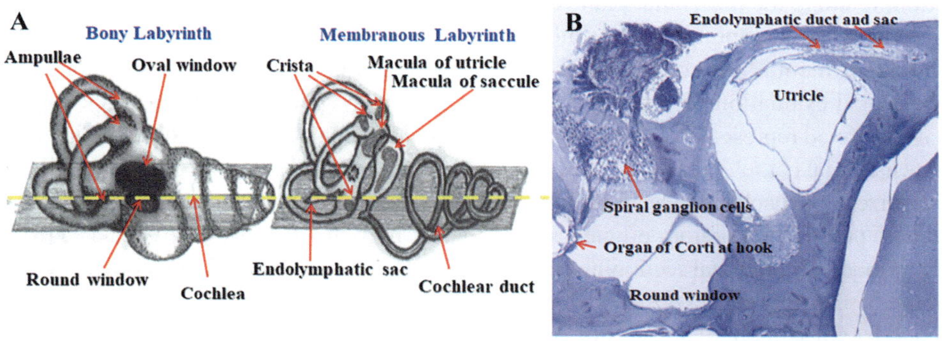

Fig. 2.4 Standardized transverse section through the endolymphatic duct plane. (**A**) Schematic representation of guinea pig labyrinthine anatomy (left to right) showing the section plane (yellow dashed line) parallel to the endolymphatic duct orientation. (**B**) The histological section demonstrates the terminal portion of the endolymphatic duct and sac, providing a critical anatomical reference for evaluating potential pathological alterations in both the endolymphatic duct and sac structures. (Reproduced with permission from Ding et al. [14])

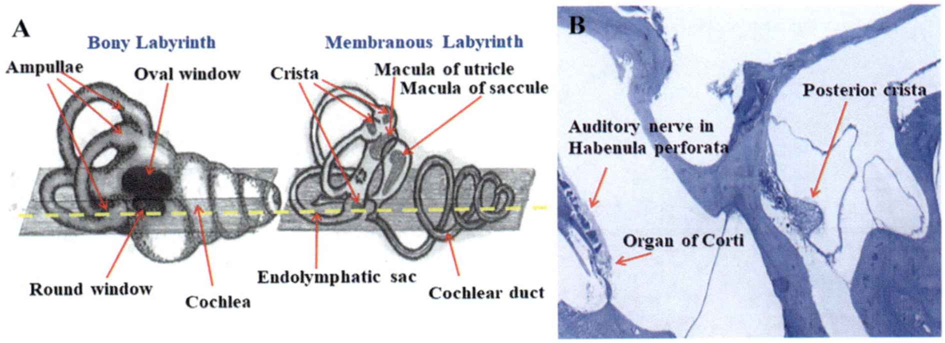

Fig. 2.5 Standardized transverse section through the posterior semicircular canal plane. (**A**) Schematic representation of guinea pig labyrinthine anatomy (left to right) with the yellow dashed line indicating the section plane corresponding to the vestibular cavity floor. (**B**) When a transverse section is made to the bottom of the vestibular cistern, a section of the posterior ampullary crista perpendicular to its crista can be observed, and the osseous spiral lamina of the cochlear basal turn can also be observed. Therefore, the hair cells on the posterior crista and the number of auditory nerve fibers in the habenula perforata in the cochlear basal turn can be evaluated within this single plane. (Reproduced with permission from Ding et al. [14])

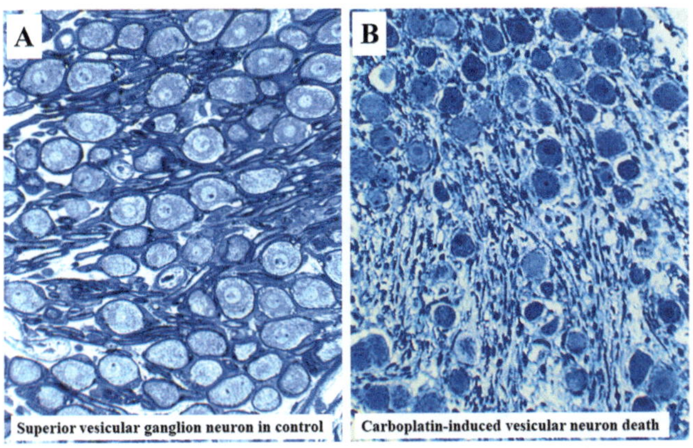

Fig. 2.6 Panel figure showing two microscopic images of neurons. (**A**) Section depicts superior vesicular ganglion neurons in a control sample, displaying a dense arrangement of cells with clear outlines. (**B**) Section shows carboplatin-induced vesicular neuron destruction, with a less dense arrangement and signs of apoptotic degradation of nuclear condensation. Both images are stained with toluidine blue in shades of blue to highlight cellular structures

organization and inferior vestibular ganglion neuron morphology (Fig. 2.8); and the fifth plane specifically examines posterior semicircular canal crista hair cells. Consequently, the pathological evaluation of the vestibular sensory epithelium and vestibular ganglion neurons can be mainly performed from the above four slice planes [14].

The inner ear's bipolar ganglion neurons establish crucial neural connections between peripheral sensory epithelia and central brainstem nuclei. These neural pathways traverse through two distinct anatomical conduits: the cochlear neuroforamen passes through the cochlear auditory nerve fibers and inferior vestibular nerve fibers, and the superior vestibular canal traverses through the superior vestibular fibers. Temporal bone sagittal sections provide optimal planes for evaluating central axonal integrity, as this orientation is perpendicular to both vestibular and auditory nerve bundles within these canals. Quantitative assessment of nerve fiber density in these canals serves as a reliable indicator of peripheral neuron survival and subsequent central input preservation [5, 9, 20] (Fig. 2.9).

Coronal or frontal slices are rarely used for temporal bone examinations. One of the reasons is that the slice angle is almost parallel to the cochlear basilar membrane and macula of utricle, as well as the superior and posterior cristae of the ampulla, which makes it difficult to obtain ideal angle of hair cell long-axis slices. Another reason is that it is impossible to cut the sensory organs in the inner ear cavity with the connecting nerve fibers and peripheral neurons on this slicing plane from coronal slice angle. Therefore, it is difficult to correlate the lesions of peripheral hair cells with the lesions of peripheral neurons for comprehensive analysis. Generally, coronal slices are deliberately selected only when it is necessary to evaluate the cilia bundles or the cuticular plate of hair cells or the type I afferent terminal surrounding the type I hair cells or the synaptic connections at the bottom of sensory hair cells [21] (Fig. 2.10A).

2.2 Slices of the Membranous Labyrinth of the Separated Vestibular End-Organs

Since long-term fixation and decalcification can lead to enzyme inactivation and loss of protein antigen-antibody reactivity, as well as complex temperature and permeability factors during embedding and dehydration, the whole temporal bone tissue sectioning technique is only suitable for routine pathological examination of the inner ear. However, it is not suitable for immunohistochemical research. If the vestibular end organs are microdissected out from the bony inner ear cavity, each vestibular end organ can be directly immunohistochemically

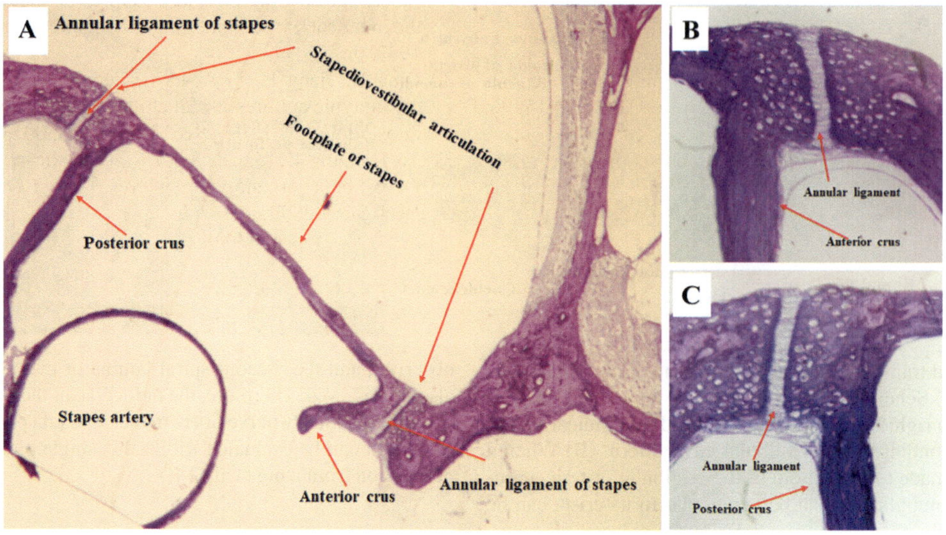

Fig. 2.7 Histological observation of stapes anatomy in rat temporal bone. This transverse section through the stapes plane demonstrates the acoustic transmission apparatus, where the stapes conducts vibrational energy from the incus to the oval window. The annular ligament's elastic properties enable stapes mobility, with pathological fibrotic or ossific changes potentially leading to complete stapes fixation—a key feature in otosclerosis models. (**A**) Overview showing the stapes footplate surrounded by intact annular ligament. (**B**) High-magnification view of anterior annular ligament morphology. (**C**) High-magnification view of posterior annular ligament morphology

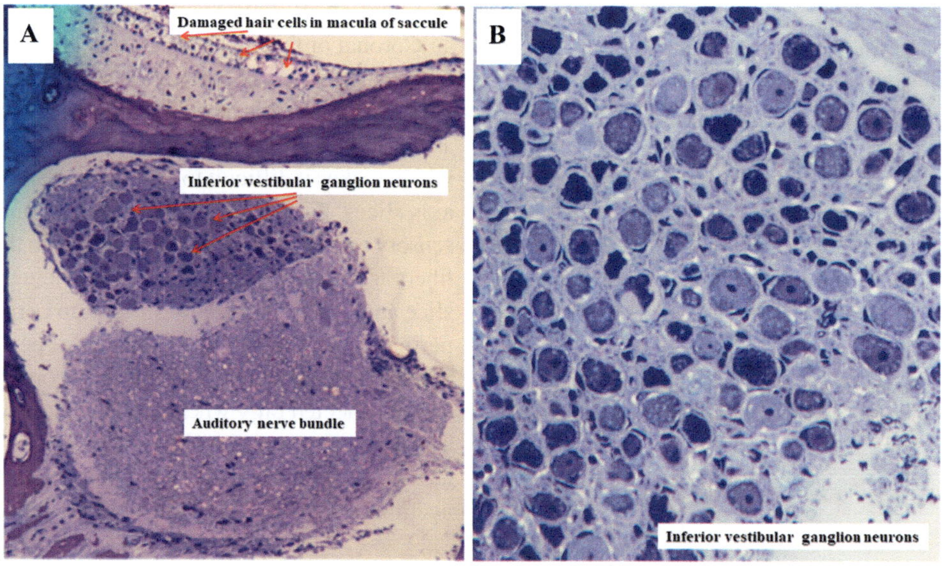

Fig. 2.8 Histopathological assessment of murine temporal bone at the middle sieve region. (**A**) This section reveals pathological changes in the macula of saccule with evident hair cell loss, while the inferior vestibular ganglion neurons at the base of the cochlear neuroforamen on the other side of the middle sieve spot zone are intact. The adjacent auditory nerve bundles in the cochlear neuroforamen also maintain normal. (**B**) A higher-magnification view provides a detailed cytological evaluation of the inferior vestibular ganglion neurons

labeled without decalcification. After completing the immunohistochemical labeling, each vestibular end organ can be sliced at an ideal cross-sectional angle. Therefore, the separated vestibular membrane labyrinth sectioning technique not only avoids the fatal drawback of long-term decalcification of the temporal bone leading to loss of tissue chemical reactivity, but also ensures the effective comparability of the pathology of each vestibular end organ slice [22–28].

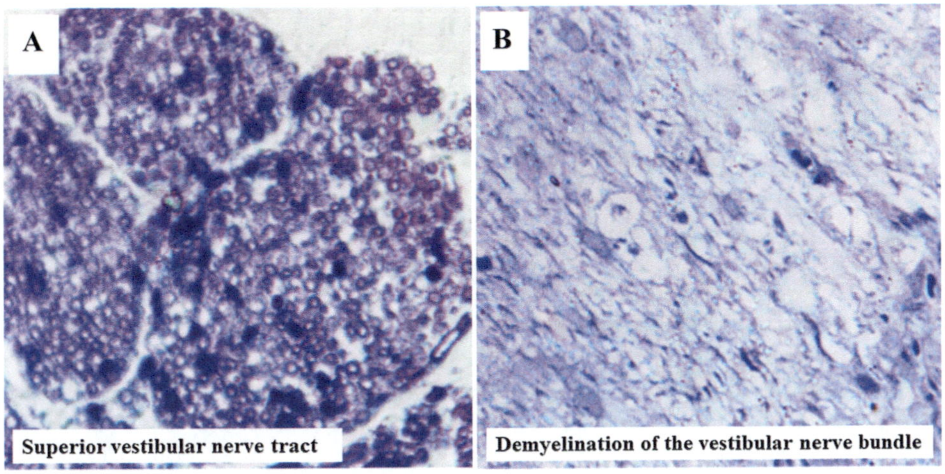

Fig. 2.9 Comparative neuropathology of vestibular nerve bundles in sagittal section. (**A**) Control micrograph demonstrates normal histological architecture of superior vestibular nerve fibers in untreated rat temporal bone. (**B**) Glycerol-treated micrograph reveals extensive axonal demyelination 24 h following glycerol injection into the superior vestibular canal, demonstrating acute neurotoxic effects on vestibular nerve integrity

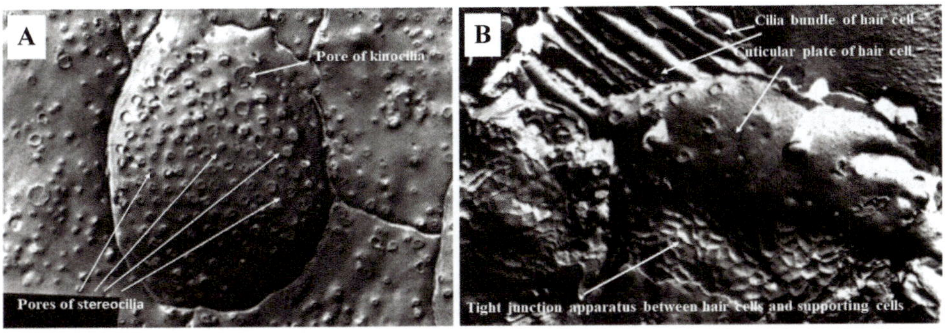

Fig. 2.10 The platinum-carbon replica film on the surface of cuticular plate of human vestibular hair cells or the lateral side of the hair cell junction device was observed under the transmission electron microscope using the freeze-etching technique. (**A**) From the plane parallel to the cuticular plate of hair cells, there is one hair root of thicker kinocilium at one end of the cuticular plate of vestibular hair cell, while many hair roots of relatively thin stereocilia are inserted into the cuticular plate of hair cell in turn along the root of the kinocilium. (**B**) The longitudinal section of vestibular hair cells on the crista ampullae reveals developmental specialization at 11 weeks, showing seven to nine parallel striated tight junctions at the hair cell neck region that form functional barriers with adjacent supporting cells

2.2.1 Perfusion Fixation of the Inner Ear Cavity

Perfusion of the inner ear cavity is an effective fixation method particularly useful for the preparation of the vestibular membranous labyrinth in smaller experimental animals, such as guinea pigs, rats, and mice. Using murine specimens as an example, the procedure is as follows. Under deep anesthesia, the neck of the mouse was pulled to cause cervical dislocation. The temporal bone of the mouse is removed within 2 min and immersed in the fixative. Under a dissection microscope, the footplate of stapes was removed and the lateral wall of the vestibular cistern was opened to fill the vestibular cavity with the fixative quickly. In order to ensure that the vestibular sensory epithelium does not undergo autolysis, the tympanic membrane of the anesthetized mouse can also be removed through the external auditory canal to expose the bone promontory, then the footplate of the stapes is removed, and the fixative is injected into the vestibular cavity. In this approach, the sensory hair cells will be effectively fixed in the alive state. After the inner ear cavity was perfused and fixed, the temporal bone was removed and immersed in the fixative for further adequate fixation, thereby completely avoiding the ischemia and hypoxia-induced postmortem changes of sensory hair cells in the inner ear [2, 9, 20].

2.2.2 Pretreatment of the Vestibular Membrane Labyrinth Before Sectioning

Under a dissecting microscope, the fixed temporal bone is immersed in phosphate buffer solution. Each membranous labyrinth of vestibular end-organs is micro-dissected out from the vestibular cistern. Since each dissected vestibular end-organ

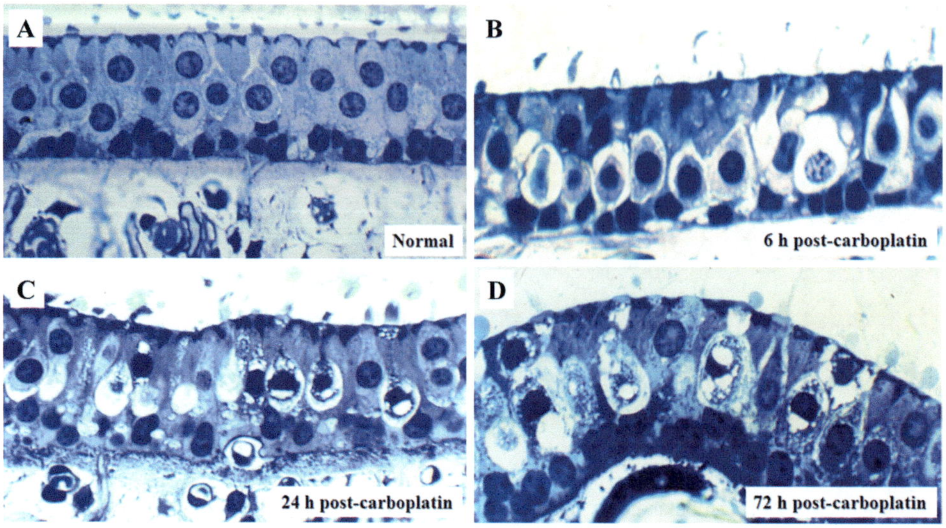

Fig. 2.11 Temporal progression of carboplatin-induced pathological changes in type I hair cells and type I afferent synapse in chinchillas. (**A**) Macular section of the utricle from a normal chinchilla showing the type I and type II hair cells and the nerve synapse and the support cells underlying the hair cells. (**B**) 6 h after subcutaneous injection of carboplatin, the gap between the type I hair cells and their type I afferent nerve endings begins to increase, and type I hair cells begin to show mild cytoplasmic condensation. (**C**) 24 h after subcutaneous injection of carboplatin, nearly all type I hair cells located at the macula of utricle in the type I calyceal afferent terminals showed marked nuclear condensation and cytoplasmic vacuolar lesions. However, type II hair cells maintain their normal structures. (**D**) Complete degeneration of type I hair cells occurs within 72 h, with only cellular debris remaining within calyceal afferent terminals. However, type II hair cells and type II afferent synapses remain intact. Therefore, it can be concluded that type I afferent synapse and type I hair cells are the major targets of carboplatin to destroy the vestibular end-organs in chinchillas

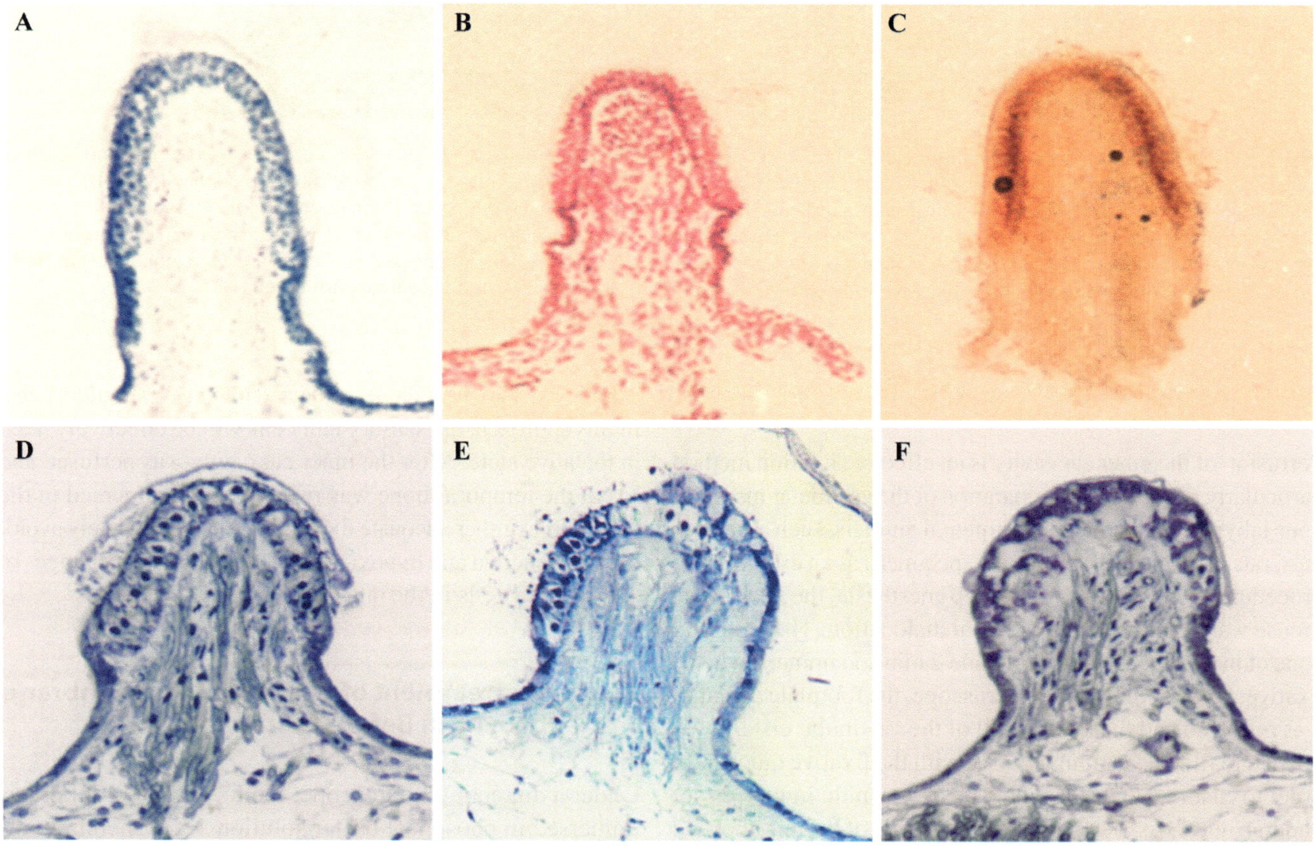

Fig. 2.12 Sections of isolated ampullary crista. (**A**) Slice of ampullary crista with hematoxylin staining in guinea pig. (**B**) Slice of ampullary crista with Feulgen reaction-labeled DNA in guinea pig. (**C**) Slice of ampullary crista with acetylcholinesterase staining in guinea pig. (**D**) Slice of ampullary crista with toluidine blue staining in mouse. (**E**) Focal sensory hair cell loss was detected in toluidine blue-stained slice of murine ampullary crista. (**F**) Toluidine blue-stained murine ampullary crista section revealing total sensory hair cell depletion

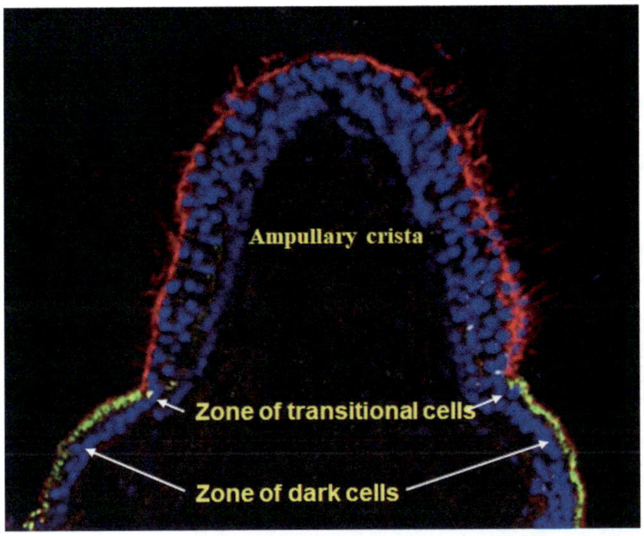

Fig. 2.13 Triple fluorescent labeling on a cryosection of the ampullary crista of chinchilla. In this micrograph, TRITC-phalloidin reveals F-actin distribution in hair cell ciliary bundles and cuticular plates (red), ToPro3 visualizes nuclear morphology (blue), and EGFP expression (green) marks successful transfection via hydroxyapatite nanocarriers. 48 h after the transfection of hydroxyapatite nanocarriers carrying the EGFP gene via the round window membrane, EGFP expression is observed in dark cells within the crista's crescent-shaped regions. This may suggest that the dark cells internalize nanocarriers through phagocytic mechanisms similar to otolith absorption, and the EGFP gene sequence carried by the nanocarrier was successfully synthesized the green fluorescent protein in the dark cells through the phagocytic function of dark cells

is membranous structure without bony tissue, there is no need for decalcification. The surface of each vestibular end-organ is covered with a gelatinous-like substance, which can bend of the ciliary bundles of the vestibular hair cells through relative movement. The surface of the maculae of saccule and utricle is covered with otolith membrane, and the top of the ampullary cristae is covered with the cupula. Under a dissection microscope, the otolith membrane on the surface of maculae of saccule and utricle is gently removed using forceps, and the cupula on ampullary cristae is removed by perfusion of running PBS rinse. Afterwards, the membrane of vestibular end-organs is removed to expose the surface of vestibular end-organs. Since the thickness of the removed vestibular end-organs is only a few layers of cells, which is equivalent to just a relatively thick section, the vestibular end organs can be directly put into various enzyme histochemical staining or immunohistochemical labeling procedures. After histochemical labeling, the sample for frozen section can be directly immersed in 10% gelatin for permeation embedding, the sample for paraffin section can be immersed in paraffin for permeation embedding after dehydration, and the sample for ultrathin section can be dehydrated and then immersed in resin permeation embedding [6, 8, 19, 23, 26, 29–31] (Fig. 2.11).

2.2.3 Slice of the Separated Vestibular End-Organs

The planar morphology of saccular and utricular maculae facilitates optimal cross-sectional analysis when sectioning perpendicular to their epithelial surface (Fig. 1.11). Ampullary cristae present distinct anatomical orientations, with their saddle-shaped sensory epithelia positioned perpendicular to the semicircular canal arc along the convex margin of the ampullary cavity. Consequently, sectioning parallel to the semicircular canal axis yields ideal crista cross-sections [11, 26, 32–34] (Figs. 2.12 and 2.13). For vestibular neuronal analysis, the superior vestibular nerve bundle adjacent to the superior sieve zone and the inferior vestibular bundle near the middle sieve zone can be directly harvested from the internal auditory canal base without decalcification. These neural tissues are suitable for histochemical processing prior to sectioning (Figs. 2.14 and 2.15).

The frozen sections embedded with gelatin or OCT are directly mounted in glycerol drop on glass slide, cover slipped, and sealed with neutral gum around the cover glass to store permanently. The semi-thin sections using resin embedding are transferred to the distilled water droplets on a glass slide to dry with drying table. The sections are fully expanded in the heating water and pasted on the glass slide. Sections that have been stained can be directly mounted with neutral gum for observation. The sections for regular pathological examinations can be stained with 1% toluidine blue on the drying table for about 1 min. After rinsing with distilled water, the slices can be sealed with neutral gum for observations [6, 11, 29, 35]. Routine pathological analysis involves 1% toluidine blue staining for approximately 60 s on a warming plate, followed by distilled water rinsing and final neutral balsam sealing [9, 20, 26] (Figs. 1.27A and 1.28; Figs. 2.6, 2.8, 2.9, 2.11, and 2.12D–F).

Following identification of optimal semithin sections from resin-embedded vestibular membranous labyrinth specimens, the tissue block is carefully trimmed to a pyramidal form. Ultrathin sections of approximately 50 nm thickness are then prepared using a glass knife-equipped ultramicrotome. Sections exhibiting silver interference colors are collected from the distilled water surface in the knife boat using copper grids. The grids are subsequently placed on filter paper to absorb excess moisture from the reverse side, ensuring proper flattening and adhesion of sections. For conventional ultrastructural analysis, grid-mounted sections undergo standard electron-dense staining prior to transmission electron microscopy examination (Figs. 2.16–2.19). In immunohistochemical studies where reaction products possess inherent electron density, omission of heavy metal counterstains (lead/uranium) permits unambiguous localization of the immune reactive products at organellar levels [4, 13, 24, 25, 28, 34, 36–38] (Figs. 2.20–2.22).

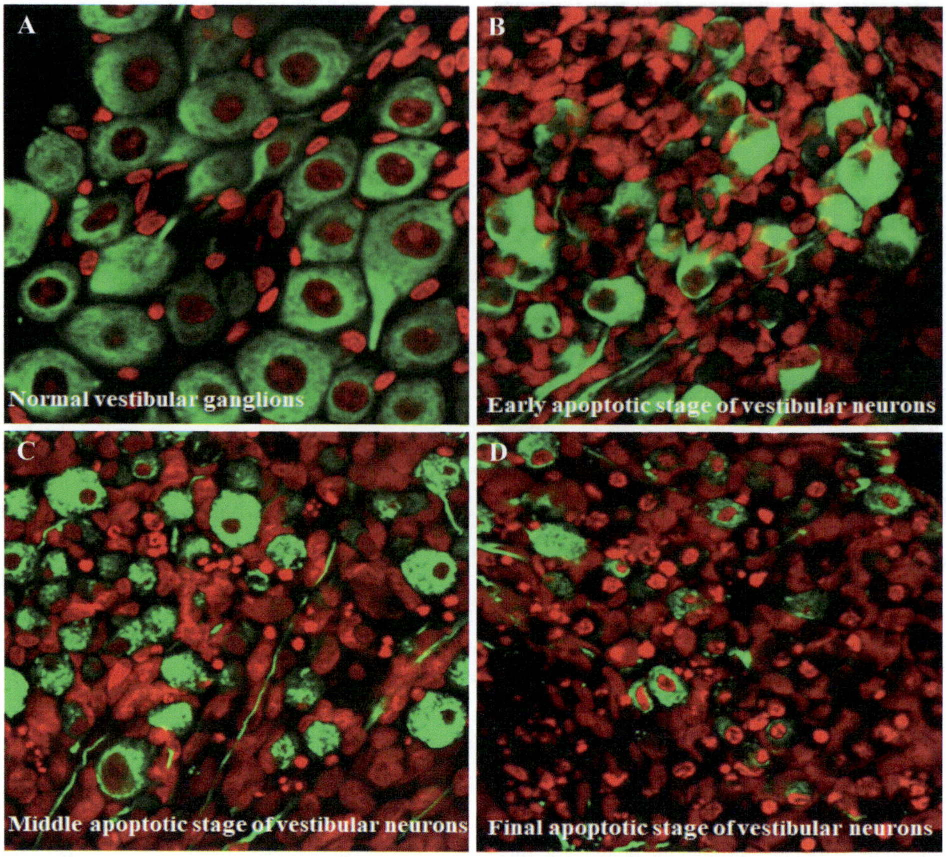

Fig. 2.14 Double staining of rat superior vestibular ganglion neurons reveals morphological changes during apoptosis, with anti-β -tubulin antibody labeling ganglion soma and processes (green) and ToPro-3 staining nuclei (red). (**A**) The superior vestibular neurons in a normal rat exhibit characteristic morphology with spherical nucleus with robust cytoplasmic volume. (**B**) The early apoptotic changes of vestibular neurons are manifested as nuclear and somatic shrinkage. (**C**) The intermediate stage of apoptotic changes of vestibular ganglion neurons demonstrates marked chromatin condensation in both nuclear and cytoplasmic compartments. (**D**) The terminal apoptosis of vestibular ganglion neurons presents with extensive neuronal loss and pronounced nuclear fragmentation in remaining neurons

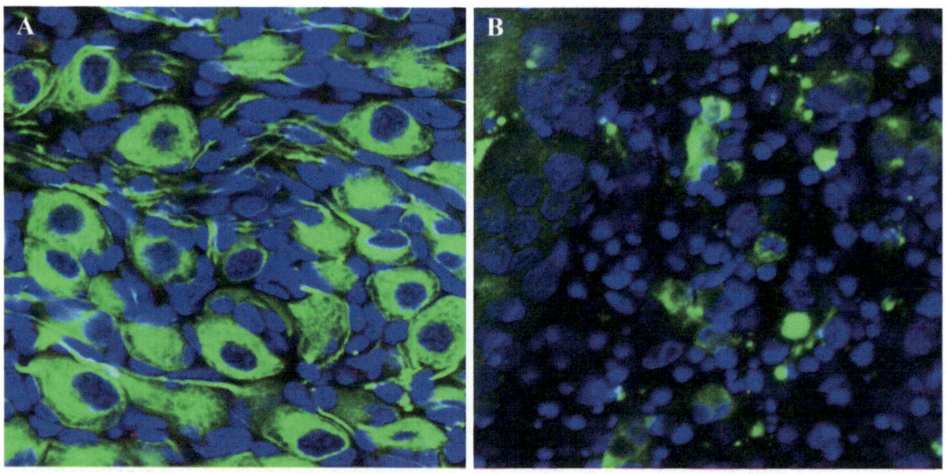

Fig. 2.15 Bilirubin-induced neurotoxicity in rat inferior vestibular ganglion. Dual-label fluorescence microscopy demonstrates cellular pathology in the inferior vestibular ganglion, with β-tubulin immunolabeling (green) delineating neuronal morphology and ToPro-3 (blue) revealing nuclear architecture. (**A**) The inferior vestibular neurons in normal rat present spherical nucleus and large body, while the surrounding glial supporting cells present smaller oval nuclei. (**B**) Bilirubin treatment causes severe condensation and fragmentation in both vestibular ganglion neurons and surrounding glial cells, confirming that bilirubin-induced destruction in both vestibular neurons and surrounding glial cells has the typical apoptotic characteristics

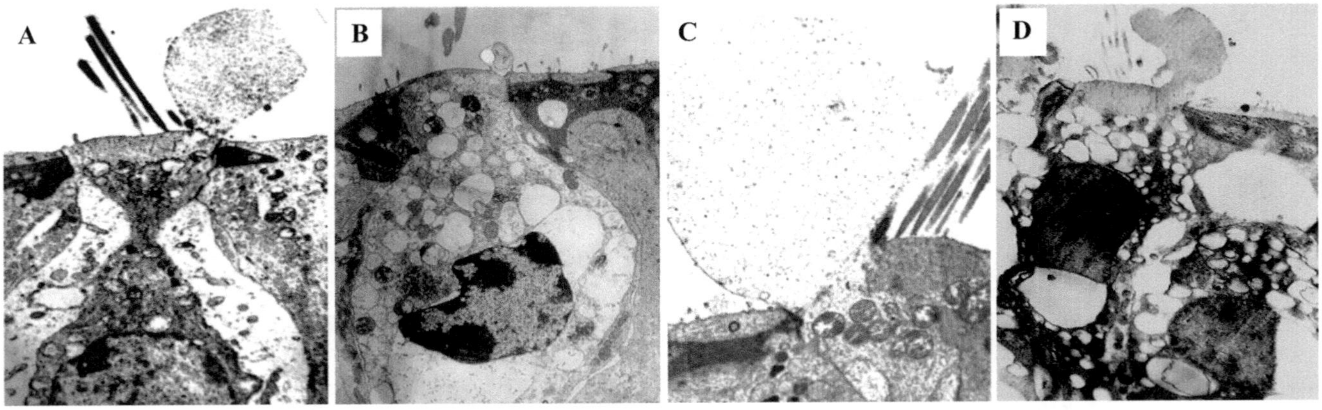

Fig. 2.16 Ultrastructural pathological changes of vestibular hair cells induced by ototoxic chemicals. (**A**) Kanamycin toxicity induces mitochondrial vacuolization in type I hair cells, with subsequent exocytotic expulsion of cellular contents through the cuticular plate. (**B**) Gentamicin exposure results in mitochondrial degeneration and intracellular edema formation, reflecting impaired cellular energy metabolism. (**C**) Gentamicin-damaged hair cells demonstrate cytoplasmic extrusion through cuticular plate perforations, containing both normal and swollen mitochondria. (**D**) Carboplatin-induced vestibular hair cell destruction exhibits the formation of massive intracellular hydrophobic cavities and the formation of abnormally large vacuoles under the nuclear membrane

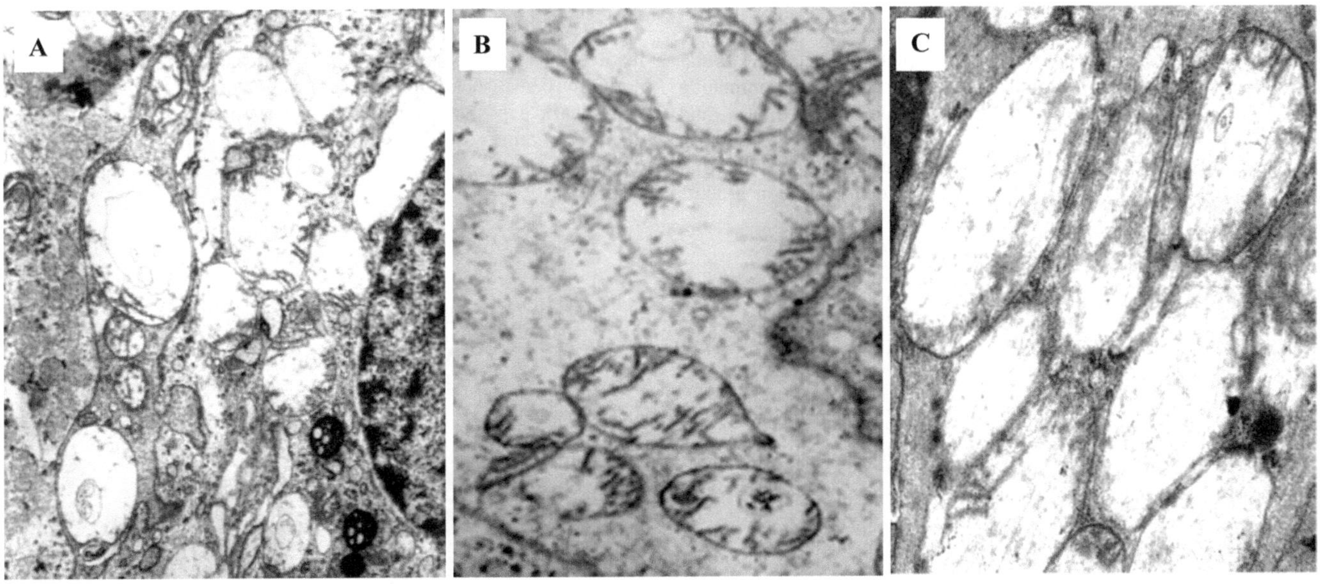

Fig. 2.17 Sequential ultrastructural changes in kanamycin-induced mitochondrial pathology. (**A**) Initial kanamycin toxicity manifests as mitochondrial cristae fragmentation, representing the primary ultrastructural alteration. (**B**) Progressive cristae dissolution leads to complete mitochondrial vacuolization, with organelles transforming into fluid-filled cavities. (**C**) Advanced mitochondrial damage demonstrates extreme swelling due to impaired osmotic regulation, ultimately disrupting cellular energy production. These findings establish that kanamycin-induced hair cell degeneration primarily results from mitochondrial dysfunction, causing critical energy deficits that impair essential cellular processes

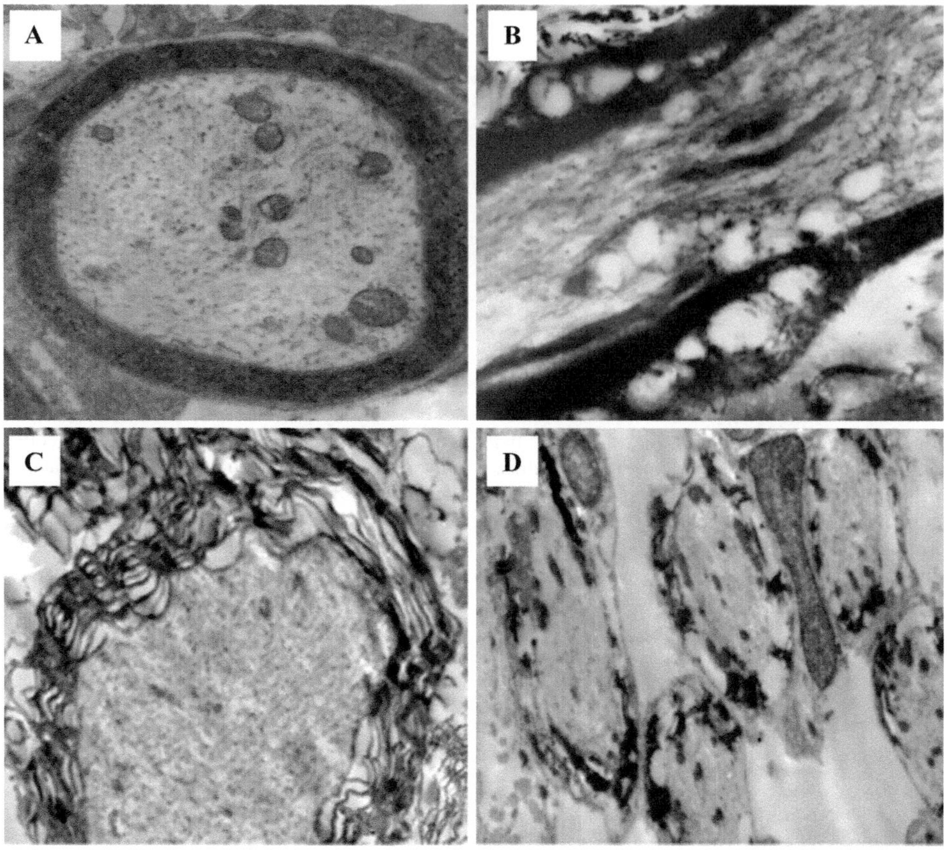

Fig. 2.18 Temporal progression of carboplatin-induced vestibular nerve demyelination. (**A**) Vestibular nerve fibers in normal chinchilla demonstrate characteristic ultrastructure with uniform axoplasm and compact, multilamellar myelin sheaths. (**B**) Initial neurotoxic effects at 24 h post-carboplatin manifest as axoplasmic vacuolization with adjacent intramyelinic vesicle formation. (**C**) The demyelination process involves progressive separation of myelin lamellae, transforming the normally dense sheath into spaced, fragmented layers within 24 h of carboplatin exposure. (**D**) 48 h post-carboplatin injection, advanced demyelination exposes naked axons following complete myelin sheath disintegration

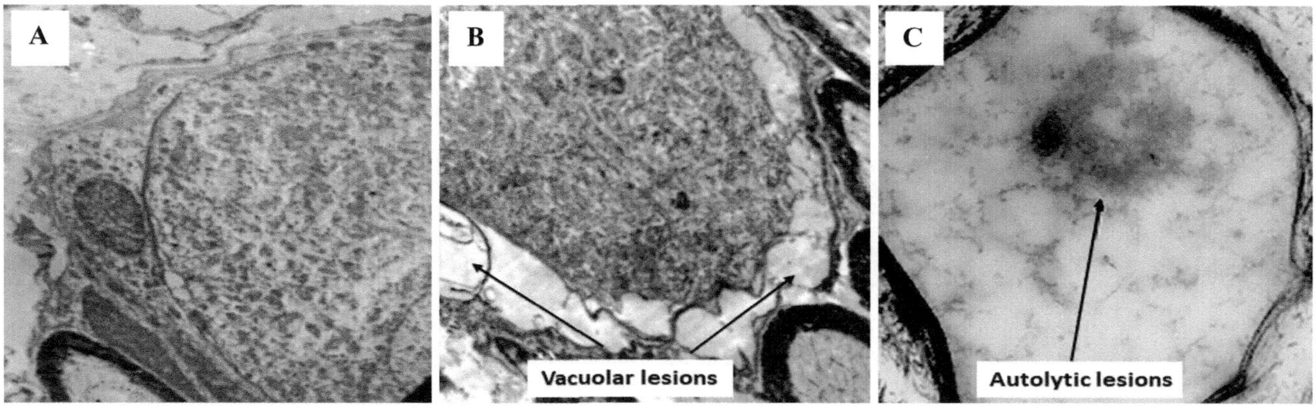

Fig. 2.19 Transmission electron micrograph shows carboplatin-induced destruction of vestibular ganglion neurons. (**A**) Normal vestibular ganglion neuron in chinchilla displays intact plasma membrane and cytoplasmic organization. (**B**) Initial neurotoxic effects observed at 24 h post-carboplatin administration include subplasmalemmal vacuolization and early cytoplasmic cavitation. (**C**) 22 h after carboplatin injection, the soma of the vestibular ganglion neuron developed extensive autolytic changes with complete disruption of cellular architecture

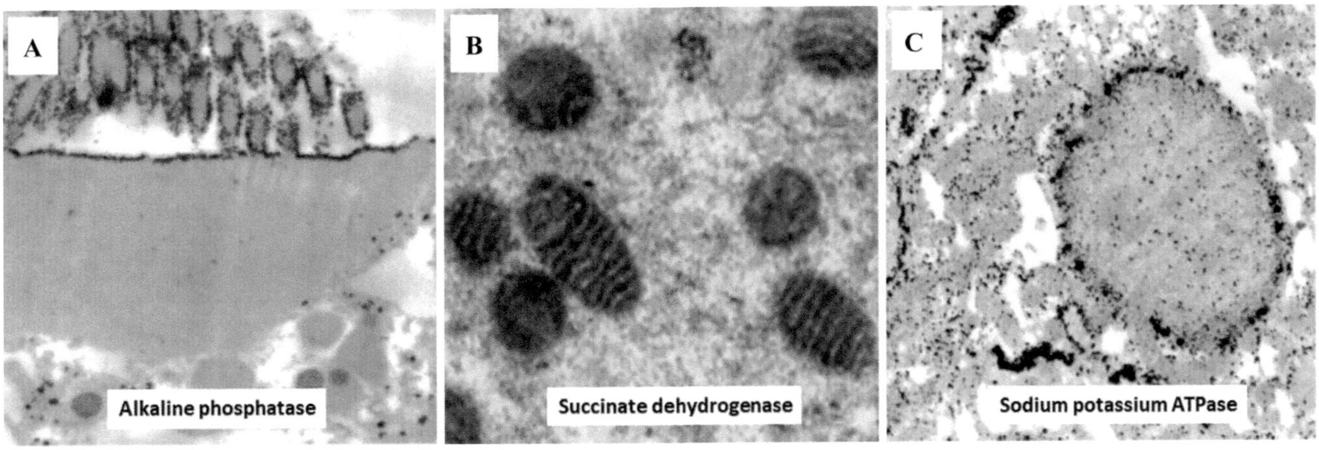

Fig. 2.20 Enzymatic ultrastructural localization in vestibular hair cells. (**A**) Alkaline phosphatase is localized on the surface of cilia membrane and cuticular plate of vestibular hair cells in normal guinea pig. (**B**) Succinate dehydrogenase is located in the mitochondrial cristae of vestibular hair cell. (**C**) Sodium-potassium ATPase is located in the plasma and intracellular membrane system of vestibular hair cells

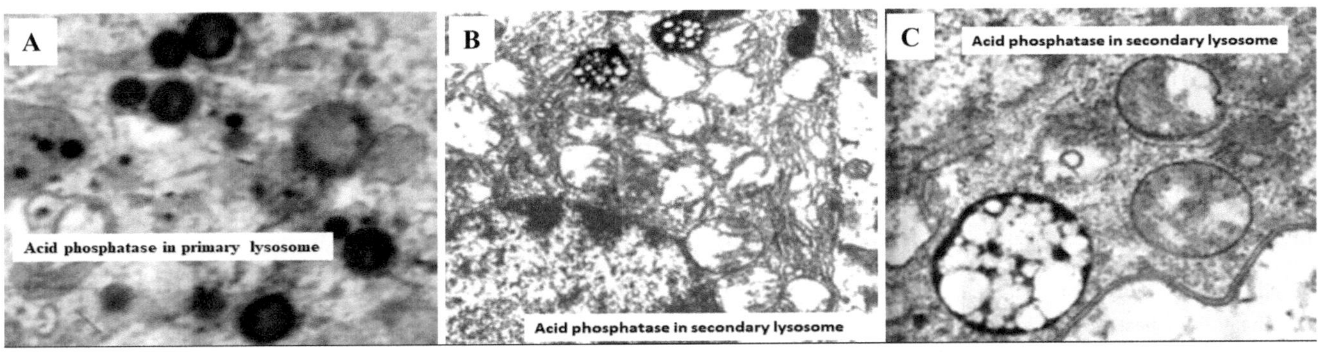

Fig. 2.21 Kanamycin-induced ultrastructural changes of acid phosphatase in lysosomes of vestibular hair cells. (**A**) Acid phosphatase in the primary lysosomes in normal vestibular hair cells exhibits uniformly high electron density. (**B**) During chronic kanamycin ototoxicity, acid phosphatase labeling shows that the primary lysosomes in vestibular hair cells are transformed into multivesicular secondary lysosomes due to phagocytosis of large numbers of denatured organelles, such as destroyed mitochondria. (**C**) When secondary lysosomes are overloaded by engulfing destroyed mitochondria, acid phosphatase-labeled secondary lysosomes undergo severe expansion. This eventually results in lysosomal membrane rupture and subsequent cellular autolysis

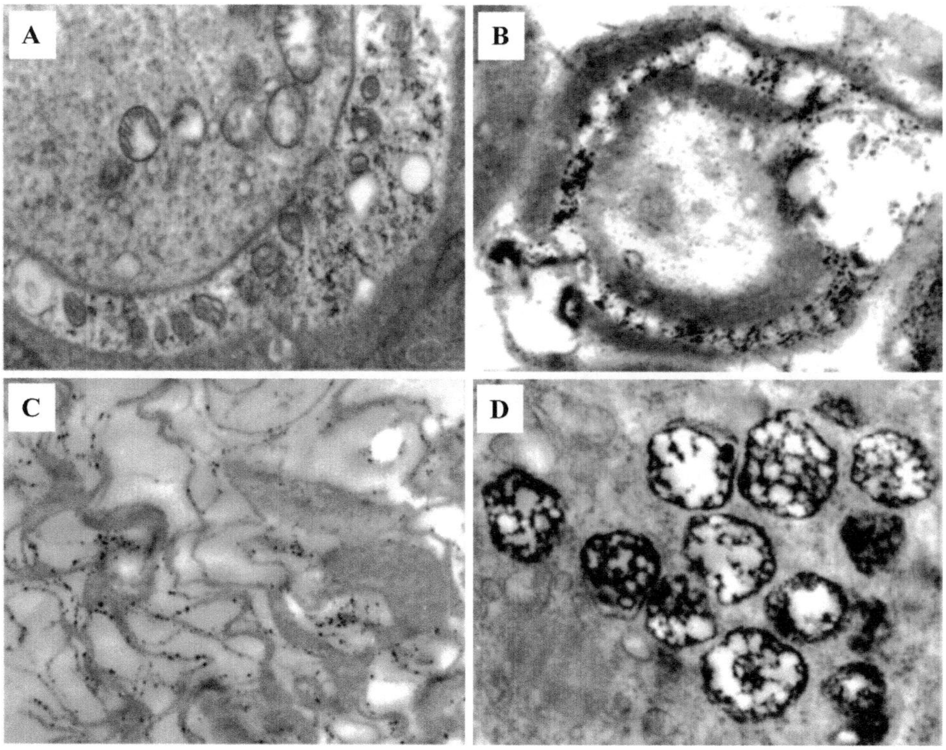

Fig. 2.22 Temporal-spatial distribution of calpain activation in carboplatin-induced vestibular neurotoxicity. (**A**) 12 h post-carboplatin, electron-dense calpain immunoreactive products accumulate preferentially within the type I afferent calyceal terminals, suggesting type I vestibular synaptic vulnerability to initial carboplatin toxicity. (**B**). 24 h after injection of carboplatin, a large number of granular calpain immunohistochemical products can be detected in the site of vestibular nerve demyelination, indicating that demyelination is closely related to the activation of calpain. (**C**) 24 h after carboplatin injection, the separated space appeared within the layers of myelin sheath around the vestibular nerve axon, and granular calpain also appeared in the decomposed myelin sheath. This may suggest that the activity of calpain was responsible for the disintegration of the myelin sheath. (**D**). 72 h after carboplatin treatment, a large number of vacuoles filled with calpain reactive products appeared in the soma of vestibular ganglion neuron, indicating that calpain plays an important role in the carboplatin-induced destruction of vestibular ganglion neurons

References

1. Schuknecht H. Histological method. In: Pathology of the ear. 1st ed. Cambridge: Harvard University Press; 1974. pp. 1–20.
2. Ding D, Jiang S. Chapter 5: Fixation techniques for inner ear specimens. In: Ding D, editor. Manual of anatomical examination of the inner ear of the guinea pig. Shanghai: Xuelin Publishing House; 1989. pp. 36–48.
3. Ding D, Jiang H, Wang J, et al. Carboplatin-induced vestibular damage: quantitative measurement of type I hair cell loss and ganglion cell loss. J Audit Speech Pathol. 2002;10:170–3.
4. Wang J, Ding D, Salvi RJ. Carboplatin-induced early cochlear lesion in chinchillas. Hear Res. 2003;181:65–72. https://doi.org/10.1016/s0378-5955(03)00176-x.
5. El-Badry MM, Ding DL, McFadden SL, Eddins AC. Physiological effects of auditory nerve myelinopathy in chinchillas. Eur J Neurosci. 2007;25:1437–46. https://doi.org/10.1111/j.1460-9568.2007.05401.x.
6. Ding D, Jiang S. Chapter 7: Slicing techniques of the inner ear. In: Ding D, editor. Manual of anatomical examination of the inner ear of the guinea pig. Shanghai: Xuelin Publishing House; 1989. pp. 61–66.
7. Ding D, Qi W, Qu Y, Salvi R. Chapter 6: Research techniques of the inner ear morphology. In: Ding D, editor. Science of the inner ear. Beijing: China Science and Technology Press; 2010. pp. 50–88.
8. Ding D, Shi L, Xing Y, et al. Sagittal sectioning of temporal bones and quantitative measurement of neural densities in the inner ear in normal mice. Chin J Otorhinolaryngol Skull Base Surg. 2024;30:69–75. https://doi.org/10.11798/j.issn.1007-1520.202424331.
9. Ding D, Shi L, Xing Y, et al. Secondary neural damage in the inner ear induced by intratympanic gentamicin injection. Chin J Otorhinolaryngol Skull Base Surg. 2024;30:11–19. https://doi.org/10.11798/j.issn.1007-1520.202424356.
10. Ding D, Qi W, Yang K, et al. Technical evolution of pathology in the inner ear. Chin J Otorhinolaryngol Skull Base Surg. 2016;22:169–78. https://doi.org/10.11798/j.issn.1007-520.201603001.
11. Ding D, Huangfu M, Jin X. Frozen sections of the inner ear. J Bengbu Med Coll. 1987;12:222.
12. Ding D, Luo D, Huangfu M. Embryonic development of the inner ear in guinea pigs. Shanghai Lab Anim Sci. 1991;11:45–46.
13. Ding D, Li M, Jiang C, Salvi R. Chapter 6: Sectioning of the inner ear. In: Ding D, editor. Morphology of the inner ear. Harbin: Heilongjiang Science and Technology Press; 2001. pp. 38–54.
14. Ding D, Yu J, Li P, et al. Standardization of experimental animals temporal bone sections. J Otol. 2015;10:66–71. https://doi.org/10.1016/j.joto.2015.08.001.
15. Ding D, Wang J, Zhang XY, Sun H, Salvi R. Quantitative analysis of hair cells, spiral ganglion neurons, and nerve fibers in the same cochlea. Chin J Otorhinolaryngol Skull Base Surg. 1998;4:200–4.

16. Ding D, Zheng X, Wang J. [Quantitation of nerve fibers in habenula perforata in chinchilla]. Zhonghua Er Bi Yan Hou Ke Za Zhi. 1998;33:30–31.
17. Ding D, Jiang H, McFadden SL, Salvi RJ, Li M. Quantitative analysis of hair cells, spiral ganglion neurons and nerve fibers in knock out mice lacking SOD 1 gene. Acta Otolaryngol Sin. 1999;30:1693–705.
18. Ding D, Li P, Qi W, et al. Study on delayed secondary lesions in the cochlea triggered by cochlear hair cell death. Chin J Otorhinolaryngol Skull Base Surg. 2022;28:1–10. https://doi.org/10.11798/j.issn.1007-1520.2022221001.
19. Ding D, Li P, Qi W, Zhang J. Quantitative observation of vestibular sensory hair cells in experimental animals. Chin J Otorhinolaryngol Skull Base Surg. 2022;28:11–18. https://doi.org/10.11798/j.issn.1007-1520.202290001.
20. Ding D, Manohar S, Kador PF, Salvi R. Multifunctional redox modulator prevents blast-induced loss of cochlear and vestibular hair cells and auditory spiral ganglion neurons. Sci Rep. 2024;14:15296. https://doi.org/10.1038/s41598-024-66406-1.
21. Zhou L, Ding D, Huangfu M, et al. Observation of the connecting apparatus between cells of human embryonic vestibular epithelium. Chin J Otorhinolaryngol. 1993;28:134–5.
22. Ding D, Luo S, Jin X. Microdissection of the vestibular end-organs in guinea pigs. Shanghai Med. 1986;9:153–4.
23. Ding D, Zhao J, Huangfu M, Jin X. Microdissection of the whole membranous labyrinth in guinea pigs. J Clin Otorhinolaryngol. 1987;1:9–11.
24. Ding D, Jiang S. Chapter 8: Preparation techniques for electron microscopy of inner ear specimen. In: Ding D, editor. Manual of anatomical examination of the inner ear of the guinea pig. Shanghai: Xuelin Publishing House; 1989. pp. 67–74.
25. Ding D, Jiang S. Chapter 10: Electron microscopic cytochemical techniques of hair cells in the inner ear. In: Ding D, editor. Manual of anatomical examination of the inner ear of the guinea pig. Shanghai: Xuelin Publishing House; 1989. pp. 100–5.
26. Ding D, Wang J, Salvi RJ. Early damage in the chinchilla vestibular sensory epithelium from carboplatin. Audiol Neurootol. 1997;2:155–67. https://doi.org/10.1159/000259238.
27. Ding D, McFadden SL, Salvi RJ. Calpain immunoreactivity and morphological damage in chinchilla inner ears after carboplatin. J Assoc Res Otolaryngol. 2002;3:68–79. https://doi.org/10.1007/s101620020004.
28. Ding L, McFadden SL, Salvi RJ. Calpain immunoreactivity and morphological damage in chinchilla inner ears after carboplatin. J Assoc Res Otolaryngol. 2002;3:68–79. https://doi.org/10.1007/s101620020004.
29. Ding D, Zhu X, Chen H, Zhao J, Huangfu M. Study on acid phosphatase in the cochlea of guinea pigs with kanamycin ototoxicity. Zhonghua Er Bi Yan Hou Ke Za Zhi. 1986;21:121–2.
30. Ding D, Jiang H, Fu Y, et al. Ototoxic effects of carboplatin in organotypic cultures in chinchillas and rats. J Otol. 2012;7:92–101. https://doi.org/10.1016/S1672-2930(12)50023-1.
31. Ding D, Jiang H, Zhang J, et al. Cisplatin-induced vestibular hair cell lesion-less damage at high doses. J Otol. 2018;13:115–21. https://doi.org/10.1016/j.joto.2018.08.002.
32. Wu X, Ding D, Jiang H, et al. Transfection using hydroxyapatite nanoparticles in the inner ear via an intact round window membrane in chinchilla. J Nanopart Res. 2012;14:708. https://doi.org/10.1007/s11051-011-0708-1.
33. Qi W, Ding D, Zhu H, et al. Efficient siRNA transfection to the inner ear through the intact round window by a novel proteidic delivery technology in the chinchilla. Gene Ther. 2014;21:10–18. https://doi.org/10.1038/gt.2013.49.
34. Ding D, Jiang H, Chen GD, et al. N-acetyl-cysteine prevents age-related hearing loss and the progressive loss of inner hair cells in gamma-glutamyl transferase 1 deficient mice. Aging (Albany NY). 2016;8:730–50. https://doi.org/10.18632/aging.100927.
35. Ding DL, McFadden SL, Wang J, Hu BH, Salvi RJ. Age- and strain-related differences in dehydrogenase activity and glycogen levels in CBA and C57 mouse cochleas. Audiol Neurootol. 1999;4:55–63.
36. Ding D, Luo D, Huangfu M, Gong Z. Enzyme cytochemistry of the inner ear under electron microscopy. J Clin Otorhinolaryngol. 1989;3:183–84.
37. Ding D, Li M, Jiang S, Salvi R. Chapter 9: Electron microscopic cytochemical techniques of inner ear cells. In: Ding D, editor. Morphology of the inner ear. Harbin: Heilongjiang Science and Technology Press; 2001. pp. 125–127.
38. Ding D, Li M, Jiang C, Salvi R. Chapter 3: Anatomy of temporal bone and inner ear. In: Ding D, editor. Morphology of the inner ear. Harbin: Heilongjiang Science and Technology Press; 2001. pp. 10–17.

3 Vestibular Micro-Dissection and Surface Preparations

The microdissection of the inner ear under a dissecting microscope represents a critical methodological approach for the precise isolation of the membranous labyrinth from the encasing bony labyrinth, enabling direct access to its delicate neuroepithelial structures. Surface preparation, a key observational technique derived from this method, involves mounting the dissected membranous labyrinth onto a glass slide in a flattened orientation, thereby permitting comprehensive topographical analysis of its cellular architecture under optical or electron microscopy. Mastery of this microdissection technique not only facilitates structural and pathological evaluation through both en face (surface preparation) and cross-sectional (slice angle) perspectives but also serves as a foundational step for integrating advanced analytical modalities. Notably, this approach is highly compatible with histochemical and cytochemical labeling for subcellular localization studies, organotypic culture systems for functional and regenerative investigations, and molecular biology techniques to decipher mechanistic pathways underlying inner ear pathologies such as cochlear degeneration or vestibular dysfunction. By bridging anatomical precision with multidisciplinary experimental strategies, microdissection-based analyses have significantly contributed to elucidating the etiopathogenesis of inner ear lesions, as evidenced by seminal studies [1–6], solidifying its role as an indispensable tool in both basic and translational otological research [4, 5, 7–15].

3.1 Fixation and Exposure of the Vestibular Membranous Labyrinth

3.1.1 Fixation of Vestibular End-Organs

The initial step in the processing of vestibular end-organs involves careful dissection of the temporal bone from the skull, followed by immediate immersion in fixative solution to ensure optimal tissue preservation. Under a dissecting microscope, the stapes footplate is gently displaced into the vestibular cavity, creating an entry through the oval window that permits rapid and complete perfusion of fixative throughout the vestibular cistern. This method ensures instantaneous fixation of all vestibular end-organs within the vestibular cistern by allowing the preservative solution to fully penetrate the membranous labyrinthine structures without delay, thereby maintaining structural integrity and minimizing postmortem artifacts for subsequent histological or ultrastructural evaluations.

3.1.2 Vestibular-Related Skeletal Landmarks on the Temporal Bone

Using the guinea pig temporal bone as a model, key vestibular anatomical landmarks can be clearly identified: the convexities of the superior and lateral semicircular canals are visible at the base of the superior tympanic chamber (Fig. 3.1A), while the posterior semicircular canal's bony prominence is located centrally within the posterior depression, positioned inferior to the round window (Fig. 3.1B). The osseous walls forming these semicircular canal protrusions are notably thin, allowing for efficient surgical exposure of the underlying membranous ampullae through careful removal of the overlying bony structures, thereby providing direct access to these critical components of the vestibular system while preserving their delicate anatomical integrity.

The medial wall of the guinea pig temporal bone's posterior fossa reveals three distinct neural canal openings adjacent to the vestibular cavity's anterior portion: the facial nerve canal opening positioned anterosuperiorly, the superior vestibular nerve canal opening located posterior to the facial nerve canal, and the auditory nerve canal situated inferior to both (Fig. 3.1C). Posterior to the cochlear afferent nerve bundles, the cochlear efferent and inferior vestibular nerve bundles converge within the cochlear neuroforamen, with inferior vestibular neurons occupying the floor of cochlear neuroforamen. These inferior

D. Ding et al., *Histopathological Atlas of the Inner Ear*,
https://doi.org/10.1007/978-981-95-6338-8_3

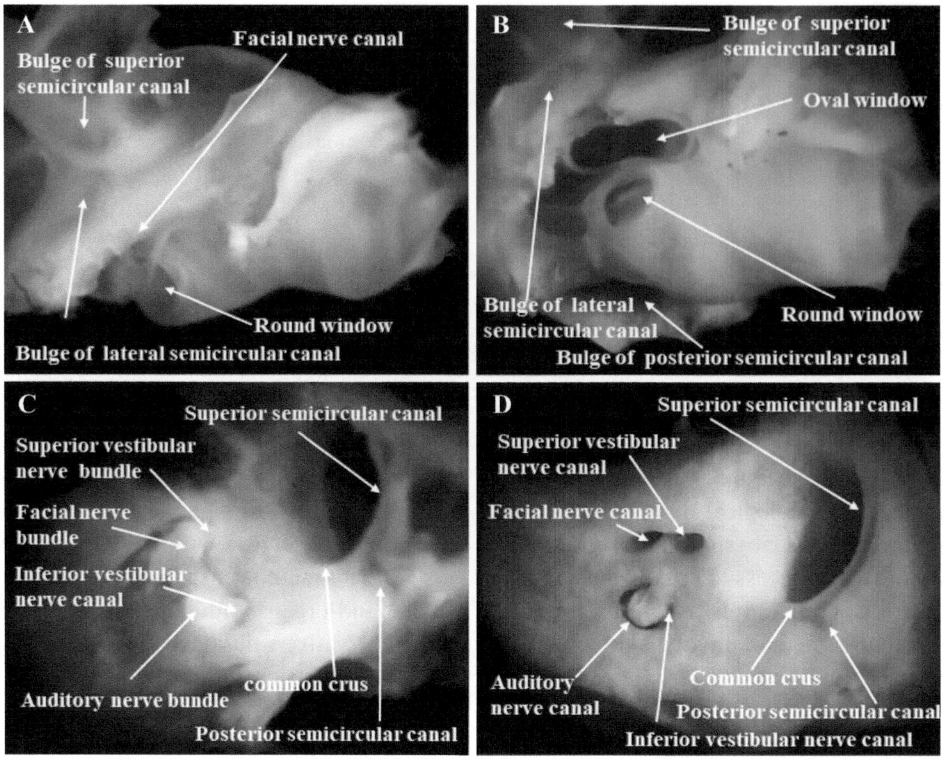

Fig. 3.1 Anatomical Landmarks of the Chinchilla Temporal Bone. (**A**) The superior tympanic chamber reveals two distinct osseous protrusions at its base corresponding to the bulges of the superior (medial) and lateral (external) semicircular canals. (**B**) The stapes footplate was removed to fully expose the oval window located in the center of the lateral wall of the vestibular cistern. (**C**) Viewed from the posterior cranial fossa, the temporal bone wall exhibits three distinct neural foramina: the facial nerve canal (anterosuperior), superior vestibular nerve canal (posterior), and cochlear nerve canal (inferior), each transmitting the corresponding nerve bundles toward the brainstem. (**D**) Following removal of the nerve tracts, the precise spatial position of the facial nerve canal, superior vestibular neuroforamen, and cochlear neuroforamen is clearly exposed

vestibular fibers project posteriorly through the middle and inferior cribriform areas to innervate the saccular macula and posterior ampullary crista [4–7, 15–20]. The cochlear efferent pathway follows the afferent fibers through the cochlear neuroforamen, traverses the modiolar perforations to enter Rosenthal's canal, and ultimately reaches the cochlear hair cells via the habenula perforata.

Posterior to these neural canals, a spherical cavity bounded by the three semicircular canals houses the cerebellar flocculus, with the superior semicircular canal forming its posterior border. The junction of superior and posterior canals creates the common crus at the cavity's inferior margin, beneath which lies the endolymphatic canal and sac within a bony fissure [18, 21, 22] (Fig. 3.1C, D). This anatomical arrangement demonstrates the precise spatial relationship between neural structures and vestibular components in the guinea pig model.

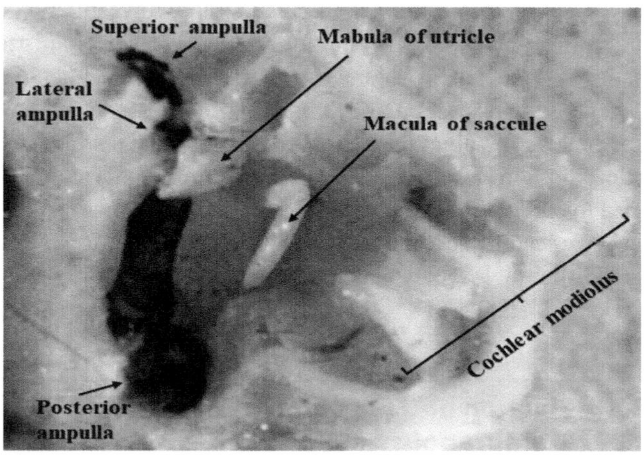

Fig. 3.2 Exposure of the vestibular membranous labyrinth within the vestibular cistern following removal of the tympanic-side bony wall of the osseous labyrinth of pigmented guinea pig

3.1.3 Exposure of Each Vestibular End-Organs

The surgical exposure of vestibular end-organs begins with extraction of the facial nerve bundle and opening of the lateral bony wall of the facial nerve canal to reveal the oval window, followed by micro-dissection of the superior and posterior bony walls of the oval window to completely expose the vestibular cistern. Upon full removal of the lateral osseous wall of vestibular cistern, the maculae of the saccule and utricle become clearly visible due to their distinctive white otolithic

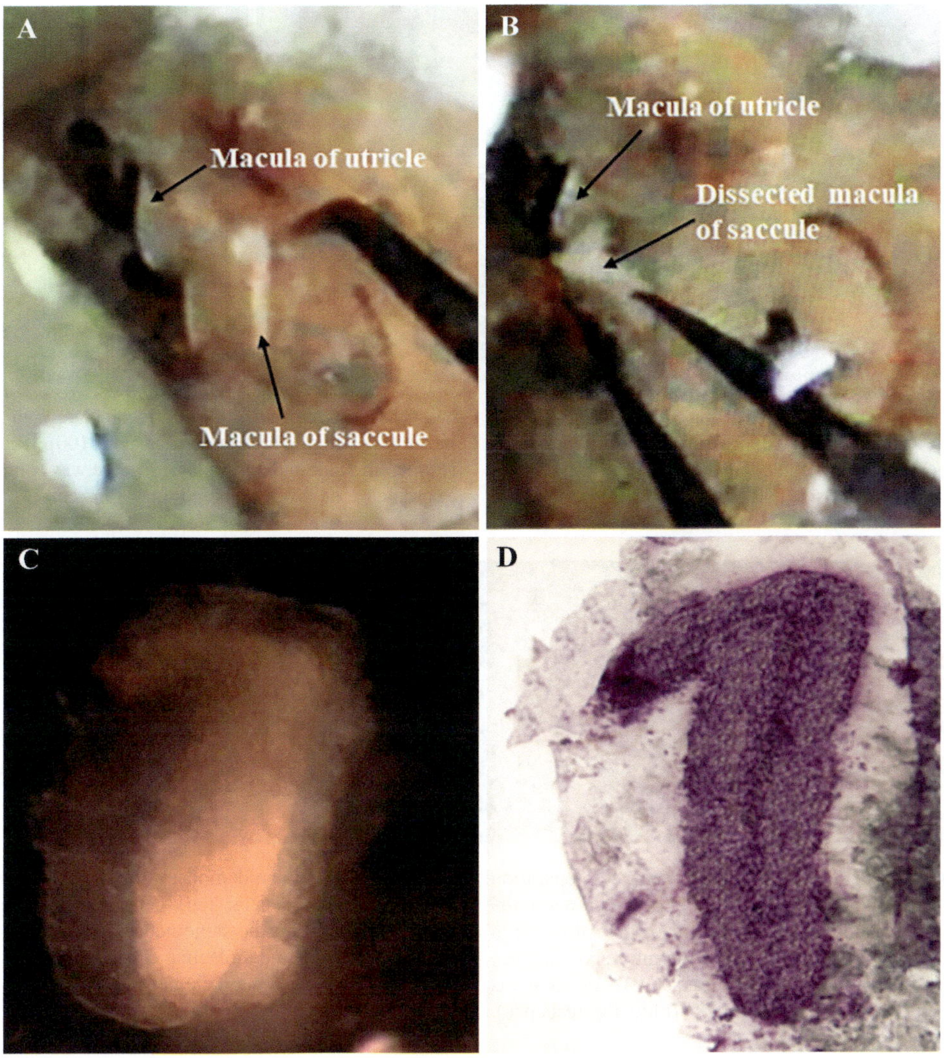

Fig. 3.3 Microdissection procedure for isolating macula of saccule in guinea pigs. (**A**) Initial separation of the saccule is performed by carefully advancing a dissection needle along the anterior margin of the macula of saccule against the bony medial wall of the vestibular cistern. (**B**) The entire saccule is then removed from the vestibular cistern using ultra-fine forceps. (**C**) The membranous wall of the saccule is torn open to expose the entire macula of saccule. (**D**) After removal of the otolith membrane, the macula of saccule was stained with succinate dehydrogenase and mounted on glass slide as a flat surface preparation

membranes adhering to the surface of maculae. The ampulla of lateral semicircular canal is positioned posterolateral to the macula of utricle and the ampulla of superior semicircular canal is located above the posterior aspect of the utricle macula, while the ampulla of posterior semicircular canal located anterior to the inferior portion of utricle [4, 5, 7, 8, 12, 15, 23] (Fig. 3.2). This systematic approach ensures optimal visualization of all major vestibular sensory epithelia while preserving their anatomical relationships.

3.2 Microdissection and Surface Preparation of the Macula of Saccule

Under a dissecting microscope, the macula of saccule is meticulously isolated by severing its nerve fibers and vasculature that traverse the middle and inferior sieve spot zones using a fine dissection needle along the vestibular cistern's medial bony wall (Fig. 3.3A), followed by complete detachment of the saccular macula from its osseous attachment (Fig. 3.3B). The freed saccule is then extracted using microforceps (Fig. 1.17; Fig. 3.3C), after which its membranous wall is carefully opened to expose the underlying otolithic membrane. This otolith membrane is then peeled off and removed using a fine needle. The isolated macula of saccule can then undergo standard histochemical staining before being flat-mounted in glycerol for light or fluorescence microscopic examination [4, 5, 12, 15] (Figs. 3.3D, 3.4, and 3.5). For ultrastructural observations, specimens are processed through graded alcohol dehydration, critical point drying, and gold sputtering to enable detailed scanning electron microscopic visualization of the surface ultrastructure of hair cells on the macula of saccule [12, 24–28] (Figs. 3.6 and 3.7).

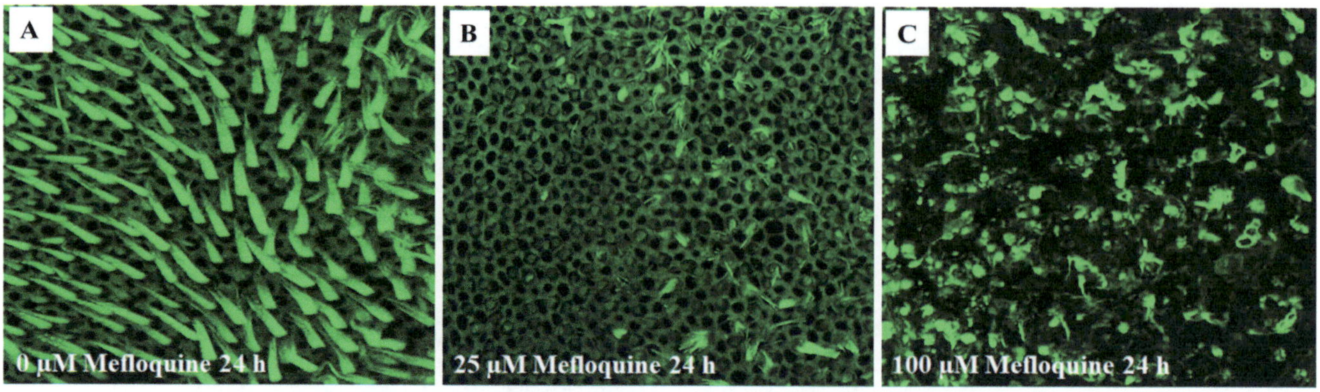

Fig. 3.4 Mefloquine-induced hair cell destruction in macula of saccule. (**A**) A normal explant of macula of saccule in serum-free medium for 24 h maintained intact surface structure of ciliary bundle. (**B**) After 24 h of incubation with 25 μM mefloquine, massive loss of bundles and destruction of hair cells were detected, but the cuticular plate of supporting cells remained intact. (**C**) After 24 h of incubation with 100 μM mefloquine, all sensory neuroepithelium in the macula of saccule was completely destroyed, with a complete loss of hair cells and supporting cells

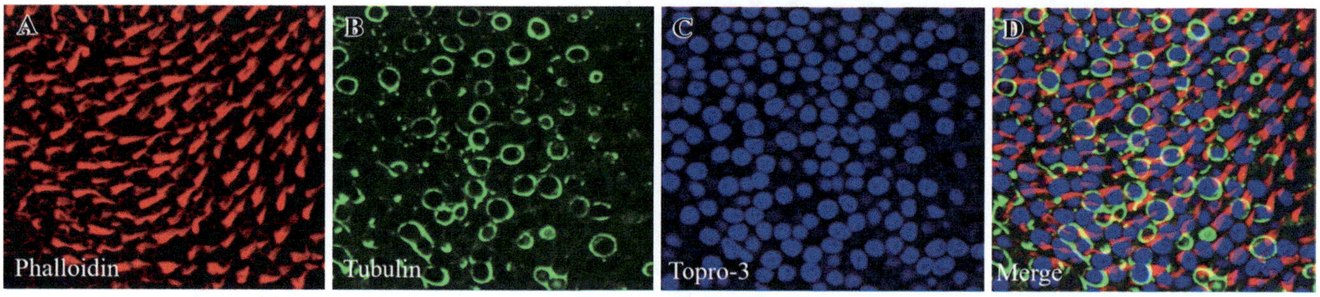

Fig. 3.5 Multiplex fluorescent staining imaging of surface preparation of macula of saccule in rats. (**A**) Phalloidin staining reveals F-actin distribution in hair cell ciliary bundles (red fluorescence). (**B**) Anti-tubulin antibody immunolabeling identifies Type I afferent nerve calyces enveloping Type I hair cells (green fluorescence). (**C**) To-Pro-3 stains the nuclei of hair cells in macula of saccule (blue fluorescence). (**D**) Composite image demonstrating spatial relationships between ciliary bundles of hair cells (red), neural innervation (green), and cellular nuclei (blue) within the same neuroepithelial field, providing comprehensive structural and molecular characterization of vestibular hair cells and their associated neural elements

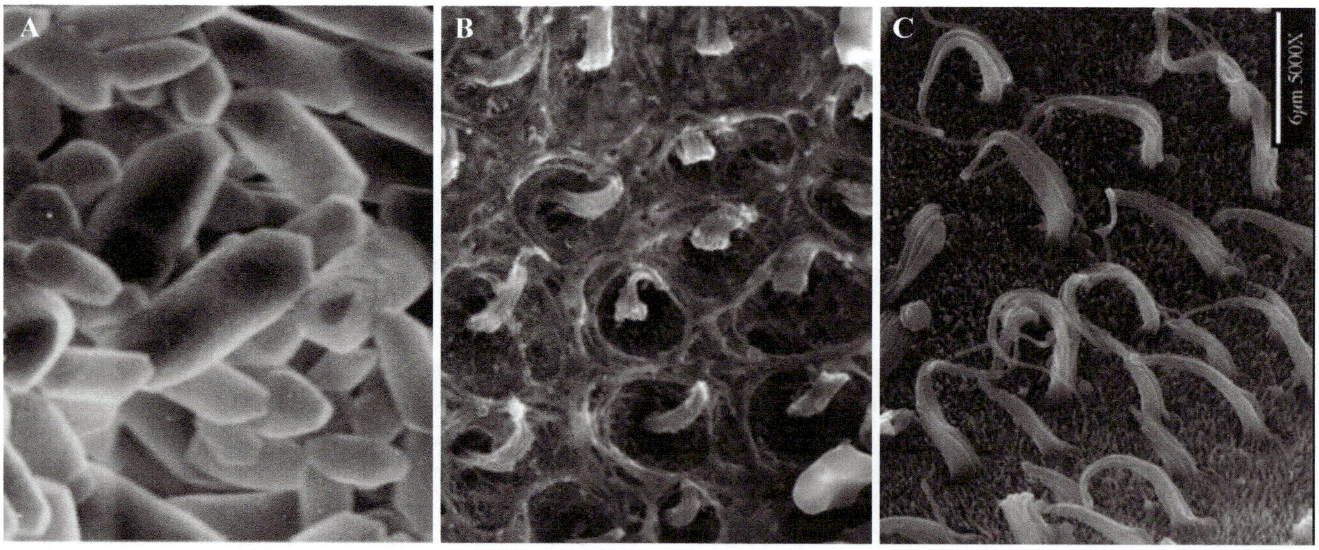

Fig. 3.6 Images of scanning electron microscopy of the surface ultrastructure of the macula of saccule. (**A**) Superior view reveals the dense otolithic membrane layer overlying the macula of saccule. (**B**) Following otolith removal, the underlying gelatinous layer is exposed, showing multiple hair cell ciliary bundles penetrating its matrix. (**C**) Complete removal of the gelatinous layer fully exposes the organized array of ciliary bundles projecting from the cuticular plate of sensory hair cells, demonstrating the hierarchical organization of the otoliths-gelatinous layer-hair cell complex

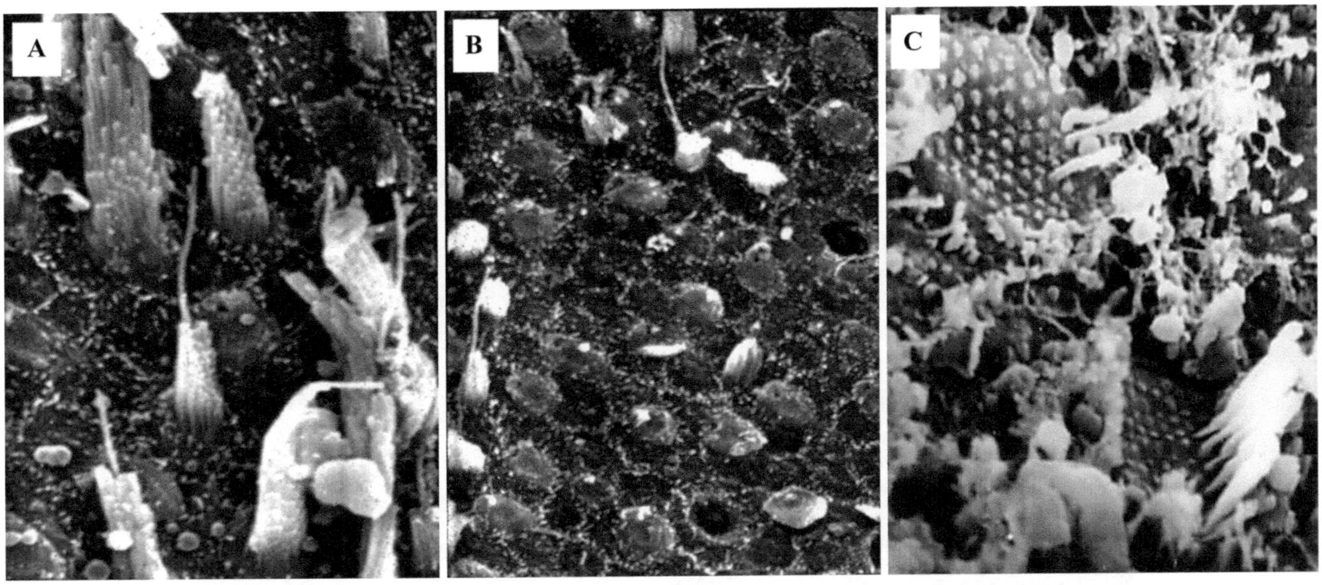

Fig. 3.7 Scanning electron microscopic observation of the pathological changes on the surface of hair cells in the macula of saccule. (**A**) Surface view demonstrates intact stereociliary bundles projecting from both Type I and Type II hair cells in normal vestibular epithelium. (**B**) Chronic kanamycin administration induces progressive hair cell damage, characterized by ciliary bundle loss while preserving the structural integrity of most cuticular plates. (**C**) Advanced ototoxic injury reveals characteristic pore-like structures on the exposed cuticular plates, representing residual insertion sites of degenerated cilia, providing ultrastructural evidence of the dynamic process of hair cell degeneration

3.3 Microdissection and Surface Preparation of the Utricular Macula

Under microscopic visualization, the macula of utricle is carefully isolated by severing its dorsal nerve fibers and vasculature at the superior sieve spot zone using a fine dissecting needle (Fig. 3.8A, B), followed by extraction of entire utricle with micro-forceps (Fig. 3.8C). The utricular membrane is then opened to expose the underlying otolithic membrane, which is subsequently removed by precision microdissection. The macula of utricle undergoes standard histochemical processing before being flat-mounted in glycerol for detailed observation of the sensory epithelium under both light and fluorescence microscopy [4–6, 12, 15, 19, 29–31] (Fig. 1.19; Figs. 3.8D, 3.9, 3.10, 3.11, 3.12, 3.13, and 3.14). For ultrastructural analysis, specimens are processed through critical point drying and sputter coating, permitting scanning electron microscopic examination of hair cell surface morphology and pathological alterations, thus facilitating comprehensive structural assessment at multiple resolution levels [24–28] (Fig. 1.15; Figs. 3.15 and 3.16).

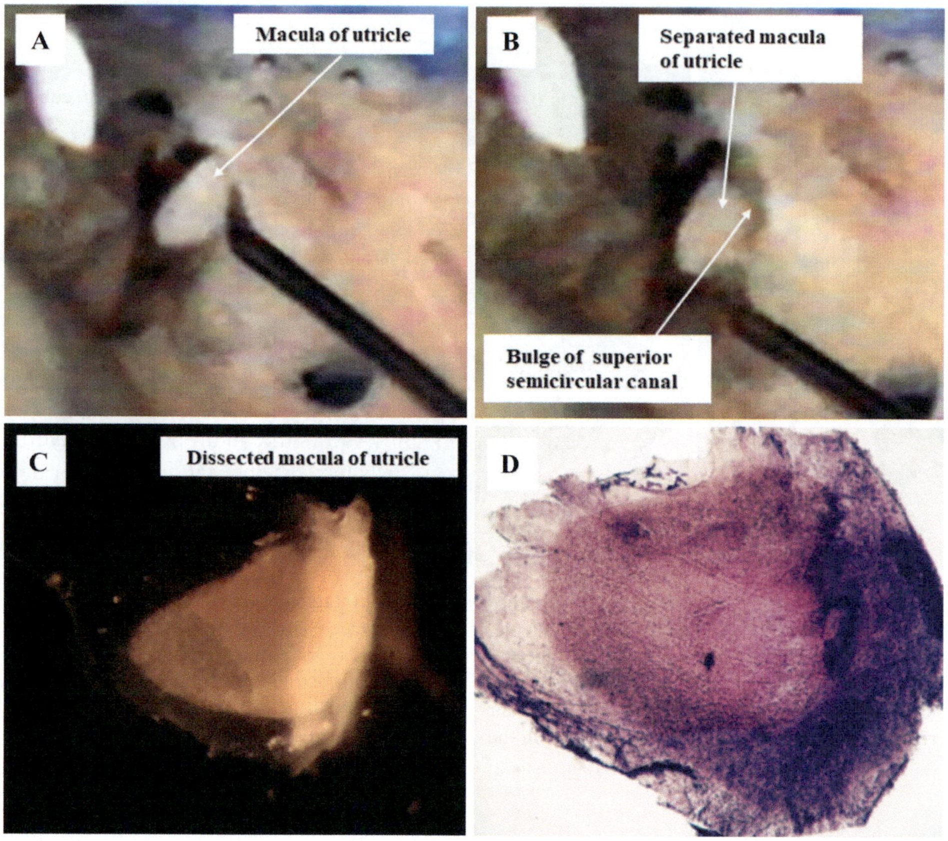

Fig. 3.8 Microanatomy and microdissection of the macula of utricle in guinea pigs. (**A**) The neurovascular supply to the macula of utricle is severed along the attachment point at the bony edge of the superior sieve spot zone using a dissecting needle. (**B**) The entire utricle is then gently detached from the vestibular cistern using microdissection technique. (**C**) The entire utricle macula was exposed by tearing open the utricle membrane. (**D**) After removing the otolith membrane covering the surface of the macula of utricle, the sample was stained with hematoxylin and then mounted on glass slide in glycerin and coverslipped as a surface preparation

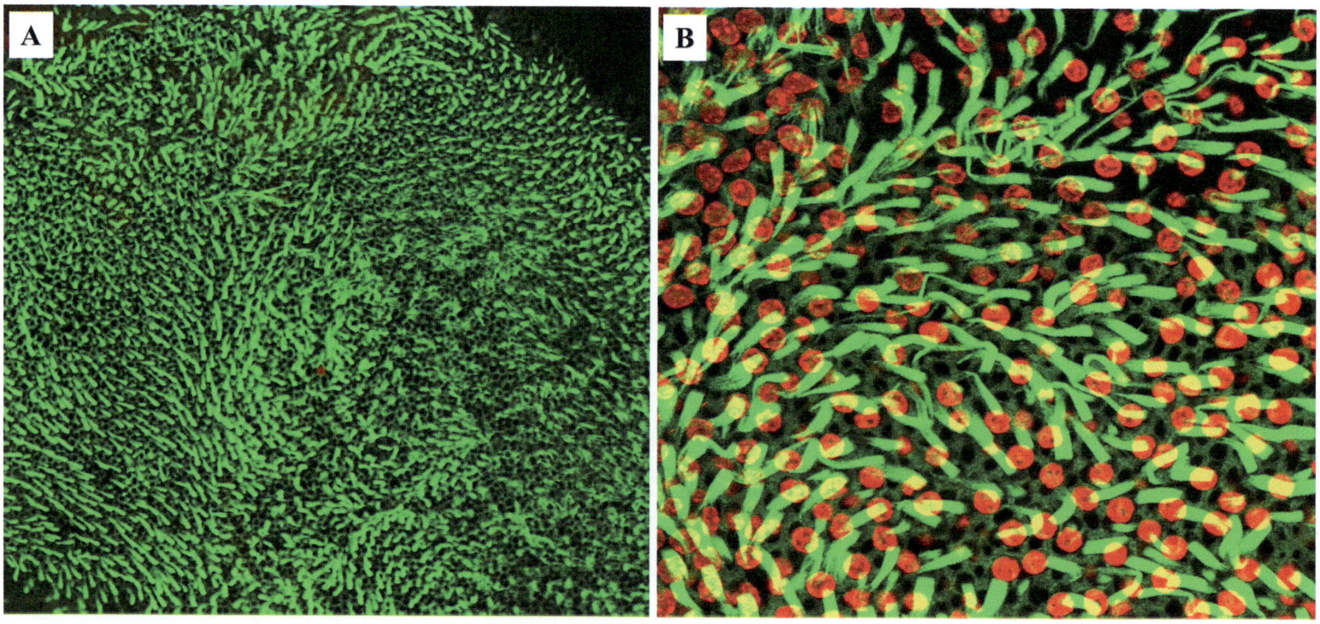

Fig. 3.9 Fluorescent staining image of the macula of utricle. (**A**) Phalloidin staining reveals the ciliary bundles (green fluorescence) on individual hair cells in the macula of utricle. (**B**) Double fluorescence staining simultaneously demonstrates phalloidin-labeled ciliary bundles (green) and To-Pro-3-stained hair cell nuclei (red). It should be explained that to improve the contrast between the two fluorescent markers, the blue nuclei shown by ToPro-3 staining were converted to red using confocal image processing software

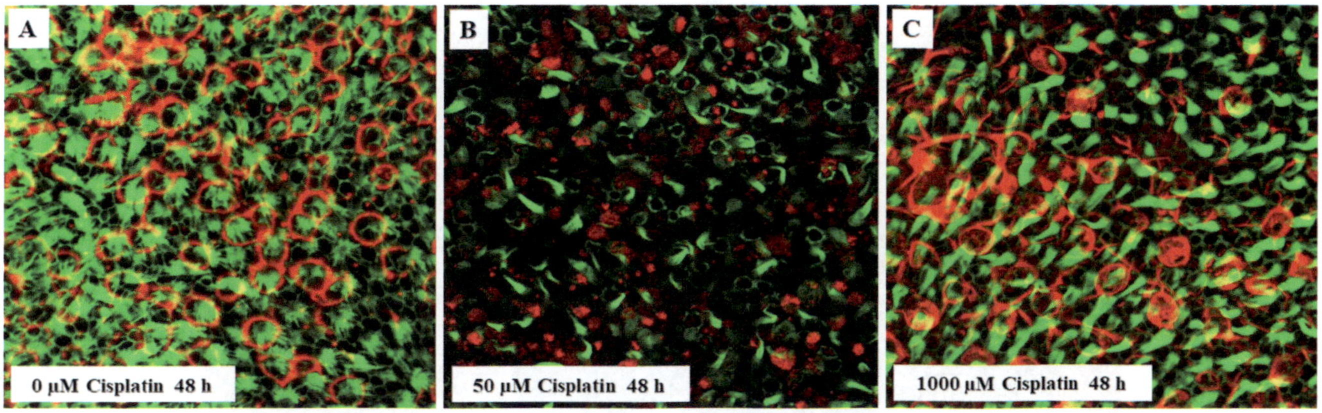

Fig. 3.10 Double fluorescence staining revealed the destructive effect of cisplatin on vestibular hair cells and their afferent nerve synapse. (**A**) A normal explant of macula of utricle cultured in serum-free medium for 48 h showed well-preserved cellular architecture, displaying intact phalloidin-labeled ciliary bundles (green) on hair cells, characteristic anti-tubulin antibody labeled annular Type I afferent terminals (red), and granular Type II afferent terminals (red). (**B**) 48 h after 50 μ M cisplatin incubation, loss of ciliary bundles of cochlear hair cells and their surrounding annular Type I afferent nerve terminals was detected. In contrast, the Type II hair cells and their granular afferent nerve terminals remained structurally intact. (**C**) Unexpectedly, 1000 μM cisplatin treatment preserves both ciliary and afferent innervations in both hair cell types, revealing a concentration-dependent paradoxical effect where low-dose cisplatin preferentially targets Type I hair cells and their calyx terminals, whereas high-dose exposure shows no significant ototoxic effects on vestibular hair cells or their afferent connections

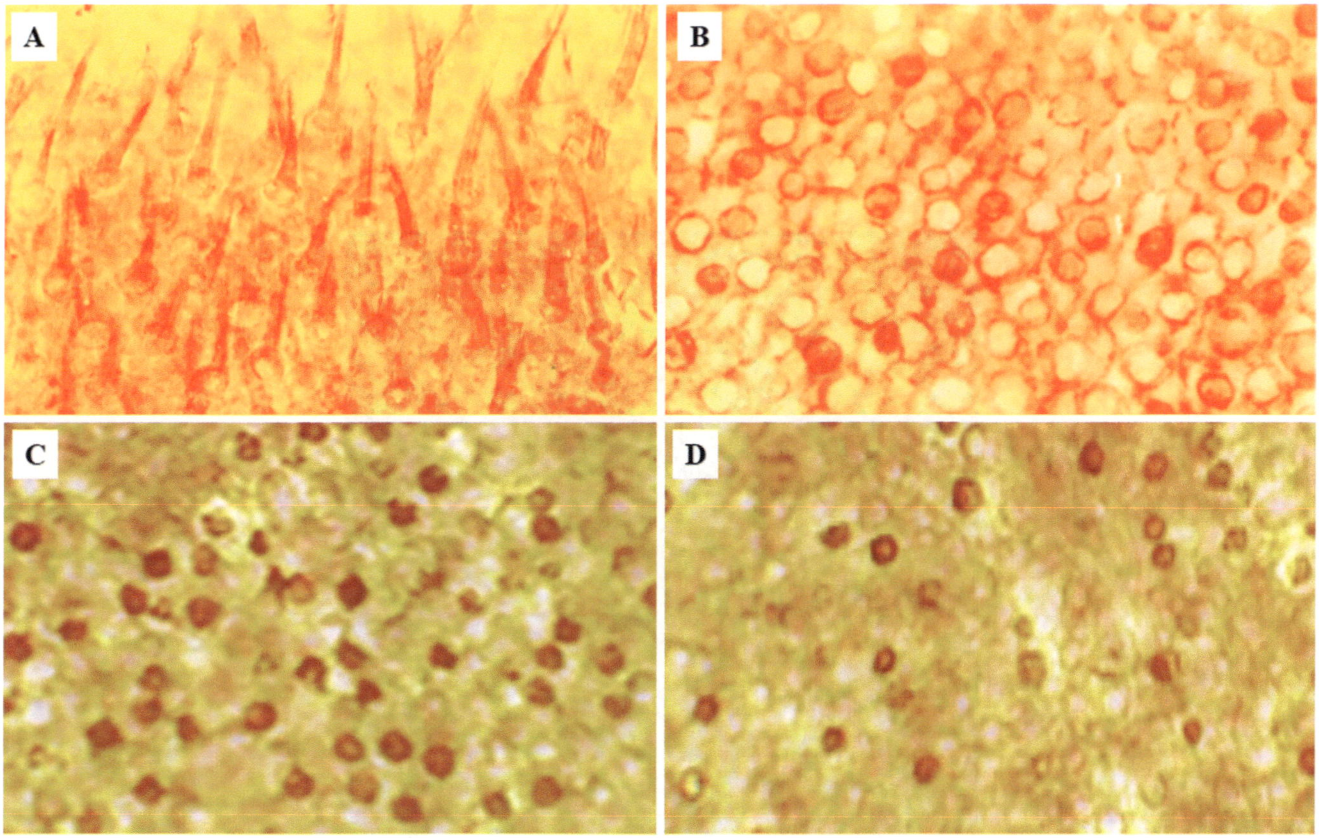

Fig. 3.11 Gentamicin-induced structural alterations on the surface of hair cells in macula of utricle. (**A**) The ciliary bundles on the hair cells of macula of utricle are labeled by precipitation of silver nitrate. (**B**) Silver nitrate infiltration reveals the polygonal boundaries of cuticular plates in normal guinea pig vestibular hair cells, demonstrating the typical mosaic pattern of the sensory epithelium. (**C**) Daily injections of gentamicin (125 mg/kg per 12 h) for seven days resulted in severe hair cell abscission, as evidenced by decreased hair cell density and disrupted epithelial organization. (**D**) Ten-day gentamicin administration (125 mg/kg per 12 h) results in near-complete degeneration of cuticular plates, with few residual cellular outlines remaining, illustrating the progressive nature of gentamicin-induced destruction of vestibular hair cells

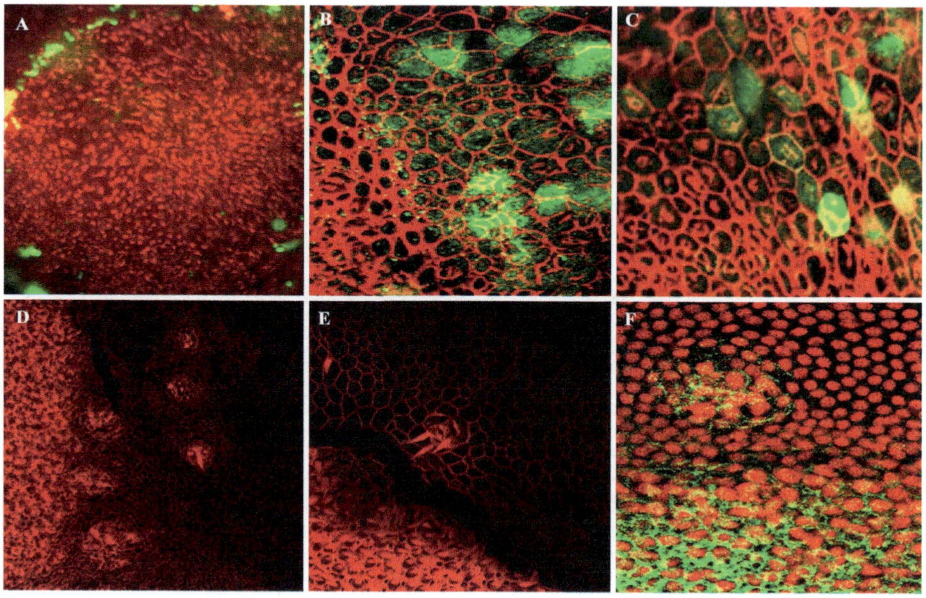

Fig. 3.12 After the adenovirus vector carrying Math1 and EGFP protein genes penetrated into the inner ear of adult chinchillas through the round window membrane, the transfected supporting cells around the macula of utricle were induced to differentiate into hair cell-like cells. (**A–C**) Three days post-transfection with adenoviral vectors carrying Math1 and EGFP transgenes, robust EGFP fluorescence (green) demonstrates successful transduction of supporting cells in both the macula of utricle (**A**) and the semilunar planum of dark cell region surrounding the bases of ampullary crista (**B**), with higher magnification revealing detailed cellular morphology of transfected supporting cells near the macula of utricle (**C**). (**D–F**) By day 10 post-transfection, discrete islands of cells exhibiting hair cell characteristics emerge within supporting cell regions: (D) shows clusters of cells developing ciliary bundles, (**E**) reveals detailed cuticular plate and ciliary bundles resembling native hair cells, while (**F**) demonstrates dual molecular evidence of cellular reprogramming through myosin VI immunoreactivity (green) in both native hair cells and converted cells, accompanied by nuclear enlargement (ToPro3, red) to hair cell-like dimensions. These findings collectively demonstrate that Math1 expression initiates a redifferentiation program in mature vestibular supporting cells, driving their transformation into phenotypically and molecularly recognizable hair cell-like cells

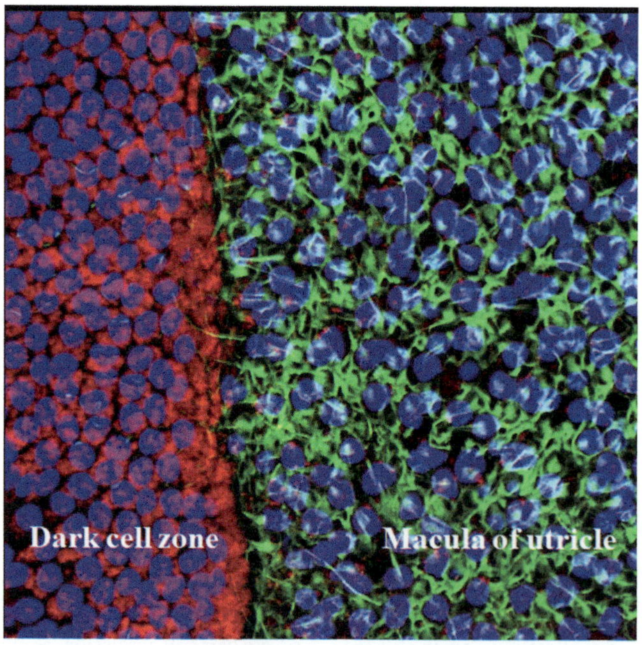

Fig. 3.13 Targeted delivery of Cy3-labeled siRNA via TAT-DRBD carriers in chinchilla vestibular system. Following transtympanic administration, Cy3-labeled siRNA complexed with TAT double-stranded RNA-binding domain (TAT-DRBD) recombinant protein vectors demonstrates selective uptake within the vestibular system, with pronounced accumulation in metabolically active dark cells (red fluorescence) surrounding the macula of utricle and semilunar planum regions of the ampullary crista, while showing minimal transfection to other cell types in the inner ear. This cell-type-specific distribution pattern suggests an active transport mechanism mediated by the enhanced phagocytic capacity of vestibular dark cells for the TAT-DRBD-siRNA complexes, highlighting their potential as privileged targets for molecular therapies in the inner ear

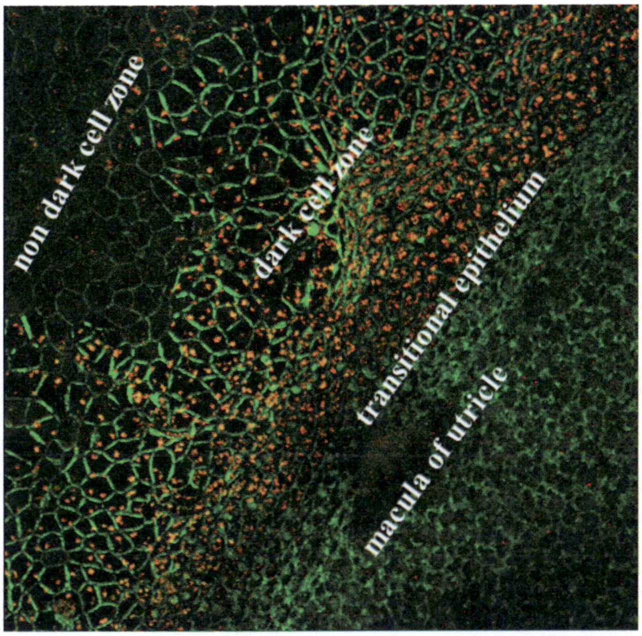

Fig. 3.14 Primate-selective siRNA transfection in vestibular dark cells mediated by TAT-DRBD carriers. The photomicrograph demonstrates successful trans-round window membrane delivery of Cy3.5-labeled siRNA complexed with TAT-DRBD recombinant proteins into primate inner ear, revealing targeted accumulation (orange fluorescence) specifically within the phagocytically active dark cell population surrounding the utricular macula, while adjacent vestibular cell types show minimal uptake, suggesting both the translational potential of this delivery platform for non-human primate models and confirming the conserved phagocytic capacity of vestibular dark cells across species for TAT-DRBD-siRNA complexes

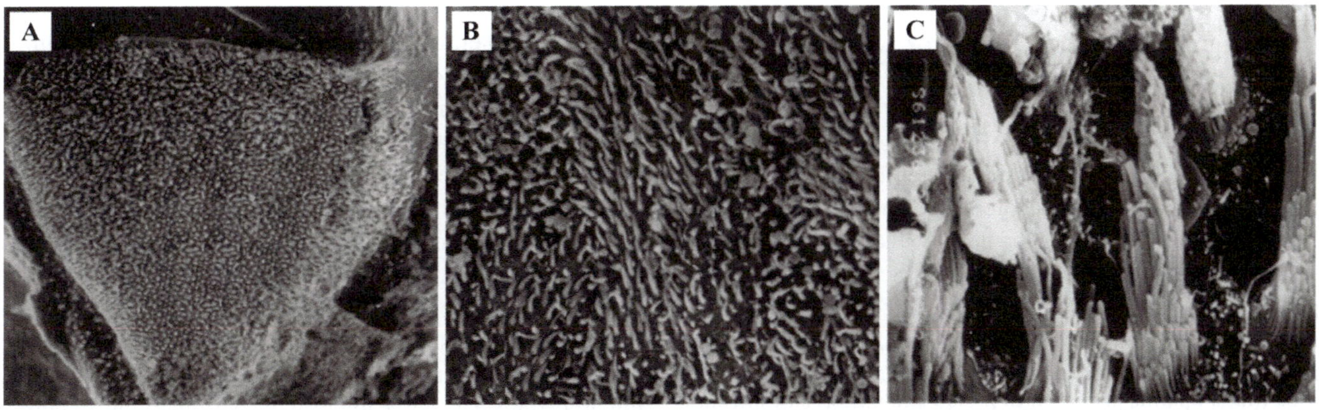

Fig. 3.15 Scanning electron microscopic observation of the surface structure of hair cells on the macula of utricle in guinea pigs. (**A**) Low-magnification overview reveals the complete sensory epithelium of the utricular macula, demonstrating the organized mosaic pattern of hair cell distribution. (**B**) Higher magnification illustrates the characteristic ciliary bundles projecting from individual hair cells, showing their precise geometric arrangement. (**C**) At maximum resolution, the ciliary bundles of Type I hair cells are arranged from tallest to shortest along the graded heights of the kinocilia

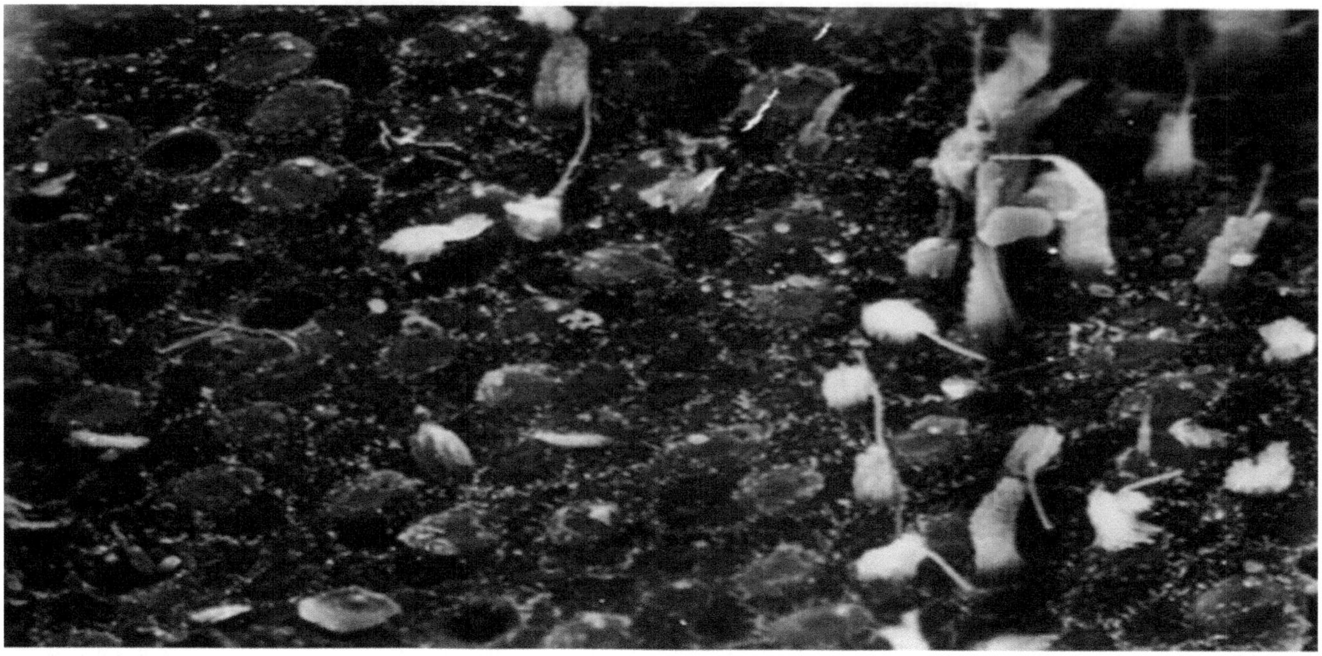

Fig. 3.16 Disruption of the ultrastructure on the surface of the sensory hair cells in the macula of utricle induced by kanamycin ototoxicity. Ten days of kanamycin administration (400 mg/kg/day) induces distinct pathological changes in the macula of utricle, where most hair cells retain their cuticular plates but show complete ciliary bundle loss, resulting in permanent mechanotransduction impairment. Notably, surviving hair cells with ciliary bundle and cuticular plate exhibit the morphology of Type II hair cells characterized by a long kinocilium with a handful of very short stereocilia, demonstrating that Type I hair cells are more vulnerable to kanamycin ototoxicity in vestibular end organs, potentially due to differences in their structural organization or molecular susceptibility

3.4 Microdissection and Surface Preparation of Semicircular Canals

Under a dissecting microscope, the neurovascular supply to the ampullary cristae of the lateral and superior semicircular canals was truncated along the bony wall at the superior sieve spots; and the neurovascular supply to the ampullary crista of posterior semicircular canal was truncated along the osseous wall at the inferior sieve spot using a dissection needle to separate the three membranous ampullae from their osseous housing, The non-ampullated end of the lateral semicircular canal and the non-ampullated ends of common crus were then also cut off with micro-rongeurs, so that both the ampullary end and the non-ampullary end of each semicircular canal were separated from the utricle (Fig. 3.17A). Use ultra-fine forceps to gently pull the end of each ampulla. When there is no elastic retraction, confirm that the tissue trabeculae that fix the membranous semicircular canal within the bony semicircular canal are completely severed, so that the intact membranous semicircular canal can be pulled out from its bony semicircular canal. Use ultra-fine forceps to gently pull the end of each ampulla until there is no elastic retraction, which indicates that the surrounding tissue trabeculae that fix the membranous semicircular canals within the bony semicircular canals have been completely disconnected. The intact membranous semicircular canals can be then pulled out from each bony semicircular canal (Fig. 3.17B). The membranous ampulla was torn open with ultra-fine forceps to fully expose the ampullary crista (Fig. 3.17C, D). The entire ampullary crista was then stained with the proposed histochemical staining procedure. The nerve fibers at the bottom of the ampullary crista was trimmed and the crista of ampulla was placed in a glycerol drop on a glass slide for observation under light microscope [4, 5, 7–9, 12, 15, 29] (Figs. 3.17E, 3.18, 3.19, 3.20, 3.21, 3.22, and 3.23). Alternatively, the ampullary crista can be routinely prepared for observation under scanning electron microscope to permit ultrastructural observations of the surface of hair cells on the ampullary crista [12, 24–28] (Figs. 3.24, 3.25, 3.26, and 3.27).

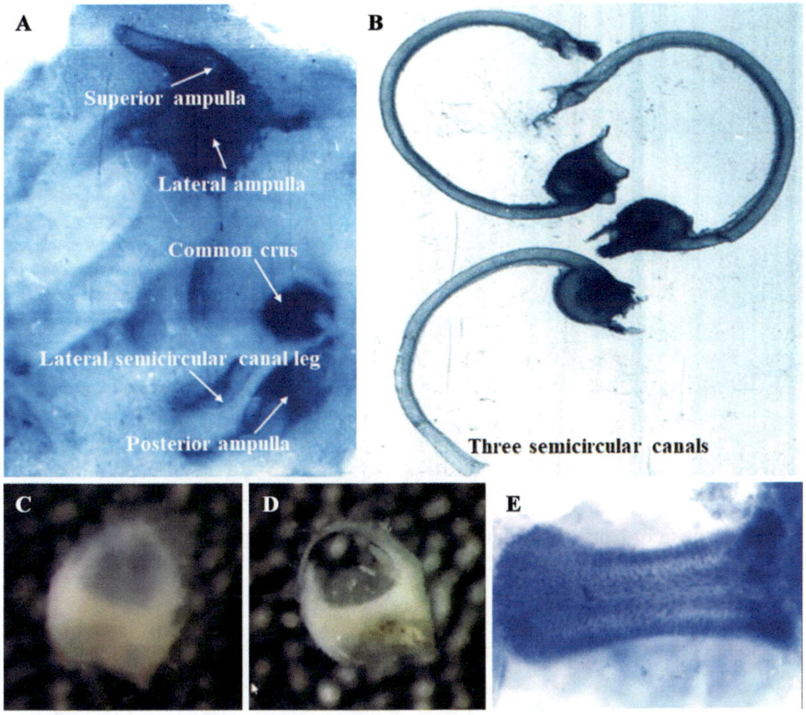

Fig. 3.17 Procedure for micro-dissection of the membranous ampullae and the surface preparations of ampullary crista under a dissecting microscope. (**A**) Surgical opening of lateral bony wall of the vestibular cistern and removal of the membranous saccule and utricle to reveal the lateral and superior membranous ampullae, as well as the posterior membranous ampulla. The non-ampulla end of the lateral semicircular canal and the common crus formed by the superior and posterior semicircular canals are also exposed. (**B**) Three membranous ampullae are in turn pulled with ultra-fine forceps respectively to gently withdraw the membranous semicircular canal from the bony semicircular canal. (**C**) The semicircular canals are dissected out to expose the entire membranous ampulla. (**D**) The membranous wall of the ampulla is ripped off to expose the entire ampullary crista. (**E**) The succinate dehydrogenase in sensory hair cells on the ampullary crista is stained in blue

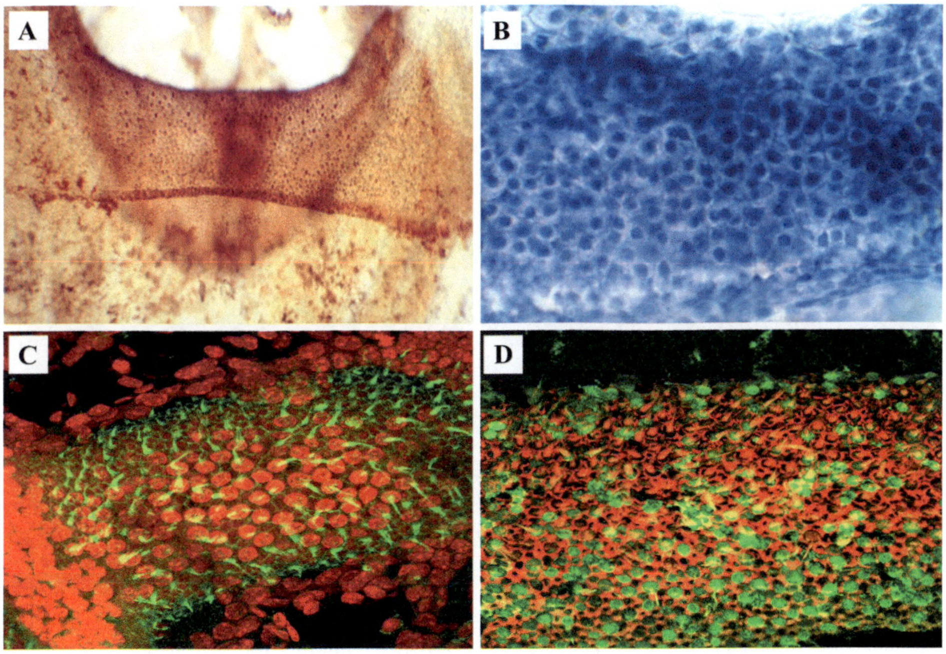

Fig. 3.18 Several histochemical staining results for the surface preparation of ampullary crista. (**A**) Silver nitrate impregnation reveals the distinct rounded boundaries of the cuticular plate of hair cells on the ampullary crista. (**B**) Hematoxylin staining shows the nuclei and density of hair cells in the ampullary crista of mouse. (**C**) Double staining of phalloidin (green) and ToPro-3 (red) to label the ciliary bundles and the nuclei of the hair cells on ampullary crista in a normal mouse. (**D**) Carboplatin induced p53-positive immunohistochemical products in green in the hair cells of the ampullary crista in chinchilla, suggesting that p53 plays an important role in carboplatin-induced apoptosis of hair cells on the ampullary crista

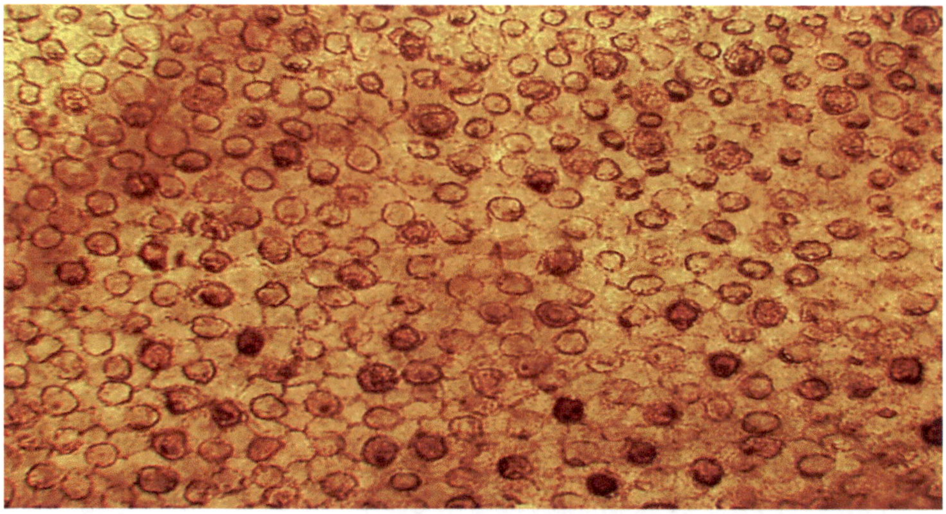

Fig. 3.19 The outline of the cuticular plate of hair cells on the ampullary crista in the normal chinchilla was stained with silver nitrate to form the silver precipitate shadow so that the cuticular plate of each hair cell was clearly displayed.

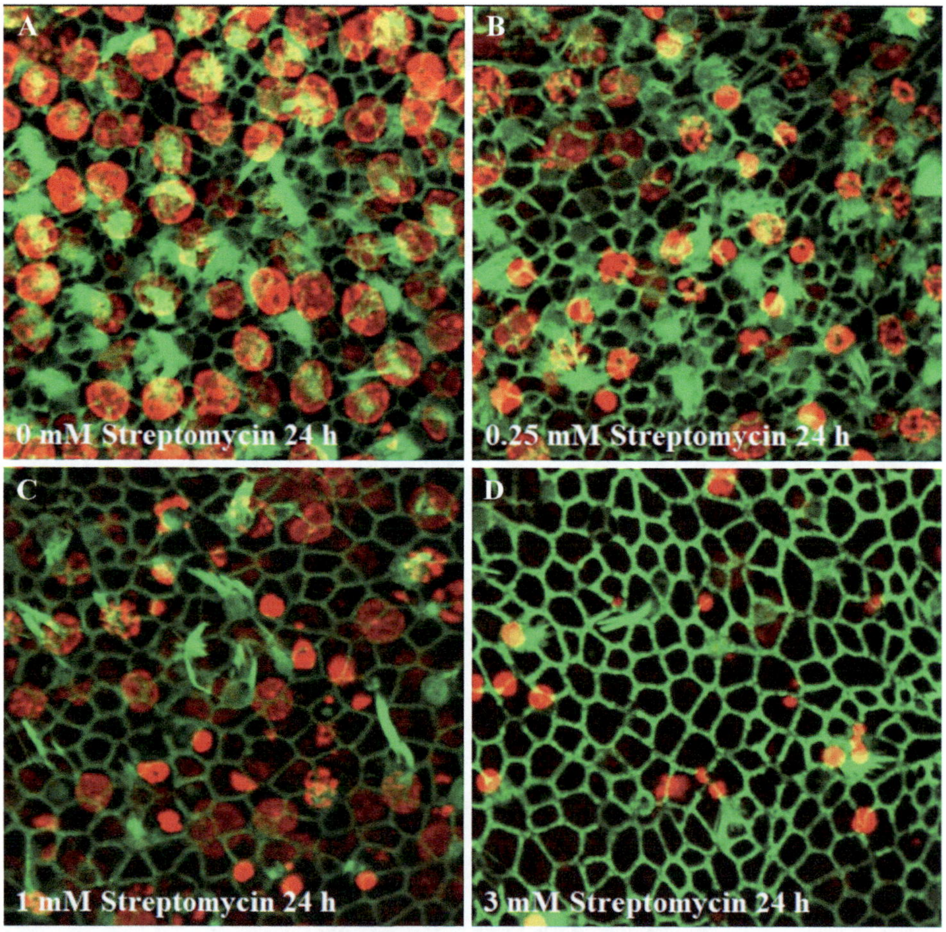

Fig. 3.20 Dose-dependent ototoxic effects of streptomycin to sensory hair cells on explants of ampullary crista. (**A**) The ciliary bundles and nuclei of hair cells in the ampullary crista in a normal rat appear normal after 24-h culture in standard serum-free medium without streptomycin. (**B**) After culturing for 24 h in serum-free medium containing 0.25 mM streptomycin, nearly 50% of hair cells on the ampullary crista were destroyed. The nuclear staining showed that the nuclei of the remaining hair cells were mostly accompanied by chromatin agglutination. (**C**) After culturing for 24 h in serum-free medium containing 1 mM streptomycin sulfate, the nuclei of the remaining hair cells showed obvious nuclear condensation or nuclear fragmentation. (**D**) After culturing for 24 h in serum-free medium containing 3 mM streptomycin sulfate, most of the hair cells on the ampullary crista were completely destroyed

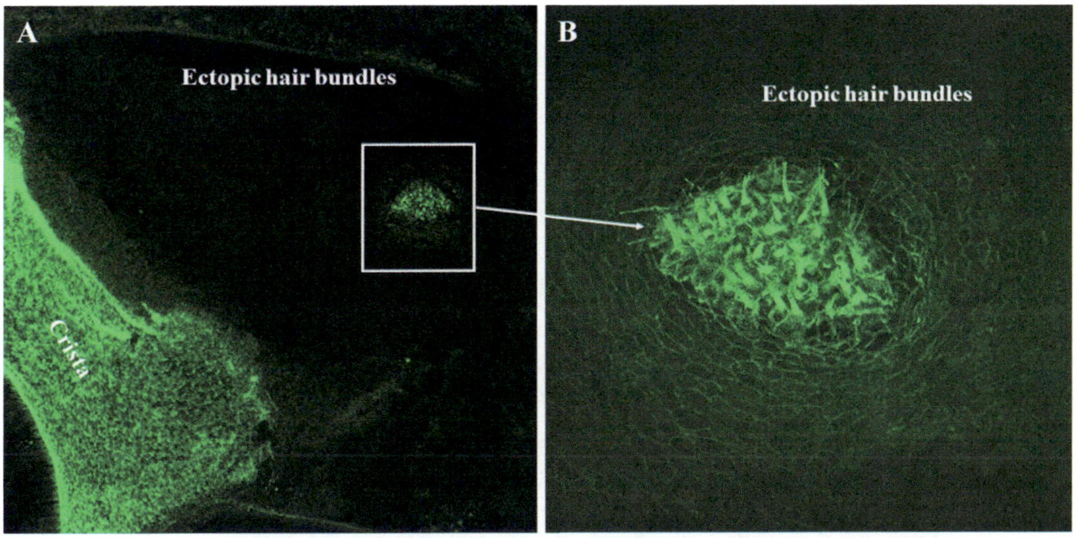

Fig. 3.21 An ectopic hair cell colony appears in the supporting cell area adjacent to the ampulla cavity of an adult chinchilla ten days after transfection with an adenoviral vector carrying the Math1 gene. (**A**) Ten days post-transfection with Math1-expressing adenoviral vectors, a distinct ectopic cluster of hair cells emerges at the ampullary base. (**B**) High-magnification shows that these ectopic cells, which appear at the floor of the ampullary cavity, display the morphology of hair cells with ciliary bundles

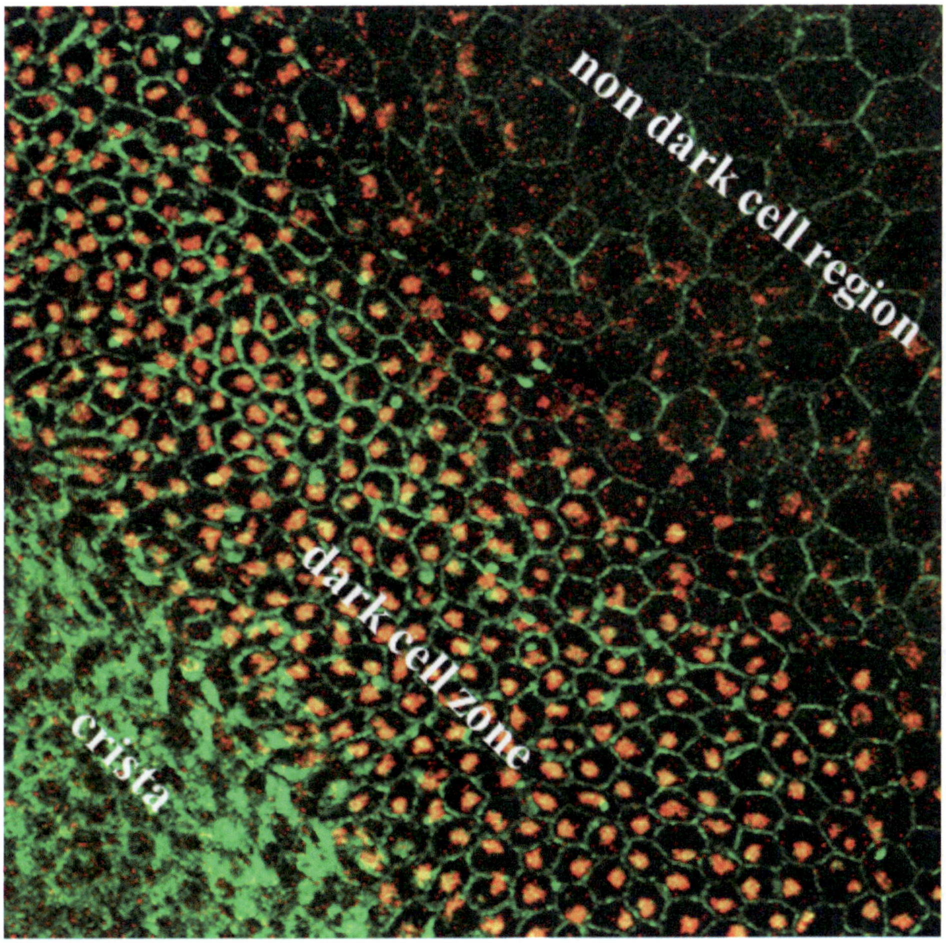

Fig. 3.22 Cy3.5-labeled siRNA is transfected into the dark cells at the semilunar plane zones surrounding the base of the ampullary crista. This micrograph reveals the accumulation of Cy3.5-labeled siRNA (orange fluorescence) within dark cells located in the semilunar planum region surrounding the crista ampullaris base, while adjacent cell types show minimal fluorescence, suggesting that these dark cells can ingest the siRNA through their robust phagocytic activity

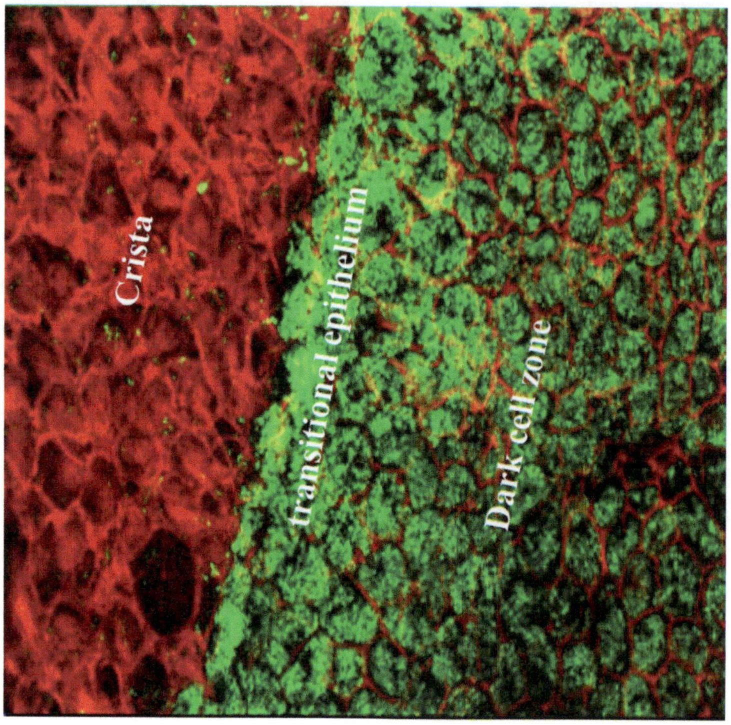

Fig. 3.23 The green fluorescent protein gene carried by hydroxyapatite nanocarriers showed green fluorescence in the dark cells at the crescent-shaped areas in both sides of crista 48 h after transfection. This phenomenon suggests that these special dark cells are able to actively internalize the nanocarriers and subsequently express the delivered transgenes, as evidenced by the abundant production of EGFP in their cytoplasm

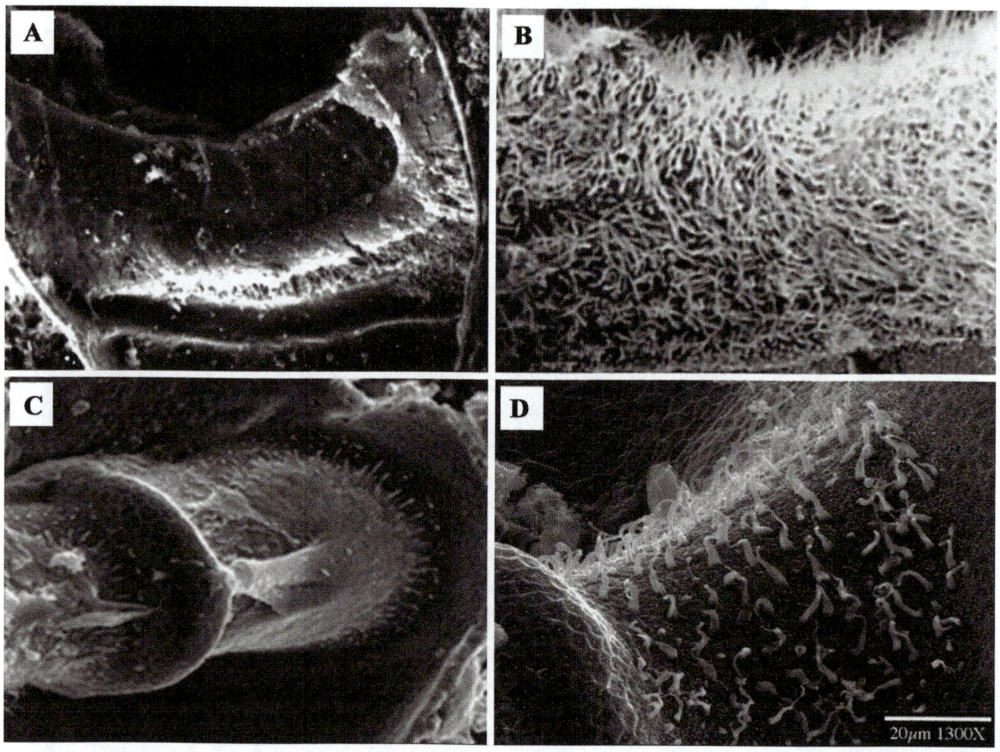

Fig. 3.24 Surface ultrastructure of the ampullary crista under a scanning electron microscope. (**A**) The gelatinous cupula on the surface of the ampullary crista of the guinea pig has almost completely covered the ciliary tuft of the hair cells after critical point dry. (**B**) Irrigation of the saline through the cavity of ampulla to effectively remove the gelatinous cupula prior to fixation to ensure adequate exposure of the surface ultrastructure of the hair cells. (**C**) The gelatinous cupula on the surface of the superior ampullary crista of rat was not rinsed before fixation. After critical point drying, the ciliary bundles of the hair cells on the crista could not be seen due to the coverage of the gelatinous cupula cap. (**D**) After pre-rinsing the ampullary cavity with saline to remove the gelatinous cupula, the cilia tuft of the hair cells on the crista of ampulla is fully exposed

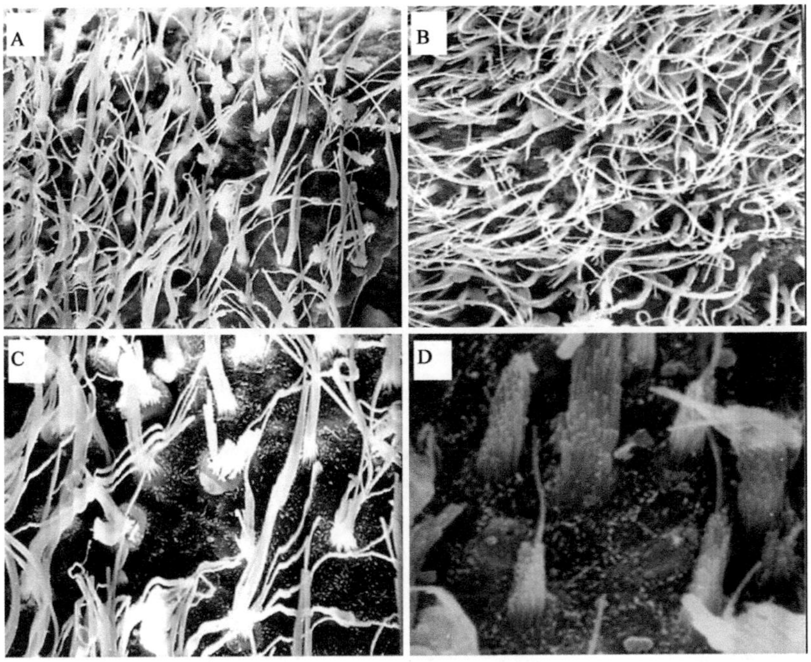

Fig. 3.25 Scanning electron micrograph showing that the cilia bundle of sensory hair cells on ampullary crista is thin and curved. (**A**) The crista ampullaris displays characteristically slender and curved ciliary bundles. (**B**) The cuticular plate of hair cells in a normal guinea pig is often obscured by their slender and curved cilia bundles. (**C**) The diameter of cilia bundles of the hair cells on ampullary crista is approximately 100–150 nm that may enhance mechanical sensitivity to endolymph flow. (**D**) In contrast, the diameter of the ciliary bundles of the hair cells on the macula of utricle is approximately 200–300 nm, which is significantly thicker than that of the hair cells on the ampullary crista, perhaps reflecting their functional adaptation to different mechanical transduction requirements

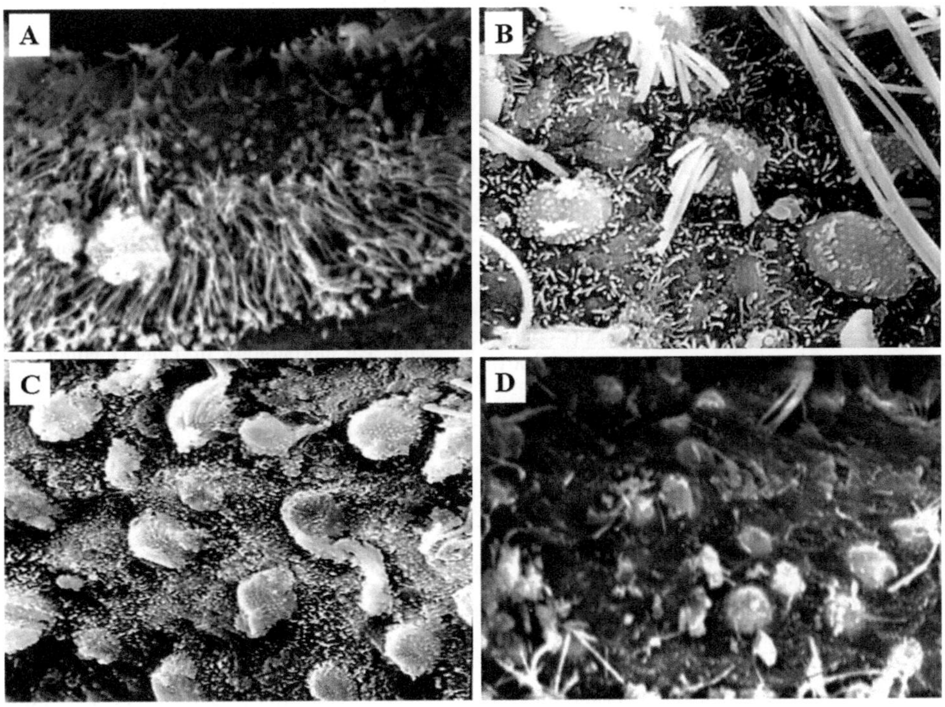

Fig. 3.26 Gentamicin-induced damage to the surface ultrastructure of hair cells on the ampullary crista. (**A**) Gentamicin-induced damage to the hair cells on the crista of ampulla first appears on the top of the crista of ampulla. (**B**) The hair cells on the ampullary crista first undergo shedding of the ciliary bundles before cellular destruction occurs. (**C**) After the ciliary bundles of hair cells on the ampullary crista are shed, the cuticular plate of the hair cells shows signs of outward bulge, suggesting that intracellular swelling or swelling of the nerve terminals may constitute pressure on the cuticular plate of the damaged hair cells. (**D**) In the late stage of gentamicin ototoxicity, the cuticular plate of hair cells is lost starting from the top of the ampullary crista and replaced by scar tissue

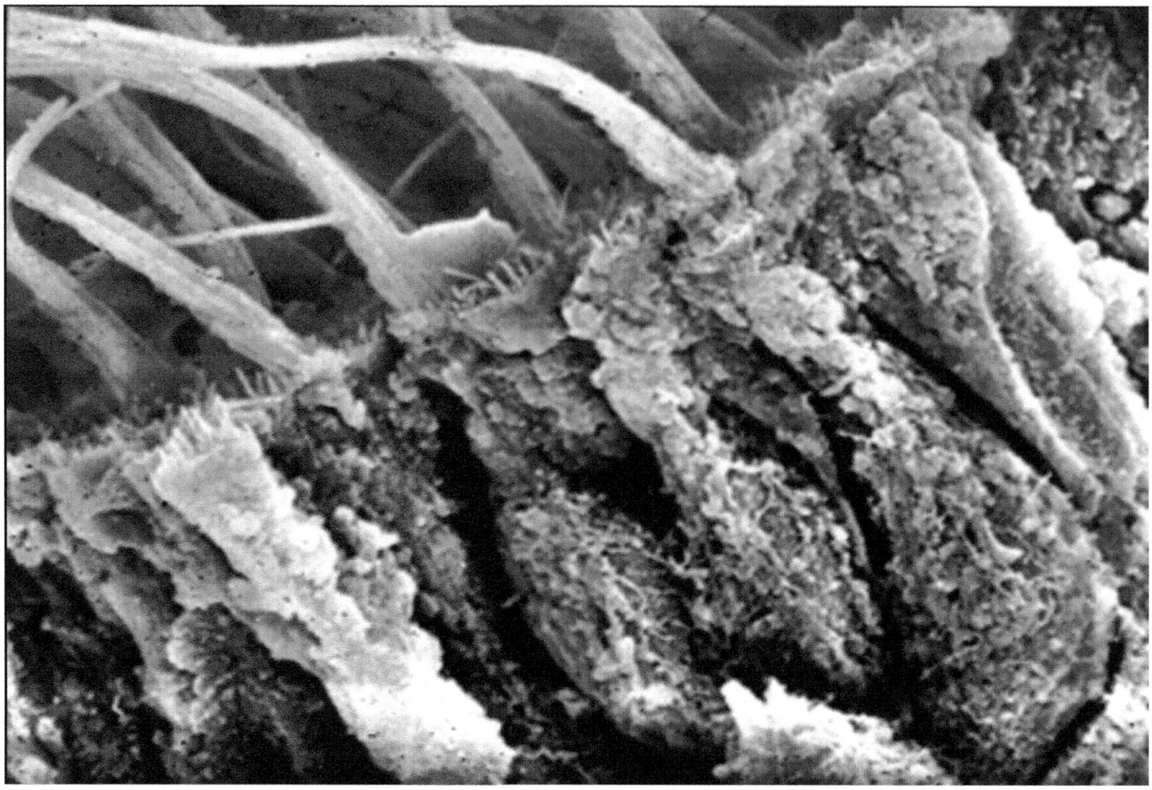

Fig. 3.27 Surface and cross-sectional ultrastructural display of ampullary crista hair cells. After the ampullary crista was truncated from the middle of crista, the ultrastructure of the surface (ciliary bundles and cuticular plates) and the basolateral cellular morphology (cell bodies and afferent nerve calyces) of the hair cells along the edge of the severed end of the ampullary crista can be observed under a scanning electron microscope. This might provide a comprehensive three-dimensional observation of the vestibular hair cells

References

1. Lim DJ, Lane WC. Vestibular sensory epithea. A scanning electron microscopic observation. Arch Otolaryngol. 1969;90:283–92. https://doi.org/10.1001/archotol.1969.00770030285007.
2. Lindeman HH. Studies on the morphology of the sensory regions of the vestibular apparatus with 45 figures. Ergeb Anat Entwicklungsgesch. 1969;42:1–113.
3. Engstrom H, Bergstrom B, Rosenhall U. Vestibular sensory epithelia. Arch Otolaryngol. 1974;100:411–18. https://doi.org/10.1001/archotol.1974.00780040425002.
4. Ding D, Luo S, Jin X. Microdissection of the vestibular end-organs in guinea pigs. Shanghai Med J. 1986;9:153–54.
5. Ding D, Zhao J, Huangfu M, Jin X. Microdissection of the whole membranous labyrinth in guinea pigs. J Clin Otorhinolaryngol. 1987;1:9–11.
6. Ding D, Chen X, Jin X. Quantitative observation technique in a small field of view in vestibular end organs. Zhonghua Er Bi Yan Hou Ke Za Zhi. 1992;27:202–3.
7. Ding D, Jiang S. Chapter 6: Surface preparation techniques of the inner ear. In: Ding D, editor. Manual of anatomical examination of the inner ear of the guinea pig. Shanghai: Xuelin Publishing House; 1989. pp. 49–60.
8. Ding D, Li M, Jiang C, Salvi R. Chapter 5: Surface preparation techniques of membranous labyrinth. In: Ding D, editor. Morphology of the inner ear. Harbin: Heilongjiang Science and Technology Press; 2001. pp. 24–37.
9. Lii M, Ding D, Zheng XY, Salvi R. Vestibular destruction by slow infusion of gentamicin into semicircular canals. Acta Otolaryngol Suppl. 2004;553:35–41. https://doi.org/10.1080/03655230410017102.
10. Desai SS, Ali H, Lysakowski A. Comparative morphology of rodent vestibular periphery. II. Cristae ampullares. J Neurophysiol. 2005;93:267–80. https://doi.org/10.1152/jn.00747.2003.
11. Desai SS, Zeh C, Lysakowski A. Comparative morphology of rodent vestibular periphery. I. Saccular and utricular maculae. J Neurophysiol. 2005;93:251–66. https://doi.org/10.1152/jn.00746.2003.
12. Ding D, Qi W, Qu Y, Salvi R Chapter 6: Research techniques of the inner ear morphology. In: Ding D, editor. Science of the inner ear. Beijing: China Science and Technology Press; 2010. pp. 50–88.
13. Taylor RR, Jagger DJ, Saeed SR, et al. Characterizing human vestibular sensory epithelia for experimental studies: new hair bundles on old tissue and implications for therapeutic interventions in ageing. Neurobiol Aging. 2015;36:2068–84. https://doi.org/10.1016/j.neurobiolaging.2015.02.013.
14. Ye H, Xing Y, Zhang L, et al. Bilirubin-induced neurotoxic and ototoxic effects in rat cochlear and vestibular organotypic cultures. Neurotoxicology. 2019;71:75–86. https://doi.org/10.1016/j.neuro.2018.12.004.
15. Ding D, Li P, Qi W, Zhang J. Quantitative observation of vestibular sensory hair cells in experimental animals. Chin J Otorhinolaryngol Skull Base Surg. 2022;28:11–18. https://doi.org/10.11798/j.issn.1007-1520.202290001.
16. Schuknecht H. 2. Anatomy. In: Pathology of the ear. 1st ed. Cambridge: Harvard University Press; 1974. pp. 40–96.
17. Ding D, Jiang S. Chapter 8: Preparation techniques for electron microscopy of inner ear specimen. In: Ding D, editor. Manual of

anatomical examination of the inner ear of the guinea pig. Shanghai: Xuelin Publishing House; 1989. pp. 67–74.
18. Ding D, Qi W, Qu Y, Salvi R Chapter 15: Animal model of intra-labyrinthal hydrops. In: Ding D, editor. Science of the inner ear. Beijing: China Science and Technology Press; 2010. pp. 183–188.
19. Ding D, Jiang H, Zhang J, et al. Cisplatin-induced vestibular hair cell lesion-less damage at high doses. J Otol. 2018;13:115–21. https://doi.org/10.1016/j.joto.2018.08.002.
20. Ding D, Shi L, Xing Y, et al. Sagittal sectioning of temporal bones and quantitative measurement of neural densities in the inner ear in normal mice. Chin J Otorhinolaryngol Skull Base Surg. 2024;30:69–75. https://doi.org/10.11798/i.issn.1007-1520.202424331.
21. Li P, Ding D, Gao K, Salvi R. Standard surgical approaches to ear surgery in rats. Chin J Otol. 2015;13:13–17. https://doi.org/10.1016/j.joto.2015.03.004.
22. Li P, Gao K, Ding D, Salvi R. Characteristic anatomical structures of rat temporal bone. J Otol. 2015;10:118–24. https://doi.org/10.1016/j.joto.2015.11.002.
23. Ding D, Manohar S, Kador PF, Salvi R. Multifunctional redox modulator prevents blast-induced loss of cochlear and vestibular hair cells and auditory spiral ganglion neurons. Sci Rep. 2024;14:15296. https://doi.org/10.1038/s41598-024-66406-1.
24. Jin X, Ding D, Luo S. Scanning electron microscopic observation of vestibular end-organs in guinea pigs. Acta Univ Med Secondae Shanghai. 1986;6:287–89.
25. Xu F, Yan L, Sun Y, Jin X, Ding D. An electron microscopic scanning examination of vestibular end-organs of guinea pigs. Shanghai Med J. 1986;9:405–6.
26. Ding D, Jiang S. Chapter 4: Inner ear anatomy and structure. In: Ding D, editor. Manual of anatomical examination of the inner ear of the guinea pig. Shanghai: Xuelin Publishing House; 1989. pp. 24–35.
27. Ding D, Li M, Jiang C, Salvi R. Chapter 3: Anatomy of temporal bone and inner ear. In: Ding D, editor. Morphology of the inner ear. Harbin: Heilongjiang Science and Technology Press; 2001. pp. 10–17.
28. Ding D, Li M, Jiang C, Salvi R. Chapter 7: Preparation technology of inner ear specimens for electron microscopy. In: Ding D, editor. Morphology of the inner ear. Harbin: Heilongjiang Science and Technology Press; 2001. pp. 55–85.
29. Ding D, Jiang S. Chapter 9: Staining techniques of the inner ear specimen. In: Ding D, editor. Manual of anatomical examination of the inner ear of the guinea pig. Shanghai: Xuelin Publishing House; 1989. pp. 75–99.
30. Ding D, Jiang H, Fu Y, et al. Ototoxic effects of carboplatin in organotypic cultures in chinchillas and rats. J Otol. 2012;7:92–101. https://doi.org/10.1016/S1672-2930(12)50023-1.
31. Yu D, Ding D, Yin S, Salvi R. Ototoxic effects of streptomycin in vestibular organotypic cultures. Chin J Otorhinolaryngol Head Neck Surg. 2009;44:207–9.

4 Organotypic Culture of the Vestibular End-Organs

The organotypic culture technique has emerged as a valuable in vitro model for investigating cellular mechanisms in the vestibular system. This approach offers significant advantages for studying both the sensory epithelium and peripheral ganglion neurons of vestibular end-organs under controlled culture conditions. Over the past two decades, a series of studies have demonstrated the effectiveness and practicality of this technique, establishing it as an important research tool in vestibular neuroscience. Therefore, there has been a growing interest in using the organotypic culture techniques to study the sensory epithelium and peripheral ganglion neurons of the vestibular end-organs in culture conditions [1–11].

4.1 Procedures for Vestibular Organotypic Cultures

4.1.1 Preparation of Culture Medium

The preparation of serum-free culture medium for vestibular organotypic cultures involved combining the components in the following proportions: 190.8 mL of 1× Basal Medium Eagle (Sigma B-1522) served as the base solution, supplemented with 2 g Bovine Serum Albumin (Sigma A-4919), 2 mL serum-free supplement (Sigma I-1884), 4.8 mL 20% glucose (Sigma G-2020), 0.4 mL Penicillin G (Sigma P-3414), and 2 mL of 200 mM L-glutamine (Sigma G-7029) to create an optimized medium for culturing the explants of the inner ear under controlled in vitro conditions [1, 2, 5, 12–14].

4.1.2 Preparation of Rat Tail Collagen Gel

Prior to vestibular explant dissection, a collagen substrate was prepared by combining Type I rat tail collagen (Collaborative Biomedical Products, Cat#40236), 10× Basal Medium Eagle (Life Technologies, Cat#41100-017), and 2% sodium carbonate (Sigma, Cat#S-2127) in a 9:1:1 ratio. A 10 μL aliquot of this collagen mixture was placed at the center of a culture dish with a diameter of 35 mm and allowed to polymerize for approximately 15 min to form a gel matrix. Subsequently, 1.4 mL of pre-made serum-free medium was carefully added to the dish, ensuring the liquid level reached equilibrium with the upper surface of the collagen gel to maintain optimal culture conditions for the subsequent explant placement [1, 2, 5, 12–14].

4.1.3 Culture Procedure of Vestibular Explants

The dissection procedure began by immersing the temporal bone in Hank's balanced salt solution. Under a dissecting microscope with sterile conditions, each vestibular end-organ was carefully micro-dissected out from the vestibular cistern (Figs. 1.4B, 1.8, 1.15, 1.17, 1.19, 1.23, 3.2, 3.3, 3.8, and 3.14; Fig. 4.1). The otolithic membrane covering the maculae of saccule and utricle was meticulously removed using ultra-fine forceps to fully expose the surface of sensory hair cells on maculae of saccule and utricle (Figs. 3.3 and 3.8; Fig. 4.2A–D). Simultaneously, the membranous ampulla was torn with forceps to expose the ampullary crista (Fig. 3.14; Fig. 4.2E). In some cases, the macula of the utricle and the superior/lateral ampullary cristae can be dissected out en bloc with their associated superior vestibular ganglions and the nerve tracts. This can maintain the interconnection between the sensory hair cells of the vestibular system and their nerves, which is helpful for evaluating the mutual influence between sensory hair cells and their innervated nerves under experimental culture conditions (Fig. 1.23; Fig. 4.3). The isolated end-organs were then transferred onto the pre-formed collagen gel matrix and allowed to adhere for 60 min in a 37°C, 5% CO_2 incubator. Following adhesion, 600 μL of serum-free culture medium was gently added to completely submerge the specimens. After overnight incubation, experimental treatments (including ototoxic compounds, neurotoxic agents, or heavy metals) were administered

D. Ding et al., *Histopathological Atlas of the Inner Ear*,
https://doi.org/10.1007/978-981-95-6338-8_4

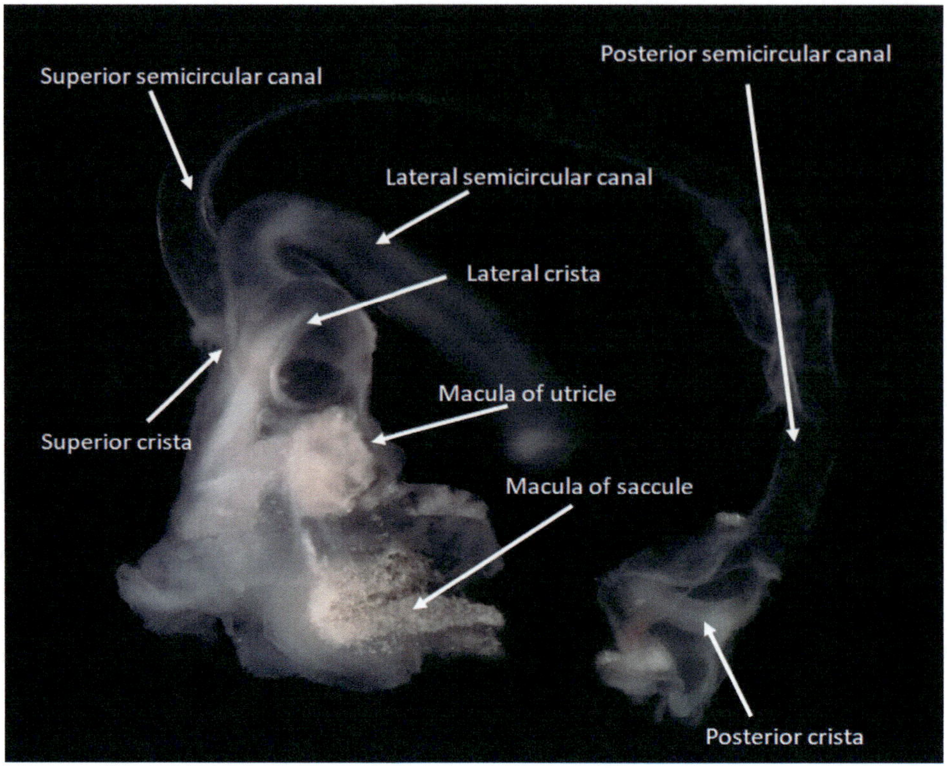

Fig. 4.1 Microdissection of the entire vestibular labyrinth

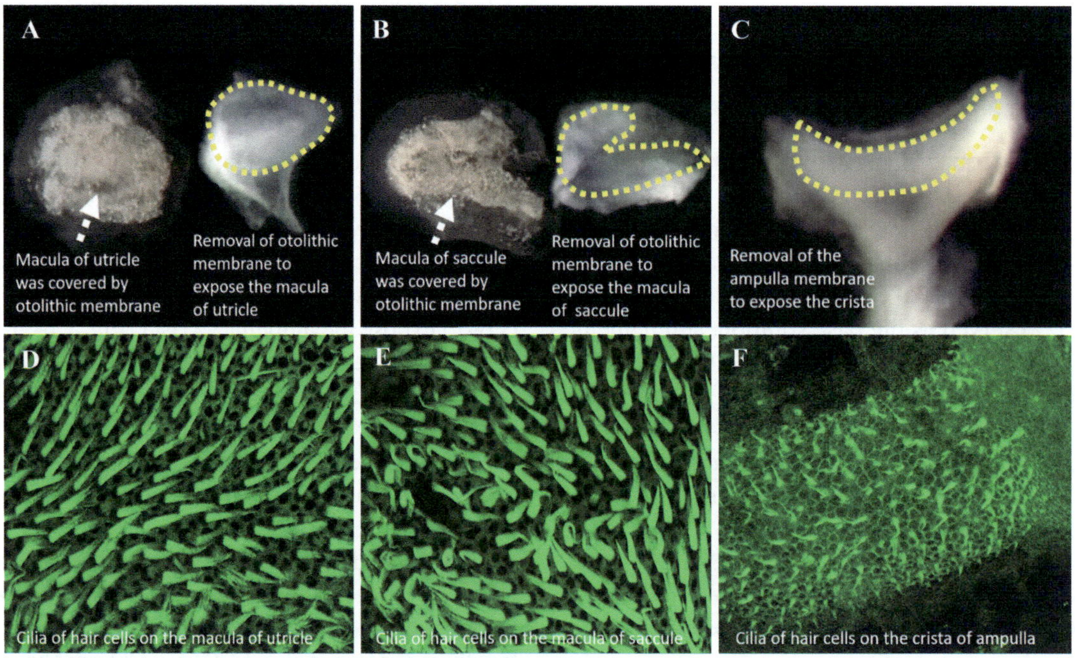

Fig. 4.2 Sample preparation steps for vestibular sensory organs. (**A**) The macula of the utricle with its overlying otolithic membrane is first exposed under microscopic visualization, followed by removal of the otolithic membrane to reveal the complete sensory epithelium, where the yellow dashed line demarcates the hair cell region in the macula of the utricle. (**B**) Similarly, the macula of the saccule is exposed, and its overlying otolithic membrane is removed, with the hair cell region outlined by yellow curves. (**C**) The membranous ampulla was torn open to expose the ampullary crista, with the hair cell region indicated by yellow dashed lines. (**D**) The ciliary bundles of the hair cells on the macula of the utricle were stained with phalloidin. (**E**) Surface preparation of the macula of the saccule with phalloidin-staining shows the ciliary bundles of the sensory hair cells. (**F**) The ciliary bundles of the hair cells on the ampullary crista were stained with phalloidin. (Reproduced with permission from Yu et al. [8])

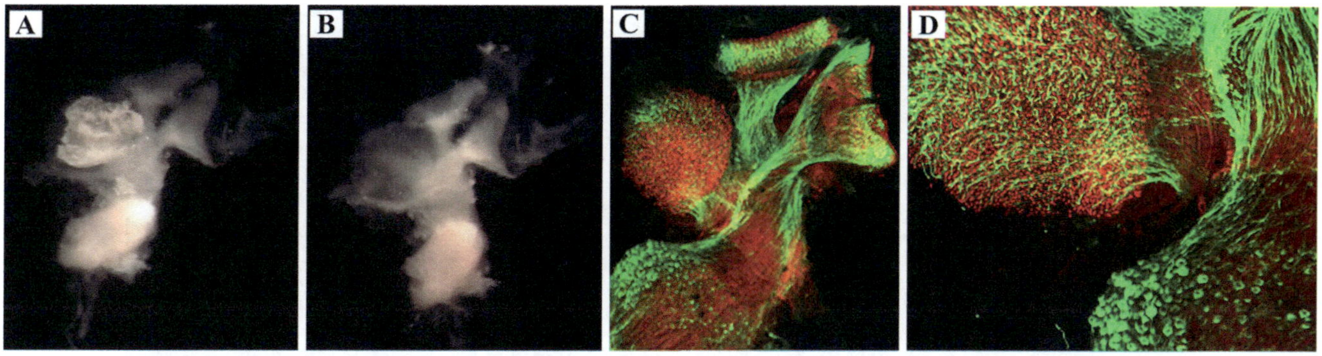

Fig. 4.3 Sample preparation for the entire macula of the utricle and the lateral and superior ampullary cristae along with the superior vestibular nerve bundles. (**A**) The entire superior vestibular nervous system, consisting of the macula of utricle, lateral/superior ampullary cristae, and superior vestibular nerve bundles, was carefully micro-dissected out from the vestibular cistern. (**B**) Microscopic removal of the otolithic membrane to expose the underlying utricular sensory epithelium. (**C**) The vestibular ganglion neurons and their nerve fibers were stained in green with anti-Tubulin antibody, and ciliary bundles of hair cells were stained in red with phalloidin. (**D**) High-power magnification shows the ciliary bundle of hair cells in red and the nerve fibers and terminals distributed at the base of the hair cells in green. (Reproduced with permission from Jiang et al. [10])

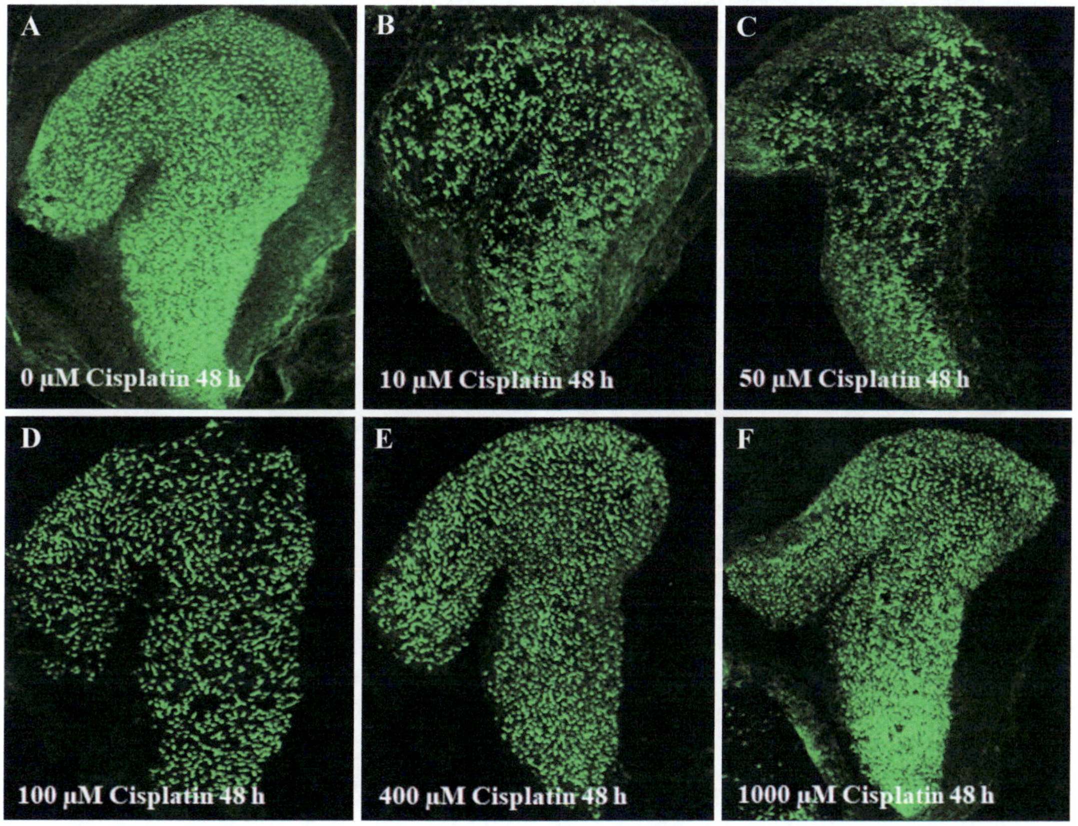

Fig. 4.4 Sample preparation of the macula of the saccule in the rat vestibular organotypic culture system and the nonlinear damage pattern caused by cisplatin. (**A**) The explant of the macula of the saccule presents normal morphology 48 h after culturing in serum-free medium without cisplatin. (**B**) 48 h after culturing in serum-free medium containing 10 μM cisplatin, the hair cells on the macula of the saccule were obviously damaged. (**C**) 48 h after culturing in serum-free medium containing 50 μM cisplatin, most hair cells on the macula of the saccule were severely destroyed. (**D**) 48 h after culturing in serum-free medium containing 100 μM cisplatin, the number of surviving hair cells in the sacculus began to increase. (**E**) 48 h after culturing in serum-free medium containing 400 μM cisplatin, the hair cells on the macula of the saccule were largely undamaged. (**F**). 48 h after culturing in serum-free medium containing 1000 μM cisplatin, the hair cells on the macula of the saccule were intact. This non-linear drug dose response supports the hypothesis that low concentrations of cisplatin can easily enter the hair cells via copper transporter channels to exert its cytotoxic effects, while high concentrations of cisplatin may cause active block of copper transporter channels, thereby preventing cellular uptake and enabling self-protection. (Reproduced with permission from Ding et al. [9])

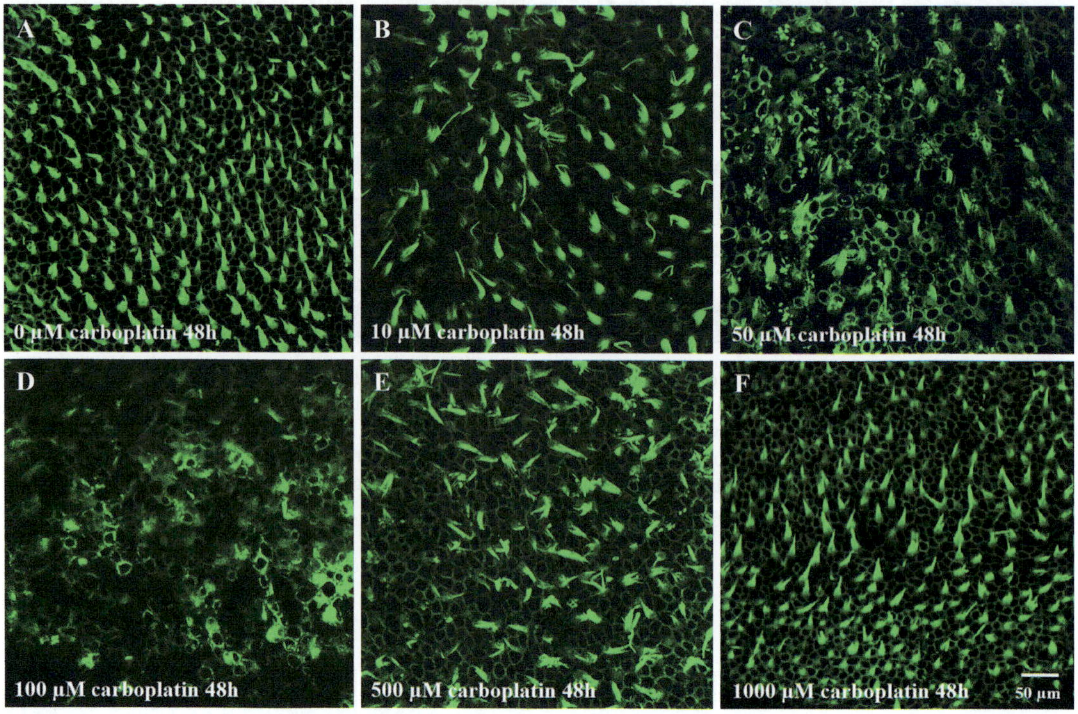

Fig. 4.5 Sample preparation of the macula of utricle in the rat vestibular organotypic culture system and the nonlinear damage pattern caused by carboplatin. (**A**) The hair cells on the macula of the utricle present intact ciliary bundles 48 h after culturing in serum-free medium without carboplatin. (**B**) 48 h after culturing with 10 μM carboplatin, the intact ciliary bundles of the hair cells started to be reduced. (**C**) 48 h after 50 μM carboplatin treatment, a large number of hair cells were damaged with cilia missing. (**D**) 48 h after culturing with 100 μM carboplatin, most hair cells were completely destroyed. (**E**) Surprisingly, 48 h after culturing with 500 μM carboplatin, it was found that many hair cells were not damaged. (**F**) 48 h after 1000 μM carboplatin treatment, most hair cells on the macula of the utricle were intact. This may suggest that a similar copper transport channel closure mechanism may block the entry of platinum drugs into cells, thereby achieving cellular self-protection. (Reproduced with permission from Ding et al. [7])

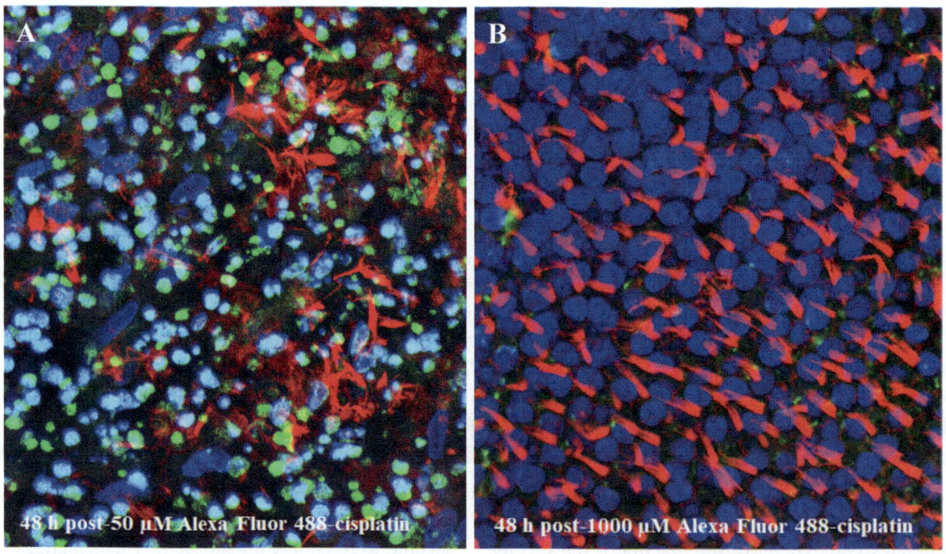

Fig. 4.6 Differential cellular uptake and cytotoxic effects of Alexa Fluor 488-conjugated cisplatin in hair cells on the macula of the utricle. (**A**) Following 48-h exposure to 50 μM Alexa Fluor 488 conjugated cisplatin, intense intracellular fluorescence accumulation correlates with morphological evidence of apoptosis (nuclear condensation/fragmentation) were detected, confirming active drug uptake and subsequent cytotoxicity. (**B**) In contrast, 1000 μM Alexa Fluor 488 conjugated cisplatin treatment for 48 h results in minimal fluorescent signal within hair cells and preserved cellular integrity, providing direct visual evidence that supraphysiological cisplatin concentrations inhibit cellular uptake. This may suggest that high concentrations of cisplatin indeed have difficulty crossing copper transport channels into hair cells. (Reproduced with permission from Ding et al. [9])

according to the study protocol. Following the designated treatment period (typically several days), cultures were terminated by replacing the medium with appropriate fixative solutions. Subsequent histological processing involved various staining protocols tailored to visualize specific cellular components and structures within the vestibular tissues (Figs. 1.23, 1.24, 2.14, 2.15, 3.4, 3.5, 3.9, 3.10, 3.20; Figs. 4.2–4.6).

References

1. Zheng JL, Gao WQ. Overexpression of Math1 induces robust production of extra hair cells in postnatal rat inner ears. Nat Neurosci. 2000;3:580–6. https://doi.org/10.1038/75753.
2. Ding D, Stracher A, Salvi RJ. Leupeptin protects cochlear and vestibular hair cells from gentamicin ototoxicity. Hear Res. 2002;164:115–26. https://doi.org/10.1016/s0378-5955(01)00417-8.
3. Ding D, Seigel GM, Salvi RJ. Migration of R28 retinal precursor cells into cochlear and vestibular organs. J Otol. 2006;1:51–56. https://doi.org/10.1016/S1672-2930(06)50009-1.
4. Yu D, Ding D, Yin S, Salvi R. Ototoxic effects of streptomycin in vestibular organotypic cultures. Chin J Otorhinolaryngol Head Neck Surg. 2009;44:207–9. https://doi.org/10.3760/cma.j.issn.1673-0860.2009.01.014.
5. Ding D, Qi W, Qu Y, Salvi R. Chapter 5: In vitro organotypic culture techniques of the inner ear. In: Ding D, editor. Science of the inner ear. Beijing, China: China Science and Technology Press; 2010. p. 39–49.
6. Yu D, Ding D, Jiang H, Stolzberg D, Salvi R. Mefloquine damage vestibular hair cells in organotypic cultures. Neurotox Res. 2011;20:51–58. https://doi.org/10.1007/s12640-010-9221-z.
7. Ding D, Jiang H, Fu Y, et al. Ototoxic effects of carboplatin in organotypic cultures in chinchillas and rats. J Otol. 2012;7:92–101. https://doi.org/10.1016/S1672-2930(12)50023-1.
8. Yu J, Ding D, Li P, et al. Technical details of sample preparation for inner ear organotypic cultures. Chin J Otol. 2015;13:64–70. https://doi.org/10.3969/j.issn.1672-2922.2015.01.011.
9. Ding D, Jiang H, Zhang J, et al. Cisplatin-induced vestibular hair cell lesion-less damage at high doses. J Otol. 2018;13:115–21. https://doi.org/10.1016/j.joto.2018.08.002.
10. Jiang H, Ding D, Zhang J, Salvi R. Development of vestibular organ cultures of utricle, saccule and crista ampullaris in which hair cells are attached to the superior and inferior vestibular ganglia [abstract]. Abstr Assoc Res Otolaryngol. 2018;41:272.
11. Ye H, Xing Y, Zhang L, et al. Bilirubin-induced neurotoxic and ototoxic effects in rat cochlear and vestibular organotypic cultures. Neurotoxicology. 2019;71:75–86. https://doi.org/10.1016/j.neuro.2018.12.004.
12. Ding D, Li M, Jiang C, Salvi R. Chapter 10: Explant culture techniques of the inner ear. In: Ding D, editor. Morphology of the inner ear. Haerbin, China: Heilongjiang Science and Technology Press; 2001. p. 139–42.
13. Ding D, Qi W, Yu D, Jiang H, Salvi R. Ototoxic effects of mefloquine in cochlear organotypic cultures. J Otol. 2009;4:76–85. https://doi.org/10.1016/S1672-2930(09)50018-9.
14. Ding D, Roth J, Salvi R. Manganese is toxic to spiral ganglion neurons and hair cells in vitro. Neurotoxicology. 2011;32:233–41. https://doi.org/10.1016/j.neuro.2010.12.003.

5 Quantitative Observations of the Vestibular Sensory Epithelium and Vestibular Nerve Fibers and Ganglion Neurons

The application of vestibular sectioning combined with surface preparation techniques provides an effective approach for localizing and qualitatively evaluating the extent and severity of lesions within the vestibular sensory epithelium. However, when precise quantitative assessment of vestibular hair cell damage is necessary for experimental purposes, we recommend incorporating specialized quantitative observation methodologies specifically designed for vestibular end-organ analysis to ensure accurate and reliable data collection. This comprehensive approach enables precise qualitative and quantitative assessment of pathological changes in the vestibular neuroepithelium [1–9].

Quantification of vestibular peripheral nerve fibers, vestibular ganglia, and vestibular central nerve fibers in the vestibular neuroforamen and cochlear neuroforamen provides crucial insights into the integrity of the vestibular nervous pathway, as these two specialized channels serve as important conduits connecting the vestibular sensory hair cells with the central vestibular nucleus in the brain stem. Sagittal sections of the vestibular neuroforamen and cochlear neuroforamen are ideal for quantitatively observing pathological changes in the vestibular nervous system [8, 9].

5.1 Quantitative Observation of Sensory Hair Cells from Vestibular Slices

Under the assumption of a 5 μm slice thickness, approximately 200 consecutive sections perpendicular to the maculae of the saccule and utricle, and about 100 sections perpendicular to an ampullary crista can be obtained from mouse vestibular tissue. Histological analysis reveals that a single cross-section perpendicular to the largest diameter of either the macula of saccule or utricle typically contains around 80 detectable hair cells (Fig. 5.1), while a section through the midpoint of an ampullary crista generally yields approximately 25 hair cells (Fig. 5.2). Although it is theoretically possible to sum hair cell counts across serial sections to estimate total number of hair cells in each vestibular end-organ, this approach is significantly limited by practical challenges including frequent section loss, inconsistent midsection cuts, and/or potential errors from repeated cell counting. These methodological constraints, combined with the labor-intensive nature of the technique, explain why quantitative analysis of vestibular hair cells through serial sectioning has seen limited application in practice [10], despite its conceptual validity for complete hair cell population assessment in vestibular sensory epithelia.

5.1.1 Questioning the Quantitative Conversion Formula of Sensory Hair Cells in Vestibular Sections

Abercrombie first established a conversion formula for double-counting correction based on the original hair cell count results on the slice in 1946. This conversion formula is $Hi = hi \times t/(t + d)$. In this formula, Hi refers to the correction value of hair cells, hi refers to the actual count of hair cell density, t refers to the thickness of the slice, and d refers to the diameter of the nucleus. From this formula, the corrected density of vestibular hair cells is equal to the density of the hair cell count times the thickness of the slice divided by the sum of the thickness of the slice and the diameter of the nucleus [11]. While this mathematical correction theoretically accounts for the overestimation arising from nuclei appearing in consecutive sections, its practical application to vestibular hair cell quantification warrants careful consideration. The fundamental premise of applying this correction to already obtained density measurements raises questions about its necessity, as the formula essentially adjusts empirical data through a theoretical model that may not fully capture the complex three-dimensional distribution of hair cells in vestibular epithelia. Since the density of the actual viable hair cells has been obtained from the slice before being substituted into the formula, why

D. Ding et al., *Histopathological Atlas of the Inner Ear*,
https://doi.org/10.1007/978-981-95-6338-8_5

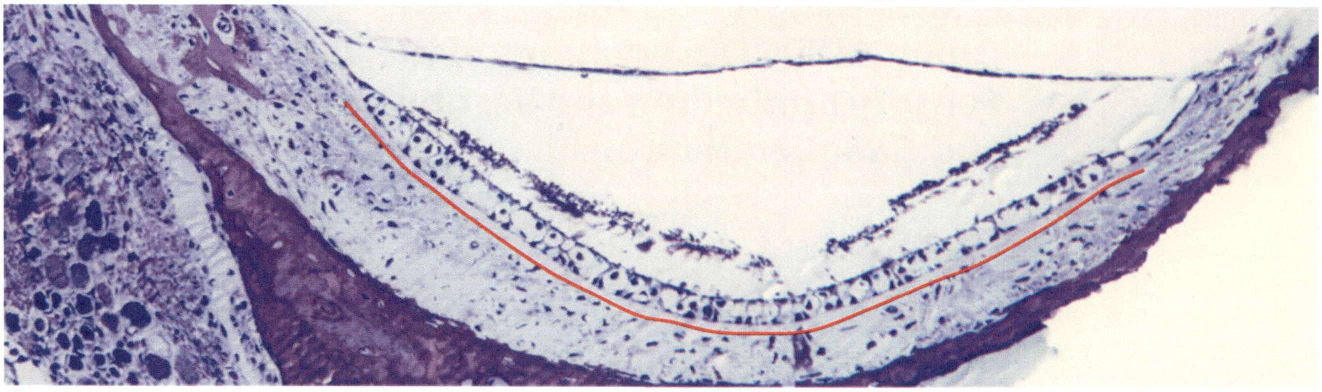

Fig. 5.1 The slice perpendicular to the macula of the saccule shows the cross-section of the sensory hair cells. This image demonstrates the characteristic histological organization of the neuroepithelium, allowing for estimation of hair cell density by correlating the number of visible hair cell profiles with the measured linear length of the macula in this sectional plane. Therefore, this morphological presentation provides both a qualitative assessment of the sensory epithelium structure and a basis for quantitative evaluation of hair cell density along the macula

even plug the actual density into the formula to multiply by the slice thickness and divide it by the slice thickness plus the diameter of the nucleus? Does the corrected hair cell density provide more accurate information than the actual vestibular hair cell density? This seems to be debatable. It has also been suggested to count hair cells every 50 μm in serial sections of each vestibular end-organ, adding the results and multiplying by 25 to obtain the total number of hair cells in each vestibular end-organ. Can this conversion method of recording one slice per 10 slices and multiplying by 25 really reflect the actual total number of hair cells on each vestibular end-organ? Such formulas proposing extrapolation from sparse sampling present significant methodological concerns regarding their ability to accurately represent total hair cell populations, as such approaches rely heavily on assumptions of uniform distribution while potentially missing regional variations in cellular density. Therefore, this formula conversion method, which lacks actual counting, is also questionable. Above quantification strategies, while mathematically elegant, may introduce systematic errors that could compromise the validity of the resulting estimates, particularly in vestibular organs where hair cell distribution patterns may exhibit significant topographical variations. The scientific community continues to debate the relative merits of these correction methods compared to direct counting approaches, with particular attention to their respective abilities to preserve the biological reality of hair cell distribution patterns in complex three-dimensional sensory epithelia.

5.1.2 A Proposal for Direct Hair Cell Counting Per Unit Length in Vestibular Slices

We advocate a more biologically grounded approach for quantifying vestibular hair cells that begins with precise measurement of the actual length unit occupied by the sensory epithelium in a section of the vestibular end-organs first, followed by direct counting of hair cells within the defined unit length (Fig. 2.1A; Fig. 5.1). This method involves systematically sampling hair cell counts from representative sections throughout the vestibular end-organ, converting these counts into linear density values (cells per unit length), and using the mean of these empirically derived densities as the most reliable estimate of the organ's overall hair cell density. While this direct measurement approach likely provides a more accurate representation of true hair cell distribution than formula-based corrections, it nevertheless carries inherent limitations since it relies on sampling rather than complete enumeration of all hair cells. The selective nature of this counting method, combined with potential sectioning artifacts and regional variations in cell density, means that even this improved technique can only provide an approximate assessment of vestibular hair cell density rather than an exact quantification. Consequently, while our proposed method offers practical advantages over purely computational corrections by maintaining closer ties to biological reality, researchers should recognize that all current histological approaches for hair cell quantification from temporal bone sections ultimately yield estimations rather than absolute counts, with each method presenting unique trade-offs between practicality and precision in assessing the complex three-dimensional architecture of vestibular sensory epithelia.

5.1.3 A Proposal for Quantitatively Assessing Hair Cell Structure and Function

While quantitative assessment of surviving vestibular hair cells serves as a reliable indicator of cellular loss in experimental studies due to their non-regenerative nature, this approach presents considerable limitations when evaluating cases of selective ciliary damage in otherwise viable hair cells. Conventional

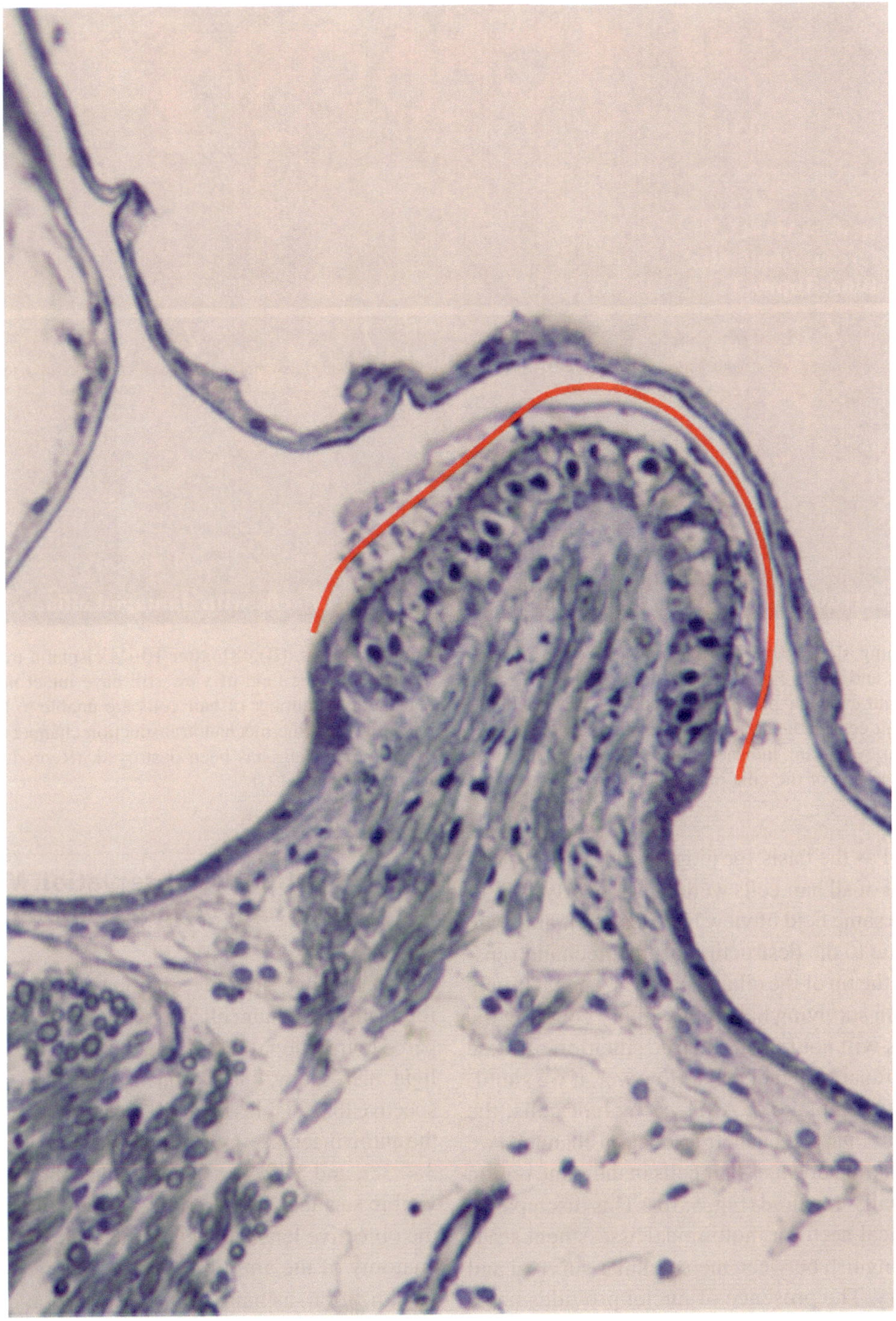

Fig. 5.2 Photomicrograph of the cross-section of the mouse ampullary crista demonstrates the section plane oriented perpendicular to the long axis of the sensory crest. The image reveals the characteristic cytoarchitecture of the neuroepithelium on the ampullary crista, demonstrating both type I and type II hair cells within their typical morphological context. By quantifying the number of observable hair cell profiles relative to the measured linear extent of the crista in this sectional plane, the micrograph provides a foundation for estimating regional hair cell density while simultaneously illustrating the histopathological changes of the vestibular hair cells

counting methods, which typically rely on nuclear staining to identify surviving cells, fail to capture the functional impairment of hair cells that retain their cell bodies but have lost their ciliary bundles. This methodological shortcoming prompted us to try to develop an assessment method that combines structural and functional markers. As demonstrated in Fig. 5.3, the choice of pathological markers dramatically influences diagnostic outcomes. In Fig. 5.3B, if the absence of hair cell nuclei were used as the basis for judging lesions, there were obviously no hair cells missing in this field of view. However, if the uptake

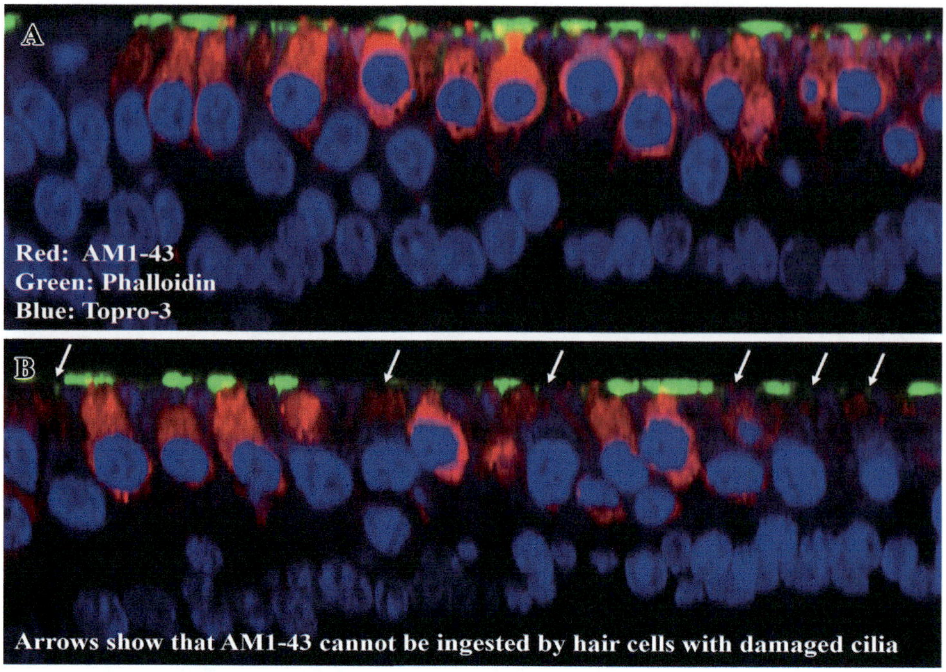

Fig. 5.3 Triple staining shows AM1-43 dye uptake (red), ToPro-3-stained nuclei (blue), and Alexa Fluor 488-phalloidin labeled F-actin (green, ciliary tufts and cuticular plate) in hair cells of the macula of the utricle. (**A**) The hair cells in the normal macula of the utricle take up AM1-43 dye into their cytoplasm, indicating that the mechanical transduction channels at the tips of the cilia of these normal hair cells are fully functional. (**B**) 48 h after 10 μM cisplatin treatment, although the hair cells in this field of view still have intact nuclear morphology, a considerable number of hair cells are unable to take up AM1-43 dye, indicating that the mechanotransduction channel at the tips of the cilia of these hair cells has been destroyed. (Reproduced with permission from Ding et al. [12])

of AM1-43 is used as the basis for judging hair cell lesions, although the nuclei of all hair cells were intact, nearly 40% of the hair cells in the same field of view have lost their ability to absorb AM1-43 due to the destruction of the mechanotransduction channel at the tip of the cilia. It can be seen that if only cilia are damaged in surviving hair cells, simply counting the nuclei of hair cells will not reflect the true situation of these damaged and non-functional hair cells. However, if we simultaneously observe the uptake of AM1-43 by hair cells, the sensitive indicator of intact mechanotransduction channels, we may find that approximately 40% hair cells in the same region have been functionally impaired (Fig. 5.3B). This discrepancy highlights the critical need for multimodal assessment strategies that can distinguish between mere cellular survival and functional integrity. The presence of nuclei provides basic information about cell viability, whereas functional markers like AM1-43 uptake offer a more comprehensive evaluation by assessing both cellular survival and sensory transduction capability [12]. Consequently, incorporating functional assessment tools such as AM1-43 labeling significantly enhances pathological evaluation by correlating morphological observations with physiological dysfunction, thereby providing a more accurate representation of the vestibular end-organ's functional status that transcends simple cellular counts and better reflects the complex spectrum of hair cell pathology.

5.2 Quantitative Observation Methods for Vestibular Surface Preparations

The surface preparation technique offers superior visualization for quantitative hair cell analysis in vestibular end-organs compared to traditional sectioning methods. When examined under light microscopy, this approach provides an optimal en face perspective that enables clear observation of every hair cell across the entire maculae of saccule and utricle [7–9, 13] (Figs. 1.18A, 3.4, 3.5, and 3.12A), as well as those hair cells located on the visible surface of the saddle-shaped ampullary crista facing the objective lens. However, the complex three-dimensional anatomy of the ampullary crista inherently limits complete visualization, as hair cells positioned on the lateral and posterior aspects parallel to the viewing plane remain obscured [7] (Figs. 1.23, 1.24, 3.17E, 3.18, and 3.19). While the surface preparation method permits a comprehensive assessment of all macular hair cells, this limitation means complete enumeration of crista hair cells remains technically challenging. Although some researchers have proposed flattening the sensory epithelium through microdissection to create a complete surface preparation [14], this approach presents significant technical difficulties in practice, particularly regarding tissue integrity preservation and reliable quantification of the entire hair cell population. The inherent trade-offs between visualization completeness and methodological feasibility must therefore be carefully considered when selecting analytical approaches for different vestibular end-organs.

5.2.1 Questioning the Formula for Converting the Surface Area of Maculae of Saccule and Utricle by Weighing Experimental Animals

Crile's 1940 power function formula (A = aBWb) established a theoretical relationship between vestibular sensory epithelium dimensions (surface area and hair cell number) and experimental animal body weight [15]. This mathematical model proposes that the morphological parameters of each vestibular end-organ can be derived by multiplying two experimentally determined coefficients (a and b) by the animal's body weight. For subjects under 4 kg, the saccular and utricular maculae exhibit coefficients of $a = 0.045 \pm 0.01$ and $b = 0.45 \pm 0.03$ for both surface area and hair cell number calculations, while the ampullary crista yields distinct parameters of $a = 0.025 \pm 0.013$ and $b = 0.44 \pm 0.07$. In larger specimens exceeding 4 kg body weight, the power-law relationships maintain similar but slightly differentiated scaling exponents, with the saccular macula showing a slope of 0.45 and the utricular macula 0.44 when plotted against body weight [15]. These empirically derived coefficients represent early attempts to establish allometric relationships between vestibular morphology and overall body size across different mammalian species. While Crile's formula offers a seemingly convenient method for estimating vestibular morphology through simple body weight measurements, critical examination reveals significant biological implausibility in its fundamental assumptions. Consider the developmental trajectory of a guinea pig: its body weight increases approximately eightfold (from 100 to 800 g) between 1 and 12 months of age, yet application of the formula's constant coefficients would paradoxically suggest a proportional expansion of vestibular hair cell numbers—a physiological impossibility given that mammalian inner ear hair cells complete their differentiation prenatally and exhibit no postnatal proliferation capacity. This contradiction highlights the formula's failure to account for basic principles of vestibular neurobiology, particularly the static nature of hair cell populations after birth, which can only decrease through pathological processes rather than increase with somatic growth. Furthermore, the model's inherent logic breaks down when considering pathological scenarios: ototoxic damage causing permanent hair cell loss produces no corresponding change in body weight, demonstrating the absence of any causative relationship between these parameters. Although some contemporary studies continue to employ this weight-based estimation method [14, 16], we maintain that such approaches have negligible scientific validity for quantitative vestibular pathology assessment, as they disregard established biological realities in favor of mathematical convenience. Direct morphometric analysis rather than allometric extrapolation remains essential for accurate evaluation of vestibular end-organ structure and pathology.

5.2.2 Area Measurement of Vestibular Sensory Epithelial Regions

Accurate measurement of hair cell density in vestibular end-organs requires precise determination of each sensory epithelium's total surface area. As previously discussed, the planar morphology of the saccular and utricular maculae allows for complete surface preparation, enabling direct microscopic measurement of their entire epithelial area [7]. In contrast, the complex saddle-shaped geometry of the ampullary crista presents significant technical challenges to complete flattening and area measurement. Consequently, the following methodological description will focus specifically on techniques for area measurement of the saccular and utricular maculae, as these structures' anatomical characteristics permit reliable and comprehensive surface area quantification when properly prepared. This distinction in methodological approach reflects the fundamental morphological differences between the relatively two-dimensional macular structures and the three-dimensionally complex crista ampullaris, which currently lacks a standardized technique for complete surface area measurement [7].

We employed ImageJ software image measurement capabilities to conduct precise morphometric analyses of saccular and utricular maculae across multiple species, including mice, nude mice, rats, guinea pigs, chinchillas, sheep, and monkeys. To illustrate our standardized measurement protocol, we present the methodology using a guinea pig saccular macula surface preparation as an example. Initial calibration was performed by capturing a reference image of a 1 mm micrometer scale under identical optical conditions (Fig. 5.4A). Using the line tool, we traced the micrometer's 1 mm demarcation, obtaining a pixel length reading of 1012.03. This calibration data was then input into the software by entering "1" in the known distance field, specifying millimeters as the unit of measurement, and applying these parameters globally to ensure consistent scaling for all subsequent measurements (Fig. 5.4B). This rigorous calibration process establishes traceable measurement standards that maintain dimensional accuracy across all specimens and experimental conditions.

Following calibration, the macula's boundaries were precisely delineated using ImageJ's freehand selection tool to trace along the transitional zone between hair cells and supporting cells on the saccular macula surface preparation (Fig. 5.4C). The area measurement was then obtained by executing the measurement command (Ctrl+M), yielding an exact value of 0.55 mm^2 for this specimen (Fig. 5.4D). Our comprehensive morphometric analysis revealed

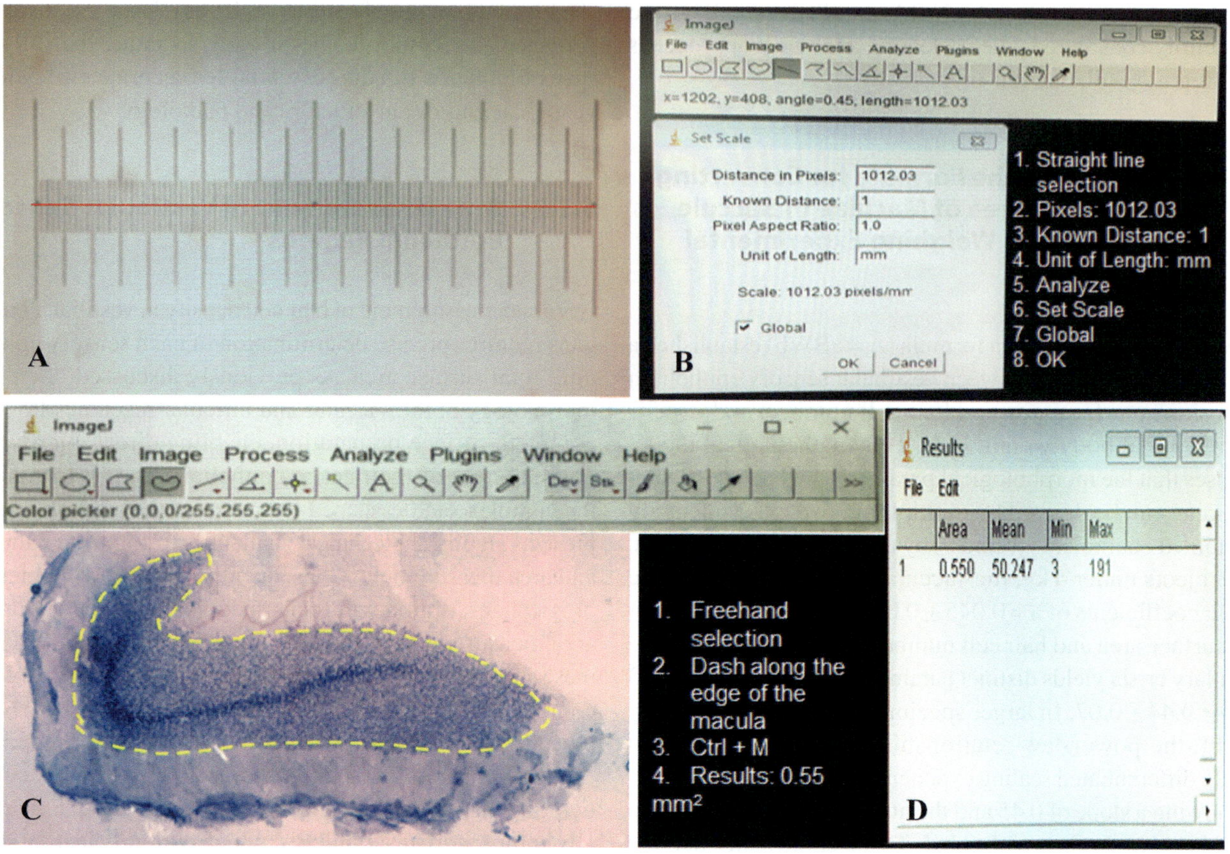

Fig. 5.4 Method for measuring the surface area of the macula of the saccule in experimental animals. Area measurement by using the ImageJ software to test the area of the macula in experimental animals. After we complete the surface preparations of the macula of the saccule and utricle, the whole picture of each macula was photographed under an optical microscope with a magnification of 100 times. (**A**) Before testing the surface preparation of the macula of the saccule, a micrometer scale with a length of 1 mm was first photographed under the same optical conditions and the same magnification. (**B**). A linear measurement tool was applied along the reference scale to obtain the pixels occupied by this length. Then fill in one in the known distance window, and fill in millimeters in the unit window, and finally select Global and click Enter to complete the setting of the measurement standard. (**C**) The manual delineation process using ImageJ's freehand selection tool to precisely trace the macular boundary along the transitional zone between the hair cell region and surrounding supporting cells, and then press the Ctrl key and the M key. (**D**). The final quantitative output, with the software automatically calculating the absolute area (0.55 mm² in this representative saccular macula specimen) following execution of the measurement command (Ctrl+M). This systematic approach ensures accurate, reproducible area measurements that account for both microscopic resolution and individual morphological variations in vestibular sensory epithelia. (Reproduced with permission from Ding et al. [7])

consistent species-specific differences in vestibular end-organ dimensions: the areas of macula of saccule in CBA/CAJ mice, nude mice, rats, guinea pigs, chinchillas, white rabbits, and monkeys were 0.193 ± 0.009, 0.216 ± 0.008, 0.323 ± 0.01, 0.528 ± 0.035, 0.687 ± 0.065, 1.237 ± 0.075, and $1.371 \pm 0.032\,mm^2$, respectively; the utricular macula areas in above animal sequence were 0.193 ± 0.02, 0.208 ± 0.013, 0.321 ± 0.011, 0.526 ± 0.034, 0.795 ± 0.017, 1.224 ± 0.082, and $1.388 \pm 0.048\,mm^2$, respectively [7] (Fig. 5.5). These measurements, obtained through standardized protocols, provide reliable reference values for comparative vestibular morphological studies across species.

5.2.3 Query Regarding the Formula for Calculating the Total Number of Hair Cells in the Maculae of Saccule and Utricle Based on the Weight of Experimental Animals

The power function formula (A = aBWb) proposed by Crile in 1940 is used to convert not only the size of the vestibular sensory epithelium, but also the total number of hair cells in each vestibular sensory epithelium area [14–16], although the accuracy and reliability of this conversion formula have been seriously questioned. Imagine if a guinea pig whose weight

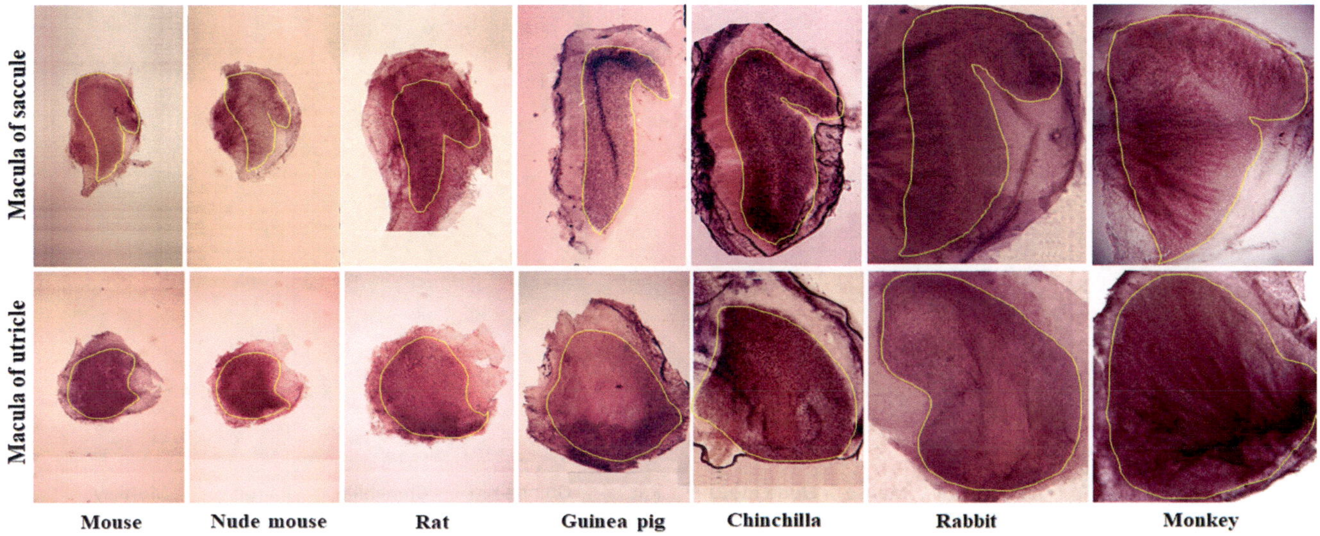

Fig. 5.5 Comparative photomicrographs of maculae of saccule and utricle from multiple commonly used experimental animal models, demonstrating the standardized morphological features and measurement methodology employed in our study. These representative images showcase interspecies variations in macular morphology while illustrating the consistent application of our area measurement protocol across different experimental models (Reproduced with permission from Ding et al. [7]). The micrographs serve both as a reference for normal macular anatomy in various species and as a visual demonstration of the measurement technique's applicability to diverse vestibular preparations, highlighting the reproducibility of our quantitative approach in comparative vestibular research

increases at least tenfold from birth to 12 months. If the coefficients a and b remain constant, but the guinea pig's weight increases tenfold, is it possible for the total number of hair cells in its vestibular sensory area to increase tenfold? Clearly, this is impossible. Assuming this weight conversion formula truly calculates the total number of hair cells in each vestibular sensory area, would the animal's weight permanently decrease if the hair cells were permanently destroyed? Of course, this is absolutely impossible. This scenario demonstrates that mathematical formulas that estimate the total number of hair cells in each vestibular sensory area based solely on the animal's weight are completely inaccurate and unreliable, and they can only bring us wrong information that has no scientific basis [7].

5.2.4 Determination of the Total Number of Hair Cells in the Maculae of Saccule and Utricle

As previously established, it is possible to count the total number of hair cells on the maculae of the saccule and utricle under a light microscope, but it is impossible to count the total number of hair cells on the ampullary cristae. Therefore, we only describe the method for hair cell counting on the maculae of the saccule and utricle as follows. Following precise measurement of macular surface areas, we conducted systematic quantification of hair cell populations in the saccular and utricular maculae across seven experimental animal species. To ensure counting accuracy, we implemented a grid-based analytical approach where each macular photomicrograph was subdivided into multiple standardized sampling squares (Fig. 5.6A). Individual hair cells within each grid unit were meticulously counted under high magnification (Fig. 5.6B), with the summation of all grid counts yielding the total hair cell population in this macula (Fig. 5.7). Our comprehensive hair cell counts revealed species-specific variations of total hair cell number in maculae of saccule and utricle: the total number of hair cells in the macula of saccule in CBA/CAJ mice, nude mice, rats, guinea pigs, chinchillas, white rabbits, and monkeys were 2476.3 ± 64.4, 2389.8 ± 47.8, 3135.3 ± 191.6, 4882.2 ± 208.7, 6128.5 ± 242.9, 10572.2 ± 464.4, and 10992.7 ± 397.4, respectively; the utricular macula counts in the same animal sequence were 2491.4 ± 54.8, 2368.0 ± 46.1, 3218.8 ± 82.9, 4925.3 ± 271.1, 7794.0 ± 386.1, 11347.4 ± 435.7, and 11114.5 ± 410.6, respectively [7]. This rigorous quantitative method provides reliable, standardized data on total vestibular hair cell counts and reveals differences in total hair cell counts in the saccular and utricular maculae between different animal species. The grid-based counting technique ensures methodological consistency while accounting for potential regional differences in hair cell density within each macular epithelium.

5.2.5 Possible Reasons for Discrepancies in Hair Cell Count Results Under the Microscope

As mentioned in the previous discussion, simply weighing the body weight of experimental animals and converting the weight using a mathematical formula to determine the total number of hair cells in the saccule and utricle without actually counting the hair cells in the vestibular sensory epithelium

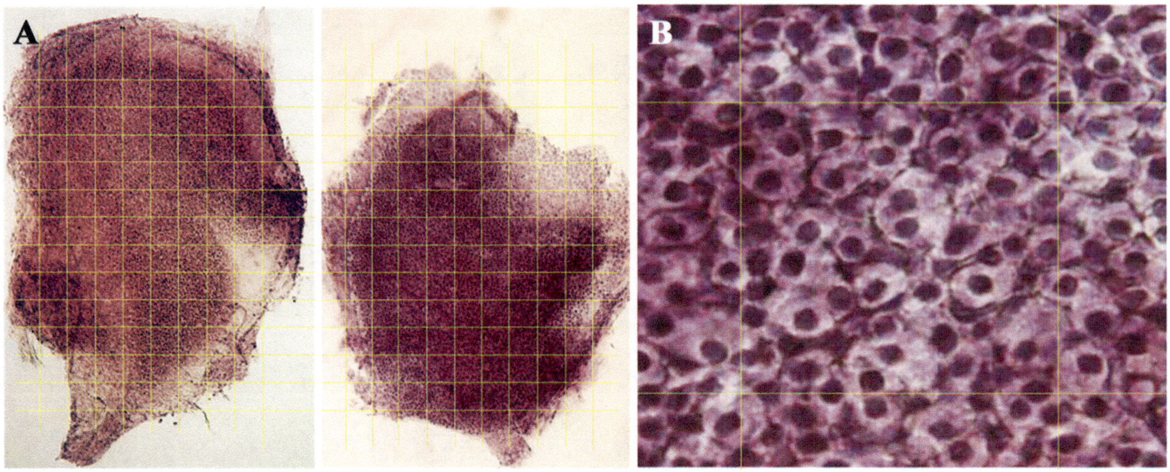

C

	Mouse	Nude mouse	Rat	Guinea pig	Chinchilla	Rabbit	Monkey
Area of macula of saccule (mm^2)	0.193±0.009	0.216±0.008	0.323±0.010	0.528±0.035	0.687±0.065	1.237±0.075	1.371±0.032
Area of macula of utricle (mm^2)	0.193±0.020	0.208±0.013	0.321±0.011	0.526±0.034	0.795±0.017	1.224±0.082	1.388±0.048
Number of hair cells in saccule	2476.3±64.4	2389.8±47.8	3135.3±191.6	4882.2±208.7	6128.5±242.9	10572.2±464.4	10992.7±397.4
Number of hair cells in utricle	2491.4±54.8	2368.0±46.1	3218.8±82.9	4925.3±271.1	7794.0±386.1	11347.4±435.7	11114.5±410.6

Fig. 5.6 Standardized quantification of the total number of hair cells in the maculae of the saccule and utricle. (**A**) The grid-based analytical approach was used to quantify the total hair cell number in the maculae of the saccule and utricle. The surface preparation of the macula of the saccule and utricle is systematically divided into smaller sampling units to facilitate methodical cell counting across the entire epithelial area. (**B**). The high-magnification view is essential for accurate identification and enumeration of individual hair cells within each grid unit, highlighting the cellular resolution required for precise quantification. (**C**). Measurement data of surface area and total hair cell counts in the maculae of saccule and utricle in various experimental animals (Reproduced with permission from Ding et al. [7]). This comprehensive visualization documents the complete workflow from tissue preparation to final quantitative analysis, emphasizing the importance of standardized protocols in obtaining reliable comparative data for vestibular sensory epithelia

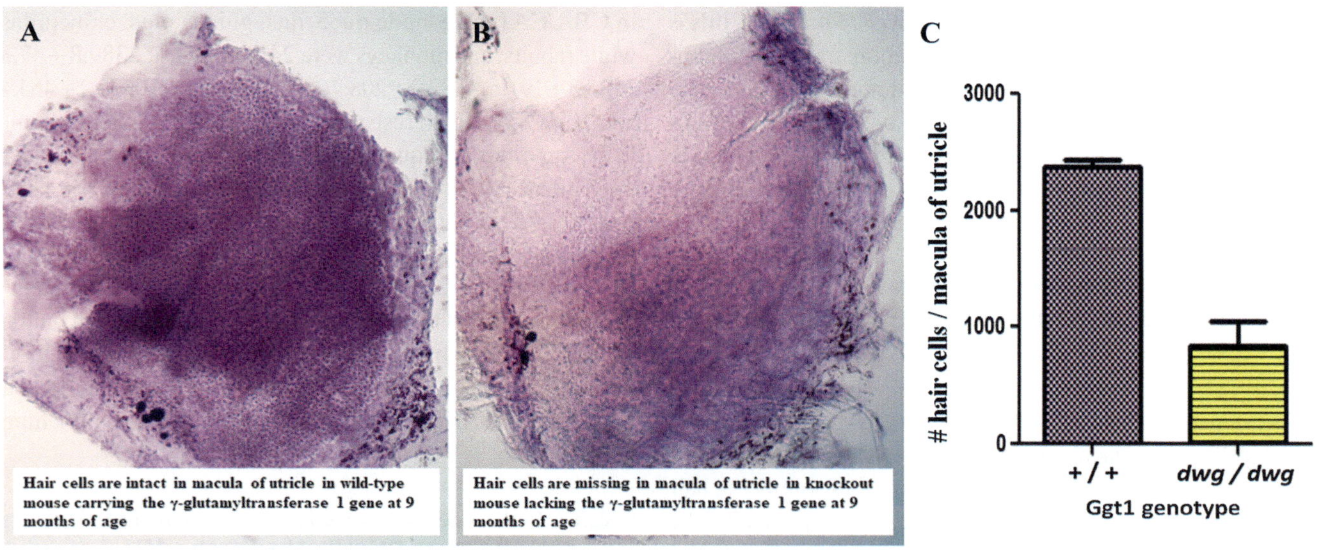

Fig. 5.7 Comparative morphological and quantitative observations of the macula of utricle in 9-month-old wild-type (+/+) and dwg/dwg mutant mice using hematoxylin-stained surface preparations. (**A**) Surface preparation of the macula of the utricle from dwg/dwg wild-type mice showed intact hair cell structure and density. (**B**). Surface preparation of the macula of the utricle in dwg/dwg-deficient mice showed a massive loss of hair cells. (**C**). Quantitative confirmation with statistical comparison demonstrates significantly reduced hair cell numbers in homozygous mutants compared to wild-type controls. These findings collectively suggest that γ-glutamyltransferase 1 plays a crucial role in maintaining vestibular hair cell viability, with its deletion potentially accelerating cellular degeneration and shortening the lifespan of vestibular sensory hair cells. The combined morphological and quantitative approach provides compelling evidence for the gene's protective function in vestibular hair cell maintenance

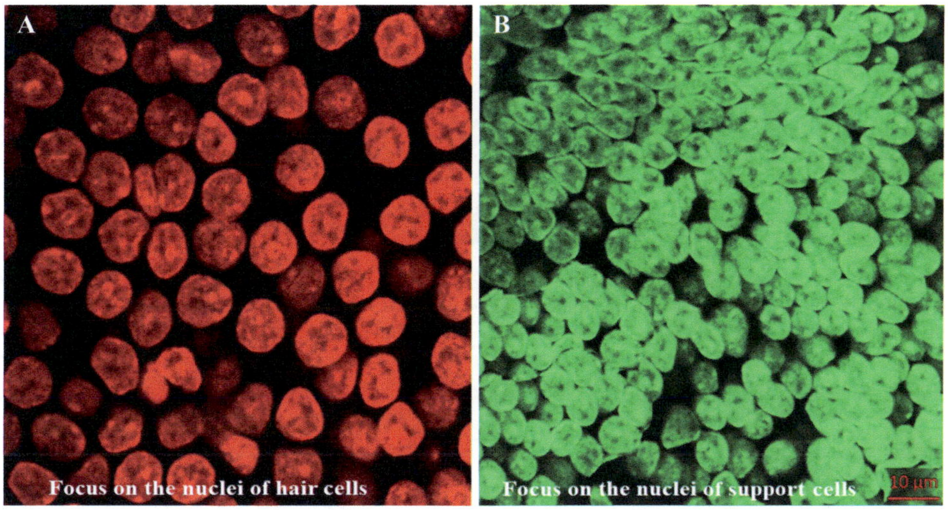

Fig. 5.8 Comparative photomicrographs of surface preparation of the macula of utricle at same field of view with identical magnification highlight critical cytological distinctions between hair cells and supporting cells under differential focusing. (**A**) The characteristic large, round nucleus of a hair cell is shown when the microscope is focused on the plane of the hair cell nucleus. (**B**). Focusing the microscope on the nuclear plane of the support cells revealed the densely packed distinctive small nuclei of the supporting cells. This direct visual comparison provides quantitative evidence that hair cell density is substantially lower than that of supporting cells within the vestibular sensory epithelium, explaining potential sources of error in historical counting methods that lacked the ability to distinguish these cellular layers (Reproduced with permission from Ding et al. [7]). The paired images exemplify how modern microscopic techniques enable precise cellular discrimination essential for accurate histomorphometric analysis of vestibular sensory epithelia

under a microscope has no scientific basis. Therefore, the data converted by a mathematical formula has no relation to the total number of hair cells in the maculae of the saccule and utricle. However, even counting cells directly under a microscope can sometimes produce significant discrepancies in the data. For example, we found that the total number of hair cells in the maculae of saccule and utricle in guinea pigs was 4882.2 ± 208.7 and 4925.3 ± 271.1, respectively [7], but the hair cell counts of the maculae of saccule and utricle in guinea pigs obtained by Lindeman in the 1960s based on phase contrast microscopy data were 7500 (6018-7983) and 9000 (7118-10760), respectively [13]. Such huge variability observed in quantitative assessments of vestibular hair cell populations prompted us to consider whether differences in sample observation methods might contribute to significant differences in hair cell count results. To understand the differences in size and density between hair cells and supporting cells, we counted the number of nuclei in the hair cell layer and the supporting cell layer, respectively, at the same region under a confocal microscope. We found that the size of the nuclei of the hair cells was much larger than that of the supporting cells, and the number of hair cells in the same area was much less than the number of supporting cells. In Fig. 5.8, we were able to identify approximately 60 hair cells at the focal length of the nuclei of hair cells and about 140 nuclei of supporting cells at the focal length of the support cells (Fig. 5.8). Therefore, the number of cells in the same area of view but at different focal lengths was not the same. In the 1960s, the surface preparation of the membranous labyrinth was routinely performed by double fixation with glutaraldehyde and osmium tetroxide without any other specific markers. The staining effect of osmium tetroxide only shows the fat droplets and myelin sheaths, while the hair cells have neither fat droplets nor nerve myelin sheaths. Therefore, the hair cells cannot be stained by osmium tetroxide at all. During that period, people had to use phase contrast microscopy to distinguish the different degrees of refraction where the cells connect to each other. In that case, as the focal length of the microscope is frequently moved up and down, the dividing refraction line between hair cells might be confused with the dividing refraction line between supporting cells, and the supporting cells may be mistakenly counted as hair cells. The high-resolution images of hair cell histochemical staining currently observed using advanced confocal microscopes are clearly more accurate and reliable than those obtained by observing unstained samples using ordinary light microscopes before the 1960s [1–9].

5.2.6 Quantification of Vestibular Hair Cells Within a Small Field of View

Comprehensive quantification of vestibular hair cell populations presents significant technical challenges that vary by end-organ type. While complete enumeration of macular hair cells is theoretically possible through meticulous microdissection and surface preparation techniques, the process remains exceptionally labor-intensive and technically demanding. The ampullary crista poses even greater difficulties, as its complex

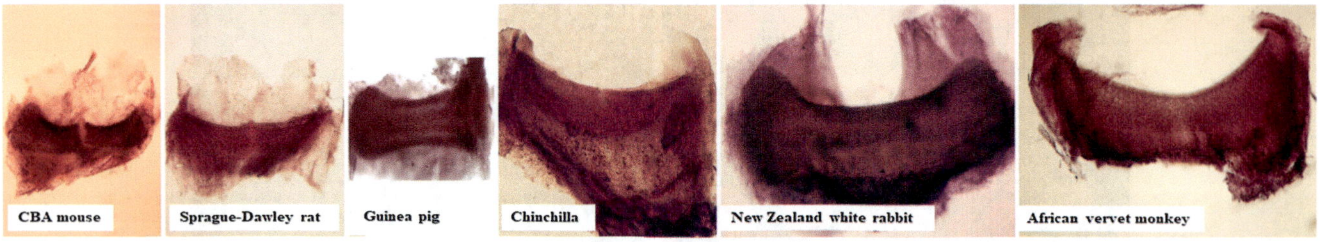

Fig. 5.9 A comparative series of surface preparation photomicrographs demonstrating the characteristic morphological features of ampullary cristae across various experimental animal models. The images highlight the inherent anatomical constraint posed by the crista's complex three-dimensional ridge-like structure, which prevents complete flattening of the sensory epithelium for comprehensive observation. Consequently, while this preparation technique allows clear visualization of hair cells on the crista's anterior surface facing the objective lens, the opposing posterior aspect remains obscured from view due to the tissue's natural curvature. This limitation fundamentally restricts complete hair cell enumeration in crista preparations, unlike the more accessible planar maculae (Reproduced with permission from Ding et al. [7]). The grouped images collectively illustrate both the technical capabilities and inherent limitations of surface preparation methodology for quantitative analysis of crista ampullaris morphology across species

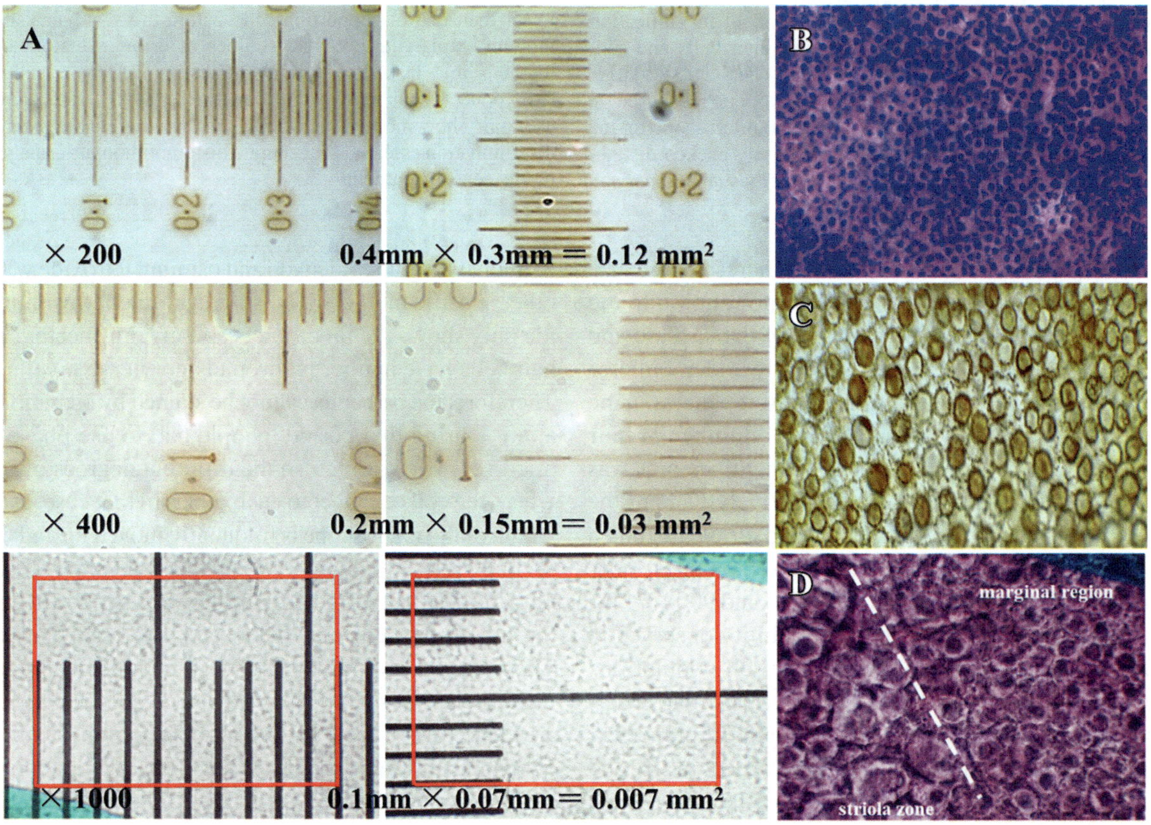

Fig. 5.10 Standardized methodology for regional hair cell density quantification in vestibular end-organs. (**A**) The critical calibration procedure showed micrometer measurements at 200× (0.12 mm² field area), 400× (0.03 mm²), and 1000× magnification (0.007 mm²), establishing precise reference scales for subsequent analyses. (**B**) A photomicrograph of the macula of the utricle of a rat with 200× magnification. (**C**) A photomicrograph of the crista of the ampulla in a chinchilla with 400× magnification. (**D**) A photomicrograph of the macula of the utricle in a rat with 1000× magnification (Reproduced with permission from Ding et al. [7]). This systematic approach ensures dimensional accuracy across magnification levels while demonstrating the technique's adaptability for both macular and crista preparations, providing a reliable framework for comparative vestibular hair cell density assessments

three-dimensional saddle-shaped structure only permits observation of the sensory epithelium facing the objective lens, leaving hair cells on the dorsal aspect inaccessible for counting [7] (Fig. 5.9). Furthermore, substantial inconsistencies in published reference data for total hair cell numbers across vestibular end-organs, stemming from fundamental methodological variations, complicate reliable comparative analyses. To address these challenges while maintaining scientific rigor,

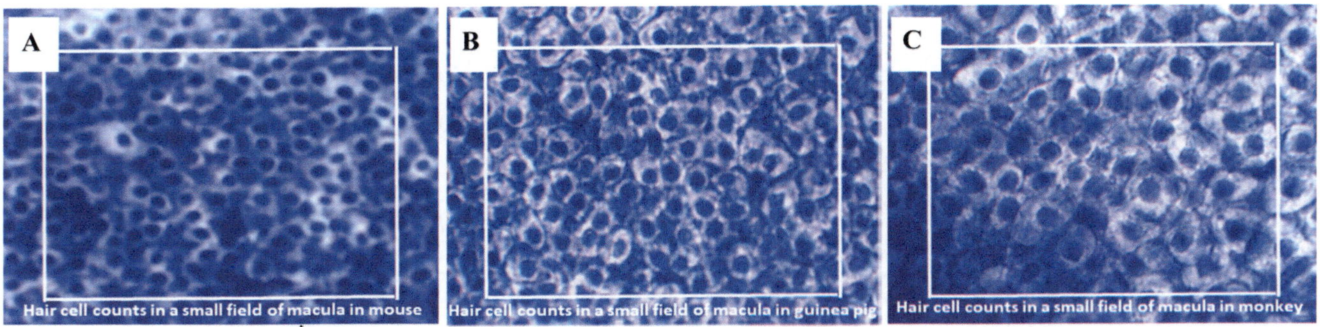

D

	Mouse	Rat	Guinea pig	Chinchilla	Rabbit	Monkey
Striola region of macula of saccule (Hair cells/0.007mm^2)	101.0±5.79	95.4±3.91	78.4±6.54	60.0±4.74	57.2±3.83	53.8±4.21
Marginal region of macula of saccule (Hair cells /0.007mm^2)	120.8±4.15	109.2±5.26	94.8±4.38	84.6±2.61	80.0±3.54	68.0±4.18
Striola region of macula of utricle (Hair cells/0.007mm^2)	103.8±5.02	91.2±2.49	74.1±3.54	60.4±4.98	57.8±1.92	54.0±2.74
Marginal region of macula of utricle (Hair cells /0.007mm^2)	119.2±3.70	106.4±4.16	90.8±3.56	81.6±2.07	77.8±3.70	66.4±2.51
Crista of ampulla (Hair cells /0.007mm^2)	112.4±6.38	105.4±3.51	95.2±3.42	84.0±7.16	78.2±2.86	70.8±2.39

Fig. 5.11 Differences in size and density of hair cells in the macula of the utricle in different experimental animal species. (**A**) The hair cells in the macula of the utricle in the mouse show a higher cell density due to their smaller size. (**B**) The size of the hair cells in the macula of the utricle in the guinea pig is slightly larger than that of the mouse, so its hair cell density is slightly lower than that of the mouse. (**C**) The size of hair cells in the macula of the utricle in monkeys is significantly larger than that of mice and guinea pigs. Therefore, the hair cell density in monkeys under the same microscope magnification is significantly lower than that of mice and guinea pigs. (**D**). The reference value of the hair cell density in the striola zone and marginal region in maculae of saccule and utricle, as well as in the ampullary cristae in 0.007 mm^2 in commonly used experimental animal species (Reproduced with permission from Ding et al. [7]). These systematic comparisons highlight important interspecies variations in vestibular sensory epithelium organization while demonstrating the reproducibility of density measurements using standardized microscopic fields

researchers have developed and validated standardized protocols for regional hair cell density assessment within defined microscopic fields of view. This practical approach has gained widespread adoption in vestibular research, as evidenced by its extensive application across numerous studies investigating various aspects of vestibular pathology and physiology [1–5, 7–9, 12, 17–20]. The field-of-view quantification method represents an optimal balance between methodological feasibility and scientific accuracy, overcoming the limitations of complete enumeration while providing reliable, reproducible data for comparative vestibular studies.

Our standardized protocol for regional hair cell density assessment involves systematic calibration of microscopic fields across multiple magnification powers. Initial calibration was performed by imaging a stage micrometer to calculate the precise viewing area for each objective lens configuration (Fig. 5.10A), establishing traceable measurement standards. Following calibration, representative regions of interest were photographed from vestibular end-organ surface preparations (Fig. 5.10B, C), and hair cells were enumerated within these defined fields. To ensure representative sampling and account for potential regional density variations, multiple non-overlapping fields were analyzed from each specimen, with the mean value derived from these replicate measurements providing the final hair cell density quantification [1, 7] (Figs. 5.11 and 5.12). This methodological approach combines rigorous calibration with systematic sampling to yield reliable, reproducible density measurements while accommodating the anatomical constraints of different vestibular end-organs.

In view of the fact that the hair cell density in the striolar area on the maculae of the saccule and utricle is much lower than that in the surrounding marginal area, when quantitatively observing the density of hair cells on the maculae of the saccule and utricle, it is sometimes necessary to evaluate the hair cell density in the striolar area and the marginal area, respectively. This will be helpful to determine whether there is a difference in the damage level of hair cells in the striolar area and the marginal area [3] (Fig. 5.13). Similarly, vestibular hair cells in different regions of the ampullary crista sometimes exhibit different patterns of vulnerability to damage. For example, hair

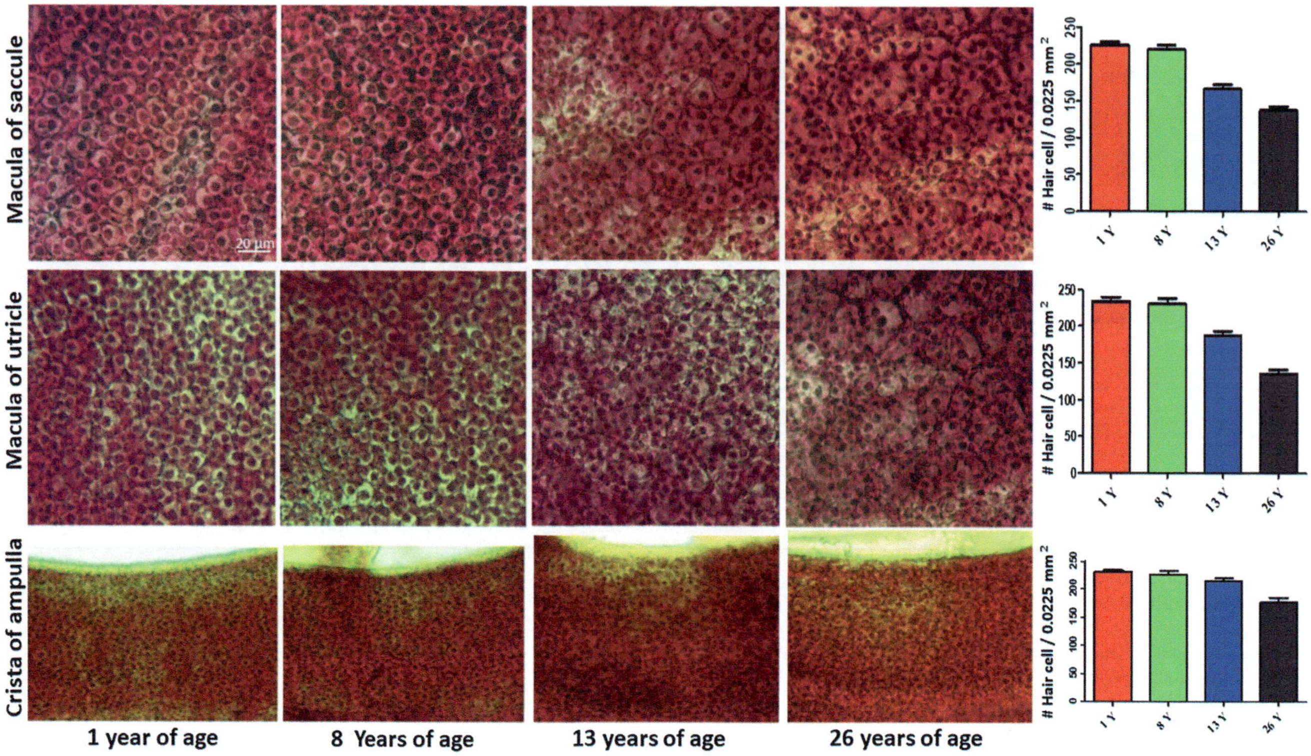

Fig. 5.12 Photomicrographs showing surface preparations of vestibular end-organs in monkeys at different ages and the results of hair cell density in the small field of view

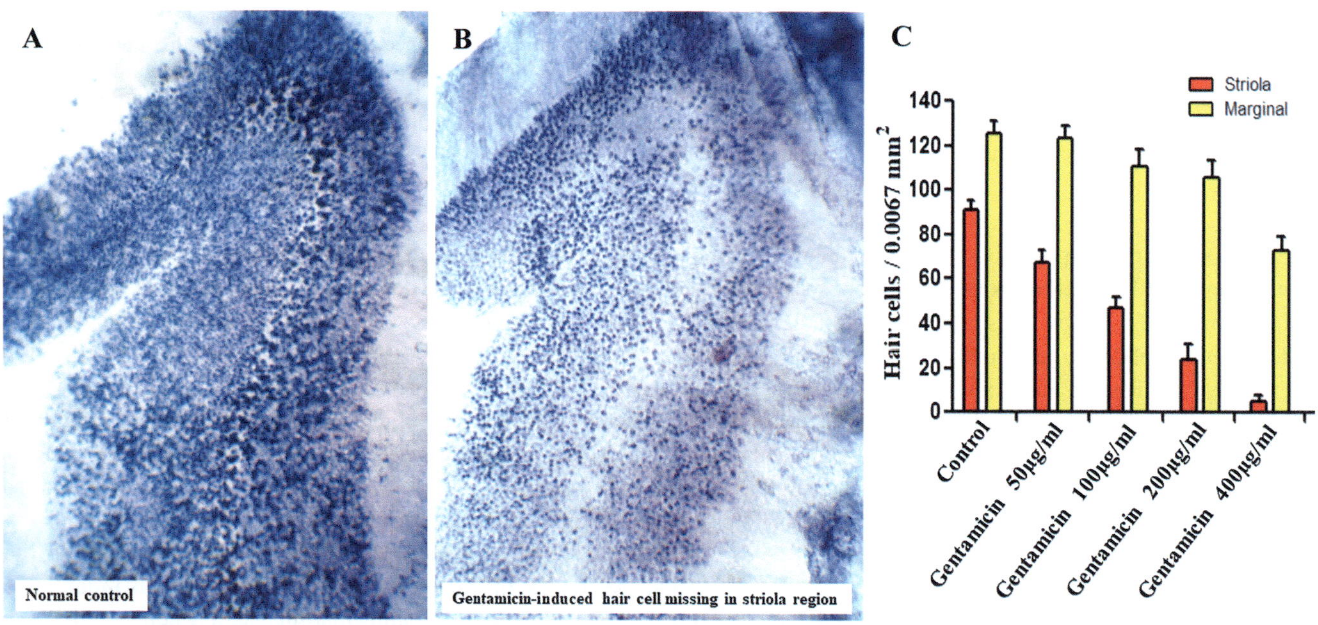

Fig. 5.13 Comparative observations of succinate dehydrogenase-stained macula of saccule in chinchilla, combining morphological and quantitative assessments of regional hair cell vulnerability. (**A**) Surface preparation of the macula of the saccule in normal chinchilla demonstrates characteristic, uniformly distributed hair cell staining patterns throughout the macular surface. (**B**) 7 days after perfusion of gentamicin (200 μg/mL) via the superior semicircular canal using a micro-osmotic pump, hair cells in the striolar region of the macula of the saccule were severely depleted, indicating that hair cells in the striolar region are highly sensitive to gentamicin-induced damage. (**C**) Quantitative comparison confirms significantly greater hair cell depletion in the striola (approximately 70% reduction) compared to marginal regions (20%–30% reduction), establishing clear topographical differences in ototoxic vulnerability within vestibular sensory epithelia. These findings underscore the necessity of region-specific analysis when evaluating hair cell damage patterns and therapeutic interventions

cells at the top of the crista ampullae are often more susceptible to ototoxic drugs than those at the base of the crista ampullae. Therefore, precise localization of the damaged hair cells on the ampullary crista is sometimes necessary to precisely locate and compare during observation and evaluation. Furthermore, different routes of ototoxic drug administration sometimes result in different damage levels of hair cells in different ampullary crista. For example, drug administration through the round window membrane tends to cause the greatest damage to hair cells on the ampullary crista of the posterior semicircular canal, whereas drug administration through the superior semicircular canal primarily damages the hair cells in the superior and lateral ampullary cristae (Fig. 5.14). Therefore, it is sometimes necessary to quantify the hair cell density in each ampullary crista separately [3]. Vestibular sensory hair cells are divided into type I and type II hair cells. Some ototoxic drugs, such as carboplatin or gentamicin, tend to preferentially destroy the type I hair cells in the vestibular end organs. In such cases, it is sometimes necessary to count the type I and type II hair cells separately within each vestibular sensory epithelium zone, as

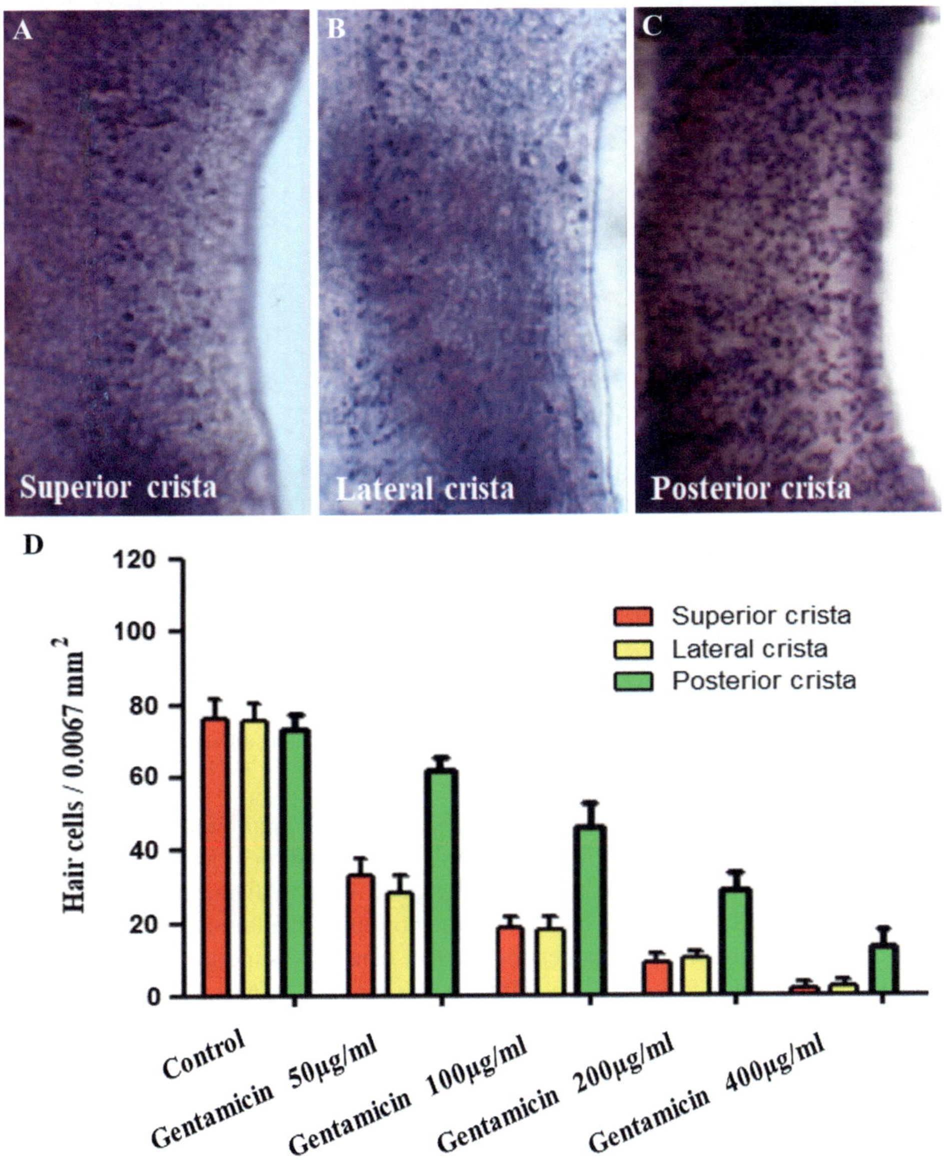

Fig. 5.14 The concentration-dependent and topographically specific effects of slow gentamicin infusion (0.5 μL/h for 7 days) via the superior semicircular canal. (**A**) The ampullary crista of the superior semicircular canal, close to the gentamicin infusion port, shows massive hair cell loss. (**B**) The lateral ampullary crista showed moderate but significant hair cell loss. (**C**) There was minimal hair cell loss on the posterior ampullary crista, distal to the gentamicin infusion site. (**D**) Quantitative comparison establishes a clear spatial pattern: superior crista (nearest infusion site) exhibits 75%–85% hair cell loss, lateral crista 50%–60%, and posterior crista 20%–30%. This confirms that ototoxic damage severity correlates inversely with distance from the drug entry point in the vestibular cistern. These findings provide compelling evidence for concentration-gradient-dependent hair cell vulnerability in semicircular canal cristae

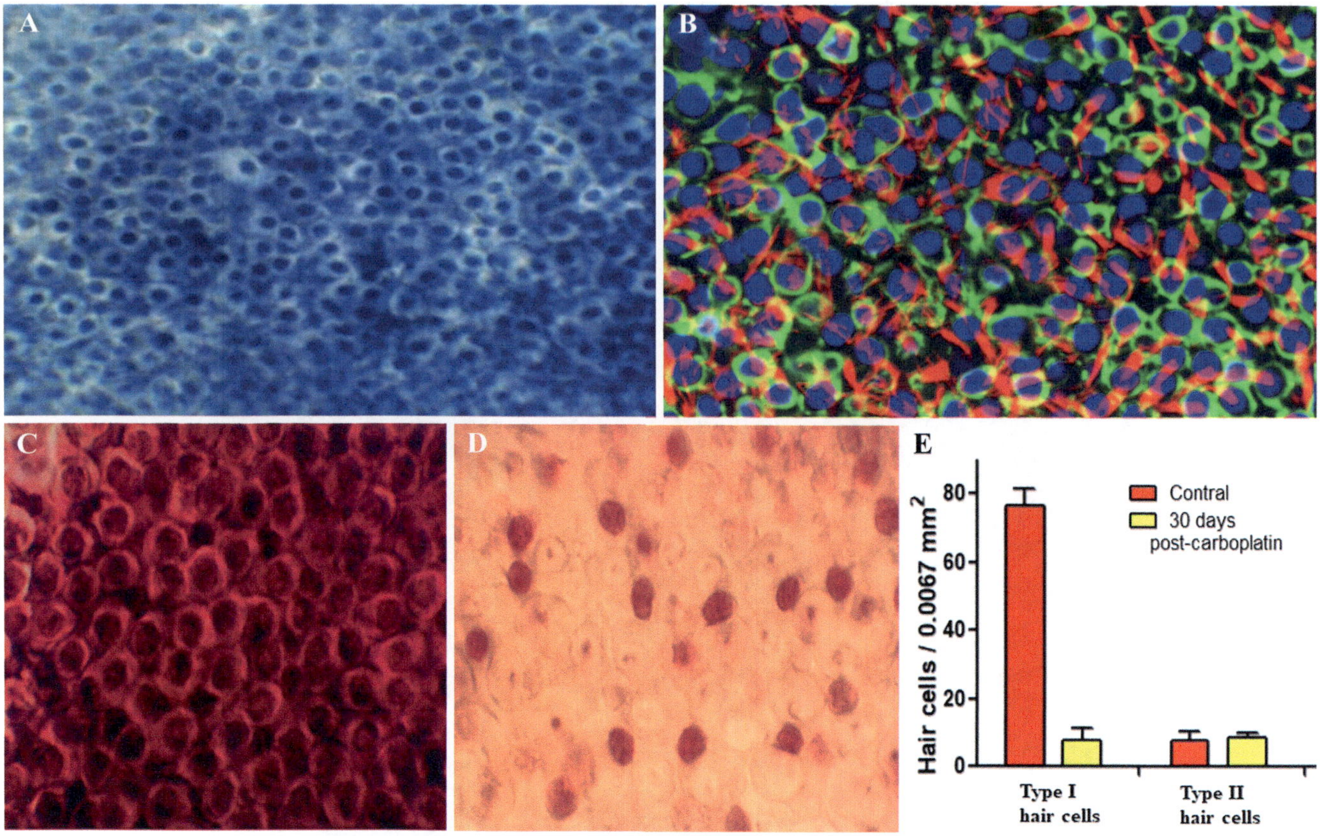

Fig. 5.15 Comprehensive methodologies for distinguishing type I and type II vestibular hair cells through combined morphological and immunohistochemical approaches. (**A**) Hematoxylin staining reveals characteristic anatomical differences: type I hair cells display distinctive annular spaces formed by calyx afferent terminals surrounding their nuclei, while type II cells lack this feature. (**B**). Anti-tubulin immunofluorescence specifically highlights the calyx terminals (green fluorescence), providing definitive identification of type I hair cells enclosed within these specialized nerve endings. (**C**) The surface preparation of the macula of the utricle in a normal chinchilla demonstrates balanced populations of both cell types, with type I cells (showing calyx formations) and type II cells (lacking calyces) clearly distinguishable. (**D**) 30 days after carboplatin treatment, selective type I hair cell loss was detected, leaving predominantly type II cells (without calyceal endings), demonstrating that carboplatin has a specific destructive effect on type I vestibular hair cells in chinchillas. (**E**) Quantitative analysis confirms carboplatin-induced preferential destruction of type I cells (85%–90% reduction) versus minimal effect on type II populations (<10% reduction), establishing its cell-type specific ototoxic profile (Reproduced with permission from Ding et al. [7]). This multimodal approach provides reliable discrimination of vestibular hair cell subtypes for investigating differential vulnerability patterns

this will help to demonstrate whether this ototoxic drug has a more specific killing effect on one type of hair cell (Fig. 5.15). These methodological considerations, substantiated by extensive experimental evidence [1, 3, 7, 18, 19, 21, 22], highlight the importance of using anatomical and cellular classification methods in vestibular pathology research to help fully understand the lesion pattern and its ototoxic damage mechanisms.

5.3 Quantitative Observation of Vestibular Nervous System

To obtain quantitative observational data on the vestibular afferent nervous system, it is first necessary to clarify the location and distribution of the vestibular nervous system. The human vestibular nervous system is anatomically different from that of commonly used mammalian experimental animals. The human vestibular nervous system is located in the internal auditory canal, which is approximately 8.5 mm long and 4 mm in diameter. There are three bony channels at the bottom of the human internal auditory canal: the facial nerve canal, the superior vestibular neuroforamen, and the cochlear neuroforamen. However, experimental animals such as mice, rats, guinea pigs, chinchillas, rabbits, and monkeys lack such a bony structure of the internal auditory canal (Figs. 3.1C, D, 6.1B, and 6.3B; Fig. 5.16). The vestibular nervous system is divided into the superior vestibular nerve pathway and the inferior vestibular nerve pathway. The superior branch of the vestibular nerve receives nerve impulse signals from the hair cells of the macula of the utricle and the upper part of the macula of the saccule, as well as the ampullary cristae of the superior and lateral semicircular canals, through the superior vestibular neuroforamen. The inferior branch of the vestibular nerve receives nerve impulse signals from the hair

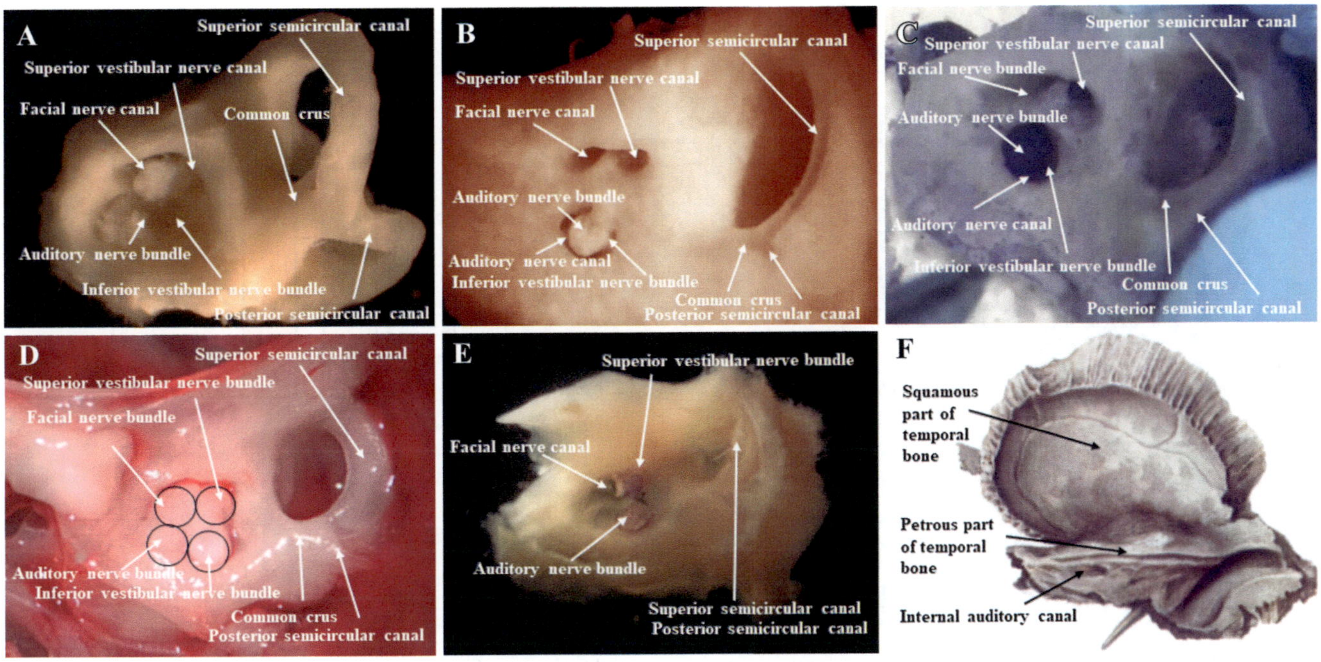

Fig. 5.16 Medial views of the lateral wall of the posterior cranial fossa of mammal showing that the facial nerve canal, superior vestibular neuroforamen, and cochlear neuroforamen are located separately within a depression on the medial surface of the temporal bone in commonly used experimental animals. However, they are not deeply hidden within the internal auditory canal as they are in humans. (**A**) Medial view of the lateral wall of the posterior cranial fossa of a monkey. (**B**) Medial view of the lateral wall of the posterior cranial fossa of the chinchilla. (**C**) Medial view of the lateral wall of the posterior cranial fossa of the guinea pig. (**D**) Medial view of the lateral wall of the posterior cranial fossa of the rat. (**E**) Medial view of the lateral wall of the posterior cranial fossa of the mouse (Reproduced with permission from Ding et al. [8]). (**F**) Medial view of the lateral wall of the posterior cranial fossa of a human

cells of the macula of the saccule and the ampullary crista of the posterior semicircular canal through the cochlear neuroforamen. Therefore, assessment of the superior vestibular system requires the collection of sagittal sections of the superior vestibular neuroforamen, while assessment of the inferior vestibular system requires the collection of sagittal sections of the base of the cochlear neuroforamen. It should be noted that most of the afferent nerve fibers passing through the cochlear neuroforamen are central nerve fibers of the auditory nerve, and the inferior vestibular nerve bundle is just a small branch located behind the auditory nerve bundle [8, 9].

5.3.1 Quantitative Observation of Vestibular Peripheral Nerve Fibers

The superior vestibular nerve fibers in the superior vestibular neuroforamen pass through the bony foramen of the superior sieve spot zone on the medial bony wall of the vestibular cistern to establish synaptic connections with the hair cells on the macula of the utricle and the upper part of the macula of the saccule and the lateral and superior semicircular canal ampullae. While the inferior vestibular nerve fibers in the cochlear neuroforamen pass through the bony foramen of the middle and inferior sieve spot zone on the medial bony wall of the vestibular cistern to establish synaptic connections with the hair cells on the macula of the saccule and the ampullary crista of the posterior semicircular canal. Therefore, in vestibular injury experiments, it is sometimes necessary to correlate the damage to the hair cells in the macula of utricle and the ampullary cristae of lateral and superior semicircular canals to the degeneration of superior vestibular nervous system in the vestibular neuroforamen, and sometimes it is necessary to correspond the lesions of the hair cells in the macula of the saccule and the ampullary crista of posterior semicircular canal to the degeneration of the inferior vestibular nervous system in the cochlear neuroforamen. To obtain quantitative data of vestibular peripheral nerve fibers, it is necessary to collect sections of the superior vestibular neuroforamen near the superior sieve spot zone and the cochlear neuroforamen near the middle sieve spot zone in the sagittal section of the temporal bone [8, 9] (Fig. 5.17).

5.3.2 Quantitative Observation of Vestibular Ganglion Neurons

The vestibular ganglion neurons were separated into two groups of neuron cell bodies in the superior group of ganglia in the vestibular neuroforamen and in the inferior group of ganglia in

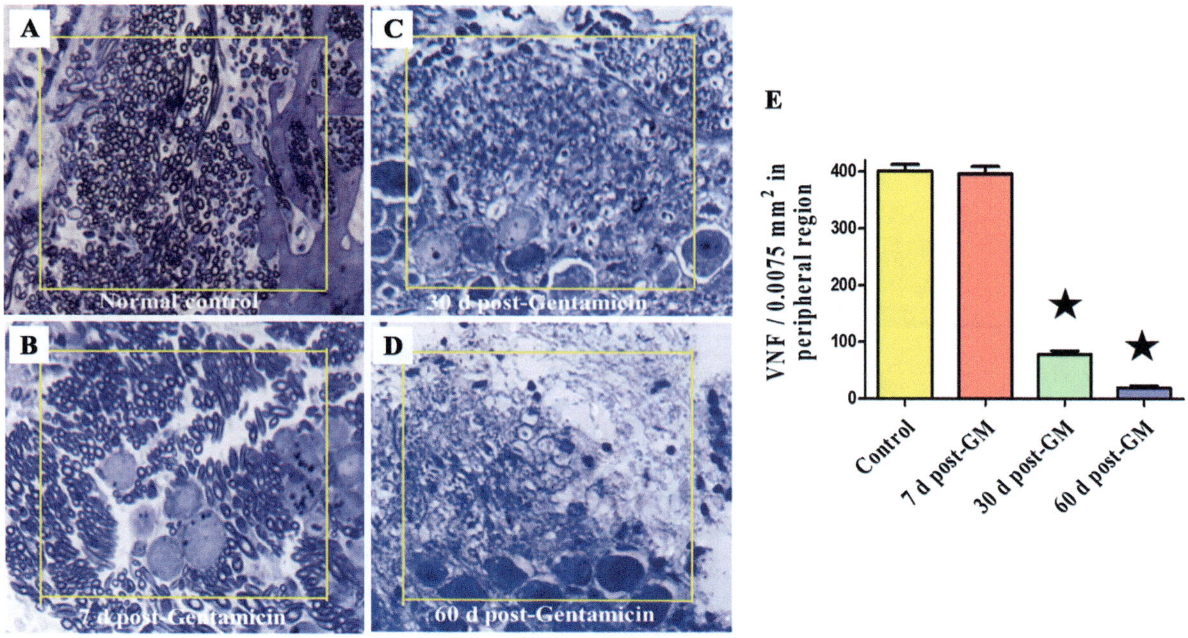

Fig. 5.17 Sagittal section of the vestibular nerve foramen of the rat shows delayed secondary destruction of peripheral superior vestibular nerve fibers induced by intratympanic injection of gentamicin. (**A**) The superior vestibular peripheral nerve fibers in a control rat are present normally. (**B**) 7 days after intratympanic injection of gentamicin, the superior vestibular peripheral nerve fibers were intact. (**C**) 30 days after intratympanic injection of gentamicin, significant demyelinating changes occur in the superior vestibular peripheral nerve fibers. (**D**) 60 days after intratympanic injection of gentamicin, the superior vestibular peripheral nerve fibers were completely destroyed. (**E**) Quantitative analysis of the density of the superior vestibular peripheral nerve fibers showed that delayed secondary destruction of the superior vestibular peripheral nerve fibers began to occur about 30 days after intratympanic injection of gentamicin to destroy the hair cells on the macula of utricle and the ampullary cristae of lateral and superior semicircular canals (Reproduced with permission from Ding et al. [8]). This indicates that the vestibular peripheral nerve fibers develop secondary lesions within 30 days after the complete destruction of vestibular hair cells

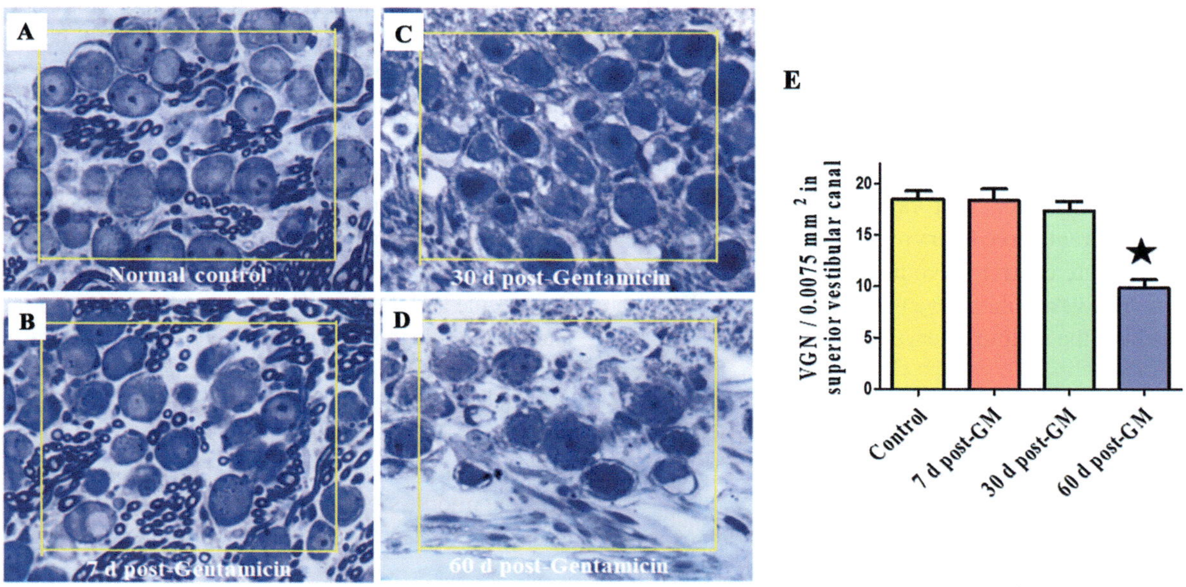

Fig. 5.18 Sagittal section of the vestibular nerve foramen of the rat shows delayed secondary destruction of superior vestibular ganglion neurons induced by intratympanic injection of gentamicin. (**A**) The vestibular ganglion neurons in the superior vestibular neuroforamen of a control rat are present normally. (**B**) 7 days after intratympanic injection of gentamicin, the vestibular ganglion neurons in the superior vestibular neuroforamen were intact. (**C**) 30 days after intratympanic injection of gentamicin, the vestibular ganglion within the vestibular neuroforamen began to develop very mild, small vacuoles with obvious demyelination of nerve fibers. (**D**) 60 days after intratympanic injection of gentamicin, the vestibular ganglion neurons in the superior vestibular neuroforamen were severely degenerated. (**E**) Quantitative analysis of the density of the vestibular ganglion neurons in the superior vestibular neuroforamen showed that delayed secondary destruction of the vestibular ganglion neurons occurs 60 days after intratympanic injection of gentamicin to destroy the hair cells on the macula of the utricle and the ampullary cristae of lateral and superior semicircular canals. (Reproduced with permission from Ding et al. [8])

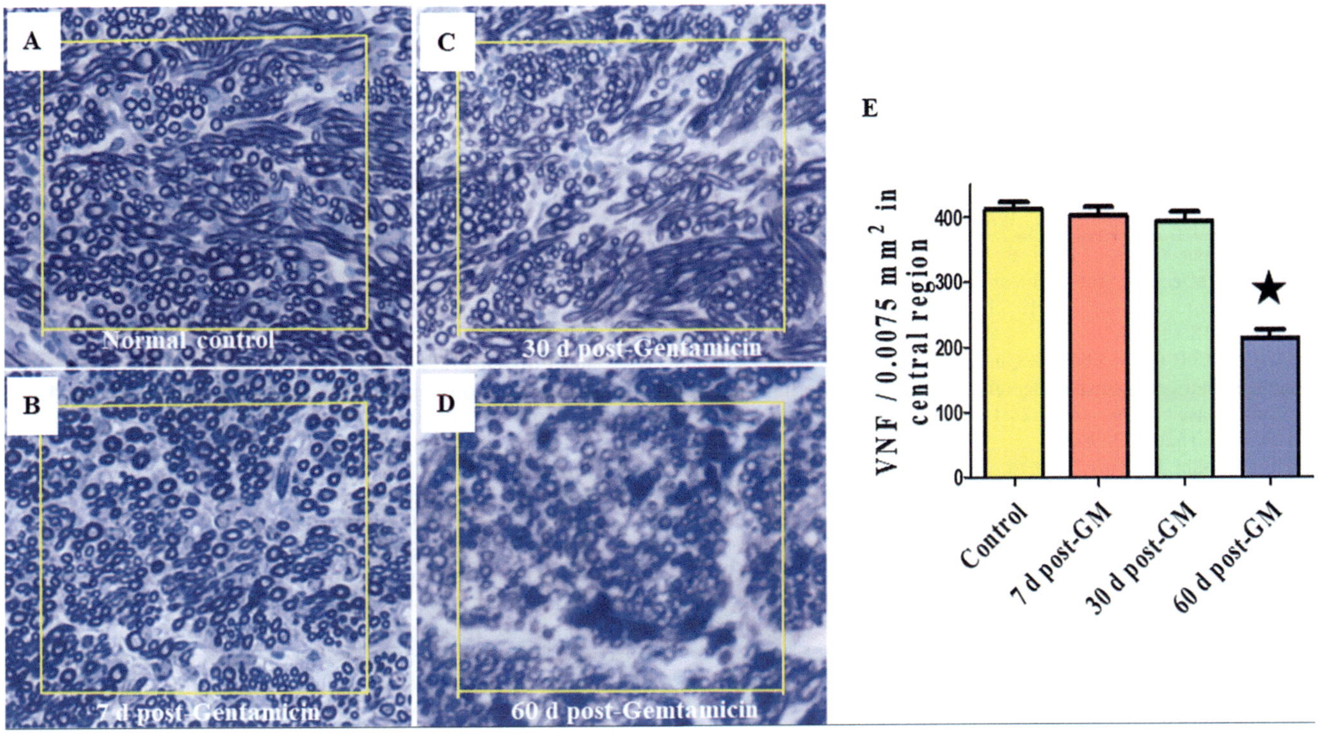

Fig. 5.19 Sagittal section through the vestibular nerve foramen of the rat shows the delayed secondary lesions in superior vestibular afferent fibers leading to the central nervous system caused by intratympanic injection of gentamicin. (**A**) The superior vestibular afferent nerve fibers leading to the central nervous system in a control rat appear normal. (**B**) 7 days after intratympanic injection of gentamicin, the superior vestibular afferent nerve fibers leading to the vestibular central nervous system expressed normal structure. (**C**) 30 days after intratympanic injection of gentamicin, the superior vestibular afferent nerve fibers leading to the vestibular central nervous system maintained their intact morphology. (**D**) 60 days after intratympanic injection of gentamicin, massive destruction of superior vestibular afferent nerve fibers leading to the vestibular central nervous system was detected. (**E**) Quantitative analysis of the density of superior vestibular nerve fibers leading to the vestibular central nervous system showed that about 60 days after the intratympanic injection of gentamicin to destroy the hair cells of the utricle macula and the lateral and superior semicircular canals, the superior vestibular nerve fibers leading to the central end began to show delayed secondary destruction (Reproduced with permission from Ding et al. [8]). A comprehensive analysis of the experimental result from Figs. 5.17–5.19 shows that after severe damage of vestibular hair cells, the peripheral vestibular nerve fibers first suffer delayed secondary damage, while secondary damage to the vestibular ganglia and central end of nerve fibers occur later. This suggests that the delayed secondary damage to the vestibular nervous system caused by gentamicin destroying vestibular hair cells has a tendency to gradually spread from the periphery to the central nervous system

the cochlear neuroforamen. The bipolar neurons of the superior vestibular neurons send peripheral nerve fibers outward through the superior cribriform area to establish synaptic connections with the hair cells on the utricle, external ampulla, and superior ampulla. The bipolar neurons of the inferior vestibular neurons send peripheral nerve fibers outward through the middle and inferior ethmoid plaques to establish synaptic connections with the hair cells on the saccule and posterior ampulla. The central axons of these bipolar neurons project medially through the vestibular or cochlear foramina to the vestibular nuclei in the brainstem. The vestibular ganglion cell group located in the superior vestibular neuroforamen is very close to the superior sieve spot zone, and the vestibular ganglion cell group located at the bottom of the cochlear neuroforamen is very close to the middle sieve spot zone. Therefore, after obtaining the slices of the vestibular peripheral nerve fibers, the accumulation site of the vestibular ganglion cell group is reached [8, 9] (Fig. 5.18).

5.3.3 Quantitative Observation of Vestibular Central Nerve Fibers

After obtaining slices of the vestibular ganglion and crossing the area where the vestibular ganglion cells accumulate, continuous sectioning continues to collect the slices of the central terminal nerve fibers projecting to the vestibular nucleus [8, 9] (Fig. 5.19).

References

1. Ding D, Chen X, Jin X. Quantitative observation technique in a small field of view in vestibular end organs. Zhonghua Er Bi Yan Hou Ke Za Zhi. 1992;27:202–3.
2. Ding D, Jiang H, Wang J, et al. Carboplatin-induced vestibular damage: quantitative measurement of type I hair cell loss and ganglion cell loss. J Audit Speech Pathol. 2002;10:170–3.

3. Lii M, Ding D, Zheng XY, Salvi R. Vestibular destruction by slow infusion of gentamicin into semicircular canals. Acta Otolaryngol Suppl. 2004;Suppl:35–41. https://doi.org/10.1080/03655230410017102.
4. Yu D, Ding D, Yin S, Salvi R. Ototoxic effects of streptomycin in vestibular organotypic cultures. Chin J Otorhinolaryngol Head Neck Surg. 2009;44:207–9.
5. Yu D, Ding D, Jiang H, Stolzberg D, Salvi R. Mefloquine damage vestibular hair cells in organotypic cultures. Neurotox Res. 2011;20:51–58. https://doi.org/10.1007/s12640-010-9221-z.
6. Ye H, Xing Y, Zhang L, et al. Bilirubin-induced neurotoxic and ototoxic effects in rat cochlear and vestibular organotypic cultures. Neurotoxicology. 2019;71:75–86. https://doi.org/10.1016/j.neuro.2018.12.004.
7. Ding D, Li P, Qi W, Zhang J. Quantitative observation of vestibular sensory hair cells in experimental animals. Chin J Otorhinolaryngol Skull Base Surg. 2022;28:11–18. https://doi.org/10.11798/j.issn.1007-1520.202290001.
8. Ding D, Shi L, Xing Y, et al. Secondary neural damage in the inner ear induced by intratympanic gentamicin injection. Chin J Otorhinolaryngol Skull Base Surg. 2024;30:11–19. https://doi.org/10.11798/j.issn.1007-1520.202424356.
9. Ding D, Manohar S, Kador PF, Salvi R. Multifunctional redox modulator prevents blast-induced loss of cochlear and vestibular hair cells and auditory spiral ganglion neurons. Sci Rep. 2024;14:15296. https://doi.org/10.1038/s41598-024-66406-1.
10. Merchant SN, Velazquez-Villasenor L, Tsuji K, et al. Temporal bone studies of the human peripheral vestibular system. Normative vestibular hair cell data. Ann Otol Rhinol Laryngol Suppl. 2000;181:3–13. https://doi.org/10.1177/00034894001090s502.
11. Abercrombie M, Johnson ML. Quantitative histology of Wallerian degeneration; nuclear population in rabbit sciatic nerve. J Anat. 1946;80:37–50.
12. Ding D, Jiang H, Zhang J, et al. Cisplatin-induced vestibular hair cell lesion-less damage at high doses. J Otol. 2018;13:115–21. https://doi.org/10.1016/j.joto.2018.08.002.
13. Lindeman HH. Studies on the morphology of the sensory regions of the vestibular apparatus with 45 figures. Ergeb Anat Entwicklungsgesch. 1969;42:1–113.
14. Desai SS, Ali H, Lysakowski A. Comparative morphology of rodent vestibular periphery. II. Cristae ampullares. J Neurophysiol. 2005;93:267–80. https://doi.org/10.1152/jn.00747.2003.
15. Crile G, Quiring D. A record of the body weight and certain organ and gland weights of 3690 animals. Ohio J Sci. 1940;40:219–59.
16. Desai SS, Zeh C, Lysakowski A. Comparative morphology of rodent vestibular periphery. I. Saccular and utricular maculae. J Neurophysiol. 2005;93:251–66. https://doi.org/10.1152/jn.00746.2003.
17. Ding D, Stracher A, Salvi RJ. Leupeptin protects cochlear and vestibular hair cells from gentamicin ototoxicity. Hear Res. 2002;164:115–126. https://doi.org/10.1016/s0378-5955(01)00417-8.
18. Zhou Y, Ding D, Kraus KS, et al. Functional and structural changes in the chinchilla cochlea and vestibular system following round window application of carboplatin. Audiol Med. 2009;7:189–99. https://doi.org/10.3109/16513860903335795.
19. Yu J, Ding D, Wang F, Jiang H, Sun H, Salvi R. Pattern of hair cell loss and delayed peripheral neuron degeneration in inner ear by a high-dose intratympanic gentamicin. J Otol. 2014;9:126–35. https://doi.org/10.1016/j.joto.2014.12.001.
20. Ding D, Jiang H, Salvi R. Cochlear spiral ganglion neuron degeneration following cyclodextrin-induced hearing loss. Hear Res. 2021;400:108125 https://doi.org/10.1016/j.heares.2020.108125.
21. Ding D, Manohar S, Jiang H, Salvi R. Hydroxypropyl-beta-cyclodextrin causes massive damage to the developing auditory and vestibular system. Hear Res. 2020;396:108073 https://doi.org/10.1016/j.heares.2020.108073.
22. Ding D, Jiang H, Chen GD, et al. N-acetyl-cysteine prevents age-related hearing loss and the progressive loss of inner hair cells in gamma-glutamyl transferase 1 deficient mice. Aging (Albany NY). 2016;8:730–50. https://doi.org/10.18632/aging.100927.

6 Anatomy of the Cochlear System

The cochlea is a cone-shaped spiral structure located in the temporal bone. The bony labyrinth of the cochlea is composed of the bony cochlear lateral walls surrounding the cochlear cavity and the bony cochlear modiolus located in the center of the cochlear cavity. The membranous structure with a spiral cone-shaped cavity similar to the bony labyrinth of the cochlea is the cochlear membranous labyrinth, which is located within the cochlear cavity between the bony volute and the bony modiolus. The space between the bony cochlear labyrinth and the membranous cochlear labyrinth is filled with perilymph, while the interior of the membranous cochlear labyrinth is filled with endolymph [1–9]. This compartmentalized arrangement with distinct fluid environments is crucial for the auditory function of the cochlea.

6.1 Cochlear Bony Labyrinth

The shape of bony cochlear labyrinth in mammals is like a spiral snail shell (Fig. 1.4A; Figs. 6.1–6.3). The base of the cochlea lies posteromedially, while its apex projects anterolaterally. A central conical structure, the modiolus, forms the bony axis of the cochlear cavity and extends horizontally along its length. The modiolus is thickest at the cochlear base, where the spiral canal is widest, and the modiolus is narrowest at the cochlear apical turn, where the spiral canal is narrowest (Fig. 6.4). As the cochlear cavities spiral from the base to the apex, the bony spiral lamina surrounding the modiolus extends from the cochlear axis toward the lateral walls, dividing the cochlear cavity into a spiral bony tube. This structural arrangement forms a continuous spiral bend, giving the cochlea its characteristic coiled shape to be a helical shape and spirals into several turns (Fig. 6.4). The spiral bony tube conforms to the curvature of the modiolus, maintaining the continuity of the lumen throughout its course.

The cochlear labyrinth's volute bone wall exhibits a trilaminar structure, comprising an outer periosteal layer of compact bone, a middle endochondral layer containing chondrocytes, and an inner thin endosteal layer. Considerable interspecies variation exists in the length of the cochlear basilar membrane and the convolution of the cochlea in mammals, with humans possessing a cochlear length of approximately 35 mm and 2.63 turns, guinea pigs exhibiting about 20 mm length and 4 turns, chinchillas demonstrating 18.4 mm length and 3 turns, rats showing 9.2 mm length and 2.4 turns, and mice displaying the smallest dimensions at 6 mm length and 2 turns [1–4, 6–12]. These anatomical differences reflect species-specific adaptations in auditory physiology while maintaining the fundamental cochlear architecture. The consistent trilaminar osseous organization across species provides structural integrity to the spiral cochlear canal while accommodating variations in length and turns that influence frequency resolution capabilities.

6.2 Cochlear Membranous Labyrinth

The cochlear membranous labyrinth, suspended within the bony labyrinth and bathed in perilymph, consists of epithelial and connective tissues that span between the modiolus and the cochlear lateral wall, with its interior containing endolymph. This delicate structure can be fully exposed by carefully removing the surrounding lateral bony wall [3, 5, 7, 9, 13–17] (Fig. 1.4B; Figs. 6.5 and 6.6). Anatomically, the basal end of the cochlear duct connects to the saccule via the *ductus reuniens* at the anteroinferior aspect of the vestibular cistern, while its apical portion spirals along the modiolus before terminating blindly in the cupular cecum. This arrangement creates a continuous endolymph-filled system that is critical for auditory transduction while maintaining structural stability through its suspension within the perilymphatic space.

The cochlear basilar membrane spans from the tympanic lip of the osseous spiral lamina to the basilar crest of the spiral ligament, creating a division that separates the cochlear cavity into the superior cavity and inferior cavity (scala tympani).

D. Ding et al., *Histopathological Atlas of the Inner Ear*,
https://doi.org/10.1007/978-981-95-6338-8_6

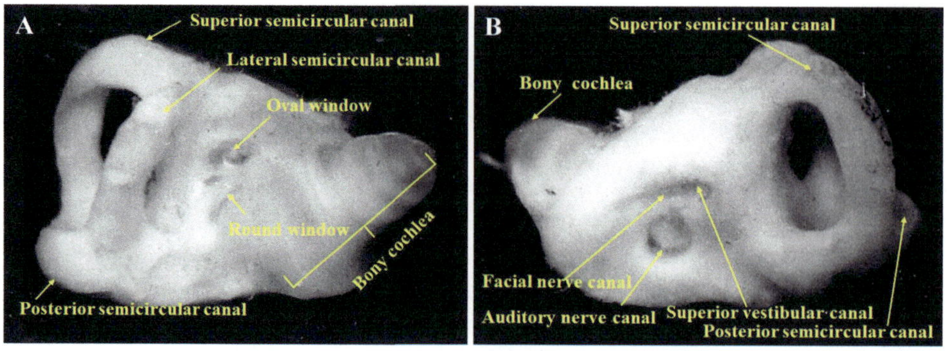

Fig. 6.1 The bony labyrinth in guinea pig. (**A**) Tympanic lateral view of the bony labyrinth of the inner ear. (**B**) Lateral intracranial view of the bony labyrinth of the inner ear

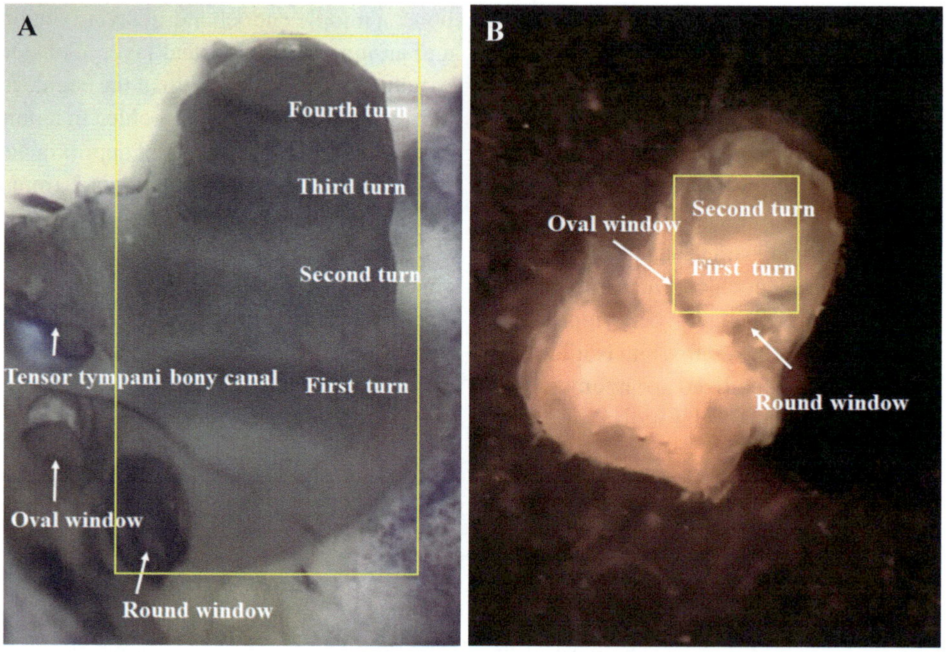

Fig. 6.2 Comparative morphology of the osseous cochlea in rodents. (**A**) Guinea pig cochlea demonstrating characteristic spiral architecture. (**B**) Rat cochlea showing species-specific anatomical features

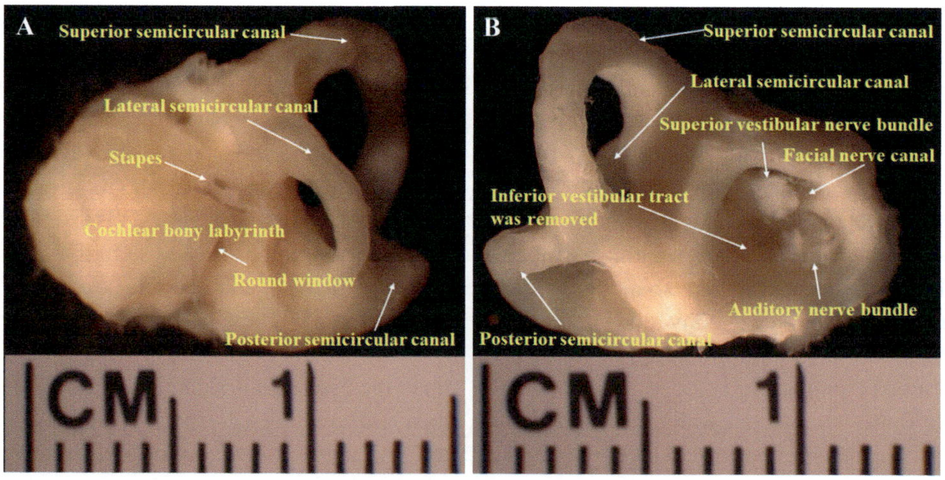

Fig. 6.3 The morphology of the bony labyrinth in primate. (**A**) Tympanic (ventral) aspect showing cochlear orientation and vestibular relationships. (**B**) Intracranial (dorsal) view demonstrating semicircular canal architecture and osseous cochlear features

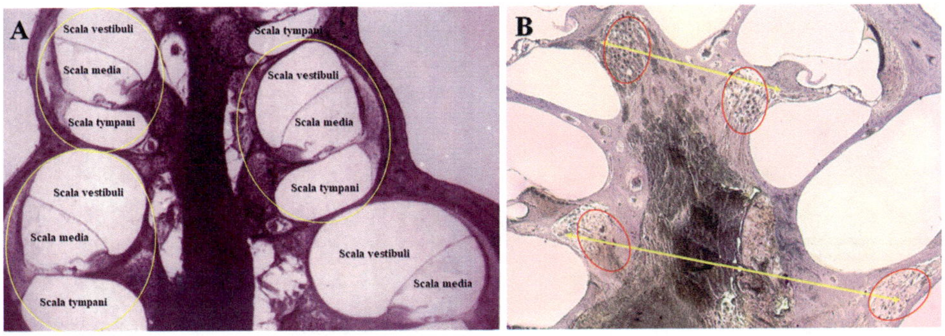

Fig. 6.4 Comparative cochlear histology following ouabain administration. (**A**) The cochlear cross-section from a normal guinea pig. The yellow circles indicate spiral bony canal profiles across cochlear turns. (**B**) The cochlear cross-section from a rat. Yellow double-headed arrows demonstrate the diameter differential between basal (wider) and second (narrower) turns. Red circles delineate Rosenthal's canal profiles. Note that 7 days after 10 mM ouabain was placed in the round window niche, with near-complete neuronal loss in the basal turn, partial preservation in the second turn, and intact apical turn neurons. This indicates that the spiral ganglion neurons in the cochlear basal turn near the round window niche suffer the most severe damage caused by ouabain, because ouabain infiltrates from the round window membrane into the basal turn of the cochlea first

Complementing this structure, Reissner's membrane (vestibular membrane) extends from the vestibular lip at the medial edge of the spiral limbus to the vestibular crest of the spiral ligament, further subdividing the upper cavity. This arrangement results in three distinct chambers: cochlear cross-sectional view shows from superior to inferior, the scala vestibuli, cochlear duct (containing endolymph), and scala tympani (Fig. 6.4). The scala vestibuli communicates with the vestibular cistern at the base of the cochlea, while the scala tympani connects to the intracranial subarachnoid space through the cochlear aqueduct near the round window. The perilymph-filled chambers of scala vestibuli and scala tympani are interconnected by the spiral foramen of helicotrema at the apex of the cochlea, forming a continuous fluid circuit within the cochlea for the conduction of basilar membrane vibrations caused by the flow of lymph fluid [1, 2, 4, 6, 9]. The precise anatomical relationships between these membranous partitions and their osseous supports create the structural foundation for cochlear micromechanics.

6.2.1 The Basal Boundary of the Cochlear Duct

The triangular cochlear duct in cross-section is delineated by three structural components: Reissner's membrane superiorly, the spiral ligament laterally, and the basilar membrane inferiorly which forms its floor. This basilar membrane exhibits precise anatomical relationships, with its medial aspect overlying the spiral limbus of the osseous spiral lamina and its lateral margin inserting at a near-right angle (approximately 90°) into the basilar crest of the spiral ligament (Figs. 6.4A and 6.7A). The organ of Corti is narrowest at the basal turn of the cochlea and gradually widens toward the apex, creating a structurally graded platform that is fundamental to the cochlea's tonotopic organization. Its fibrous composition, featuring radially oriented filaments embedded in an amorphous ground substance, provides both the mechanical resilience and elasticity required for sound-induced vibrations while maintaining firm attachments at both the osseous and ligamentous junctions.

In cross-section, the cochlear basilar membrane reveals a precisely organized architecture with the organ of Corti positioned centrally, flanked medially by the inner sulcus and laterally by the outer sulcus. The sensory epithelium of the organ of Corti comprises mechanosensory inner hair cells, outer hair cells, and specialized supporting cells that maintain structural integrity. A distinctive triangular space—the tunnel of Corti—is formed by the interlocking arrangement of single rows of inner and outer pillar cells, whose apical cuticular plates overlap while their basal foot processes remain separated, creating a rigid scaffolding system. This pillar cell complex provides both mechanical support and compartmentalization within the organ of Corti, with the inner pillar cells' heads articulating with the outer pillar cells' plates to form a stable triangular prism structure [1, 2, 4, 6, 18]. The geometric precision of this cellular architecture facilitates the micromechanical properties essential for sound transduction while maintaining the tonotopic organization along the cochlear spiral.

The organ of Corti demonstrates a highly organized cellular arrangement, with the inner hair cell row positioned medial to the inner pillar cells' cuticular plates that form the Corti tunnel boundary. These inner hair cells are surrounded by specialized supporting cells: inner phalangeal cells providing direct structural support, border cells creating a transitional zone, and inner sulcus cells extending toward the medial spiral sulcus—a space partially covered by the overhanging tectorial membrane originating from the vestibular lip. Laterally, three rows of outer hair cells align adjacent to the outer pillar cells' cuticular plates, supported by Deiters' cells (outer phalangeal cells) that cup their basal poles, with successive layers of Hensen's cells, Claudius cells, and Boettcher cells (present in the basal turn) completing the lateral cellular array [1, 2, 4, 6, 18] (Figs. 6.7A, D, 6.8, and 6.9).

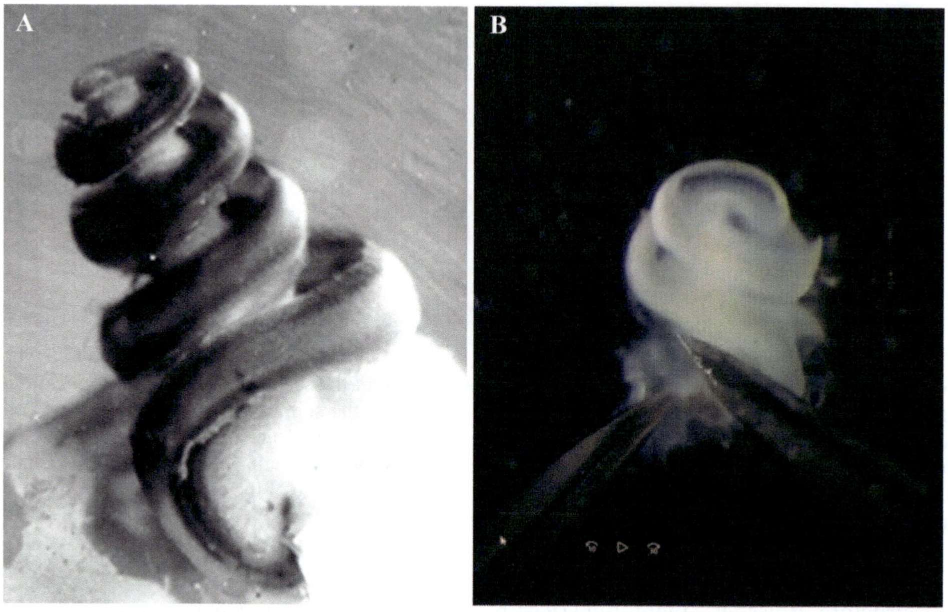

Fig. 6.5 The volute of the cochlear bony labyrinth was peeled off to expose the entire cochlear membrane labyrinth. (**A**) After removing the entire cochlear volute, the intact spiral structure of the cochlear membranous labyrinth of guinea pig is fully exposed. (**B**) Remove the entire cochlear shell to expose the cochlear membranous labyrinth of the mouse. The delicate structure of the cochlear membranous labyrinth remains suspended between the modiolus and lateral attachment points, preserved within their native spatial configuration

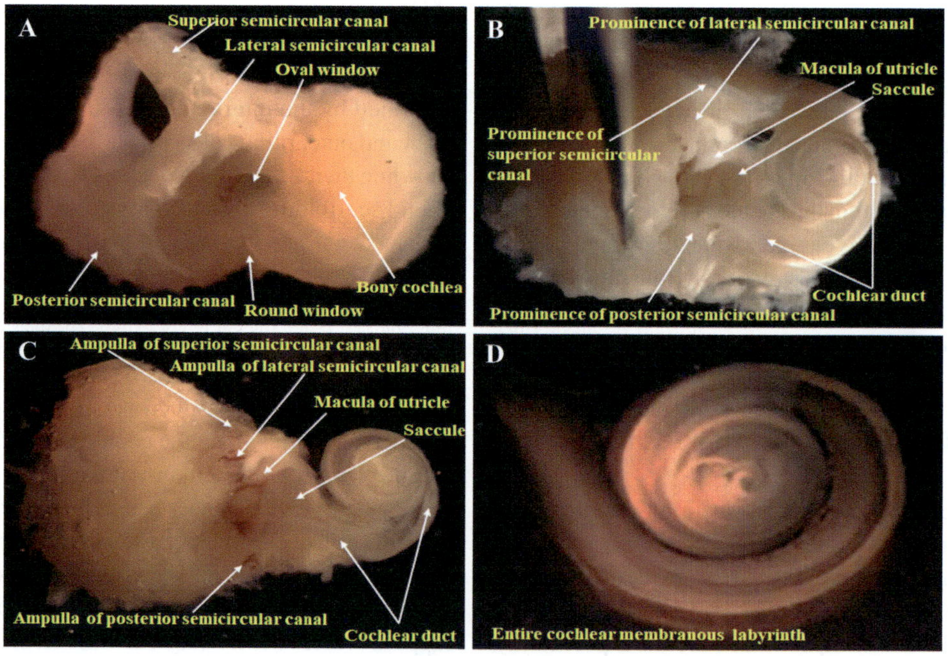

Fig. 6.6 Microdissection steps of the primate cochlear membranous labyrinth. (**A**) Initial exposure of the osseous cochlear labyrinth. (**B**) Removal of the bony shell revealing the intact membranous labyrinth of the cochlea. (**C**) Surgical separation of the basilar membrane from the modiolus. (**D**) Final isolation of the complete cochlear membranous labyrinth demonstrating preservation of its spiral architecture and neural connections. This sequential dissection technique maintains the structural integrity of critical cochlear components while allowing for detailed examination of their anatomical relationships

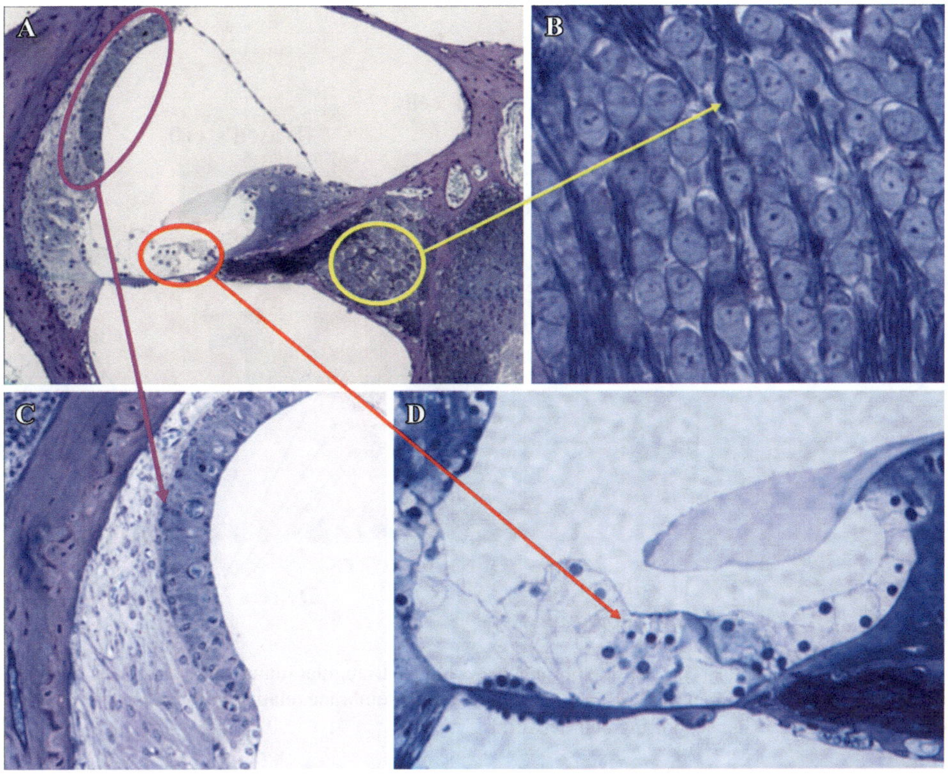

Fig. 6.7 Histological features of rat cochlear architecture in semi-thin section. (**A**) Cross-sectional view demonstrating the spatial relationship among the basilar membrane, spiral ligament, and Rosenthal's canal within the cochlear structure. (**B**) High-magnification detail of spiral ganglion neurons residing within Rosenthal's canal, showing their characteristic clustering pattern along the cochlear spiral. (**C**) Lateral wall morphology featuring the composite structure of the spiral ligament with adjacent stria vascularis, illustrating their vascular and connective tissue organization. (**D**) Organ of Corti resting on the basilar membrane platform, displaying preserved cellular architecture of the sensory epithelium. This composite figure systematically presents the key functional microanatomical units of the mammalian cochlea in their native spatial orientations.(Reproduced with permission from Ding et al. [17])

All hair cells and supporting cells maintain critical barrier functions through specialized junctions in their cuticular plates and apical membranes, effectively isolating their cell bodies from the potassium-rich endolymph while permitting selective ionic exchange. The interstitial spaces within the organ of Corti, including the tunnel of Corti, contain Corti's lymph—a perilymph-like fluid that facilitates metabolic support while maintaining the electrochemical gradients essential for electromechanical conversion [1, 2, 4, 6, 9]. This precise cellular organization and compartmentalization underlie the cochlea's ability to maintain both structural stability and physiological function in the face of the endolymph-perilymph electrochemical gradient.

The frequency selectivity of cochlear hair cells is determined by systematic variations in their morphological characteristics and the width of the organ of Corti along the basilar membrane. In the basal turn's hook region, where the organ of Corti is narrowest (approximately 100–150 μm), the compact cellular architecture and shorter, stiffer hair cells are mechanically tuned to high-frequency vibrations. The middle basal turn exhibits intermediate dimensions (150–200 μm) corresponding to medium-frequency responsiveness, while the apical turn's wider organ of Corti (200–300 μm) with taller, more flexible hair cells facilitates low-frequency detection (Fig. 6.10A–C). This precise structural gradient underlies the cochlea's tonotopic organization, though a common misconception in literature erroneously attributes these width variations to the basilar membrane itself rather than specifically to the organ of Corti's cellular architecture [1, 2, 4, 6, 9, 11]. The basilar membrane's width actually remains relatively constant, while its stiffness gradient—decreasing from base to apex—works in concert with the organ of Corti's dimensional changes to create the full spectrum of frequency sensitivity. The width of the cochlear basilar membrane is anatomically defined by two distinct measurement approaches: either as the span between the inner edge of osseous spiral lamina and the basilar crest of spiral ligament, or alternatively as the vibrating portion between the nuclei of inner pillar cells and the basilar crest of spiral ligament. While professional consensus generally favors the former definition, our morphometric study in CBA mice provides definitive evidence regarding width variations along the cochlear spiral. Precise measurements from the medial border

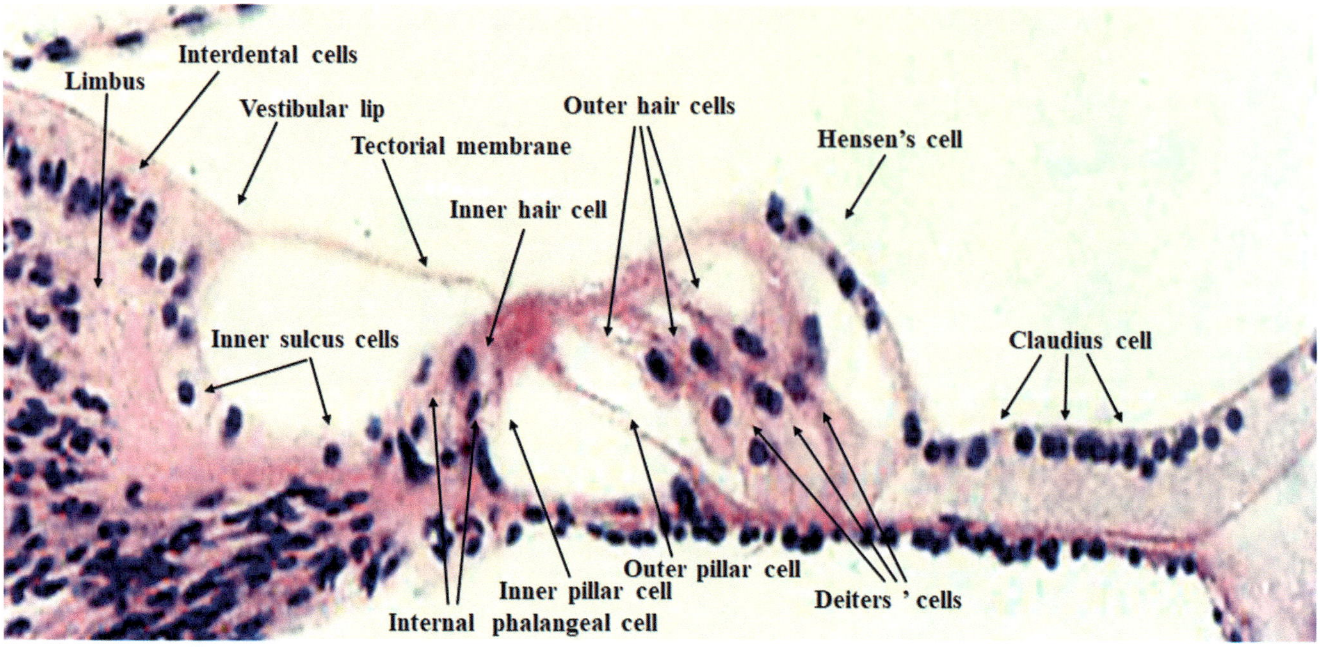

Fig. 6.8 Histological section of the cochlear basilar membrane in guinea pig. The cellular architecture of the organ of Corti includes the precisely arranged inner and outer hair cells, supporting cell network, and the triangular tunnel of Corti formed by pillar cells, with visible tectorial membrane relationships and basilar membrane structural integrity

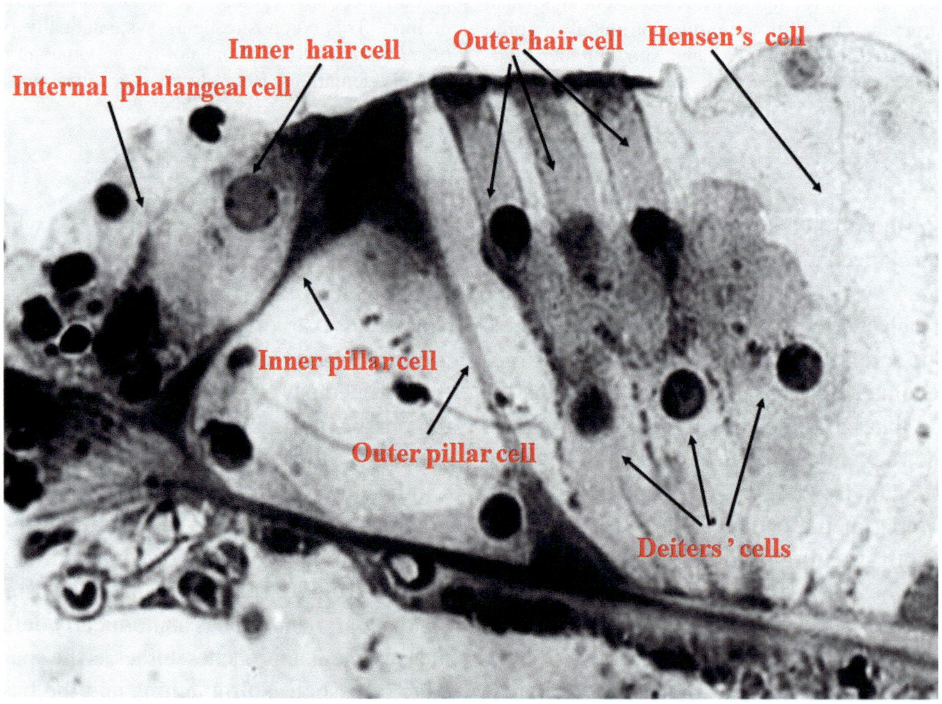

Fig. 6.9 High- magnification micrograph of a semi-thin section through the organ of Corti from a guinea pig. The characteristic cytoarchitecture of the organ of Corti includes the sensory hair cells (inner and outer rows) and the supporting cells (pillar cells, Deiters' cells, and Hensen's cells)

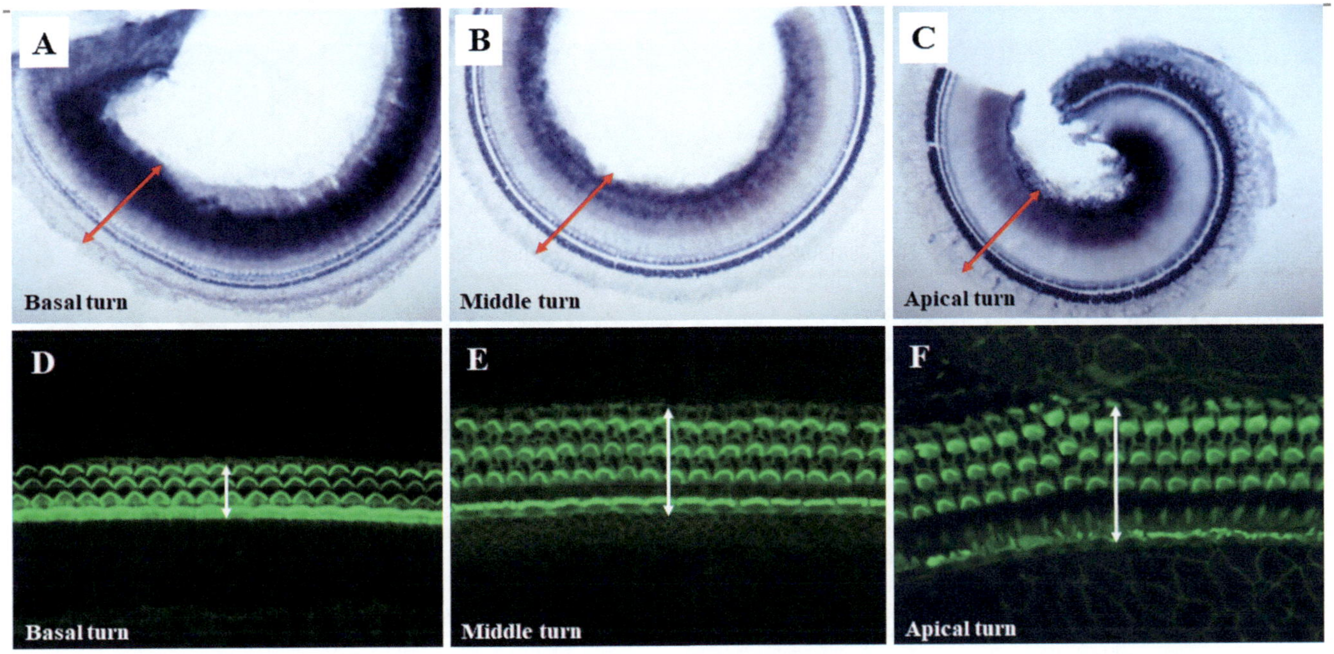

Fig. 6.10 Morphological changes of the width of the cochlear basilar membrane and the width of the organ of Corti on the surface preparation of rat cochlear basilar membrane. (**A–C**) Double-headed arrows indicate consistent basilar membrane width measurements across turns (basal, middle, and apical, respectively), revealing minimal dimensional variation along the cochlear spiral. (**D–F**) Corresponding organ of Corti measurements show progressive width expansion from the narrow basal turn (D) through intermediate middle turn (E) to the widest apical turn (F), establishing a clear inverse relationship between sensory organ dimensions and basilar membrane width. These morphological data demonstrate that frequency selectivity is determined by the organ of Corti's width gradient rather than basilar membrane dimensions, resolving a longstanding misconception in cochlear mechanics. The images provide visual confirmation that while the supporting basilar membrane maintains relatively constant width, the overlying sensory epithelium exhibits systematic variations that correlate precisely with characteristic frequency responses along the cochlear length

of osseous spiral lamina to the basilar crest of spiral ligament revealed a progressive narrowing pattern: 339.1 ± 9.87 μm at 1.5 mm from the basal turn origin, 304.5 ± 11.82 μm at 3 mm, and 300.1 ± 7.22 μm at 5 mm [11]. These findings demonstrate an inverse width of cochlear basilar membrane gradient from base to apex in murine cochleae, contradicting the conventional textbook description of basilar membrane widening toward the apex. The results clarify that while the organ of Corti shows characteristic width variations critical for frequency tuning, the basilar membrane itself exhibits an opposite dimensional trend that must be considered in cochlear biomechanical models. This distinction between membrane width and sensory organ dimensions resolves previous contradictions in the literature regarding cochlear structural gradients. Our measurements in rhesus monkeys demonstrate a consistent basilar membrane width gradient across species, with dimensions decreasing from 740.8 ± 29.63 μm in the basal turn to 690.8 ± 31.25 μm in the middle turn and 680 ± 31.45 μm in the apical turn, confirming the same narrowing trend observed in murine models. This pattern is visually evident in rat cochlear surface preparations (Fig. 6.10D–F), where both measurement methods—from the inner edge of osseous spiral lamina to the basilar crest of spiral ligament, and the functionally relevant vibrating portion between inner pillar cells and basilar crest—unequivocally show progressive width reduction from base to apex. These primate and rodent findings collectively establish that the basilar membrane's anatomical width follows an inverse gradient to the organ of Corti's dimensions, challenging conventional descriptions while providing empirical evidence for consistent cross-species structural patterns in cochlear architecture. The demonstrated width reduction correlates with known increases in membrane flexibility toward the apex, suggesting an integrated mechanical adaptation where dimensional changes complement material property variations to achieve optimal frequency-specific responsiveness along the cochlear spiral.

During embryonic development, mammalian cochlear hair cells transiently exhibit the primitive hair bundle organization seen in vestibular receptors—comprising a single kinocilium accompanied by multiple stereocilia. However, unlike vestibular hair cells which retain this configuration throughout life (Figs. 1.13 and 2.10), cochlear hair cells undergo complete kinocilium regression during late gestation, resulting in mature auditory receptors that possess only stereociliary bundles [1, 2, 4, 6]. This fundamental structural divergence raises important questions about functional specialization, as vestibular hair cells rely on their persistent kinocilium for establishing morphological polarity and directional sensitivity to mechanical stimuli [19] (Figs. 1.10 and 1.11). The absence of this polarizing organelle in cochlear hair cells suggests potential differences in stimulus transduction mechanisms and

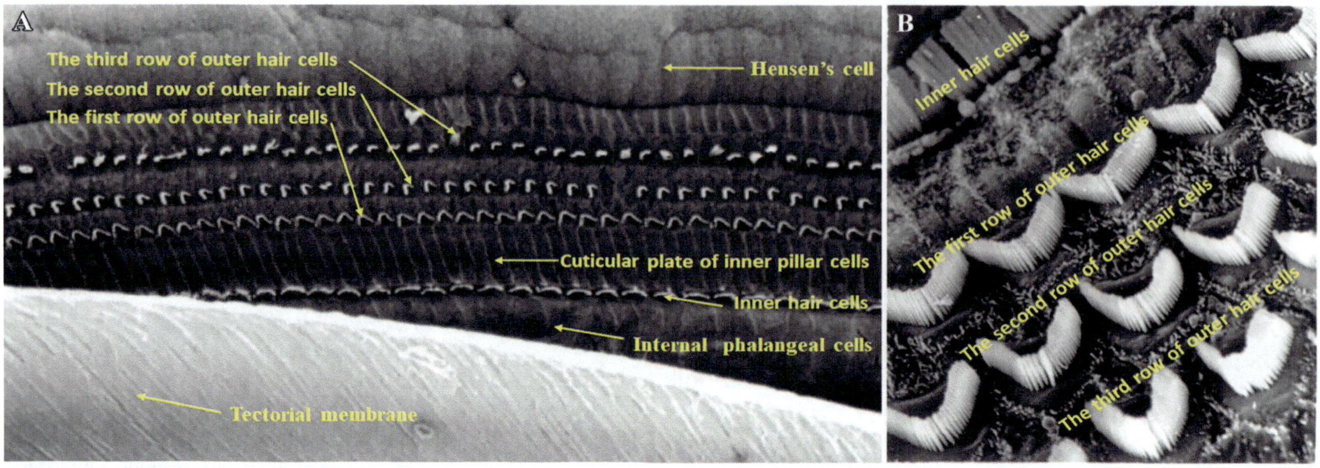

Fig. 6.11 Comparative surface morphology of cochlear sensory structures. (**A**) Scanning electron micrograph of chinchilla cochlear basilar membrane showing the characteristic arrangement of inner and outer hair cell stereociliary bundles. (**B**) High-resolution ultrastructural image of guinea pig hair cell stereocilia demonstrating the precise organization of actin-filled stereocilia and their tip links, with visible gradation in height across the bundle's rows. Both panels illustrate the species-conserved architectural specializations that facilitate mechanoelectrical transduction in the mammalian cochlea

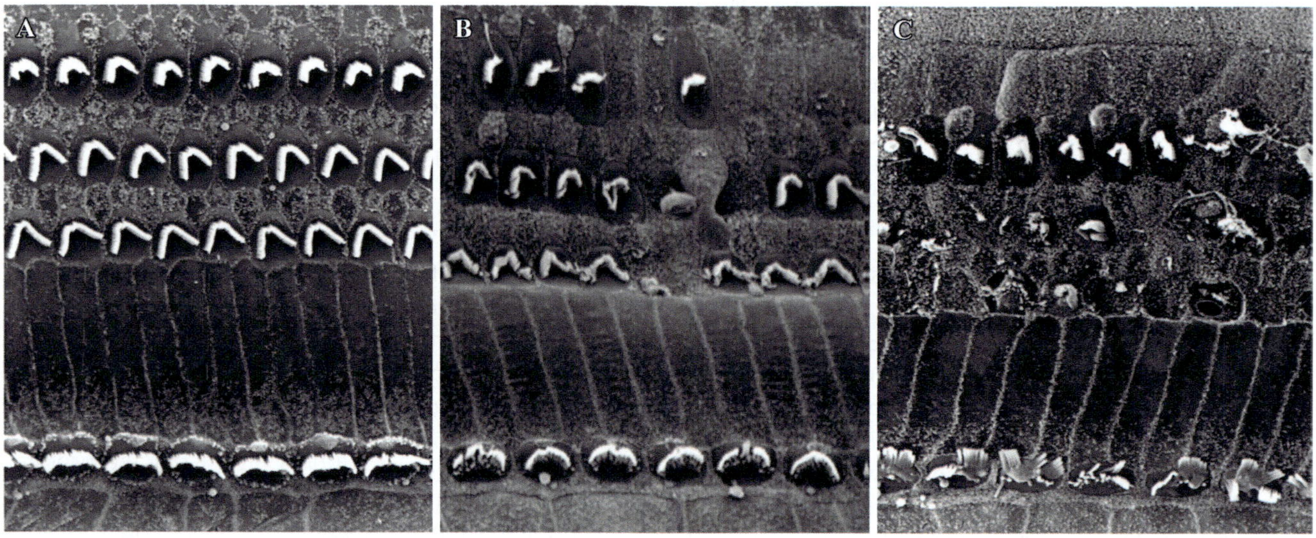

Fig. 6.12 Scanning electron micrographs of chinchilla cochlear sensory epithelium under normal and noise-exposed conditions. (**A**) Normal morphology showing intact stereociliary bundles on the cuticular plate of inner and outer hair cells. (**B**) Moderate noise-induced trauma demonstrating selective outer hair cell loss and stereocilia fusion while inner hair cells remain relatively preserved. (**C**) Severe acoustic damage revealing complete destruction of both inner and outer hair cells populations with residual scar formations, illustrating the vulnerability gradient of cochlear sensory cells to acoustic overstimulation. This series provides a progressive view of noise-induced cochleopathology from initial outer hair cell damage to complete sensory epithelium degeneration

neurotransmitter release patterns compared to their vestibular counterparts. While the kinocilium's role in vestibular mechanotransduction is well-established, whether and how cochlear hair cells compensate for its absence to achieve their exquisite frequency selectivity and rapid synaptic signaling remains an important area for future investigation, particularly regarding the potential alternative polarization mechanisms that may operate in the mature organ of Corti.

The stereociliary bundles of cochlear inner and outer hair cells exhibit distinct organizational patterns reflecting their functional specialization (Figs. 6.11 and 6.12). Inner hair cells display two arched rows of stereocilia on their oval cuticular plates, with the row adjacent to the inner pillar cells demonstrating greater height compared to the shorter row near the inner phalangeal and border cells (Fig. 6.13). In contrast, outer hair cells feature three rows of W-shaped stereocilia in a precisely graded staircase configuration on their circular cuticular plates, showing progressive height variation from the tallest row proximal to Hensen's cells to the shortest row facing the outer pillar cells [1, 2, 4, 6, 9] (Fig. 6.14). These stereocilia

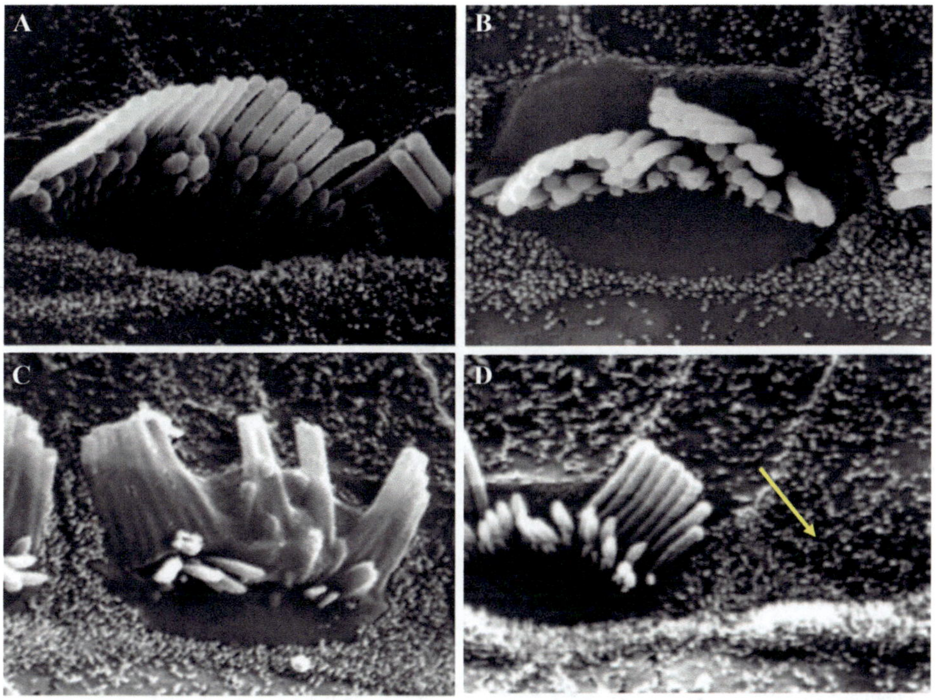

Fig. 6.13 Scanning electron micrographs of chinchilla inner hair cell stereocilia under normal and pathological conditions. (**A**) Normal morphology showing the characteristic two-rowed stereociliary bundle with height asymmetry—longer stereocilia oriented toward inner pillar cells and shorter stereocilia facing inner phalangeal cells. (**B**) Initial damage phase demonstrating early bundle disorganization while maintaining cellular integrity. (**C**) Progressive pathology featuring stereocilia fusion preferentially affecting the taller stereociliary row. (**D**) Terminal phase showing complete hair cell loss with subsequent epithelial repair through integration of the cuticular plates of inner pillar cells and the surfaces of inner phalangeal cells, illustrating the limited regenerative capacity of hair cells. This sequence documents the stereotypical progression of inner hair cell degeneration from initial stereociliary damage to final scar formation

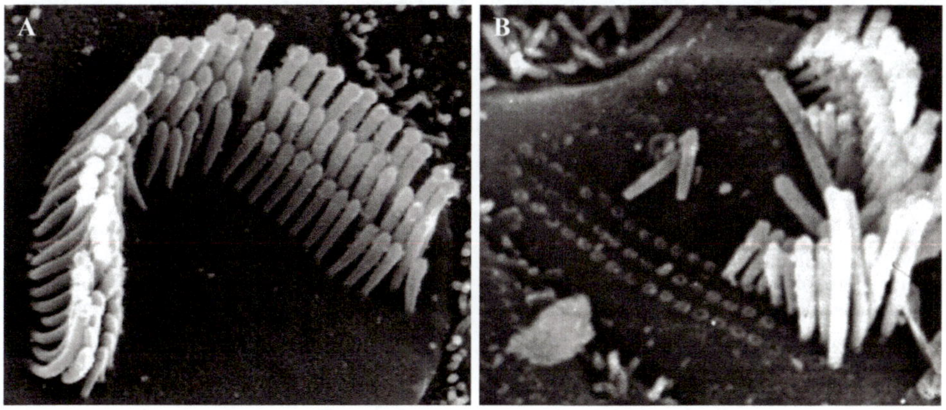

Fig. 6.14 Scanning electron micrographs of stereocilia on cuticular plate of outer hair cell under physiological and ototoxic conditions. (**A**) Normal ultrastructure demonstrating the characteristic three-rowed, W-shaped stereociliary bundle with precise staircase organization on the cuticular plate of outer hair cells in guinea pig. (**B**) Kanamycin-induced ototoxicity showing complete stereocilia loss while preserving the structural integrity of cuticular plate, with distinct residual implantation pits marking the original positions of all three stereociliary rows—providing clear morphological evidence of the selective targeting of kanamycin to the mechanosensory apparatus while sparing the cellular scaffold. This comparison highlights both the sophisticated organization of healthy outer hair cell bundles and the stereotypical pattern of aminoglycoside-induced damage that preferentially affects the stereociliary machinery essential for cochlear amplification

arrangements create mechanically tuned structures that optimize frequency-specific stimulation—the asymmetrical bundle of stereocilia on inner hair cells enhances directional sensitivity to basilar membrane displacement, while the stepped array of stereocilia on outer hair cell facilitates active cochlear amplification through coordinated bundle movement. The

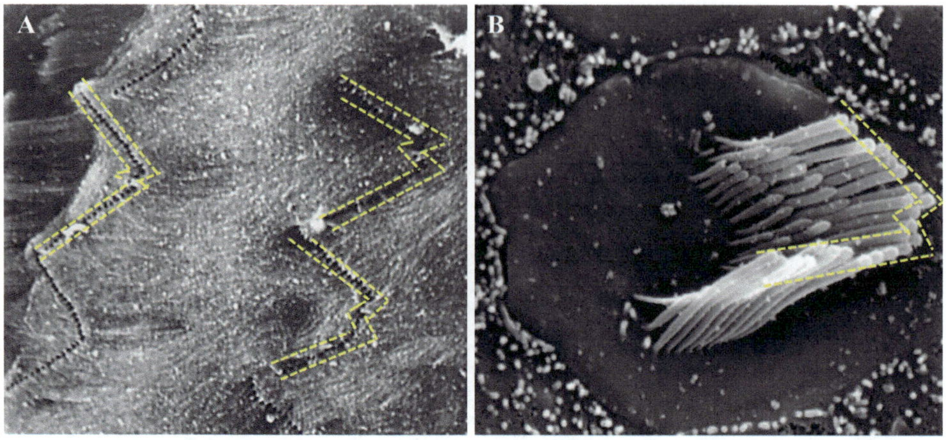

Fig. 6.15 Scanning electron micrograph showing traces of the insertion of the longest row of stereocilia of outer hair cell on the tectorial membrane. (**A**) Tectorial membrane surface showing precise linear arrays of implantation pits corresponding to the longest (third-row) stereocilia of outer hair cells. (**B**) Higher magnification revealing the one-to-one topographic relationship between these pits and the apical-most stereociliary row, indicating selective insertion of only the longest stereocilia while the shorter first and second rows remain unattached. This anatomical evidence suggests a sophisticated mechanical coupling mechanism where the tectorial membrane engages specifically with the tallest stereociliary elements to optimize frequency-specific stimulation while maintaining appropriate tension gradients across the hair bundle during cochlear micromechanics

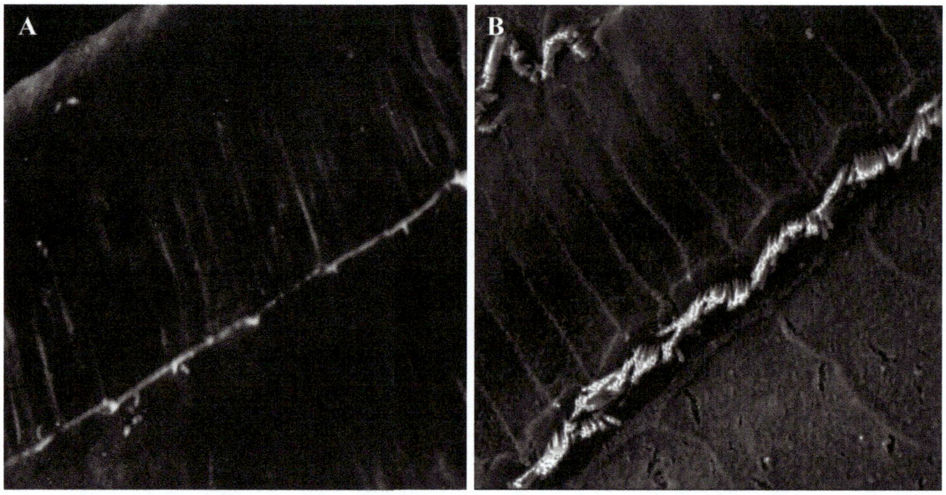

Fig. 6.16 Traces of insertion of the stereocilia of inner hair cell on the tectorial membrane. (**A**) Tectorial membrane surface showing distinct imprint patterns corresponding to the taller stereociliary row of inner hair cells. (**B**) Comparative morphology demonstrating precise alignment between these impressions and the longer stereocilia facing the inner pillar cells, confirming their physical insertion while the shorter stereociliary row remains free-standing. This anatomical relationship suggests a differential coupling mechanism where selective engagement of the taller stereocilia facilitates mechanical stimulation while maintaining appropriate bundle mobility during auditory transduction

morphological differences between the two hair cell types correspond to their distinct roles in auditory transduction, with inner hair cells primarily serving as sensory receptors and outer hair cells functioning as mechanical amplifiers.

While conventional anatomical descriptions suggest that only the stereocilia of outer hair cells are inserted into the tectorial membrane, the presence of distinct stereocilia imprint patterns of both inner and outer hair cell stereocilia was detected on the tectorial membrane surface (Figs. 6.15 and 6.16). This indicates that the long stereocilia on both inner and outer hair cells may maintain physical connections with the tectorial membrane. During acoustic stimulation, the differential motion between the basilar membrane (anchored to the osseous spiral lamina) and the tectorial membrane (attached to the vestibular lip on the spiral limbus) generates shear forces that deflect the long stereocilia of the inner and outer hair cells inserted into the tectorial membrane. This coordinated mechanical interaction facilitates simultaneous activation of both hair cell populations—outer hair cells undergoing active electromotile responses for cochlear amplification, while inner hair cells initiate afferent neurotransmission. The observed imprint patterns challenge textbook paradigms by suggesting a more

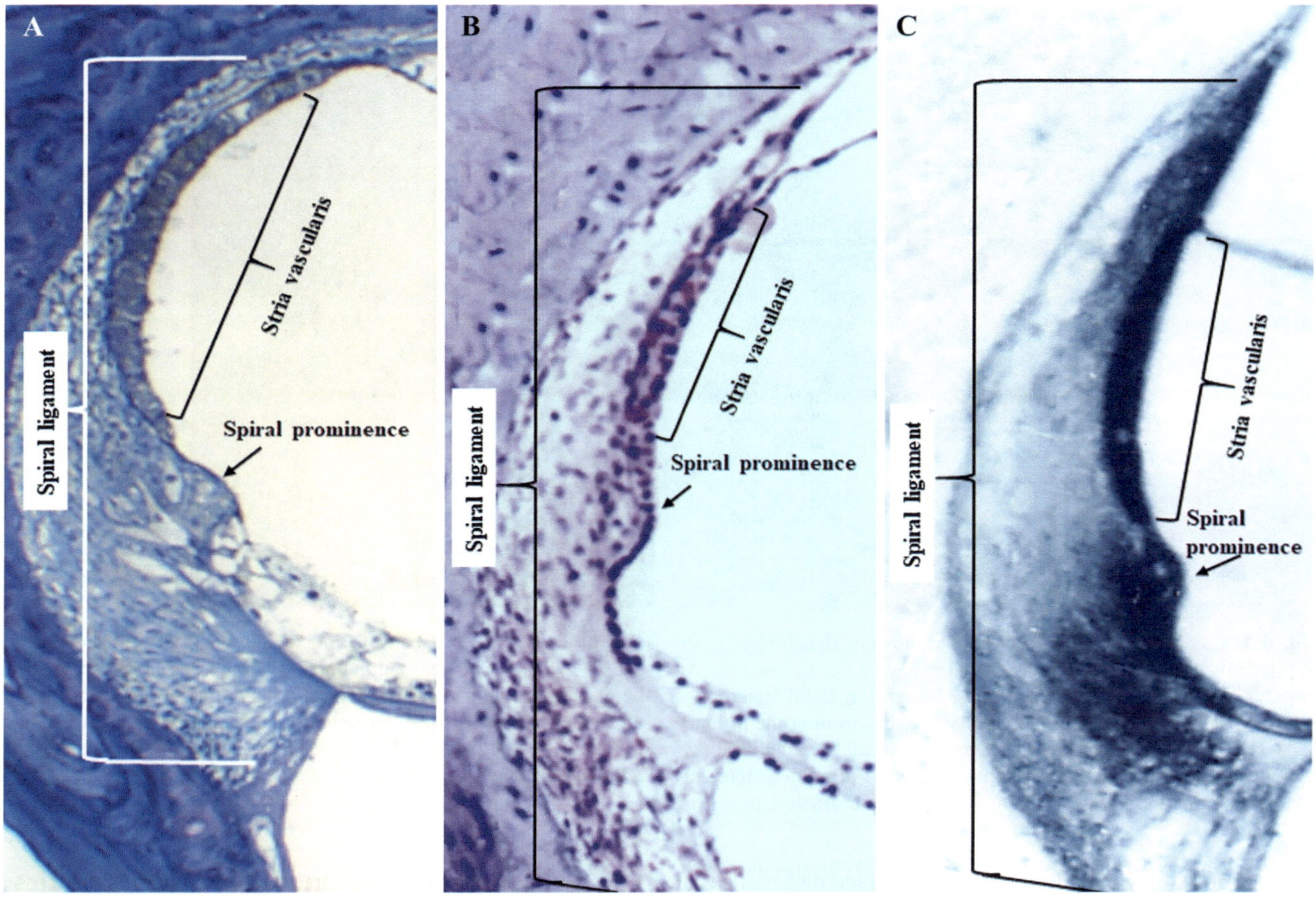

Fig. 6.17 Histological characteristics of the spiral ligament revealed by different staining methods. (**A**) Semi-thin plastic section of mouse spiral ligament demonstrating cytoarchitecture through toluidine blue staining, highlighting cellular organization and extracellular matrix components. (**B**) Collodion-embedded guinea pig specimen stained with hematoxylin-eosin revealing classical histological features of fibrocyte populations and vascular networks. (**C**) Cryosection of guinea pig tissue stained for succinate dehydrogenase activity visualization, highlighting the intense aerobic metabolic activity patterns within the epithelial cells at the stria vascularis. This multimodal presentation enables comparative analysis of structural and functional properties across different technical approaches while maintaining anatomical reference points for orientation within the lateral cochlear wall

integrated mechanical system where both hair cell types participate directly in tectorial membrane-mediated stimulation, with their stereociliary displacements being mechanically coupled during the traveling wave propagation along the cochlear partition. This revised understanding better explains the precise timing requirements for phase-locked neural responses across the auditory frequency spectrum.

6.2.2 Structural Organization of the Cochlear Duct Lateral Wall

The lateral boundary of the cochlear duct is formed by specialized epithelial and connective tissue structures extending between two critical attachment points: Reissner's membrane inserts at the vestibular crest of the spiral ligament, while the basilar membrane anchors at the ligament's basilar crest, delineating the medial surface of the spiral ligament as the duct's lateral wall. This region exhibits distinct histological specializations, including the spiral prominence—a ridge of cuboidal epithelial cells—and the stria vascularis, a stratified epithelial bed extending from the prominence to Reissner's membrane attachment. The stria vascularis displays a unique trilaminar organization: (1) endolymph-facing marginal cells with extensive basal infoldings, (2) a highly vascularized intermediate layer containing dark cells and capillary networks, and (3) a basal cell layer forming tight junctions with the underlying spiral ligament (Fig. 6.17). This structural arrangement facilitates the stria's dual functions in maintaining the endocochlear potential through ion transport and providing metabolic support to adjacent cochlear structures, with the spiral ligament serving as both mechanical support and ion reservoir. The precise spatial relationships between these components create the anatomical foundation for the cochlea's electrochemical gradients and mechanical stability. The stria vascularis exhibits cellular heterogeneity beyond its

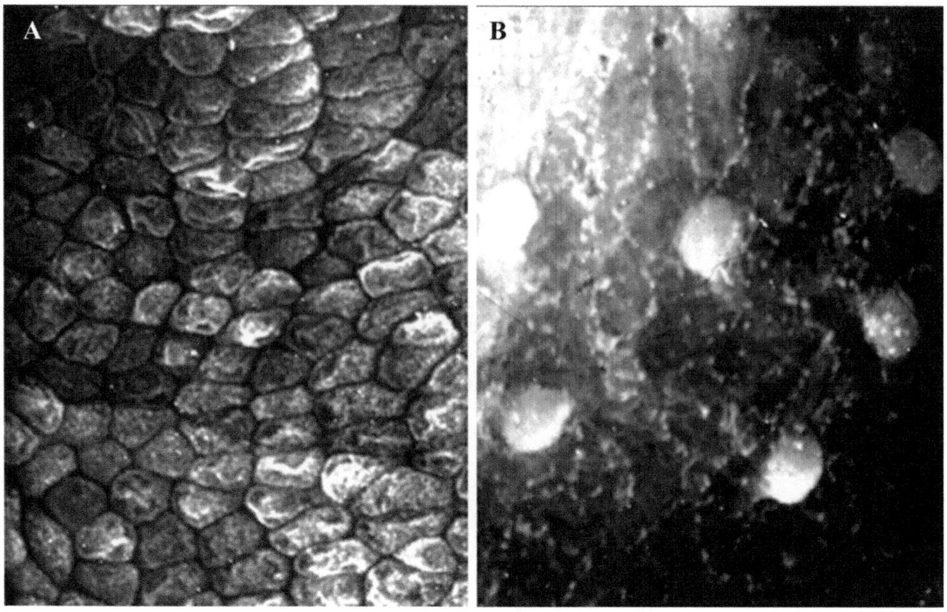

Fig. 6.18 Scanning electron micrograph showing the ultrastructure of bilateral surface of the Reissner's membrane of the guinea pig. (**A**) Endolymphatic surface (scala media aspect) revealing tightly interposed epithelial cells with minimal intercellular spaces, forming the primary barrier interface. (**B**) Perilymphatic surface (scala vestibuli aspect) showing loosely arranged mesothelial cells with prominent intercellular gaps, consistent with selective permeability characteristics. This structural asymmetry supports the membrane's functional specialization, where the dense epithelial layer maintains ionic segregation between endolymph and perilymph compartments while the porous mesothelial layer permits controlled fluid exchange, reflecting an evolutionary adaptation for simultaneous barrier function and homeostatic regulation in cochlear physiology

three principal layers, containing interspersed dark cells that span the entire epithelial thickness from the marginal cell surface to the basal cell layer [20–22]. Dark cells in black-eyed pigmented experimental animals contain melanin, while dark cells in red-eyed albino experimental animals do not. Regardless of whether they contain melanin or not, these dark cells participate in the essential functions of the stria vascularis in endolymph production, ion homeostasis, and generation of intracochlear electrical potentials. Adjacent to this secretory epithelium, the spiral prominence's cuboidal epithelial cells remain functionally enigmatic, while the external sulcus region between the prominence and basilar crest forms part of the potassium recycling pathway critical for hair cell transduction. The underlying spiral ligament comprises a specialized fibrovascular network—containing fibroblasts, extracellular matrix, and blood vessels—whose intercellular spaces communicate with the perilymphatic compartment, facilitating ion exchange between vascular and fluid systems [1, 2, 4, 6, 23]. This integrated structural complex maintains the precise electrochemical environment required for auditory transduction while providing mechanical stabilization of the cochlear partition. The presence of melanin in dark cells correlates with their proposed roles in oxidative stress protection and ion transport regulation, though the evolutionary conservation of non-pigmented variants in albino animals suggests additional, pigment-independent functions in cochlear homeostasis.

6.2.3 Structural and Functional Characteristics of Reissner's Membrane

Reissner's membrane forms the upper boundary of the cochlear duct, creating a critical partition between the endolymph-filled scala media and perilymph-containing scala vestibuli. This delicate 2 μm-thick bilayer structure consists of two layers of morphologically distinct cell layers: a densely packed squamous epithelial layer facing the endolymph with abundant microvilli, and a sparsely distributed mesothelial layer adjacent to the perilymph, separated by a well-defined basal lamina (Fig. 6.18). Functioning synergistically with the spiral ligament and basilar membrane, Reissner's membrane maintains the unique electrochemical environment essential for auditory transduction, preserving the +70–90 mV endocochlear potential through selective ionic permeability. Beyond its barrier functions, this membrane serves multiple physiological roles: (1) attenuating mechanical interference from vestibular scala vasculature, (2) facilitating perilymphatic flow between scala vestibuli and scala tympani via the helicotrema, and (3) enabling precise frequency-specific basilar membrane vibrations in response to traveling wave propagation [24–27]. The membrane's ultrastructural specialization reflects its dual capacity as both a selective ionic barrier and a mechanically compliant partition, allowing passive displacement during acoustic stimulation while maintaining the electrochemical gradients fundamental to cochlear amplification. Experimental evidence demonstrates

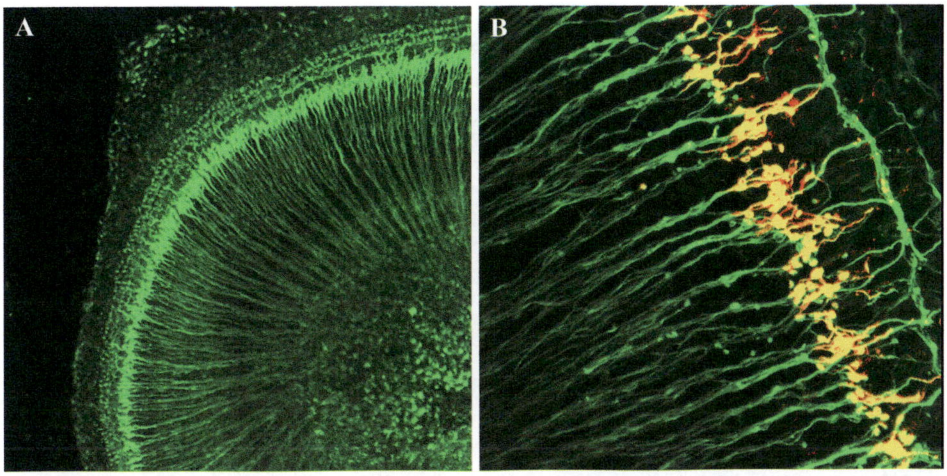

Fig. 6.19 Neuroanatomical organization of cochlear afferent innervation. (**A**) Anti-Tubulin antibody immunolabeling revealing the complete arborization pattern of auditory nerve fibers and their synaptic terminals within the organ of Corti in rat, demonstrating the dense neural network supporting hair cell connectivity. (**B**) Double immunofluorescence combining anti-neurofilament-200 antibody (axonal marker, green) and anti-synapsin antibody (presynaptic marker, orange) staining, providing simultaneous visualization of afferent fiber trajectories and their type I synaptic specializations at hair cell interfaces, highlighting the precise spatial relationship between neural processes and sensory targets in cochlear circuitry. This dual-panel presentation captures both the global distribution and molecular specialization of afferent innervation patterns essential for auditory signal transmission

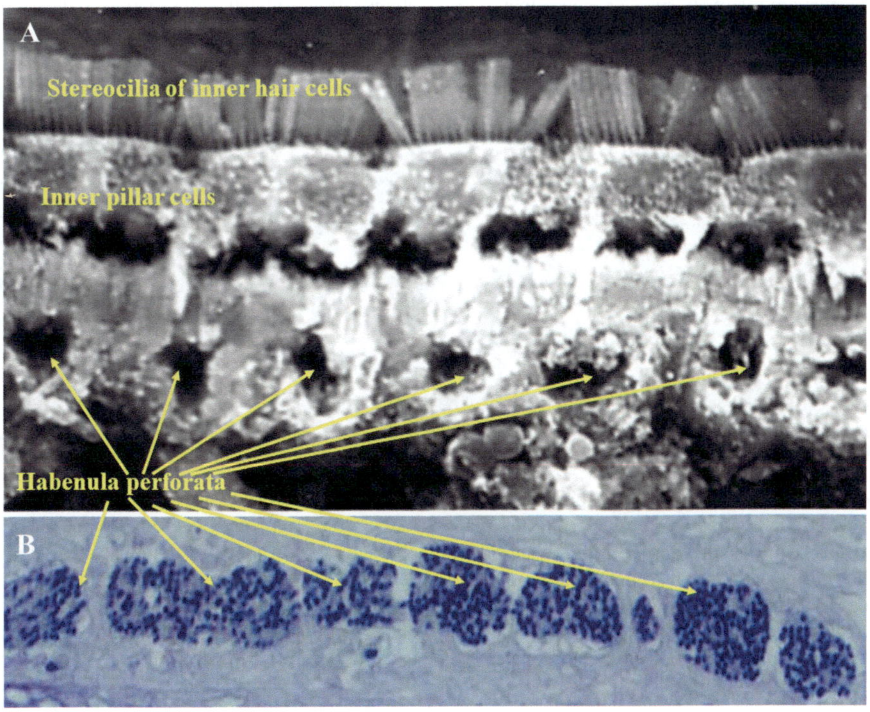

Fig. 6.20 Structural gateway for cochlear neural transmission through the habenula perforata. (**A**) Scanning electron micrograph detailing the perforated architecture of the osseous spiral lamina, showing the precise array of neural transit channels that permit passage of afferent and efferent fibers between Rosenthal's canal and the organ of Corti. (**B**) Light micrograph of a semi-thin cross-section through the habenula perforata demonstrating the auditory afferent nerve fibers of peripheral spiral ganglion neurons in Rosenthal's canal and the cochlear efferent nerve fibers within the habenula perforata, illustrating the neural connection between the spiral ganglion neurons and the sensory hair cells in the organ of Corti. Together these images reveal the specialized osteo-neural interface that coordinates the bidirectional flow of auditory information while maintaining mechanical stability of the cochlear partition

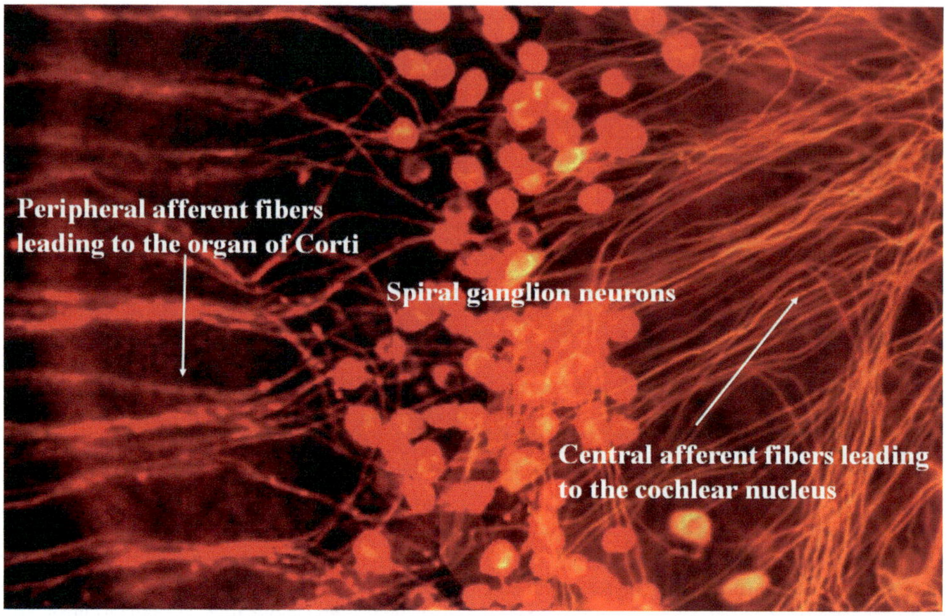

Fig. 6.21 Neural architecture of spiral ganglion neurons and their projections. Peripheral afferent fibers extending through the osseous spiral lamina to form specialized synaptic contacts with cochlear hair cells, demonstrating the precise tonotopic organization of these sensory connections. The peripheral nerve fibers of the spiral ganglion leading to the organ of Corti in the cochlea are relatively sparse because they pass through the hebanula perforata, while their central nerve fibers of the spiral ganglion leading to the central auditory pathway are relatively dense because they converge into the cochlear neuroforamen. This dual projection system highlights the spiral ganglion's pivotal role as the first neural relay in the auditory pathway, maintaining strict frequency-specific organization from hair cell synapses to the cochlear nucleus in brainstem

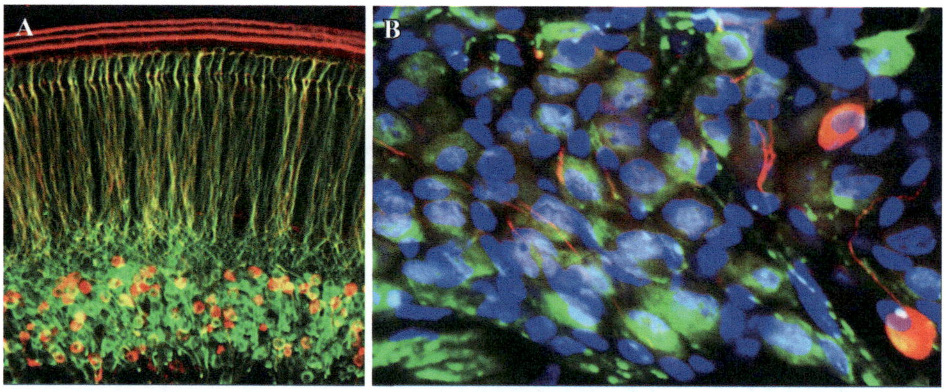

Fig. 6.22 Immunohistochemical differentiation of spiral ganglion neuron subtypes. (**A**) Selective labeling of type II spiral ganglion neurons and their peripheral fibers (red) using anti-peripherin antibody, demonstrating their distinct projection pattern to outer hair cells. (**B**) Dual-channel fluorescence revealing the complementary distribution of type I neurons (green, anti-neurofilament-200) and type II neurons (red, anti-peripherin) within Rosenthal's canal, with their respective fiber trajectories showing the type I neurons' dense innervation of inner hair cells versus type II neurons' sparse outer hair cell connections. This characterization visually demonstrates the fundamental dichotomy in spiral ganglion organization that underlies parallel auditory processing pathways—the numerically dominant type I system for precise frequency coding and the specialized type II network for cochlear feedback modulation

Reissner's membrane plays an active role in cochlear ionic regulation through selective sodium absorption from endolymph, while ultrastructural studies reveal a distinct interstitial compartment between its epithelial and mesothelial layers that may facilitate novel transport mechanisms [28]. This morphological specialization suggests the membrane participates in both established and potentially undiscovered pathways for maintaining cochlear fluid homeostasis, extending beyond its classical role as a passive barrier to include active regulation of the endolymphatic environment. The observed subcellular architecture implies the existence of sophisticated transport systems that may involve transcellular and paracellular routes working in concert to modulate the composition of cochlear fluids, though the precise molecular mechanisms underlying

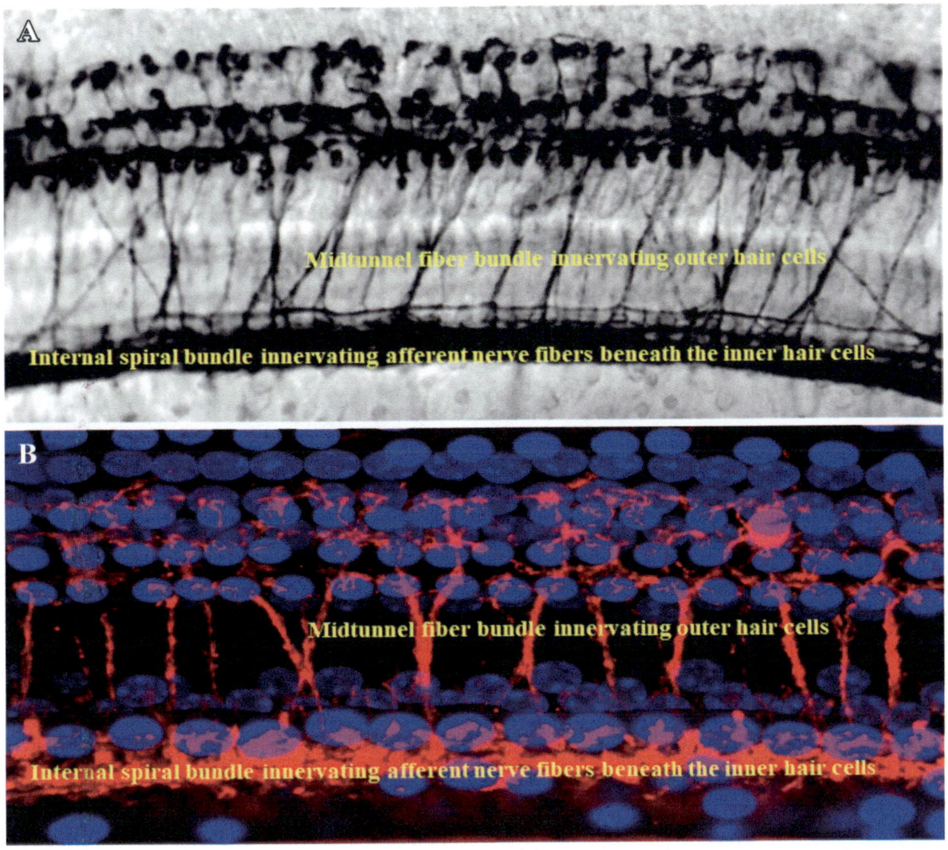

Fig. 6.23 Acetylcholinesterase staining showing the distribution pattern of cochlear efferent nerve innervation. (**A**) Acetylcholinesterase histochemistry revealing the complete trajectory of efferent fibers from habenula perforata to their terminal arborizations, highlighting the medial olivocochlear projections to outer hair cells and lateral olivocochlear fibers in the inner spiral bundle. (**B**) Immunohistochemical staining using anti-acetylcholinesterase antibody specifically marks the distribution of cochlear efferent nerve fibers in the cochlear basilar membrane. These stainings validate the distinct termination pattern of the efferent pathways while illustrating their shared cholinergic neurotransmission mechanisms in cochlear feedback regulation

these processes remain to be fully elucidated. These findings position Reissner's membrane as a dynamic interface rather than merely a structural partition, contributing to the precise ionic balance required for normal auditory function through both characterized and putative regulatory pathways.

6.3 Nervous System of the Cochlea

The cochlear nervous system comprises two functionally distinct pathways: the afferent system, which conducts mechanoelectrical signals from sensory hair cells to central auditory nuclei through spiral ganglion neurons, and the efferent system originating primarily in the superior olivary complex that provides modulation of cochlear function based on signals from the auditory center. This bidirectional neural network enables both bottom-up signal transmission and top-down control of auditory sensitivity, with type I afferent fibers (innervating inner hair cells) constituting 95% of the auditory nerve for precise sound encoding, while medial olivocochlear efferent synapses connect the outer hair cells and type I afferent nerve fibers to regulate the sensitivity of the cochlea to sound stimulation through cholinergic inhibition [1, 2, 4, 6]. The intricate spatial organization of these neural elements—including their selective hair cell connectivity patterns and tonotopic projections—forms the structural basis for both faithful sound representation and dynamic range adaptation in the auditory pathway.

6.3.1 Cochlear Afferent Nerve Pathway

The primary auditory afferents originate from bipolar spiral ganglion neurons residing in Rosenthal's canal within the cochlear modiolus. These specialized neurons extend peripheral processes that traverse the habenula perforata openings in the osseous spiral lamina to form synaptic contacts with both inner and outer hair cells on the basilar membrane [1, 2, 4, 6, 16, 17, 29–34]. Their central axons import to the auditory nerve bundle within the cochlear neuroforamen through small foramina in the medial bony wall of Rosenthal's canal, ultimately synapsing in the cochlear nuclei of the brainstem to initiate central auditory processing [16, 17, 35]. This precisely organized pathway exhibits tonotopic organization from periphery to center, with type I myelinated fibers (comprising 95% of afferents) forming specialized synapses exclusively with inner hair cells for high-fidelity signal transmission, while the remaining type II unmyelinated fibers predominantly contact outer hair cells, potentially serving protective or modulatory functions [1, 2, 4, 6, 36, 37] (Fig. 1.1; Figs. 6.19–6.21). The spatial segregation of these neural elements within Rosenthal's canal mirrors their distinct functional roles in auditory transduction and processing.

The spiral ganglion neurons exhibit dichotomous morphological and functional specialization, with type I neurons comprising 95% of the population and forming exclusive, divergent connections to inner hair cells (Fig. 6.22). Each type I neuron usually receives an auditory signal from one inner hair cell, and one inner hair cell establishes synaptic connections with about 20 type I afferent neurons, which means that one inner hair cell can send auditory signals to multiple type I spiral ganglia simultaneously, thereby achieving precise signal amplification and processing. In contrast, the smaller type II population (5%) demonstrates opposite connectivity logic—these neurons establish convergent serial connections with outer hair cells, where each type II neuron integrates input from 15 to 20 outer hair cells while each outer hair cell projects to only one type II neuron [1, 2, 4, 6]. This striking dichotomy in innervation patterns reflects fundamental differences in their functional roles: type I neurons mediate high-fidelity auditory transmission through parallel processing, while type II neurons likely serve integrative or modulatory functions through their widespread outer hair cell networks. The structural specialization extends to their myelination patterns and central projections, with type I neurons being heavily myelinated for rapid signal conduction to cochlear nuclei, whereas type II neurons remain unmyelinated, consistent with their proposed role in cochlear feedback regulation rather than primary acoustic encoding.

6.3.2 Efferent Modulation of Cochlear Function

The auditory efferent pathway originating in the superior olivary complex that mediate top-down control of auditory processing. The cochlea is innervated by two cholinergic feedback pathways. They are respectively termed the medial olivocochlear pathway and the lateral olivocochlear pathway. The olivocochlear bundles project to both the ipsilateral and contralateral cochleae. The medial olivocochlear pathway sends control signals from the brainstem to the cochlear outer hair cells, and the lateral olivocochlear pathway sends control signals from brainstem to the auditory nerve fibers beneath the inner hair cells. The cochlear efferent nerve fibers from the medial olive body enter the cochlear basilar membrane via the habenula perforata and form the upper tunnel radiation bundle to cross the tunnel of Corti to establish synaptic connections with the outer hair cells. The cochlear efferent nerve fibers from the lateral olive body enter the cochlear basilar membrane also via the habenula perforata and form the internal spiral bundle to establish synaptic connections to the type I afferent nerve fibers beneath the inner hair cells (Fig. 6.23). The function of the medial olivocochlear efferents innervating the outer hair cells is considered to inhibit the activity of outer hair cells and thereby reducing the gain of cochlear amplification. The function of the lateral olivocochlear efferent innervating the auditory afferent fibers beneath the inner hair cells is considered to reduce the chance of auditory neuropathy by inhibiting the presynaptic glutamatergic transmission and inhibiting the activity of cochlear afferent fibers [1, 2, 4, 6]. The system's bilaterality provides noise protection through contralateral suppression reflexes, while its differential terminal patterns reflect specialized mechanisms for controlling mechanical versus neural aspects of auditory transduction. This sophisticated feedback architecture demonstrates how central auditory structures dynamically regulate peripheral sensitivity to optimize signal detection in complex acoustic environments.

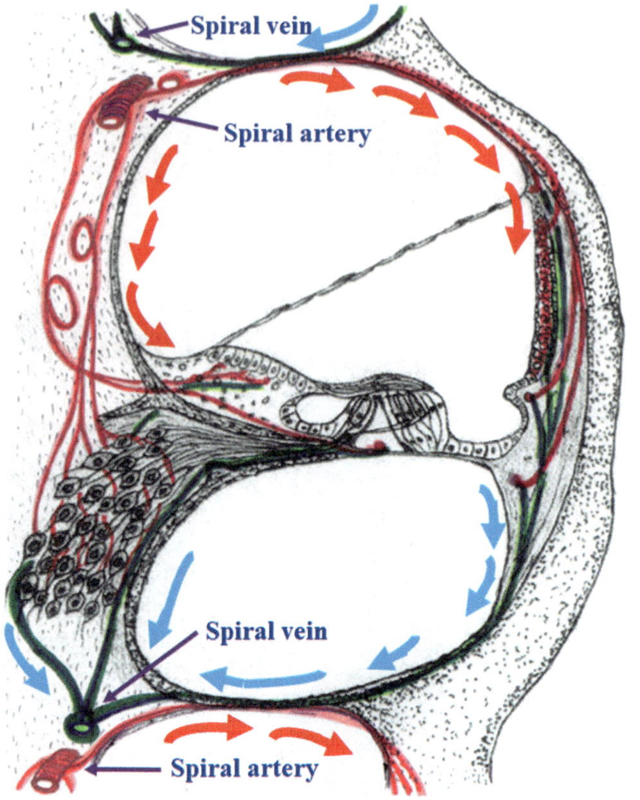

Fig. 6.24 The pattern of cochlear blood circulation

6.4 Vascular Supply and Metabolic Exchange in the Cochlea

The cochlear membranous labyrinth receives its arterial blood supply through branches of the labyrinthine artery originating from the vertebrobasilar system, with venous drainage occurring via the superior and inferior petrosal sinuses that ultimately empty into the internal jugular vein. This vascular network features a unique straight-through capillary architecture connecting arterial and venous systems, suggesting highly efficient metabolic exchange during single circulatory passes [1, 2, 4, 6]. The specialized arrangement of cochlear vasculature—particularly the stria vascularis capillary beds and spiral ligament vessels—appears optimized for rapid ion transport and endolymph homeostasis, though the precise mechanisms governing transcellular exchange between the vascular compartment and cochlear epithelial cells remain incompletely characterized. Current gaps in understanding include the molecular pathways mediating substance transfer across blood-labyrinth barriers, temporal dynamics of metabolic exchange, and regulatory mechanisms coordinating vascular perfusion with cochlear bioelectrical activity—all representing critical areas for future investigation given their implications for hearing preservation and therapeutic intervention.

6.4.1 Cochlear Artery Vascularity

The labyrinthine artery, coursing through the internal auditory canal's dura mater, bifurcates into the common cochlear artery and anterior vestibular artery at the temporal bone's canal openings. The common cochlear artery further divides into two principal branches: (1) the main cochlear branch forming spiral modiolar arteries that ascend through Rosenthal's canal to vascularize the cochlear apex and second turn, and (2) the vestibulocochlear branch emitting three subdivisions—one spiraling artery supplying the basal turn and two vestibular branches penetrating the middle/inferior sieve areas to perfuse the saccule, utricle, and posterior semicircular canal system (Fig. 1.31). This dual-origin supply creates overlapping vascular territories, with the modiolar spiral arteries (main cochlear branch) predominantly serving the apical cochlear turns while the vestibulocochlear branch's spiral artery exclusively supplies the basal turn, demonstrating both anatomical segregation and functional redundancy in cochlear perfusion [1, 2, 4, 6]. The spiral modiolar arteries maintain consistent caliber throughout their ascent, reflecting their critical role in maintaining the metabolic demands of high-frequency processing regions, while their anastomoses with vestibulocochlear branches provide collateral circulation that may protect against ischemic damage in the vulnerable basal turn.

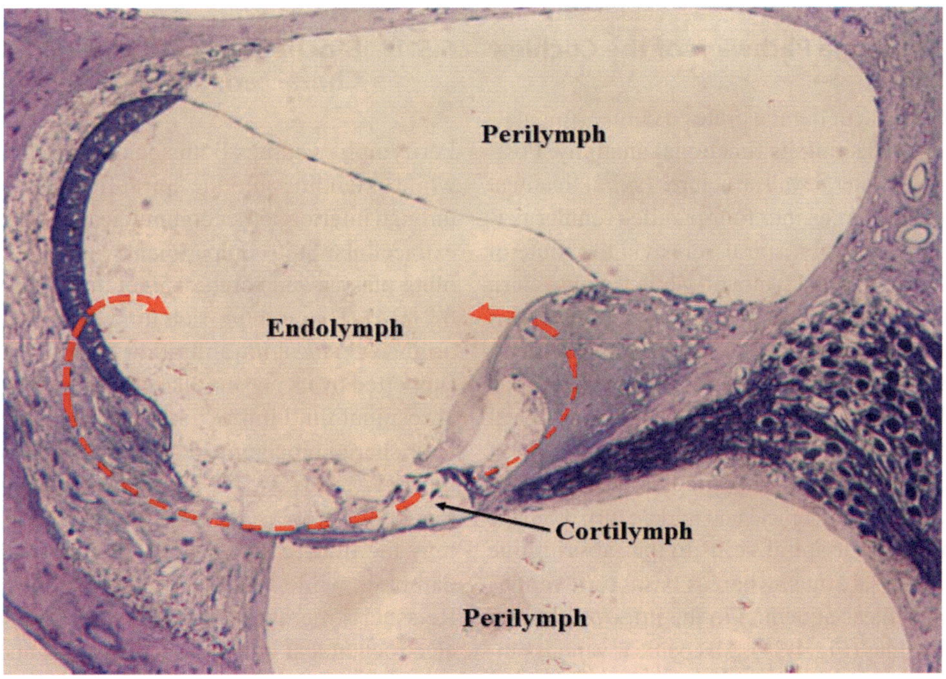

Fig. 6.25 Distribution of endolymph in the cochlear cavity and the medial and lateral pathways of endolymph circulation through the basilar membrane

6.4.2 Microvascular Architecture of the Cochlea

The spiral modiolar arteries within Rosenthal's canal emit seven distinct capillary networks that radially perfuse cochlear structures through precise vascular distributions. Lateral projections form four functional capillary beds: (1) vestibular crest capillaries supplying Reissner's membrane attachments, (2) stria vascularis capillaries maintaining endocochlear potential, (3) spiral prominence capillaries, and (4) inferior spiral ligament capillaries near scala tympani—all arterial capillaries travel along the lateral wall through the submucosal membrane of the lateral wall of scala vestibuli. Medial projections similarly divide into three specialized networks servicing the spiral limbus, tunnel of Corti vasculature, and spiral ganglion neuronal clusters. This dichotomized vascular organization creates discrete metabolic zones where arterial-venous conversion occurs immediately after capillary exchange, suggesting highly localized regulation of cochlear homeostasis [1, 2, 4, 6, 23, 38, 39] (Fig. 6.24). The stria vascularis and spiral ganglion capillary beds demonstrate particularly dense anastomoses, reflecting their high metabolic demands for endolymph production and neural activity, respectively, while the tunnel of Corti's sparse vasculature correlates with its avascular organ of Corti. This specialized angioarchitecture supports both generalized cochlear metabolism and structure-specific functional requirements through differential perfusion patterns.

6.4.3 Venous Drainage Pathways of the Cochlea

The cochlear venous system demonstrates a compartmentalized drainage pattern reflecting its functional anatomy. Post-capillary blood from the lateral wall structures (spiral ligament and stria vascularis) converges into four parallel venular networks before entering modiolar spiral veins via the route of subperiosteal capillaries of scala tympani, while venous return from basilar membrane and Rosenthal's canal regions drains directly into the modiolar spiral veins. Two principal collecting systems—the anterior spiral vein (draining spiral lamina and scala vestibuli) and posterior spiral vein (serving spiral ganglion, cochlear duct lateral wall, and scala tympani)—form the major venous return pathways. Topographic specialization exists along the cochlear spiral: apical and middle turn drainage proceeds through modiolar spiral veins to the labyrinthine vein and superior petrosal sinus, whereas basal turn venous return follows the cochlear aqueduct to the inferior petrosal sinus' lateral venous sinus (Fig. 1.34). All cochlear venous outflow ultimately converges into the internal jugular vein, completing the circulatory loop [1, 2, 4, 6, 23, 38]. This drainage architecture maintains precise pressure gradients essential for cochlear fluid homeostasis while providing multiple collateral pathways that may protect against venous congestion in this metabolically sensitive organ. The separation of scala-specific drainage routes suggests functional adaptation to the distinct biochemical requirements of various cochlear compartments.

6.5 Compartmentalization of Cochlear Lymphatic Fluids

The cochlea maintains three distinct extracellular fluid compartments with specialized ionic compositions: (1) potassium-rich endolymph filling the scala media, (2) sodium-dominated perilymph occupying both scala vestibuli and scala tympani, and (3) cortilymph—a perilymph-like fluid bathing the organ of Corti's interstitial spaces (Fig. 6.25). These fluid systems create segregated electrochemical environments essential for auditory transduction, with the endolymph's +80 mV endocochlear potential driving mechanoelectrical conversion, while perilymph and cortilymph maintain neural excitability through their neuron-friendly composition. The tight regulation of these fluid compartments occurs through multiple barrier systems, including Reissner's membrane and basilar membrane (separating endolymph from perilymph), reticular lamina of the organ of Corti (isolating endolymph from cortilymph), and basilar membrane (partitioning cortilymph from perilymph), demonstrating the sophisticated fluid management architecture in the cochlea that enables precise sound processing while preventing ionic cross-contamination.

6.5.1 Biochemical and Physiological Characteristics of Perilymph

Perilymph occupies both scala vestibuli and scala tympani while extending into the spiral ligament's interstitial spaces through inferior border communications, forming a continuous extracellular fluid compartment with ionic composition resembling plasma and cerebrospinal fluid (Na+ ≈138 mM, K+ ≈ 6.9 mM). This sodium-rich fluid demonstrates dual potential origins: (1) local ultrafiltration from scala vascular networks supported by its plasma-like electrolyte profile, versus (2) cerebrospinal fluid influx through the cochlear aqueduct given their shared biochemical signatures and anatomical connectivity [1, 2, 4, 6, 34, 40, 41]. The fluid's penetration into spiral ligament fibroblasts creates a perilymphatic continuum that may facilitate cochlear ionic homeostasis and mechanical damping, while its strategic separation from endolymph by Reissner's membrane and basilar membrane maintains the electrochemical gradients essential for auditory transduction (Fig. 6.25). Current evidence suggests both proposed sources likely contribute to perilymph production, with vascular filtration dominating basal turn homeostasis and cerebrospinal fluid exchange becoming more significant in apical regions, though the precise regulatory mechanisms governing this dual-origin system remain incompletely characterized.

6.5.2 Endolymph Composition and Physiological Significance

Endolymph, the specialized fluid within the cochlear duct (Fig. 6.25), exhibits a unique ionic composition dominated by potassium ($K+ \approx 154$ mM) with minimal sodium ($Na+ \approx 0.91$ mM), creating an electrochemical environment essential for auditory transduction. This potassium-rich solution maintains a +80–90 mV endocochlear potential relative to perilymph, which when combined with hair cells' intrinsic −70 mV resting potential, establishes a 160 mV gradient across their apical cuticular plate—the largest transmembrane potential difference in human physiology. The endolymphatic system operates through two complementary circulation pathways: (1) a radial flow system in the utricle and semicircular canals where local dark cells mediate self-contained secretion and absorption, and (2) a longitudinal flow pathway from the stria vascularis through the cochlear duct and ductus reuniens to the saccule and endolymphatic sac. This dual-system reflects anatomical constraints, as the saccule's lack of dark cells necessitates long-distance transport to the endolymphatic sac for absorption, while the stria vascularis must simultaneously supply the endolymph to the cochlear duct and the saccule [1, 2, 4, 6, 8, 41]. During sound stimulation, potassium influx through mechanically-gated channels depolarizes hair cells, triggering neurotransmitter release, with subsequent potassium recycling back to the cochlear duct occurring via two routes: the medial pathway through spiral limbus interdental cells and the lateral pathway via stria vascularis epithelial cells (Fig. 6.25). This precise ionic management system ensures maintenance of the endocochlear potential while preventing intracellular potassium accumulation, demonstrating the cochlea's sophisticated integration of mechanical, electrical, and chemical signaling processes. Therefore, the stria vascularis functioning as both the primary generator of the endocochlear potential and a critical component of the potassium recycling machinery, demonstrating the cochlea's integrated electrochemical design for sustained high-frequency signaling.

6.5.3 Functional Characteristics of Cortilymph

Cortilymph occupies the interstitial spaces within the organ of Corti, bounded superiorly by the reticular lamina and inferiorly by the basilar membrane (Fig. 6.25). This perilymph-like fluid maintains direct communication with scala tympani perilymph through porous channels at the basilar membrane's attachment zone, creating a continuous extracellular compartment that shares similar ionic composition (predominantly Na+-rich, low K+) with cerebrospinal fluid [1, 2, 4, 6, 41, 42]. The free exchange between Cortilymph and perilymph establishes an important pharmacological pathway that allows therapeutic drugs or ototoxic compounds to enter the perilymph via systemic routes or local round window infiltration quickly penetrate into the immediate microenvironment of Cortilymph that makes the hair cells and supporting cells in the organ of Corti immersed in Cortilymph quickly exposed to the drugs [39, 43–45]. This anatomical arrangement positions Cortilymph as a critical mediator in both normal cochlear physiology (maintaining ionic homeostasis for neural excitation) and drug delivery (serving as a conduit for pharmacologic agents), while its isolation from endolymph by the reticular lamina preserves the essential electrochemical gradients required for mechanoelectrical transduction. The fluid's strategic location enables it to simultaneously participate in neural metabolic support and serve as a distribution network for compounds affecting auditory function.

References

1. Schuknecht H. 2. Anatomy. In: Schuknecht H, editor. Pathology of the ear. 1st ed. Cambridge: Harvard University Press; 1974. pp. 40–96.
2. Ding D, Jiang S. Chapter 4: Inner ear anatomy and structure. In: Ding D, editor. Manual of anatomical examination of the inner ear of the guinea pig. Shanghai: Xuelin Publishing House; 1989. pp. 24–35.
3. Ding D, Jiang S. Chapter 6: Surface preparation techniques of the inner ear. In: Ding D, editor. Manual of anatomical examination of the inner ear of the guinea pig. Shanghai: Xuelin Publishing House; 1989. pp. 49–60.
4. Ding D, Li M, Jiang C, Salvi R. Chapter 3: Anatomy of temporal bone and inner ear. In: Ding D, editor. Morphology of the inner ear. Harbin: Heilongjiang Science and Technology Press; 2001. p. 10–17.
5. Ding D, Li M, Jiang C, Salvi R. Chapter 5: Surface preparation techniques of membranous labyrinth. In: Ding D, editor. Morphology of the inner ear. Harbin: Heilongjiang Science and Technology Press; 2001. p. 24–37.
6. Ding D, Qi W, Qu Y, Salvi R. Chapter 1: Anatomy of the inner ear. In: Ding D, editor. Science of the inner ear. Beijing: China Science and Technology Press; 2010. p. 1–8.
7. Ding D, Qi W, Qu Y, Salvi R. Chapter 6: Research techniques of the inner ear morphology. In: Ding D, editor. Science of the inner ear. Beijing: China Science and Technology Press; 2010. p. 50–88.
8. Ding D, Qi W, Qu Y, Salvi R. Chapter 15: Animal model of intra-labyrinthal hydrops. In: Ding D, editor. Science of the inner ear. Beijing: China Science and Technology Press; 2010. p. 183–8.
9. Hayes SH, Ding D, Salvi R, Allman BL. Anatomy and physiology of the external, middle and inner ear. In: Celesis GG, editor. Disorders of peripheral and central auditory processing. Handbook of clinical neurophysiology, vol. 10. New York: Elsevier; 2013. p. 3–23.
10. Ding D, McFadden SL, Salvi R. Cochlear hair cell densities and inner-ear staining techniques. In: Willott JF, editor. Handbook of mouse auditory research from behavior to molecular biology. Boca Raton: CRC Press; 2001. p. 189–204.
11. Liu H, Ding D, Sun H, Jiang H, Salvi R. Reference data of sensory epithelium in the inner ear in CBA mice. Chin J Otol. 2011;9:224–31.
12. Ding D, Li P, Qi W, et al. Different patterns of age-related damage to cochlear hair cells in different species of experimental animals. Chin J Otorhinolaryngol. Skull Base Surg. 2023;29:7–13. https://doi.org/10.11798/j.issn.1007-1520.202323084.

13. Ding D, Zhao J, Huangfu M. Modified cochlear surface preparations. Zhonghua Er Bi Yan Hou Ke Za Zhi. 1981;16:207–9.
14. Ding D, Wang J, He Y. Surface preparation technique of the spiral ligament of the cochlea in guinea pig. Shanghai Med J. 1984;7:657–8.
15. Ding D, Zhao J, Huangfu M, Jin X. Microdissection of the whole membranous labyrinth in guinea pigs. J Clin Otorhinolaryngol. 1987;1:9–11.
16. Ding D, Manohar S, Kador PF, Salvi R. Multifunctional redox modulator prevents blast-induced loss of cochlear and vestibular hair cells and auditory spiral ganglion neurons. Sci Rep. 2024;14:15296. https://doi.org/10.1038/s41598-024-66406-1.
17. Ding D, Shi L, Xing Y, et al. Sagittal sectioning of temporal bones and quantitative measurement of neural densities in the inner ear in normal mice. Chin J Otorhinolaryngol Skull Base Surg. 2024;30:69–75. https://doi.org/10.11798/j.issn.1007-1520.202424331.
18. Ding D, Chen GD, Zhang C, et al. Supporting cell involvement in cochlear damage and repair: novel insights from a quantitative analysis of cyclodextrin-induced ototoxicity in mice. Hear Res. 2025;459:109201 https://doi.org/10.1016/j.heares.2025.109201.
19. Ding D, Qi W, Salvi R. Antiphase stimulation model of vestibular hair cells. Chin J Otol. 2017;15:715–20.
20. Lim DJ, Freilich IW. Ultrastructure of the stria vascularis, vestibular dark cells and endolymphatic sac following acute diuretic ototoxicity. Scand Audiol Suppl. 1981;14 Suppl:139–55.
21. Ding D, Jin X, Zhang Z, Zhu Q. Study on the different susceptibility between red-eyed and black-eyed guinea pigs to gentamicin. Acta Otolaryngol. 1995;9:70–74.
22. Ciuman RR. Stria vascularis and vestibular dark cells: characterisation of main structures responsible for inner-ear homeostasis, and their pathophysiological relations. J Laryngol Otol. 2009;123:151–62. https://doi.org/10.1017/S0022215108002624.
23. Ding D, Liu H, Qi W, et al. Ototoxic effects and mechanisms of loop diuretics. J Otol. 2016;11:145–56. https://doi.org/10.1016/j.joto.2016.10.001.
24. Qvortrup K, Rostgaard J. Mesothelium of Reissner's membrane in guinea pigs: an electron microscopic study. Eur Arch Otorhinolaryngol. 1990;248:57–62. https://doi.org/10.1007/BF00634783.
25. Qvortrup K, Rostgaard J. Three-dimensional organization of a transcellular tubulocisternal endoplasmic reticulum in epithelial cells of Reissner's membrane in the guinea-pig. Cell Tissue Res. 1990;261:287–99. https://doi.org/10.1007/BF00318670.
26. Eric J. Auditory System, Peripheral. In: John D, editor. Encyclopedia of the neurological sciences. London: Academic Press; 2003. p. 305–11.
27. Krey JF, Gillespie PG. Chapter 23:Molecular biology of hearing and balance. In: Brady ST, Siegel GJ, ... Price DL, editors. Basic neurochemistry: principles of molecular, cellular, and medical neurobiology. 8th ed. London: Academic Press; 2012. pp. 916–27.
28. Maynard RL, Downes N. Chapter 23: The ear. In: Maynard RL, Downes N, editors. Anatomy and histology of the laboratory rat in toxicology and biomedical research. London: Academic Press; 2019. pp. 293–302.
29. Ding D, Wang J, Zhang XY, Sun H, Salvi R. Quantitative analysis of hair cells, spiral ganglion neurons, and nerve fibers in the same cochlea. Chin J Otorhinolaryngol. Skull Base Surg. 1998;4:200–4.
30. Ding D, Wang J, Zheng XY, Salvi RJ. Early damage of spiral ganglion caused by carboplatin in chinchilla. J Audiol Speech Pathol. 1998;6:65–67.
31. Ding D, Jiang H, Manohar S, et al. Spatiotemporal developmental upregulation of prestin correlates with the severity and location of cyclodextrin-induced outer hair cell loss and hearing loss. Front Cell Dev Biol. 2021;9:643709. https://doi.org/10.3389/fcell.2021.643709.
32. Ding D, Qi W, Jiang H, Salvi R. Excitotoxic damage to auditory nerve afferents and spiral ganglion neurons is correlated with developmental upregulation of AMPA and KA receptors. Hear Res. 2021;411:108358 https://doi.org/10.1016/j.heares.2021.108358.
33. Ding D, Li P, Qi W, et al. Study on delayed secondary lesions in the cochlea triggered by cochlear hair cell death. Chin J Otorhinolaryngol Skull Base Surg. 2022;28:1–10. https://doi.org/10.11798/j.issn.1007-1520.2022221001.
34. Cho KH, Kim JH, Honkura Y, et al. Cochlear aqueduct revisited: A histological study using human fetuses. Ann Anat. 2024;253:152236 https://doi.org/10.1016/j.aanat.2024.152236.
35. El-Badry MM, Ding DL, McFadden SL, Eddins AC. Physiological effects of auditory nerve myelinopathy in chinchillas. Eur J Neurosci. 2007;25:1437–46. https://doi.org/10.1111/j.1460-9568.2007.05401.x.
36. Liberman MC, Kujawa SG. Cochlear synaptopathy in acquired sensorineural hearing loss: manifestations and mechanisms. Hear Res. 2017;349:138–47. https://doi.org/10.1016/j.heares.2017.01.003.
37. Ding D, Jiang H, Salvi R. Cochlear spiral ganglion neuron degeneration following cyclodextrin-induced hearing loss. Hear Res. 2021;400:108125. https://doi.org/10.1016/j.heares.2020.108125.
38. Ding D, Jiang H, McFadden SL, Richard S. Ethacrynic acid is the key for opening of the blood-labyrinth barrier. Chin J Otol. 2004;2:42–47.
39. Ding D, Salvi R. Review of cellular changes in the cochlea due to aminoglycoside antibiotics. Volta Rev. 2005;105:407–38.
40. Lempert J, Meltzer PE, Wever EG, Lawrence M, Rambo JH. Structure and function of the cochlear aqueduct. AMA Arch Otolaryngol. 1952;55:134–45. https://doi.org/10.1001/archotol.1952.00710010143003.
41. Sterkers O, Ferrary E, Amiel C. Production of inner ear fluids. Physiol Rev. 1988;68:1083–128. https://doi.org/10.1152/physrev.1988.68.4.1083.
42. Engstrom H. The cortilymph, the third lymph of the inner ear. Acta Morphol Neerl Scand. 1960;3:195–204.
43. Ding D, Jin X, Zhao J. Accumulation sites of kanamycin in cochlear basal membrane cells. Zhonghua Er Bi Yan Hou Ke Za Zhi. 1995;30:323–5.
44. Ding D, Jin X, Zhao J. [Accumulation sites of kanamycin in the organ of Corti by microautoradiography]. Zhonghua Er Bi Yan Hou Ke Za Zhi. 1997;32:348–9.
45. Ding D, Shi L, Xing Y, et al. Secondary neural damage in the inner ear induced by intratympanic gentamicin injection. Chin J Otorhinolaryngol Skull Base Surg. 2024;30:11–19. https://doi.org/10.11798/j.issn.1007-1520.202424356.

Sectioning Technique of Cochlear Tissue

7

The cochlear cavity is divided into three fluid-filled spiral chambers by the cochlear basilar membrane and Reissner's membrane. These three chambers rotating around the modiolus are termed the scala vestibuli, the scala media, and the scala tympani. The scala vestibuli and the scala tympani are filled with perilymph, while the scala media is filled with endolymph. Since the cochlear basilar membrane extends from the osseous spiral lamina of the modiolus to the basilar crest of the spiral ligament, and Reissner's membrane stretches from the inner edge of the limbus of the cochlear basilar membrane located on the osseous spiral lamina of the modiolus to the upper edge of the vascular stria covering the surface of the spiral ligament located on the vestibular ridge of the spiral ligament, the scala vestibuli, scala media, and scala tympani in the cochlea can be best observed from a cross-sectional slice parallel to the modiolus [1–7] (Figs. 6.4A and 6.25; Figs. 7.1 and 7.2).

The sample preparation steps for cochlear sections are basically the same as those for traditional soft tissue sections. However, due to its unique bony shell and hollow, membranous structure, cochlear sections intended for histopathological examination require special attention to important sample preparation steps such as decalcification, infiltration, impregnation, embedding, and sectioning angles to ensure that high-quality, ideal slices are obtained that faithfully present the delicate microstructure of the cochlea.

7.1 Sample Preparation of Whole Temporal Bone Slices

7.1.1 Fixation of the Temporal Bone

Tissue fixation serves as the foundational step in inner ear pathological examination, with the primary aim of rapidly coagulating or precipitating proteins to terminate both endogenous and exogenous enzymatic activities, thereby preserving tissue morphology as close as possible to its living state. For temporal bone fixation, two primary methods are utilized: systemic cardiac perfusion under anesthesia or localized inner ear perfusion. While aldehyde fixatives are suitable for long-term storage of temporal bone intended for routine histopathological examinations, their use requires careful consideration in specialized staining applications. In enzyme histochemical studies, prolonged aldehyde fixation must be avoided due to its tendency to denature enzymatic proteins [3, 7–17]. Similarly, immunohistochemical staining is compromised by extended aldehyde fixation, as the aldehyde groups form carboxymethyl cross-links with antigenic protein amino groups, altering the three-dimensional conformation of epitopes. When these cross-linking networks obscure antigenic determinants, the epitopes lose their capacity for specific antibody binding [18–20].

7.1.2 Decalcification of the Temporal Bone

Decalcification of the temporal bone represents a critical preparatory step for cochlear sectioning, as the cochlea is entirely encased within this osseous structure. Both simple and mixed acid decalcification solutions effectively remove calcium salts from bony tissue, with hydrochloric acid-based solutions exemplifying the underlying chemical process: calcium carbonate in bone undergoes a metathesis reaction with hydrogen chloride to form water-soluble calcium chloride and unstable carbonic acid, which rapidly decomposes into carbon dioxide and water. This reaction mechanism explains the frequent formation of vacuolar artifacts within the closed cochlear cavity (Fig. 7.3), as liberated carbon dioxide accumulates in this confined space. After acid decalcification, it is often necessary to thoroughly remove the bubbles in the inner ear cavity by inner ear perfusion or vacuum aspiration to ensure that no cavitation will be formed in the inner ear cavity during the subsequent infiltration and embedding process. Beyond causing structural artifacts, acid decalcification presents significant limitations

D. Ding et al., *Histopathological Atlas of the Inner Ear*,
https://doi.org/10.1007/978-981-95-6338-8_7

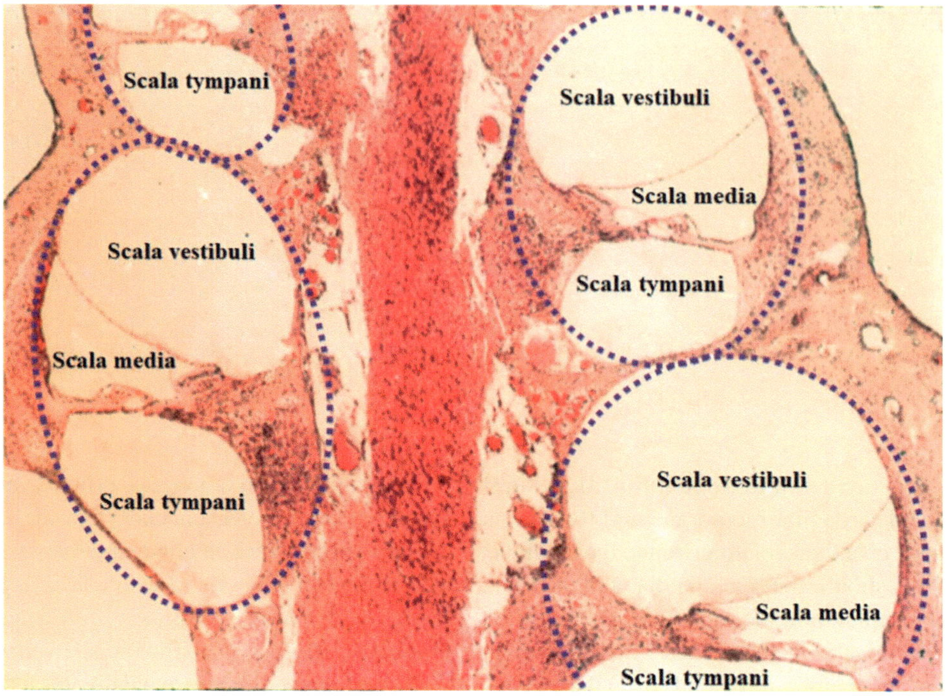

Fig. 7.1 A cochlear slice from a guinea pig. The collodion embedding section of the cochlea parallel to the modiolus clearly shows the scala vestibuli, scala media, and scala tympani separated by the cochlear basilar membrane and the vestibular membrane

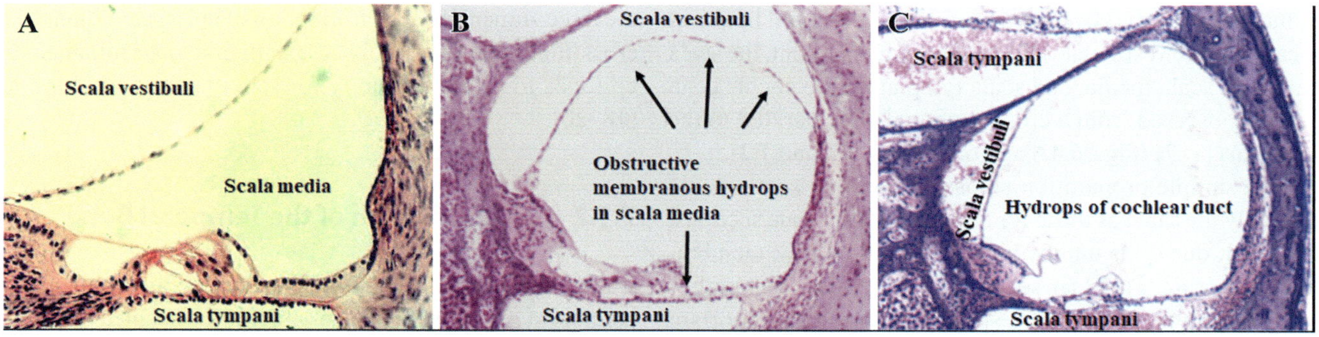

Fig. 7.2 Sections parallel to the cochlear modiolus show typical morphological changes in cochlear hydrops after surgical destruction of the endolymphatic sac. (**A**) Section of a normal guinea pig cochlea showing the triangular scala media. (**B**) 30 days after endolymphatic sac destruction, the cavity of the scala media was significantly enlarged, indicating that the increased pressure in the scala media resulted in the Reissner membrane bulging upward, while the basilar membrane bulged downward. (**C**) 30 days after the surgical destruction of the endolymphatic sac, the scala media of this guinea pig showed more severe cochlear hydrops. The expanded and bulging vestibular membrane almost completely occupied the space of the entire scala vestibuli. In addition, signs of hemorrhage were found in both the scala vestibuli and scala tympani, suggesting that the pressure changes of cochlear hydrops may also cause capillary damage in the cochlea

for specialized staining applications—it potently inhibits enzymatic activity and disrupts antigenic determinants, rendering it suitable only for routine histological staining of temporal bone specimens [2, 3, 7, 10, 16, 17, 20–23]. While ethylenediamine tetraacetate (EDTA) chelation decalcification demonstrates marginally better preservation of some enzymatic activities and antigenic epitopes compared to acid methods, its capacity to maintain biological reactivity remains substantially limited, raising legitimate concerns about the reliability of subsequent enzyme histochemical staining and immunohistochemical results obtained from EDTA-treated specimens.

7.1.3 Embedding of the Temporal Bone

To achieve optimal cochlear sections that faithfully replicate in vivo conditions, thorough infiltration with embedding medium is essential to displace interstitial fluid and provide structural

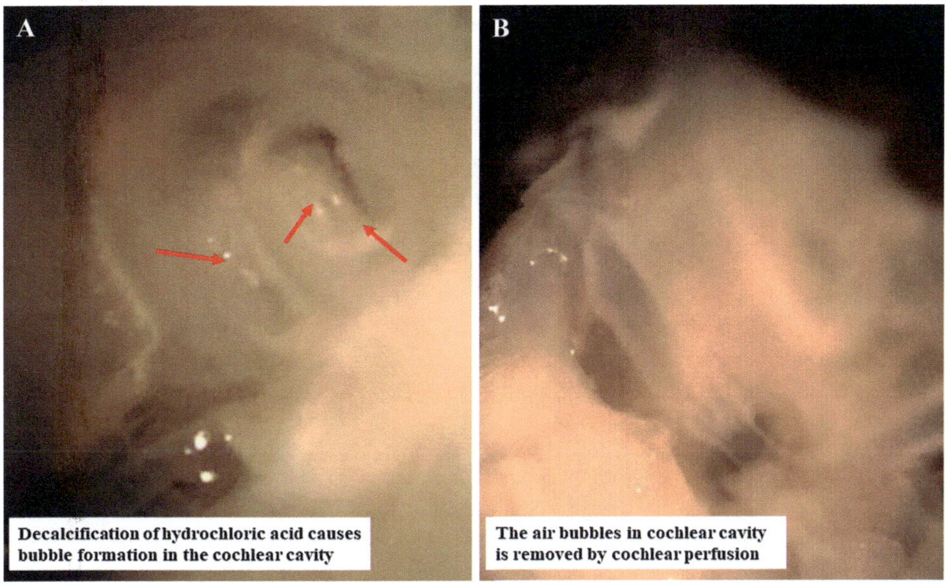

Fig. 7.3 Hydrochloric acid decalcification causes bubble formation in the cochlea, and cochlear perfusion expels bubbles in the cochlear cavity. (**A**) Decalcification using 5% hydrochloric acid for 48 h induces lots of bubbles within the cochlear cavity due to carbon dioxide liberation during the decalcification process. (**B**) Air bubbles in the cochlear cavity are effectively expelled by cochlear perfusion

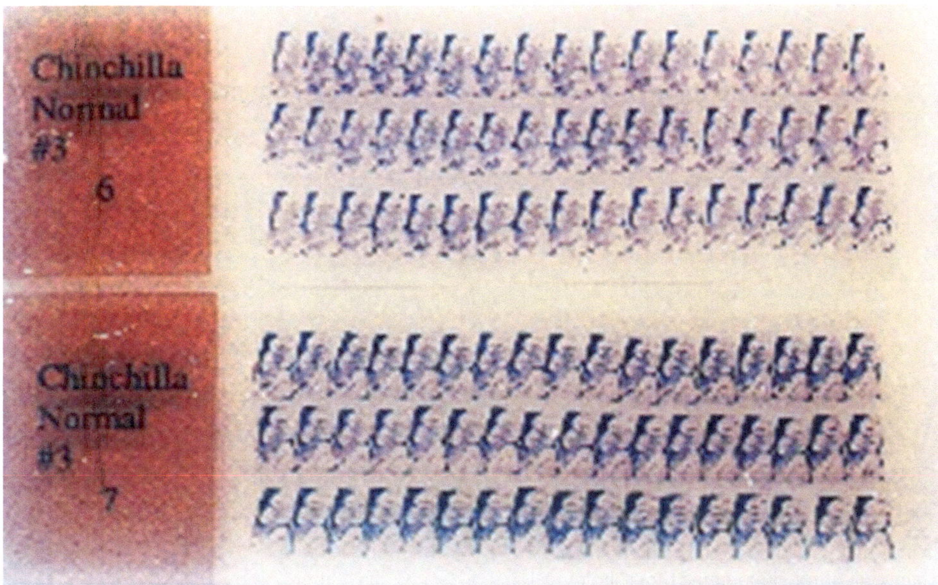

Fig. 7.4 Serial sections of the mid-axis parallel to the modiolus of the cochlea from the chinchilla

support throughout the cochlear cavities and intracellular spaces. The temporal bone frozen section illustrates this process: following decalcification and pre-staining, specimens undergo sequential immersion in progressively concentrated gelatin solutions—initially in 10% gelatin at 37°C for overnight, followed by 25% gelatin at 37°C under identical conditions for 24 h to ensure complete infiltration. The gelatin-impregnated temporal bone is then cryofixed on a microtome cooling stage to solidify the matrix prior to serial sectioning of the entire specimen [2, 3, 10, 21, 24, 25]. This methodology demonstrates the critical relationship between proper medium infiltration and the preservation of cochlear structure during histological processing.

7.1.4 Slice of Temporal Bone

Among the three main sections of the temporal bone (coronal, sagittal, and transverse), the sagittal and transverse planes

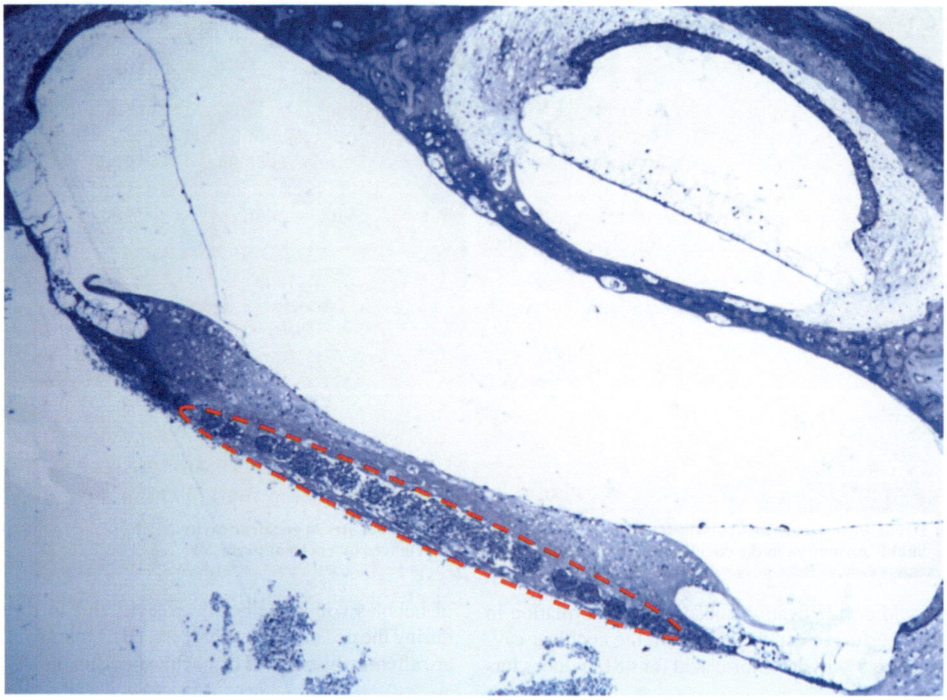

Fig. 7.5 A semithin section of epoxy resin-embedded mouse cochlea. The red-dashed circle marks one row of the habenula perforata in the spiral lamina of the cochlear basal turn. Auditory nerve fibers connecting to cochlear hair cells can be seen passing through each habenula perforata

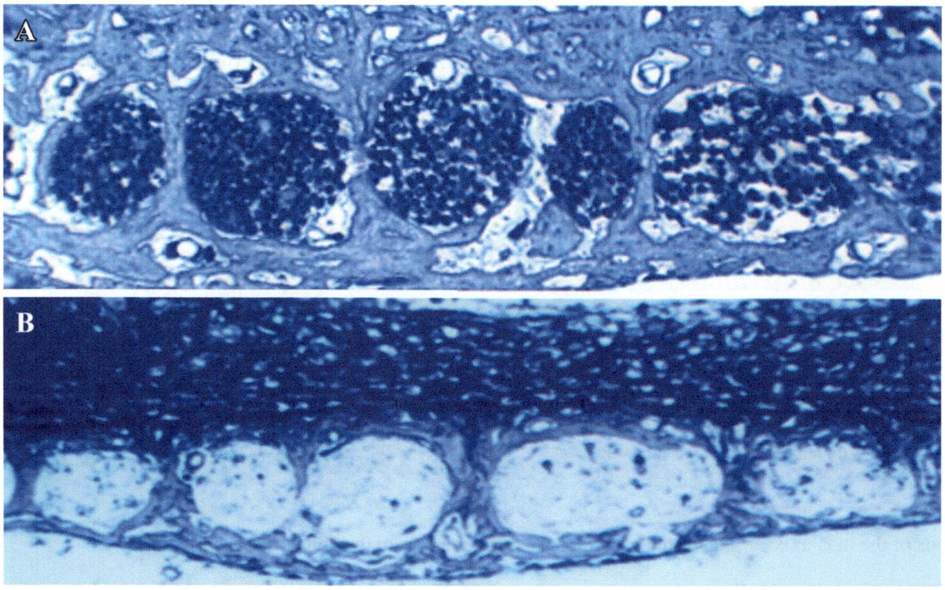

Fig. 7.6 Semithin sections of epoxy resin-embedded rat cochlea. (**A**) A slice cutting from a normal rat at the osseous spiral lamina shows the dense auditory nerve fibers in the habenula perforata. (**B**) 6 month after intense narrowband noise (115 dB SPL centered at 10 kHz for 30 min) exposure, the auditory nerve fibers in the habenula perforata are almost completely disappeared

parallel to the modiolus have become the standardized examination for cochlear lesions due to their superior anatomical appearance and diagnostic utility [2, 3, 6, 7, 16, 17, 21, 26–29] (Figs. 7.1, 7.2, and 7.4). When sectioning parallel to the modiolus, the initial landmark encountered is the habenula perforata of the cochlear basal turn—a series of bony perforations in the osseous spiral lamina (Figs. 7.5–7.7). The channels of habenula perforata in the osseous spiral lamina of the modiolus have special histological significance because this is the only pathway for auditory afferent nerve fibers connecting the

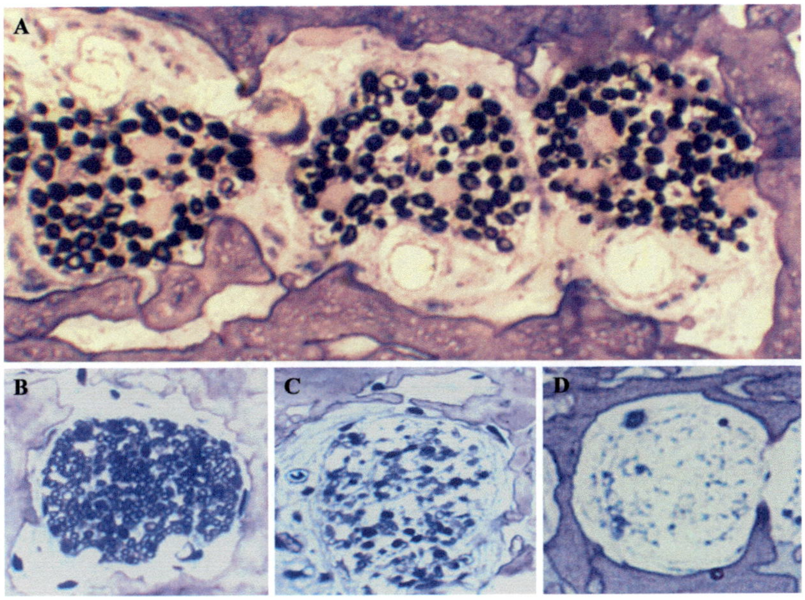

Fig. 7.7 Semithin section of epoxy-embedded osseous spiral lamina of chinchilla. (**A**) Auditory nerve fibers in the habenula perforata were stained with toluidine blue. (**B**) Slice of the osseous spiral lamina shows dense nerve fibers in the habenula perforata in a normal chinchilla. (**C**) On the third day after carboplatin injection, the number of auditory nerve fibers in the habenula perforata was greatly reduced, and demyelination of the auditory nerve fibers began to occur. (**D**) On the fifth day after carboplatin injection, the auditory nerve fibers in the habenula perforata were completely destroyed

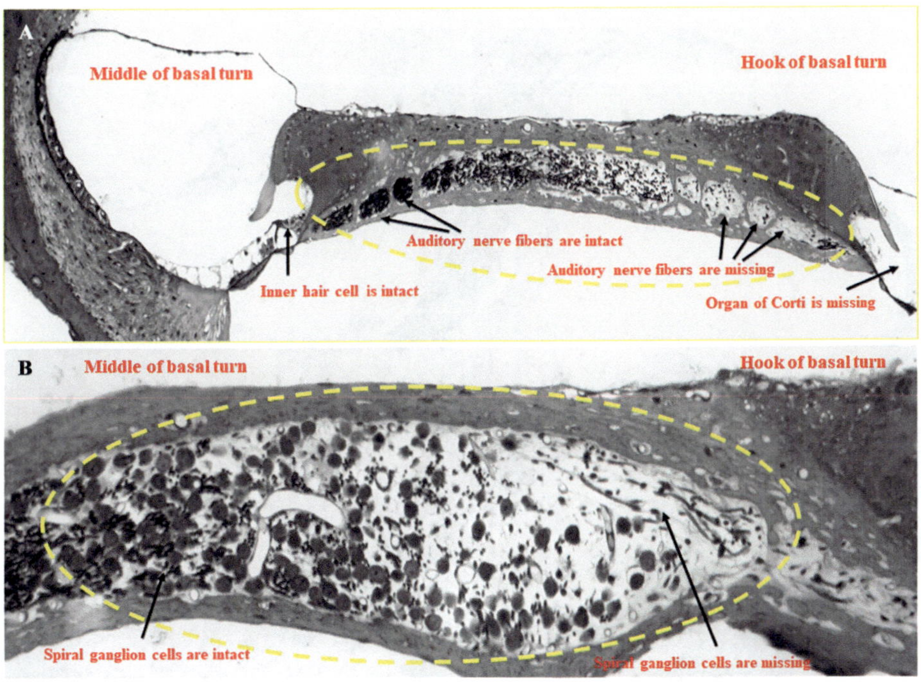

Fig. 7.8 Bone spiral lamina sections demonstrate age-related cochlear nerve degeneration in C57BL/6J mice at 6 months of age. (**A**) The hook region demonstrates complete loss of both inner and outer hair cells with corresponding degeneration of auditory nerve fibers in the adjacent habenula perforata (right side), while the mid-region of the basal turn (left side) shows selective outer hair cell loss with preserved inner hair cells and intact nerve fibers, establishing a direct correlation between hair cell viability and neural preservation. (**B**) Corresponding sections through Rosenthal's canal reveal region-specific neurodegeneration, with spiral ganglion neuron loss in the hook region (right side) contrasting with intact neurons in the mid-region of the basal turn (left side), demonstrating that inner hair cell loss triggers sequential degeneration of both auditory nerve fibers and their associated spiral ganglion neurons. These results not only demonstrate that age-related damage to cochlear hair cells and peripheral spiral ganglion neurons in C57 mice begins at the cochlear basal turn and gradually spreads to the apex, but also provide convincing morphological evidence for the hierarchical dependence of cochlear nerve survival on the integrity of sensory hair cells, among which inner hair cells are important trophic supporters of the entire afferent nerve pathway

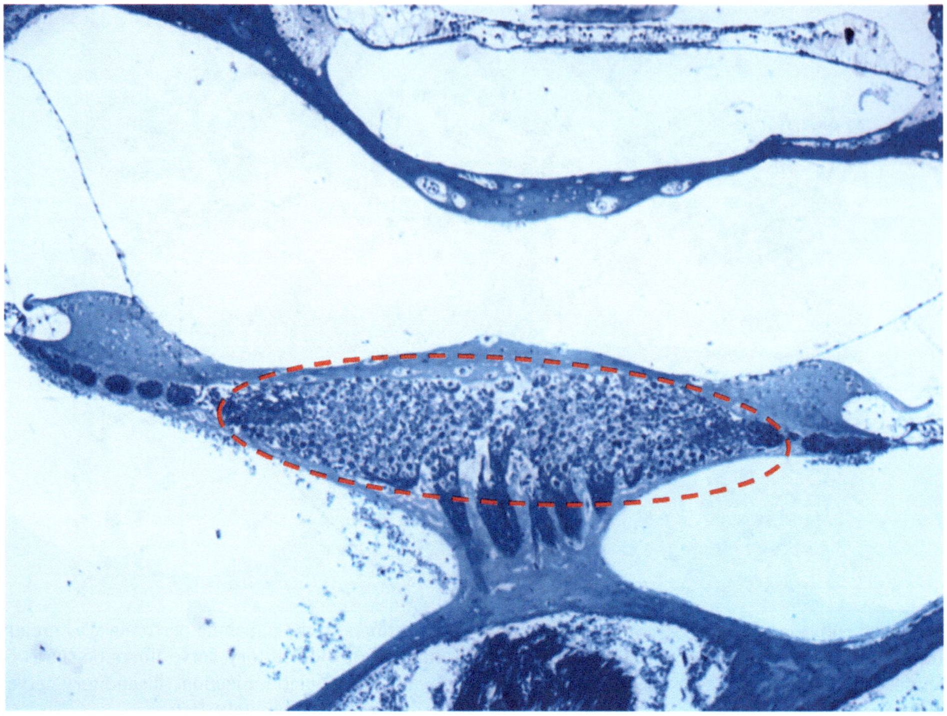

Fig. 7.9 A photomicrograph of a mouse cochlear section parallel to the modiolus. This slice just cuts through Rosenthal's canal on one side of the cochlear basal turn, exposing a large number of spiral ganglion cells in Rosenthal's canal

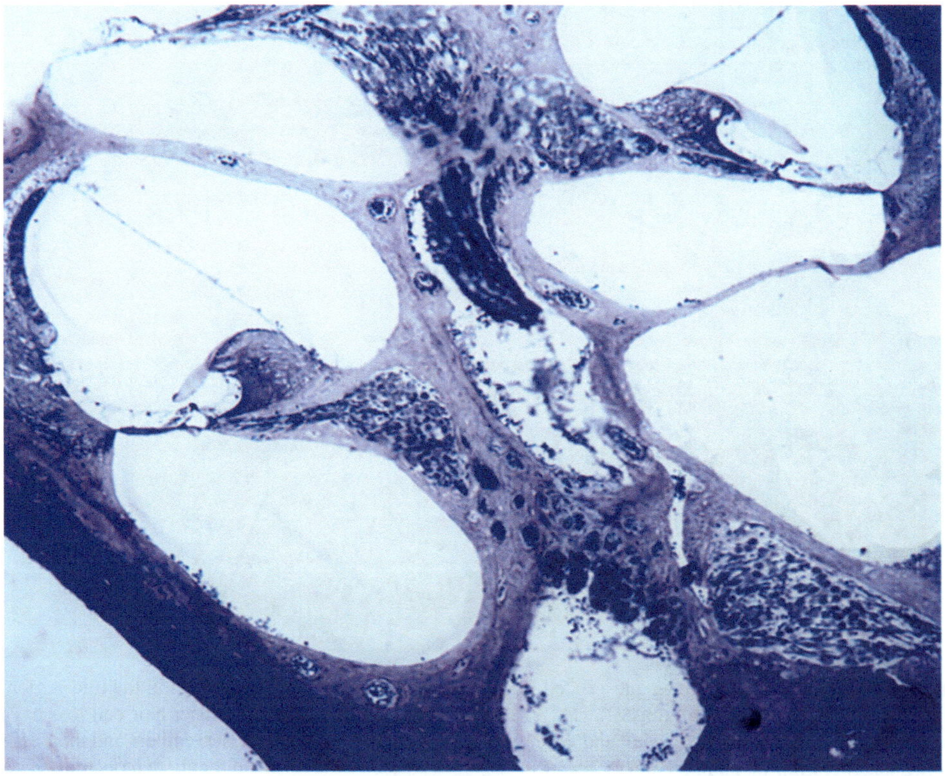

Fig. 7.10 A semithin section parallel to the cochlear modiolus from EPON 812-embedded rat temporal bone

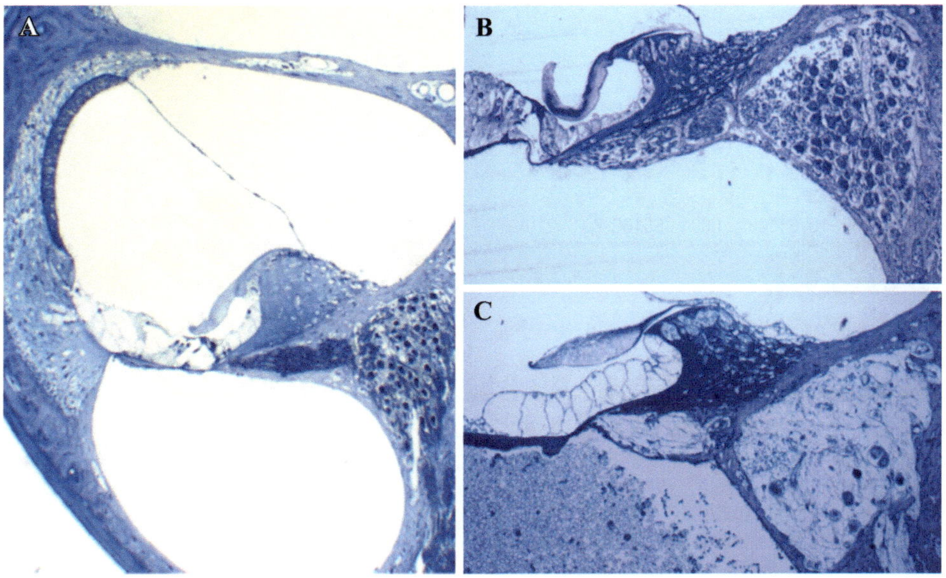

Fig. 7.11 Semithin sections of EPON 812-embedded cochleae. (**A**) A cross-sectional section of the normal mouse cochlear duct shows the entire cochlear duct structure, including the cochlear basilar membrane, spiral ligament, stria vascularis, and modiolar spiral duct. (**B**) Axial sections of the organ of Corti and spiral ganglion neurons from a rat simultaneously show the positional relationship between the organ of Corti and the spiral ganglion neurons. (**C**) After 6 months of exposure to strong narrow-band noise (115 dB SPL, center frequency of 10 kHz, for 30 min), a cross-sectional section of the mouse cochlear duct shows that the organ of Corti and spiral ganglion neurons corresponding to the 10 kHz frequency position were completely destroyed

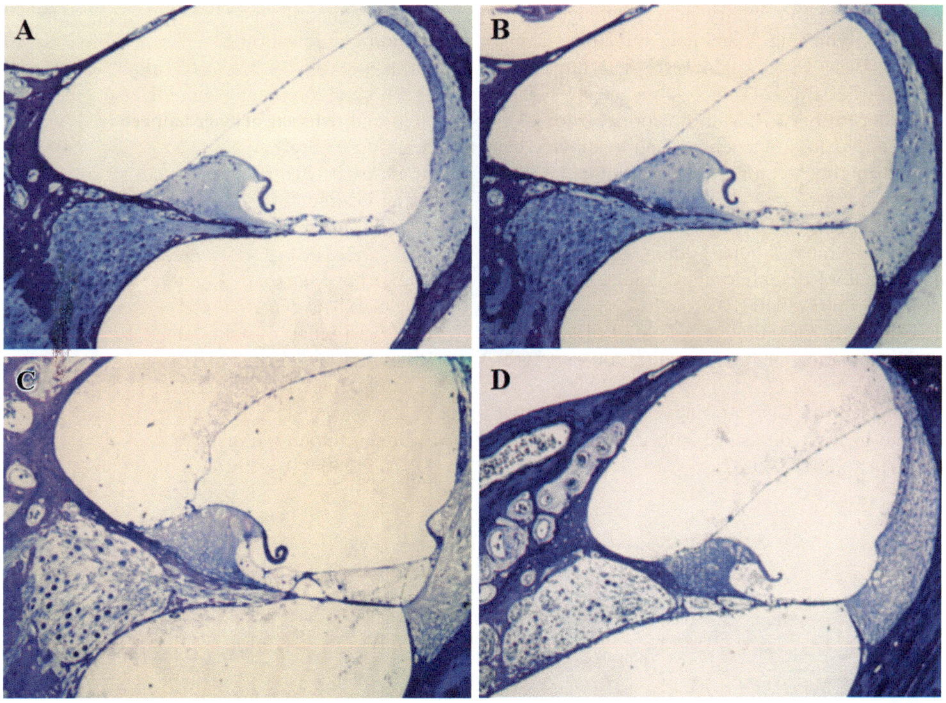

Fig. 7.12 Semithin section of Epon 812-embedded rat cochlea. (**A**) A cross-section of the cochlear duct from a normal rat was used as a control. (**B**) One week after subcutaneous injection of cyclodextrin (4000 mg/kg), only damage was detected in outer hair cells, while the inner hair cells and spiral ganglia were intact. (**C**) 4 weeks after cyclodextrin injection, secondary damage was expanded to inner hair cells and spiral ganglion neurons. (**D**) 8 weeks after cyclodextrin treatment, massive death of supporting cells on the basal membrane and secondary collapse of the structure of the organ of Corti led to the death of inner hair cells, and the spiral ganglion neurons in Rosenthal's canal also experienced obvious delayed neuronal death

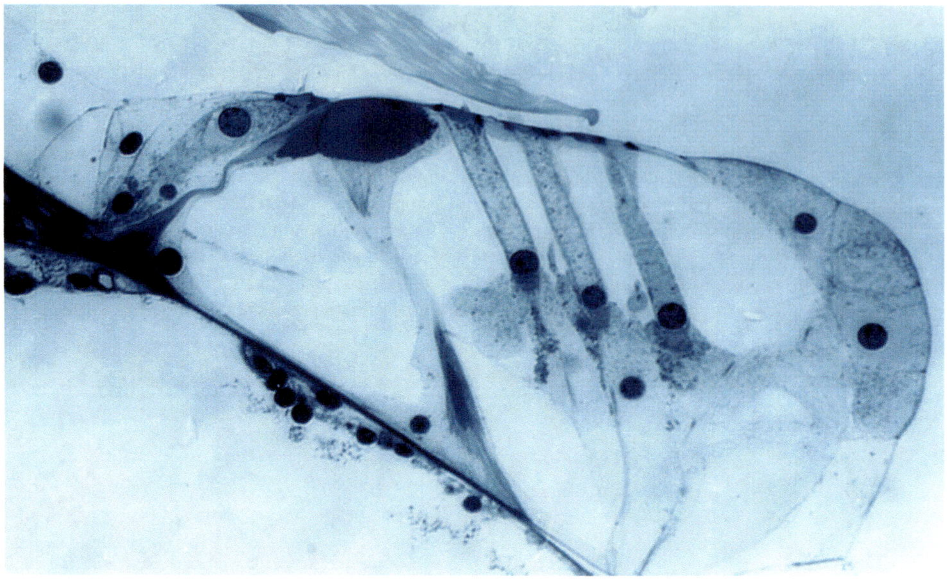

Fig. 7.13 The precise spatial structure of inner and outer hair cells and their surrounding supporting cells in a semithin section of the modiolus from a chinchilla cochlea

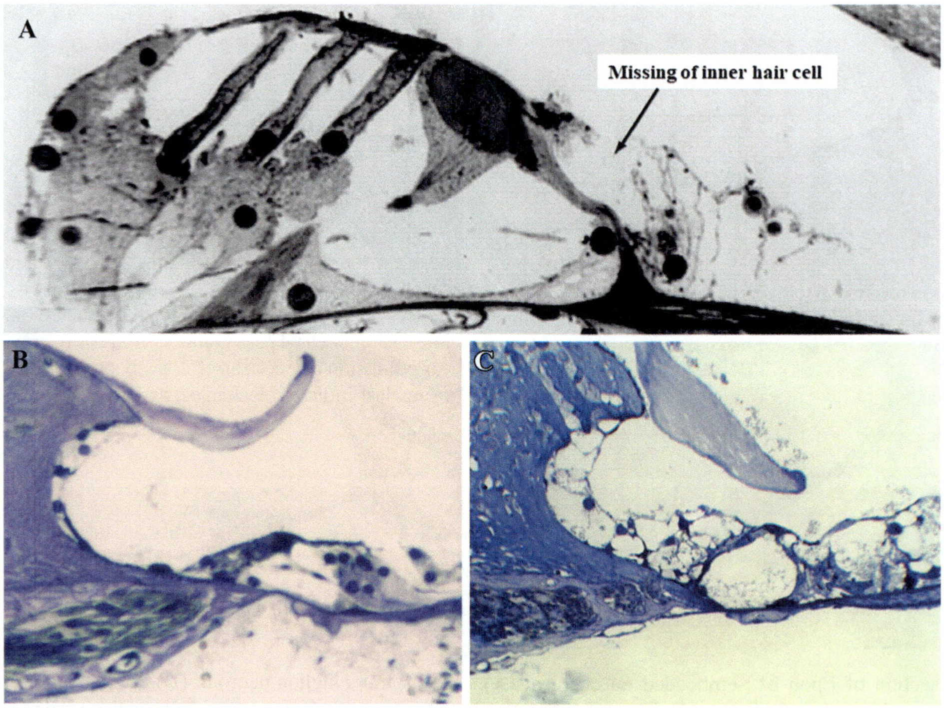

Fig. 7.14 Semithin sections of the organ of Corti cutting along a plane parallel to the cochlear modiolus. (**A**) On the third day after carboplatin injection, the inner hair cells of the chinchilla were destroyed, but the outer hair cells were intact, indicating that carboplatin selectively destroys the inner hair cells in chinchillas. (**B**) A semi-thin section of the organ of Corti from a normal rat. (**C**) The late intracochlear pathological changes occurring in aminoglycoside-injected mice showed complete destruction of the entire structure of the organ of Corti

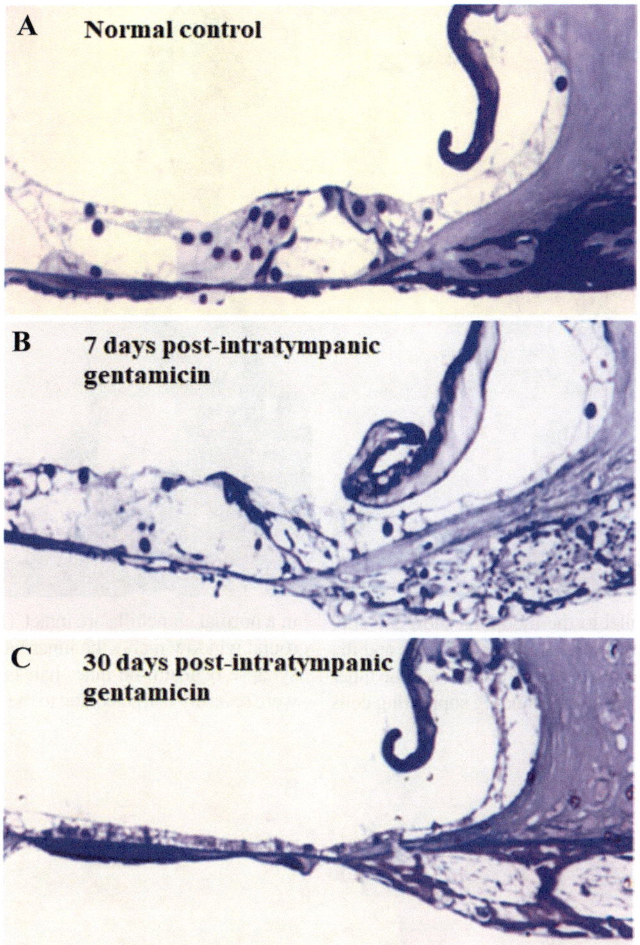

Fig. 7.15 The progression of lesions in the organ of Corti in rat cochleae caused by intratympanic administration of gentamicin. (**A**) The structure of the organ of Corti in a normal rat is normal, and the sensory hair cells and supporting cell groups are intact. (**B**) 7 days after intratympanic injection of gentamicin, the sensory hair cells on the organ of Corti were completely destroyed, and the supporting cells also began to be obviously damaged. (**C**) 30 days after intratympanic injection of gentamicin, all the hair cells on the basilar membrane of the cochlea disappeared, and most of the supporting cells were also completely destroyed. The above series of pathological changes provides important clues for understanding the dynamic pathological cascade caused by intratympanic injection of gentamicin

spiral ganglion neurons and the cochlear hair cells, and also the cochlear efferent nerves connecting the cochlear hair cells. The density of nerve fibers in the habenula perforata has become an important quantitative parameter to reflect and evaluate the state of the connection between the cochlear sensory hair cells and the nervous system [2, 3, 6, 7, 16, 17, 21–23, 28–34] (Figs. 7.5–7.8A). Both transverse and sagittal sections parallel to the modiolus can display important tissue structures, from the cochlear hair cells to the auditory peripheral nerve fibers connecting to the spiral ganglion, and from the spiral ganglion soma to the auditory nerve fibers at the central ends of the auditory nerve leading to the intracranial auditory centers. This technique has become one of the important morphological research methods for evaluating the cochlear pathological changes.

Horizontal or sagittal sectioning parallel to the modiolus enables systematic examination of cochlear neural structures at multiple anatomical levels. When this plane of slice reaches Rosenthal's canal, it reveals the characteristic morphology and distribution of spiral ganglion neuron soma (Figs. 7.8B and 7.9). Especially when the slice plane is advanced to the midline of the cochlear modiolus, the organ of Corti and its connected spiral ganglion neurons at each turn of the cochlea can be ideally demonstrated. This provides a comprehensive view of the peripheral auditory pathways in the cochlea (Figs. 7.10–7.19). Counting the number of spiral ganglion neurons in Rosenthal's canal on mid-axial sections of the cochlear modiolus has become a reliable histological parameter for assessing the integrity of peripheral cochlear neurons and has been confirmed in many experimental models of cochlear

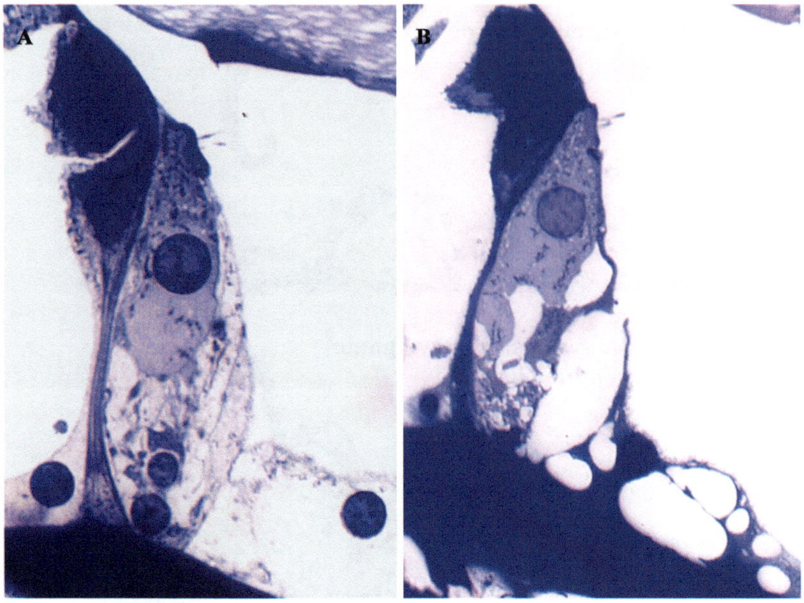

Fig. 7.16 Semithin cross-sections parallel to the modiolus show the specific destruction of type I afferent synapses beneath inner hair cells and the surrounding supporting cells by local treatment of kainic acid. (**A**) The inner hair cells, the type I afferent terminals, and the surrounding supporting cells in a normal chinchilla are intact. (**B**) 24h after kainic acid placement on the round window niche, the inner hair cells were intact, but the type I afferent synapse beneath the inner hair cells and the surrounding supporting cells were severely damaged due to the excitotoxic effect of kainic acid

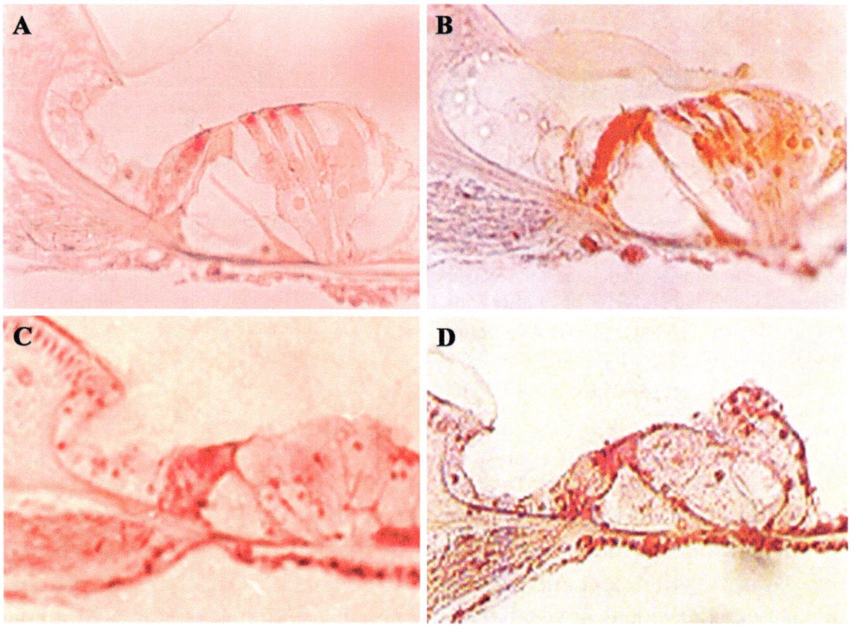

Fig. 7.17 Acid phosphatase staining in gelatin-embedded frozen sections of the organ of Corti in guinea pigs. (**A**) The labeling of acid phosphatase in normal hair cells is localized beneath the cuticular plate of the hair cells. (**B**) The guinea pig was treated with kanamycin at a daily dose of 500mg/kg for 7 days. On the last day of kanamycin treatment, although the inner and outer hair cells maintained normal morphology and structure, the expression of acid phosphatase in the inner and outer hair cells was significantly enhanced and diffused to the entire cytoplasm. Given that acid phosphatase is a marker enzyme of lysosomes, it suggests that abnormal lysosomal activity occurs before the pathological destruction of hair cells. (**C**) On the fourth day after stopping the kanamycin treatment, the outer hair cells were extremely swollen, and the staining of acid phosphatase in outer hair cells had completely disappeared. It is suggested that the acid phosphatase originally concentrated in lysosomes may have been dispersed into the cytoplasm during the destructive stage when hair cells were swollen. (**D**) On the sixth day after the last injection of kanamycin, the outer hair cells had disappeared, and the interior space of the organ of Corti was completely occupied by the swollen Deiters' cells. The swelling of inner hair cells is starting to occur, and the expression of acid phosphatase in the inner hair cells begins to weaken. This sequential pattern of lysosome-mediated heterolytic and autolytic processes contributes to kanamycin-induced hair cell necrosis. The dynamic changes of acid phosphatase can be used as a sensitive indicator of lysosome activity during the progressive cellular breakdown. The differential temporal progression of degeneration between the inner and outer hair cells highlights distinct vulnerability patterns to aminoglycoside toxicity within cochlear sensory epithelium

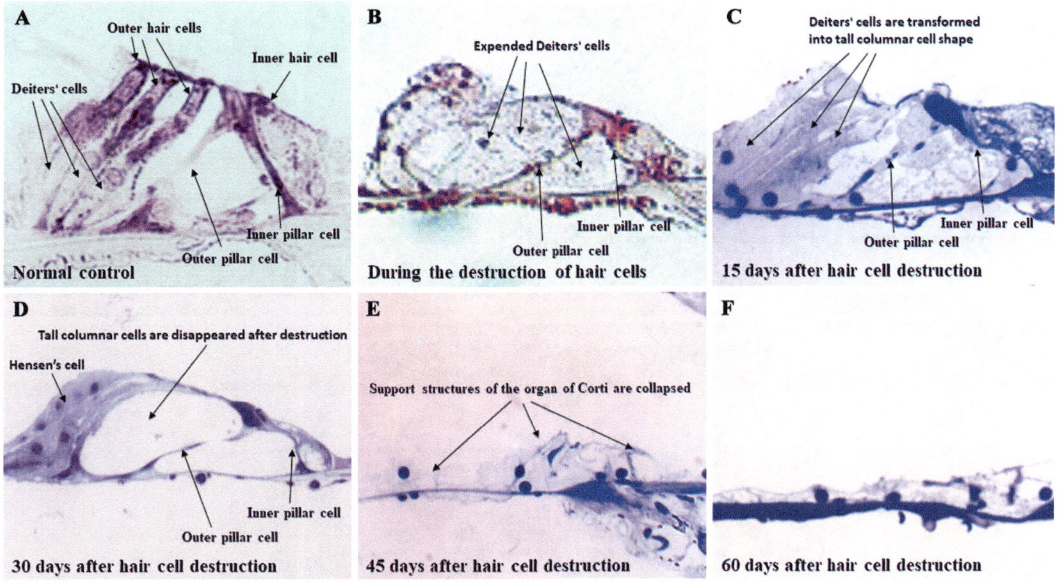

Fig. 7.18 The sequential histopathological changes in the organ of Corti following hair cell loss through a series of representative sections. (**A**) Normal cochlear section demonstrates the cellular structures of the organ of Corti. (**B**) During the outer hair cell destruction, the swollen Deiters' cells rapidly fill the Nuel's space and expel the destroyed cuticular plate of the outer hair cells into the scala media. (**C**) The swollen Deiters cells then differentiate into a tall columnar configuration to support the "ceiling" of the organ of Corti. (**D**) Deiters cells die about 30 days after differentiating into tall columnar cells, and the shape of the organ of Corti is temporarily supported by the connection between the surface of Hensen's cells and the outer pillar cells. (**E**) As the outer and inner pillar cells collapse, the inner hair cells also fall over and die, marking that all cells on the organ of Corti undergo the final stage of complete destruction due to the collapse of the supporting structure of the organ of Corti. (**F**) The final pathological destruction of the organ of Corti is that only a layer of flat squamous epithelium remains on the basilar membrane. This chronological progression illustrates the dynamic cellular reorganization and eventual failure of supporting cell compensatory mechanisms following sensory hair cell loss, providing reference pathological evidence for understanding the series of pathological processes of the cochlear Corti organ. (Reproduced with permission from Ding et al. [23])

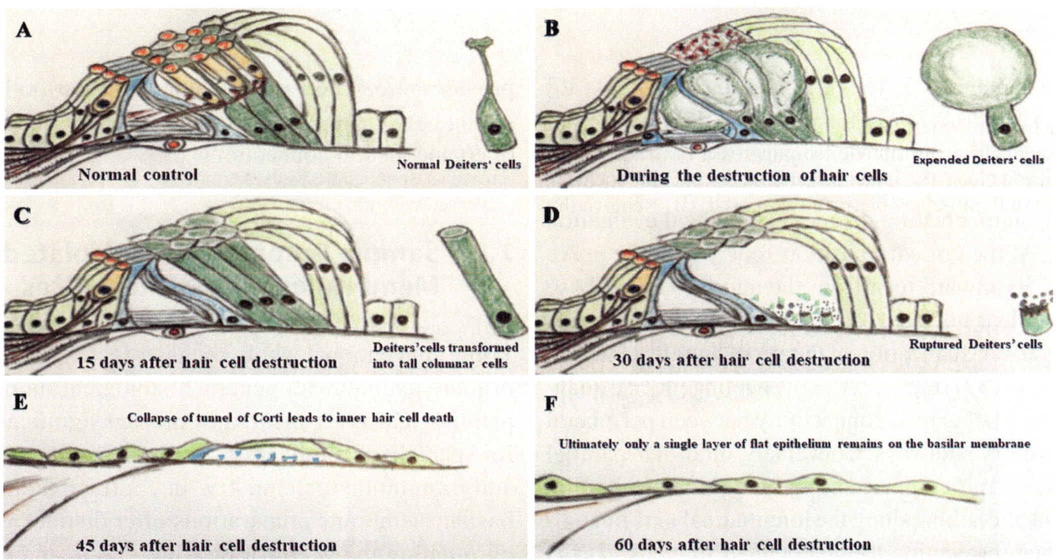

Fig. 7.19 The hand-drawn series diagrams again illustrate the entire process of primary and secondary changes in the organ of Corti. (**A**) An anatomical structural diagram of the normal organ of Corti. (**B**) In the early stages of outer hair cell destruction, Deiters cells immediately expand to fill the entire interior space of the organ of Corti. (**C**) Subsequent cellular differentiation reveals Deiters' cells transforming into tall columnar forms that provide structural support during the scarring phase. (**D**) 30 days after injury, Deiters cells that differentiate into tall columnar morphology die, and Hensen cells continue to survive for a very short period before undergoing secondary death. (**E**) The late pathological characteristics are the death of inner hair cells and the complete collapse of the organ of Corti. (**F**) The terminal stage demonstrates complete architectural flattening. This schematic effectively visualizes the temporal sequence of supporting cell plasticity and eventual failure in maintaining cochlear microstructure after outer hair cell loss, highlighting both the compensatory capacity and ultimate limitations of cochlear supporting cell responses to injury

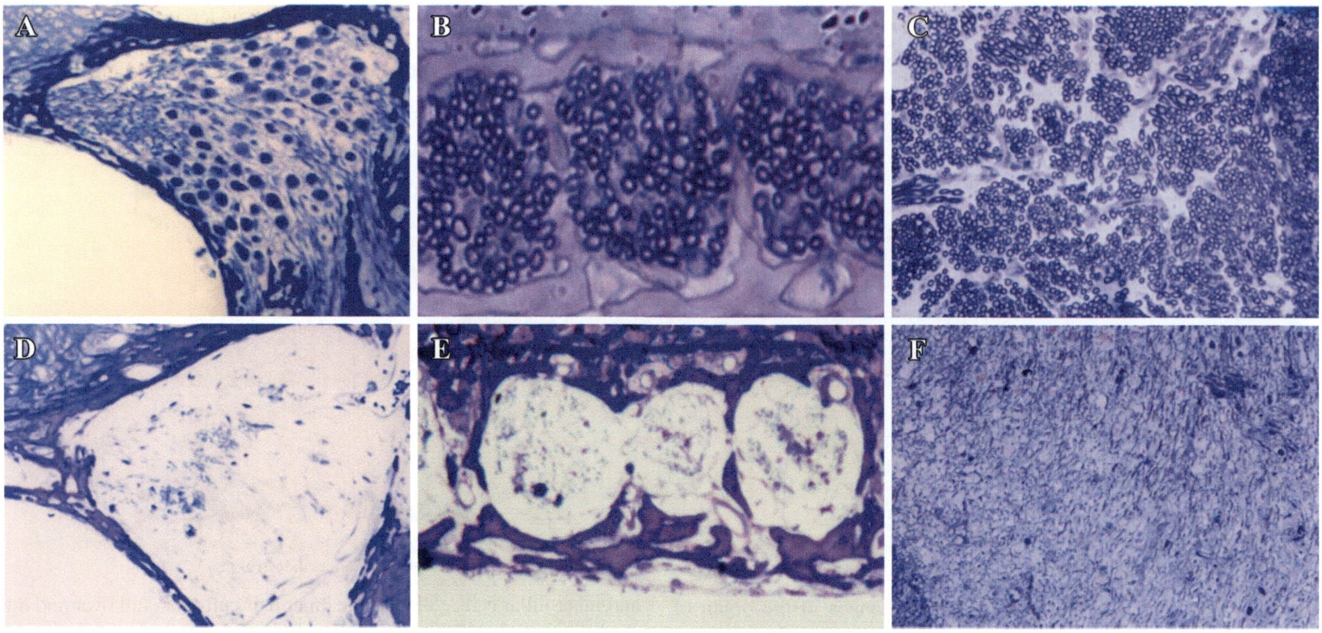

Fig. 7.20 A series of composite micrographs shows the subsequent secondary damage of the entire peripheral auditory nerve system within the cochlea after hair cell loss induced by intratympanic injection of gentamicin. (**A**) Section parallel to the modiolus shows that Rosenthal's canal contains dense spiral ganglion cells in normal rats. (**B**) The cross-sectional slice of the habenula perforata in a normal rat shows that the habenula perforata was filled with the peripheral nerve fibers connecting the organ of Corti. (**C**) The cochlear nerve foramen of a normal rat is filled with cochlear nerve fibers connecting the central auditory nervous system. (**D**) 60 days after intratympanic injection of gentamicin, there was a near-complete loss of spiral ganglion cells in Rosenthal's canal. (**E**) The peripheral auditory nerve fibers in the Habenula Perforata disappeared 60 days after intratympanic injection of gentamicin. (**F**) 60 days after intratympanic injection of gentamicin, the nerve fibers in the cochlear nerve foramen leading to the auditory center have almost completely collapsed. This temporal-spatial progression demonstrates gentamicin's capacity to induce retrograde neurodegeneration along the entire auditory pathway, from peripheral synaptic terminals to the central axons, following initial ototoxic insult to the sensory hair cells. (Reproduced with permission from Ding et al. [7, 17])

auditory nerve damage [6, 7, 16, 17, 22, 23, 28, 29, 31, 34–36] (Figs. 7.10–7.12, 7.20A, D, 7.21, and 7.22A, B).

The auditory nerve bundle demonstrates a characteristic anatomical trajectory as it extends from the cochlear modiolus to the brainstem, creating distinct histological evaluation opportunities. At the critical transition zone where the nerve bundle makes its inward turn from the auditory canal base toward the cochlear nucleus, sagittal plane sections provide optimal transverse visualization of the nerve bundle's internal architecture [7, 17, 37] (Fig. 7.22C, D), enabling precise quantitative assessment of axonal connectivity between peripheral and central auditory pathways. Conversely, modiolar-parallel cross-sections permit comprehensive qualitative evaluation of pathological alterations along the longitudinal axis of auditory nerve fibers projecting to the cochlear nucleus [7, 17] (Fig. 7.23). This dual-plane sectioning approach capitalizes on the nerve bundle's natural anatomical course to facilitate complementary assessments: sagittal sections reveal cross-sectional fiber organization and myelination patterns ideal for morphometric analysis, while modiolar-parallel sections allow tracking of axonal integrity along the nerve's entire projection pathway. The strategic orientation of these sectioning planes provides researchers with a comprehensive toolkit for investigating both the microstructural and longitudinal organization of cochleoneural connections.

7.2 Sample Preparation for Isolated Cochlear Membrane Labyrinthine Slices

While conventional whole cochlear sectioning techniques are primarily suitable for general histological staining and basic pathological assessment, they present significant limitations for specialized applications such as enzyme histochemistry and immunohistochemistry. In contrast, isolated cochlear basilar membrane preparations offer distinct advantages by eliminating the need for decalcification and its associated artifacts. This alternative methodology circumvents the technical challenges posed by acid-based decalcification, including enzyme inactivation and antigenic epitope disruption, thereby providing superior preservation of biological activity for specialized staining techniques [38–50]. The basilar membrane isolation approach thus represents an optimized preparation strategy for cochlear specimens requiring

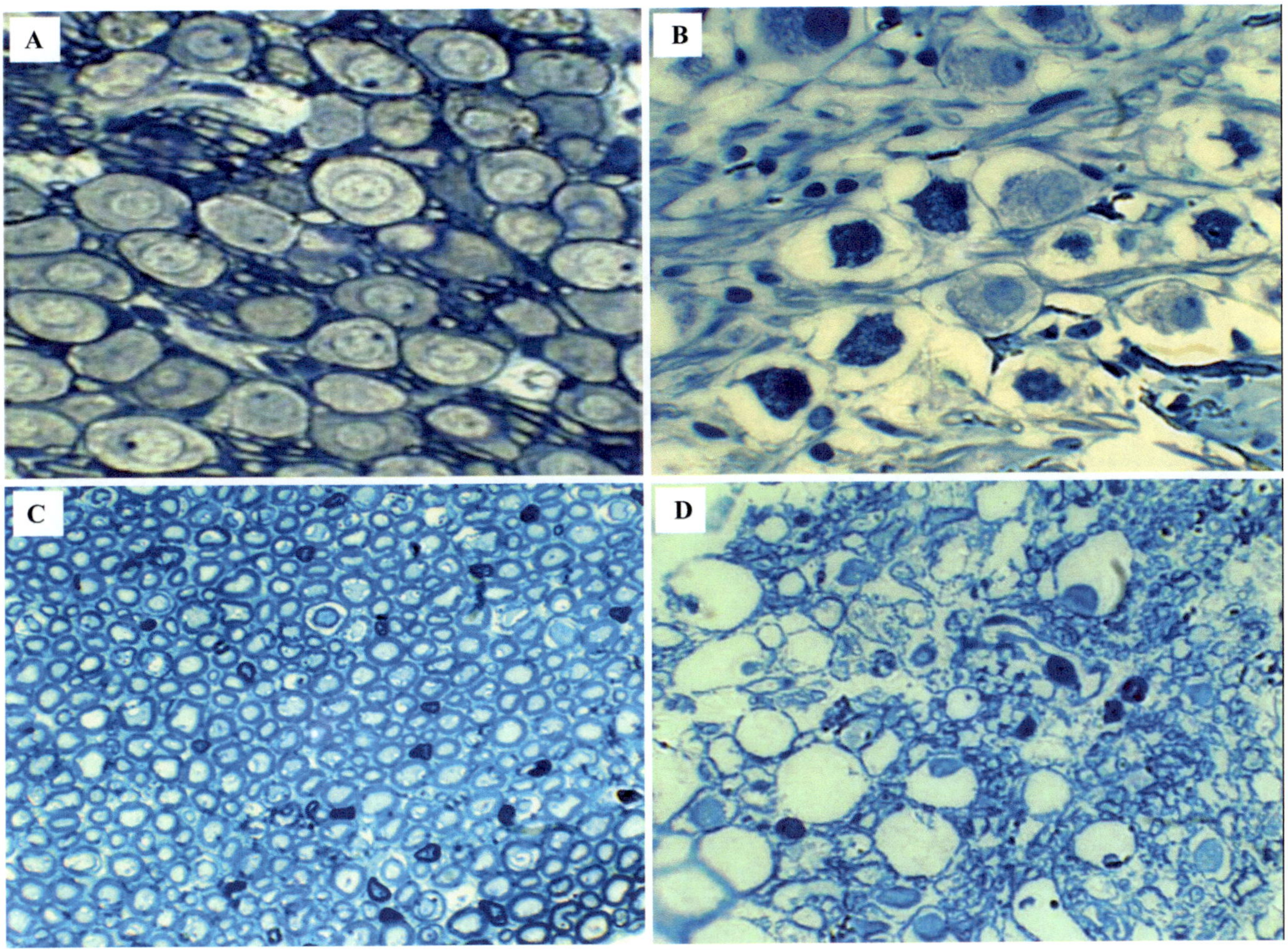

Fig. 7.21 Semithin section view showing the spiral ganglion and auditory nerve tract in chinchillas. (**A**) The intact spiral ganglion neurons were detected in Rosenthal's canal of a normal chinchilla. (**B**) 72 h after carboplatin injection, spiral ganglion cells showed obvious nuclear pyknosis, suggesting that carboplatin-induced spiral ganglion destruction exhibits typical apoptotic features. (**C**) A sagittal section through the cochlear nerve canal shows a cross-section of the auditory nerve fibers with surrounding dense myelin layers. (**D**) 24 h after injection of 10 μL of doxorubicin solution with a concentration of 37.5 μg/mL into the cochlear nerve canal, a sagittal section of the auditory nerve bundle showed severe demyelinating lesions in the auditory nerve fibers

enzymatic or immunohistochemical analysis, maintaining both structural integrity and biochemical reactivity while avoiding the confounding variables introduced by traditional decalcification processes. This technical advancement has significantly expanded the research capabilities in cochlear molecular histopathology.

7.2.1 Fixation of the Cochlea

The cochlear perfusion fixation technique represents an optimal approach for rapid tissue preservation under near-physiologic conditions. Following surgical exposure of the round and oval windows under microscopic guidance, a small apical cochleostomy enables direct perfusion of fixative through the cochlear labyrinth while allowing simultaneous outflow through both windows. This method achieves instantaneous replacement of perilymph in scala vestibuli and scala tympani with fixative solution, resulting in immediate immersion of organ of Corti cellular elements in stabilizing fixative solution while maintaining their living-state configuration. The technique's principal advantage lies in its ability to capture cellular morphology in a near-native state by minimizing the post-mortem degradation interval, making it particularly valuable for ultrastructural and molecular studies requiring high-fidelity preservation [7, 9, 12, 16, 17, 21, 38, 40, 45, 46, 49, 51, 52]. The direct perfusion methodology has been consistently demonstrated as superior to immersion fixation for preserving delicate cochlear microarchitecture and biochemical integrity [7, 12, 16, 21, 43, 45, 46, 53, 54].

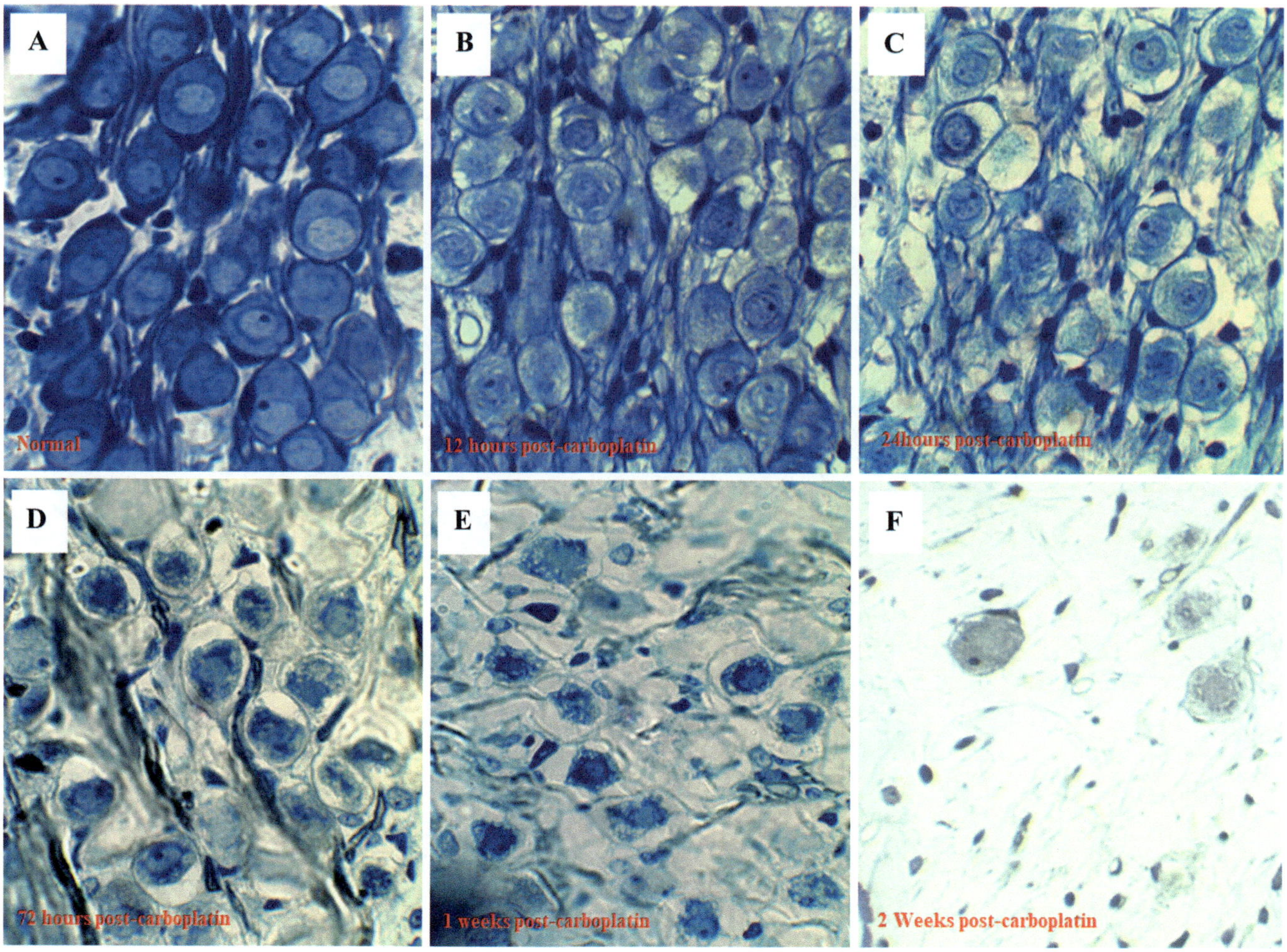

Fig. 7.22 Semithin sections of Rosenthal's canal parallel to the modiolus in chinchillas show the process of pathological changes of the spiral ganglion induced by carboplatin. (**A**) The spiral ganglion cells of normal chinchillas maintain perfect neuronal morphological structure. (**B**) 12 h after carboplatin administration, small vacuoles began to appear in a few spiral ganglion cells. (**C**) 24 h post-carboplatin administration, intracellular vacuolar degeneration appears within many spiral ganglion neurons. (**D**) 72 h after carboplatin injection, the nuclei of spiral ganglion neurons were significantly deformed due to the compression of large vacuoles. (**E**) 1 week after injection of carboplatin, the spiral ganglion showed obvious nuclear condensation and large vacuoles in the cytoplasm. (**F**) 2 weeks after carboplatin administration, the vast majority of type I spiral ganglia were completely destroyed, while the type II spiral ganglia were spared

7.2.2 Staining and Slicing of the Isolated Cochlear Basilar Membrane and Spiral Ligament

The cochlear basilar membrane and spiral ligament, being non-osseous membranous tissues, offer distinct technical advantages for histological processing. Following microdissection from the osseous spiral lamina and lateral cochlear wall, respectively, these structures can undergo direct processing without decalcification. With thicknesses ranging from 30 to 100 microns depending on species (50 µm for murine basilar membrane, 30 µm for stria vascularis), these membranes permit unimpeded dye penetration comparable to standard thick sections. This dimensional characteristic enables immediate application of enzymatic histochemical stains and immunohistochemical labeling protocols. Post-staining, the tissues can be embedded in epoxy resin for semithin sectioning (perpendicular to membrane planes) or gelatin for cryosectioning, as demonstrated in multiple methodological references [16, 34, 38, 42, 43, 45, 46, 48, 49, 53, 55–61] (Figs. 6.4, 6.7, 6.9, 6.17, 6.25, and 1.13; Figs. 7.18, 7.22, 7.23, 7.24A, B, and 7.25). Alternatively, flat-mount preparations allow confocal microscopic acquisition of z-stack image series for three-dimensional protein localization analysis through computational reconstruction [43, 45, 46, 54, 57, 58, 61, 62] (Figs. 7.26 and 7.27). For light microscopic examination, resin-embedded semi-thin sections can be toluidine blue-stained using a standardized protocol involving thermal adhesion to slides, dye application, and controlled dehydration, yielding high-resolution visualization of cochlear microstructures including the organ of Corti, stria vascularis, and neural elements [6, 7, 16, 17, 22, 23, 28, 33, 62, 63]. These membrane-specific techniques circumvent

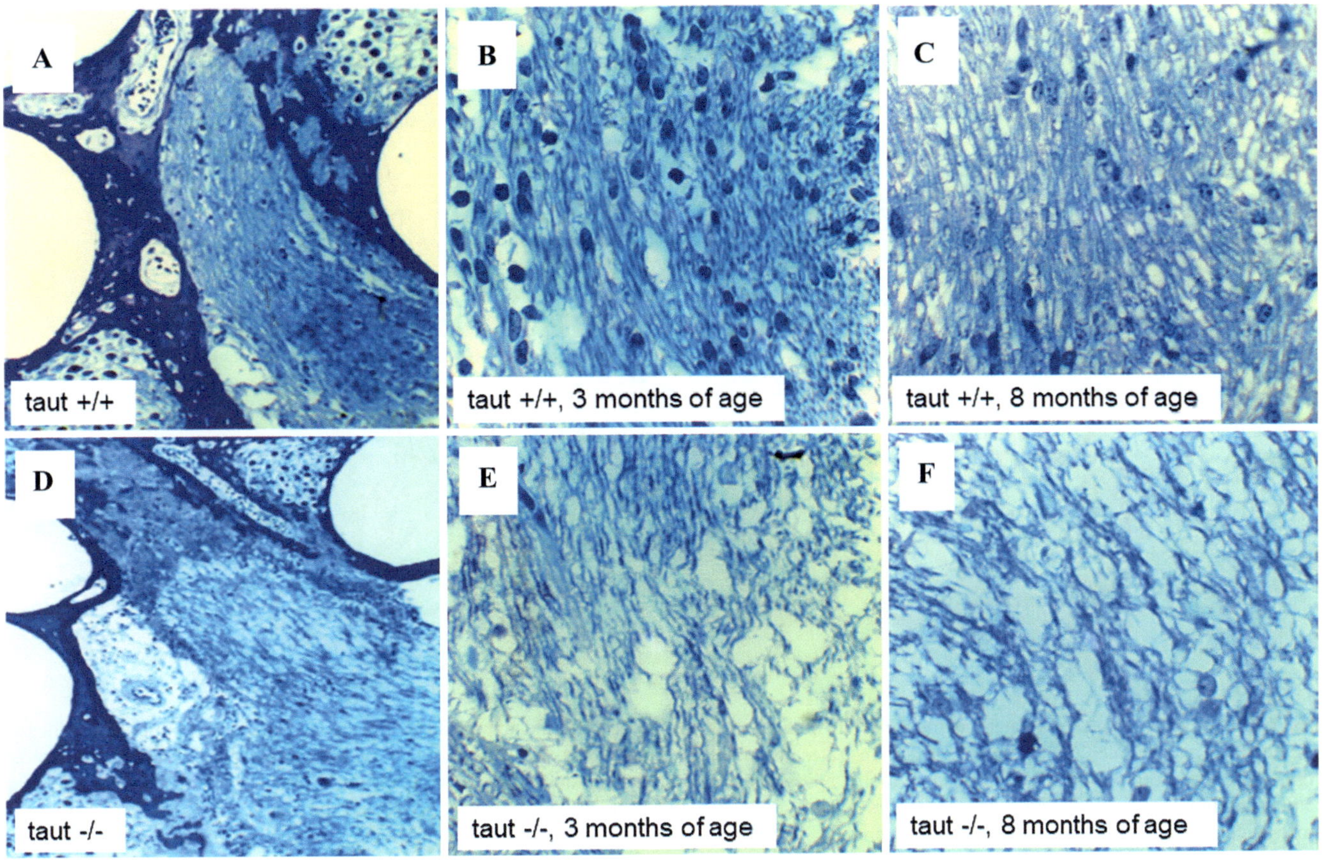

Fig. 7.23 Semithin sections parallel to the modiolus of the cochlea of wild-type TAUT mice and TAUT knockout mice were observed and compared. (**A**) The nerve fibers in the central canal of the modiolus in wild-type TAUT mice are completely wrapped by myelin, and the nuclei of glial cells can be seen in the gaps within nerve bundles. (**B**) Wild-type TAUT mice at 3 months of age maintain robust myelination with abundant glial cell nuclei interspersed among auditory nerve bundles, indicating preserved myelin sheath and neuroglial interactions. (C) 8 months after birth, the myelin sheaths of auditory nerve fibers and the nuclei of glial cells surrounding the nerve fibers in wild-type TAUT mice maintained normal structures. (**D**) Sections parallel to the central canal of the modiolus show that TAUT knockout mice exhibit fundamental myelination defects, with absent or incomplete myelin sheaths around the auditory nerve fibers. (**E**) 3 months after birth, auditory nerve fibers projecting to the cochlear nucleus lose myelin in a TAUT-deficient mouse. The nuclei of glial cells are not detected in the gaps of the auditory bundles. (**F**) 8 months after birth, the myelin sheath of the auditory nerve fibers and the surrounding glial cells in TAUT-deficient mice disappeared, suggesting that the reason why TAUT gene deficiency causes the loss of myelin sheath in auditory nerve fibers may be related to the loss of glial cells. These findings confirm that the auditory nerve fibers in the cochlear neuroforamen leading to the cochlear nucleus of taurine transporter (TAUT) gene-deficient mice were abnormal, mainly manifested by the loss of surrounding glial cells and the lesions of the myelin sheath around the cochlear nerve fibers

decalcification artifacts while providing multiple analytical options from conventional histology to advanced three-dimensional protein mapping.

After obtaining ideal positioning semi-thin sections from the Epon 812 embedded cochlear membranous labyrinth, ultrathin sections can be collected sequentially along the same plane using a glass knife for observation under transmission electron microscopy (TEM). This approach ensures accurate orientation of the sample sectioning [4, 29, 64–73] (Figs. 7.28–7.34). Beyond conventional TEM observations, advanced techniques can be employed to study molecular localization at the ultrastructural level. Radioautography using tritium-labeled kanamycin allows precise mapping of drug binding sites on ultrathin sections coated with photosensitive emulsion [68] (Fig. 7.35). Furthermore, enzyme histochemical reactions generating metal-labeled products can be directly visualized under TEM due to their characteristic high electron density, which specifically marks enzymatic proteins [69, 74–76] (Figs. 7.36 and 7.37). For immunohistochemical studies, biotin-labeled products reacted with 3,3′-diaminobenzidine (DAB) can enhance its contrast through osmium tetroxide treatment, forming electron-dense osmium-diaminobenzidine complexes that permit precise subcellular localization of antigens [71] (Fig. 7.38). These TEM-based cytochemical techniques

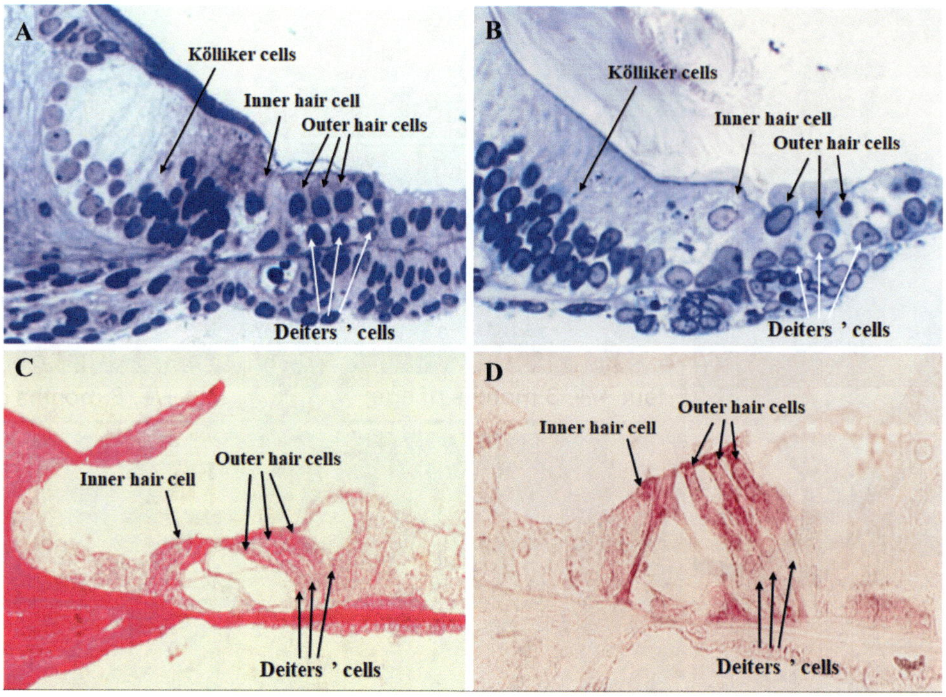

Fig. 7.24 Sections from the isolated cochlear basilar membrane. (**A**) The neonatal rat specimen (postnatal day 3) demonstrates an immature organ of Corti morphology, characterized by solid epithelial organization lacking Nuel's space and persistence of Kölliker's cells in the inner sulcus region. (**B**) Gentamicin-treated explants (0.5 mM for 24 h) reveal characteristic ototoxic changes, including outer hair cell nuclear pyknosis and cytoplasmic extrusion through the cuticular plate, representing the classic features of aminoglycoside-induced hair cell degeneration. (**C**) Glycogen staining showing the distribution of glycoproteins on the frozen section of the cochlear basilar membrane of an adult guinea pig. (**D**) Distribution of nonspecific esterase is shown on the frozen section of an adult guinea pig

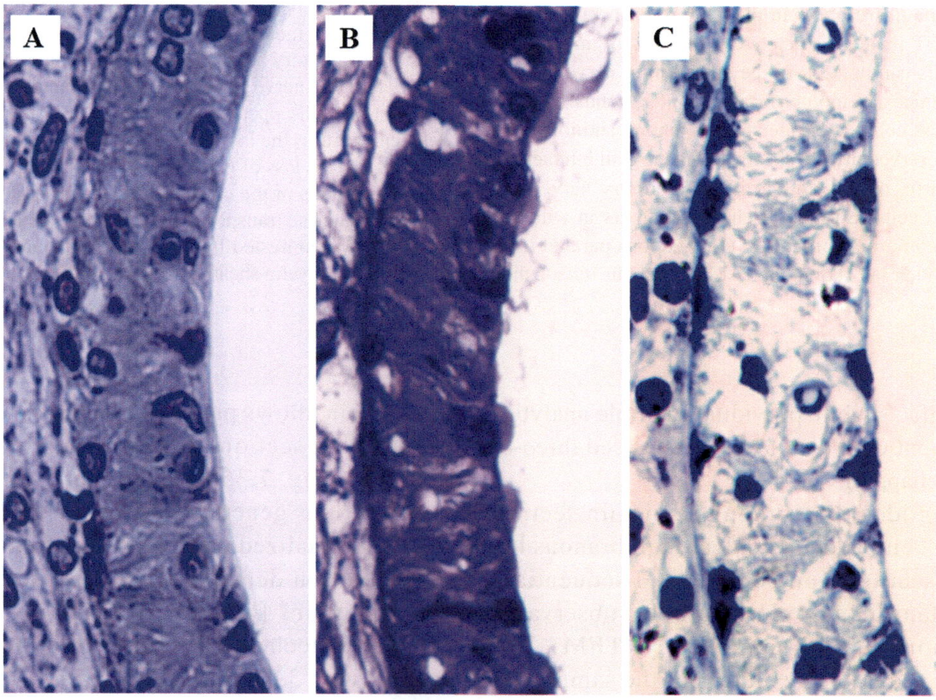

Fig. 7.25 Semi-thin sections of the spiral ligament showing pathological changes of the stria vascularis in mice induced by furosemides. (**A**) Semi-thin section of the spiral ligament from a normal control mouse shows the structural stratification of marginal cells, intermediate cells, and basal cells of the stria vascularis. (**B**) 10 min after intraperitoneal injection of furosemide (200 mg/kg), the marginal cells of the stria vascularis became uneven resulting from cellular swelling. (**C**) 60 min after injection of furosemide, all three layers of epithelial cells in the stria vascularis underwent severe vacuolar degeneration

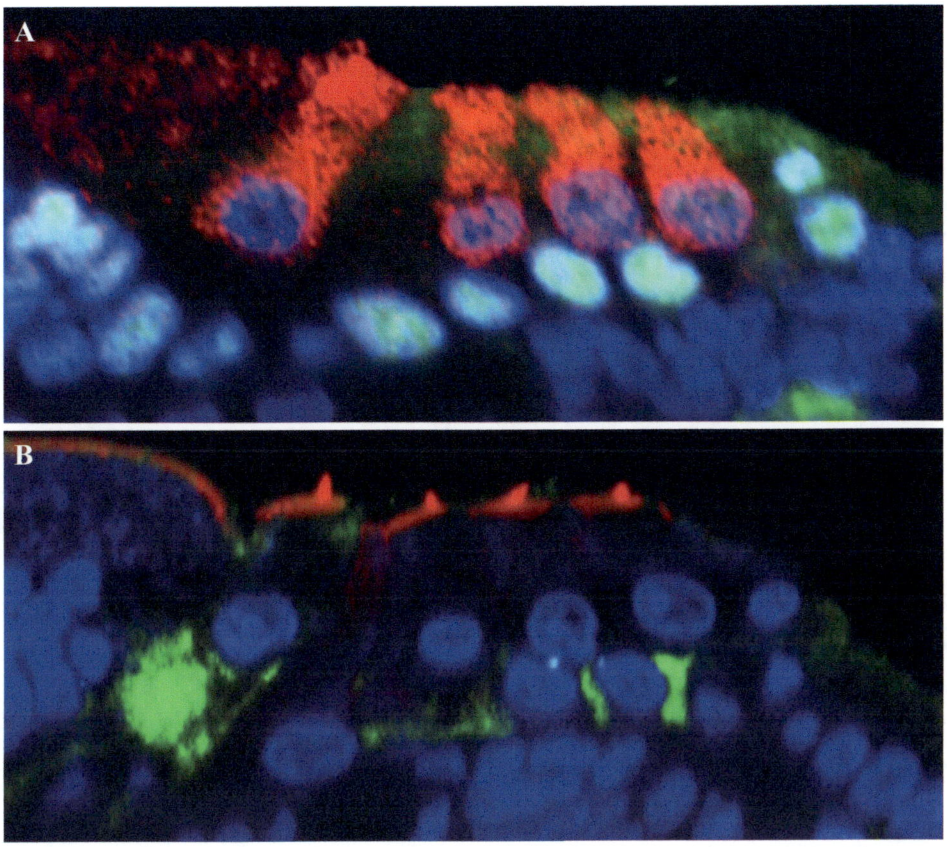

Fig. 7.26 Confocal image processing software was used to obtain Z-stack slice images of the organ of Corti. (**A**) Z-section of the organ of Corti was triple-labeled with Myosin VI, Sox2, and ToPro-3. The red fluorescence identifies the hair cells, the green fluorescence identifies the nuclei of support cells, and the blue fluorescence identifies the nuclei of cells. (**B**) Z-section of the organ of Corti was triple-labeled with Tubulin, phalloidin, and ToPro-3. The red fluorescence labels the stereocilia and cuticular plate of the hair cells, the green fluorescence labels the neuronal synapses at the bottom of the hair cells, and the blue fluorescence labels nuclei

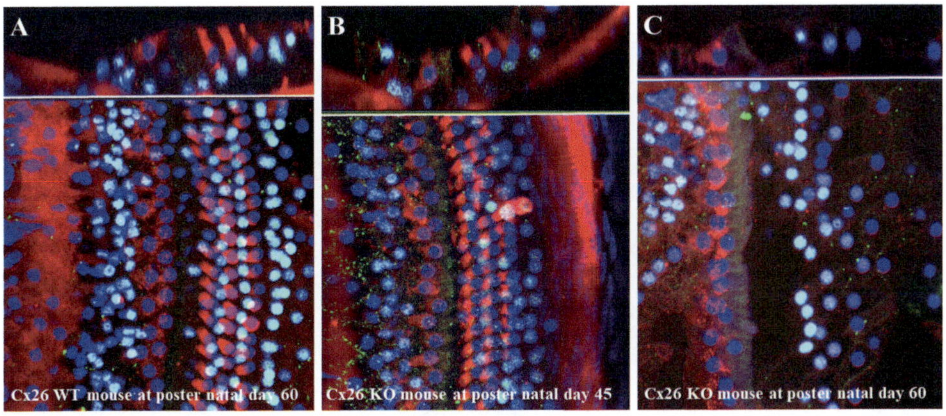

Fig. 7.27 Comparison of confocal images of the cochlear epithelium of Cx26 wild-type and Cx26-deficient mice using multiple fluorescent markers (myosin VI, Sox2, ToPro-3). Each panel combines Z-plane reconstructed cross-sections (upper) with corresponding surface preparations (lower), where red fluorescence marks hair cells (Myosin VI), green identifies supporting cell nuclei (Sox2), and blue stains all nuclei (ToPro-3). (**A**) The 60-day-old wild-type specimen demonstrates preserved cytoarchitecture of both hair cells and supporting cells, representing normal mature cochlear morphology. (**B**) Initial pathology in 45-day-old Cx26-deficient mice reveals intact hair cells but early supporting cell damage, indicating selective vulnerability of these gap junction-rich cells. (**C**) Advanced degeneration in 60-day-old mutants shows complete loss of outer hair cells and Deiters' cells, suggesting a pathogenic sequence where connexin 26 deficiency disrupts intercellular communication, leading to secondary hair cell anoikis (detachment-induced apoptosis) through gap junction dysfunction and extracellular matrix breakdown. These findings provide visual evidence for the critical role of Cx26-mediated intercellular communication in cochlear homeostasis, with the temporal progression highlighting how primary supporting cell pathology ultimately drives secondary sensory cell degeneration in this genetic model of hearing loss

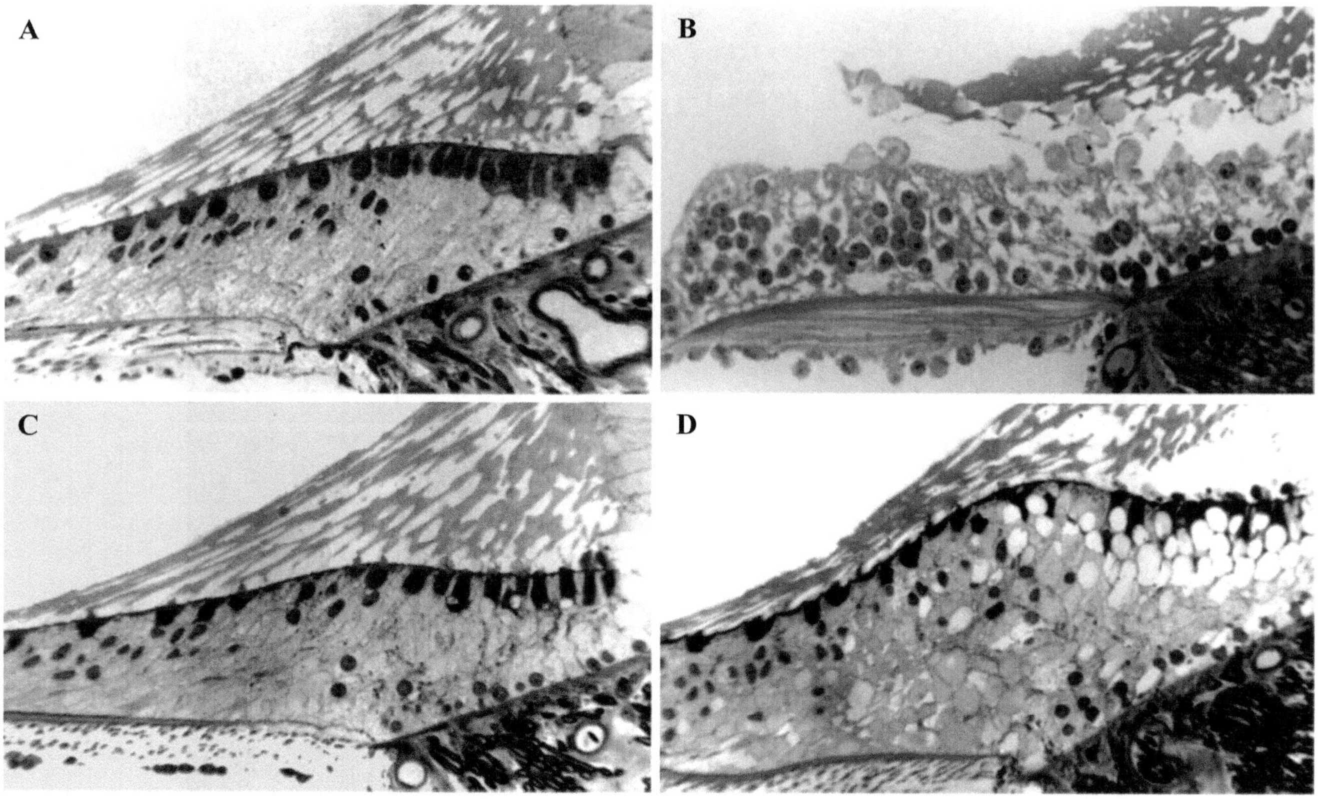

Fig. 7.28 Semi-thin sections of chicken cochlear basilar membrane. (**A**) The histological structure of the cochlear basilar membrane in control chicken present normal structure. (**B**) Complete destruction of most hair cells on the second day after the kanamycin injections (400 mg/kg/day × 10 days), showing the emergence of proliferating cells along the basilar membrane that subsequently differentiate into regenerating hair cells. (**C**) A low concentration of kainic acid (0.3 mM) application in the round window niche only results in transient mild vacuolar degeneration of afferent synapses beneath the tall hair cells. (**D**) High concentration of kainic acid (5 mM) application in the round window niche caused severe cavitation of the afferent nerve synapse beneath the tall hair cells, but the tall hair cells themselves were intact. These findings indicate that (1) Kanamycin selectively destroys the cochlear hair cells in the chicken, while the hair cell regeneration occurred naturally 10 days after injury. (2) Kainic acid specifically destroys the afferent nerve synapses beneath the tall hair cells in chicken, but does not destroy the sensory hair cells in chicken

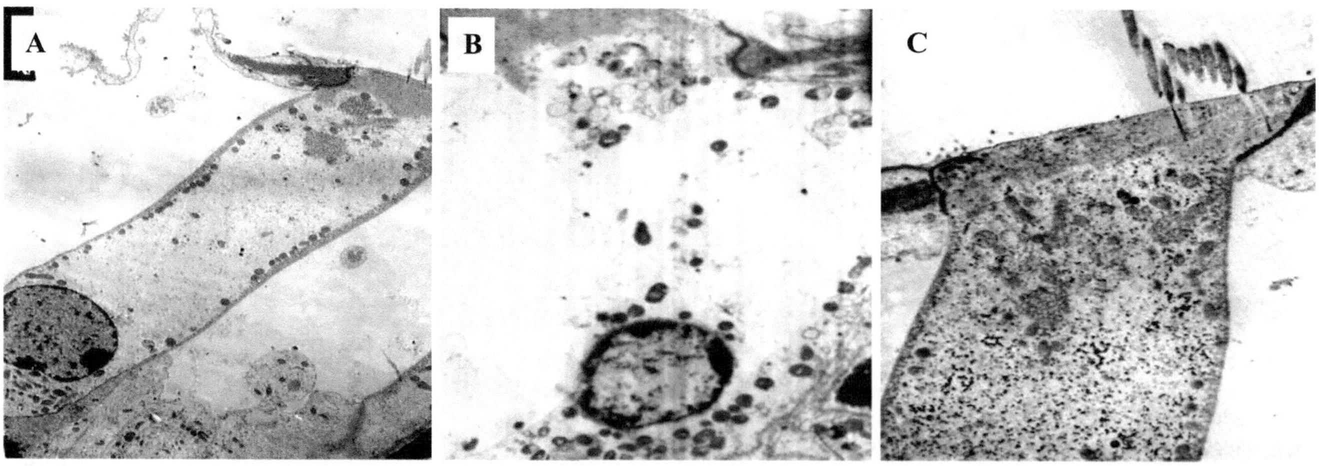

Fig. 7.29 Ultrastructural changes of outer hair cells in guinea pigs caused by different experimental conditions. (**A**) The typical morphology of outer hair cells in a normal guinea pig. (**B**) The extreme swelling of outer hair cells is caused by severe hypoxia. (**C**) 30 min after 9370 MHz high-frequency electromagnetic wave irradiation, a large number of electron-dense deposits have appeared in the outer hair cells. Although the nature of these particles is still unclear, their high electron density suggests that they may be related to oxidation products complexed with metal ions. The above observations demonstrate the sensitivity of outer hair cells to various physical and chemical interference at the ultrastructural level

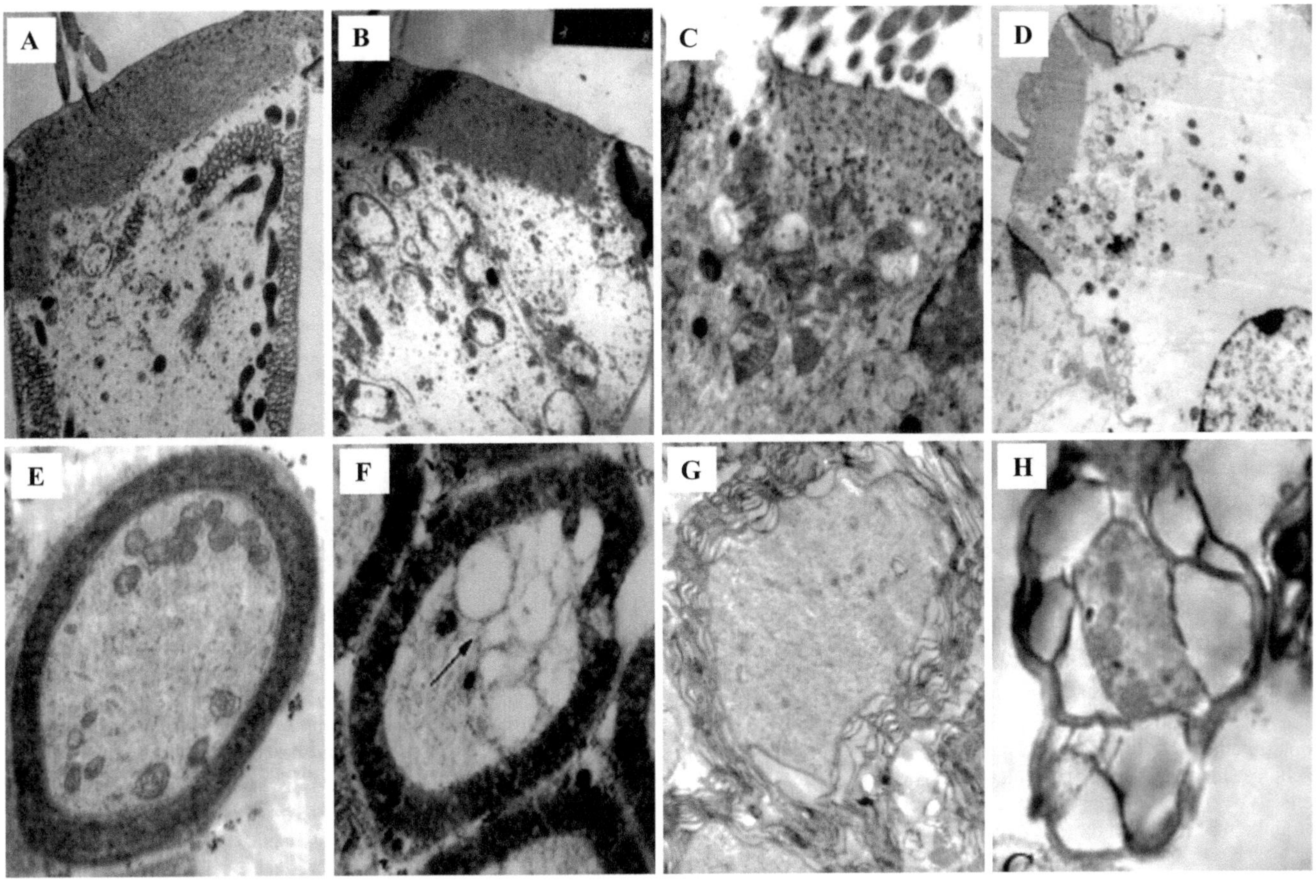

Fig. 7.30 Transmission electron microscopy (TEM) images of cochlear hair cells and auditory nerve fibers under various experimental conditions. (**A**) Normal ultrastructure of guinea pig cochlear outer hair cells serves as control. (**B**) The initial pathological change induced by kanamycin treatment (400 mg/kg/day for 7 days) manifests as mitochondrial vacuolization in outer hair cells, indicating mitochondria as primary targets of aminoglycoside toxicity. (**C**) One week after intramuscular injection of kanamycin (400 mg/kg/day × 7), progressive damage leads to perforation of the cuticular plate of hair cells, and the cellular contents overflow from the rupture of the cuticular plate. (**D**) 30 min after hypoxia, the huge hydrophobic cavities appeared in the swollen outer hair cells. (**E**) Micrograph of an ultrathin section of the auditory nerve fiber in a normal chinchilla. (**F**) Vacuolar-like lesions appeared in the axon of auditory nerve fibers in chinchilla 24 h after carboplatin injection (100 mg/kg). (**G**) 48 h after carboplatin injection, the myelin sheath around the auditory nerve fibers of the chinchilla began to separate, indicating that demyelinating lesions began to occur. (**H**) After 72 h of carboplatin treatment, large vacuoles appeared in the myelin sheath layers, which had squeezed the axonal deformation. These observations systematically document the sequence of ultrastructural alterations in both sensory hair cells and auditory nerve fibers following various ototoxic insults

provide nanometer-scale resolution of molecular distributions within cellular ultrastructure, representing true cellular-level analysis, in contrast to light or fluorescence microscopy that offer only micron-scale resolution suitable for tissue or organ-level histochemical studies.

7.2.3 Frozen Substitution and Frozen Sections of Isolated Spiral Ligaments and Enzyme Histochemical Staining

The main difficulties faced in cochlear enzyme histochemistry or immunohistochemistry research are tissue fixation, decalcification, and embedding. Although aldehyde chemical fixatives can quickly coagulate proteins, they can also inactivate a variety of enzymes to varying degrees. Some enzymes are even completely inactivated by aldehyde fixatives, such as succinate dehydrogenase. The carboxyl group formed by cross-linking the aldehyde group of the aldehyde fixative with the amino group of the antigen protein can change the three-dimensional structure of the antigenic determinant cluster, making the structurally altered antigen unable to react specifically with the antibody. In order to avoid or reduce the effects of aldehyde fixatives on enzyme activity and the structure of antigenic reaction clusters, some people advocate avoiding the use of aldehyde fixatives or shortening the fixation time of aldehyde fixatives in enzyme histochemistry and immunohistochemistry experiments.

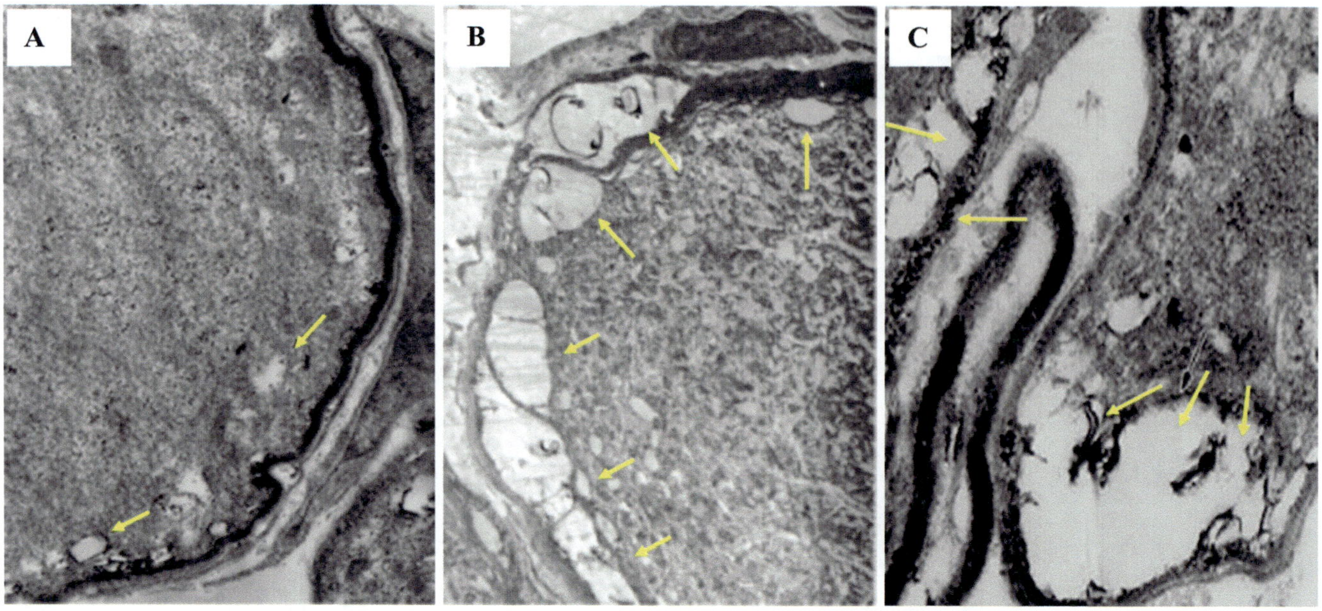

Fig. 7.31 The temporal progression of carboplatin-induced ultrastructural changes in chinchilla spiral ganglion neurons. (**A**) The earliest detectable pathology in type I spiral ganglion neurons appears as small subcapsular vacuoles (indicated by yellow arrows) within 6 h post-carboplatin administration. (**B**) 12 h post-carboplatin, these intramyelinic vacuoles undergo progressive enlargement in type I spiral ganglion cells. (**C**) 72 h following carboplatin injection, the initially discrete intramyelinic vacuoles coalesce into extensive, confluent vacuolar structures. These sequential morphological alterations provide compelling ultrastructural evidence that type I spiral ganglion neurons represent a primary target of carboplatin in the chinchilla experimental model, with the subcapsular and intramyelinic compartments showing particular vulnerability to platinum-based compounds. The observed vacuolar pathology suggests a potential mechanism of carboplatin-induced neuronal damage through progressive disruption of cellular compartmentalization

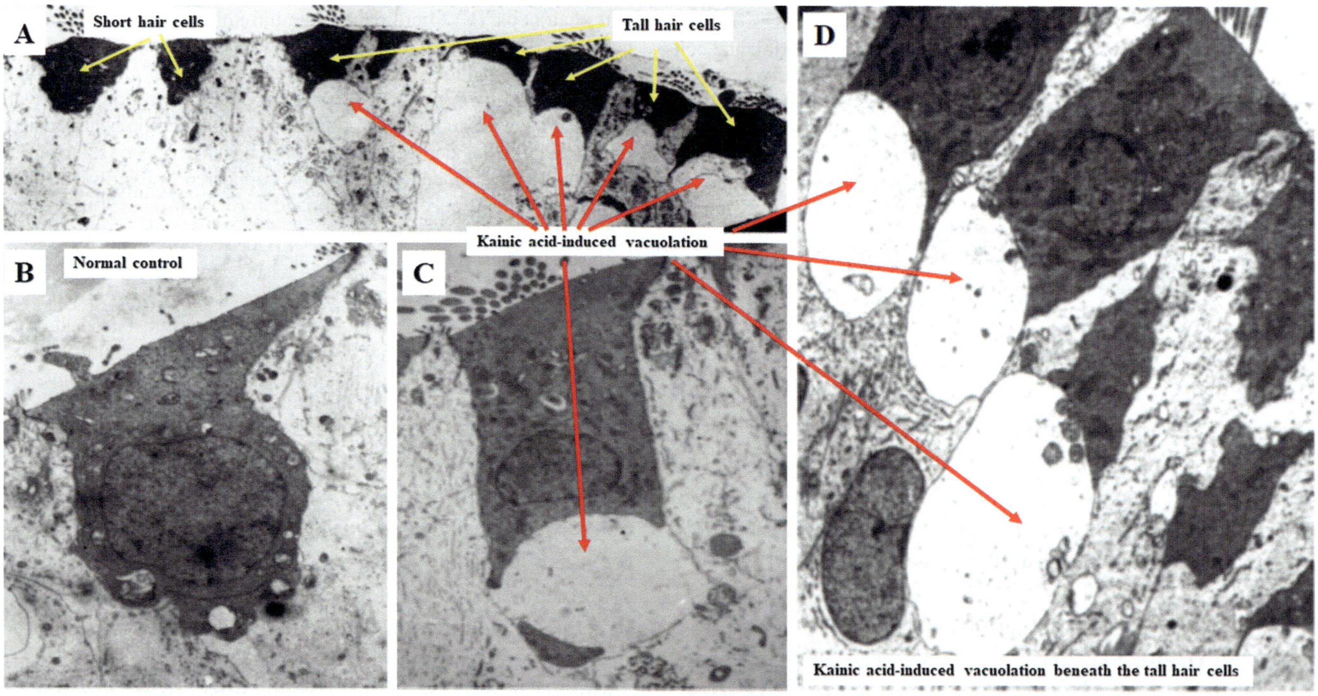

Fig. 7.32 Transmission electron microscopy (TEM) images of chicken cochlear hair cells showing various vacuolar destruction of afferent nerve terminals beneath the tall hair cells after local application of kainic acid on the round window membrane. (**A**) Local application of Kainic acid via the round window membrane induces the synapse vacuolation beneath the tall hair cells. (**B**) The high hair cells and their connecting nerve synapses in normal control chickens maintain normal morphology. (**C** and **D**) show that high concentration of Kainic acid selectively destroys the type I afferent synapse beneath the tall hair cells, suggesting that the type I afferent nerve terminals of tall hair cells contain the target of glutamate receptors. These findings provide ultrastructural evidence for the excitotoxic role of glutamate receptors in the avian cochlea, with type I afferent synapses beneath tall hair cells showing particular sensitivity to glutamatergic neurotoxicity

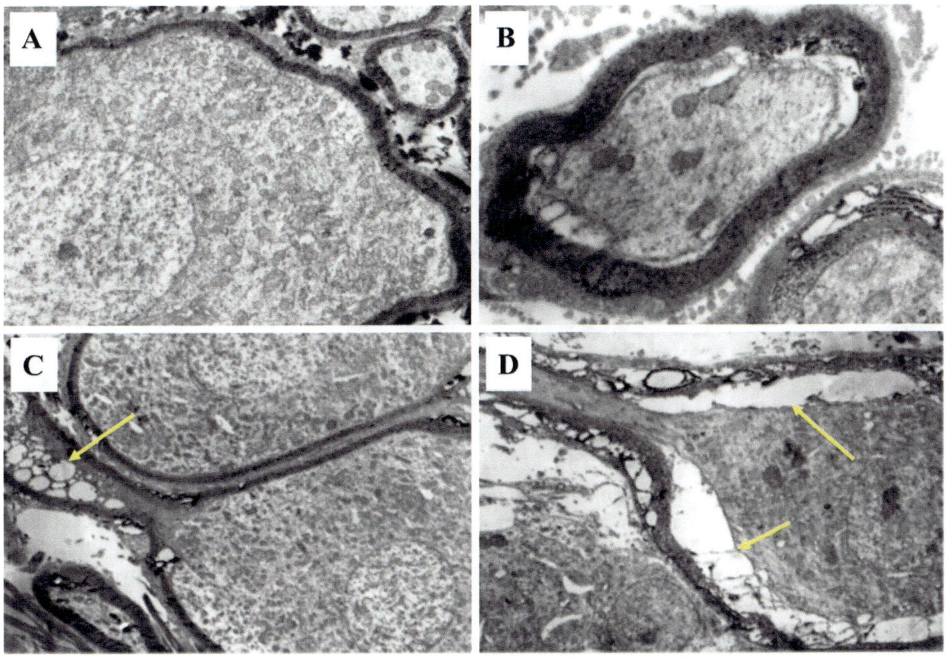

Fig. 7.33 The progressive destructive effects of kainic acid on spiral ganglion neurons and auditory nerve fibers in the chicken. (**A**) Normal ultrastructure of spiral ganglion neurons in control chickens demonstrates the baseline morphology. (**B**) After kainic acid enters the cochlea through the round window membrane of the chicken, it not only quickly destroys the afferent nerve synapse beneath the tall hair cells but also causes vacuolar degeneration and demyelination of the type I spiral ganglion. (**C**) The anatomical proximity between type I spiral ganglion neurons and tall hair cells facilitates kainic acid diffusion and enter the soma of the spiral ganglion through the connecting auditory nerve fibers, resulting in spreading damage to the type I afferent nerve fibers and ganglion cell. (**D**) With prolonged exposure and higher concentrations, kainic acid triggers severe myelin sheath disruption in spiral ganglion neurons, forming extensive intramyelinic fluid-filled cavities. These observations demonstrate a dose- and time-dependent neurotoxic cascade, where initial synaptic damage progresses to widespread axonal and neuronal pathology in the avian auditory pathway, highlighting the vulnerability of both peripheral and central components of the auditory system to excitotoxic injury

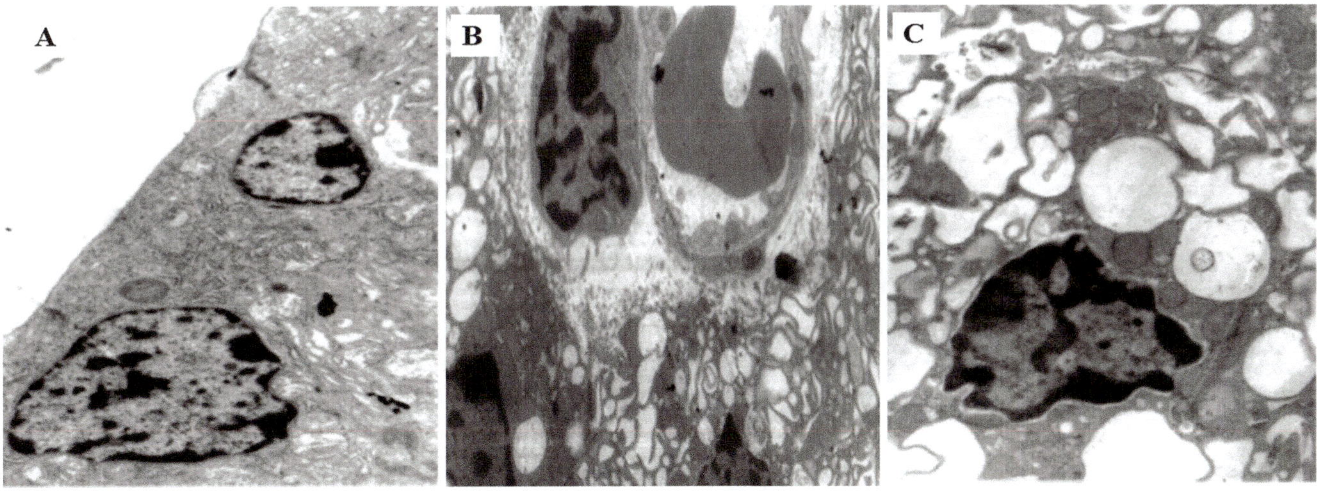

Fig. 7.34 Ultrastructural alterations in the stria vascularis of the guinea pig under various pathological conditions. (**A**) Transmission electron micrograph of stria vascularis epithelial cells from a normal guinea pig. (**B**) Transmission electron micrograph shows that hypoxia-induced ultrastructural damage in the epithelial cells of stria vascularis, indicating that stria vascularis epithelium is highly sensitive to hypoxia. (**C**) 30 min after intravenous injection of ethacrynic acid. Extremely severe hypoxic damage occurs within the epithelial cells of the stria vascularis. These comparative observations demonstrate the hypoxic lesions of stria vascular cells that occurred over time after injection of ethacrynic acid, particularly highlighting the vulnerability of stria vascular epithelial cells to both hypoxia and drug damage

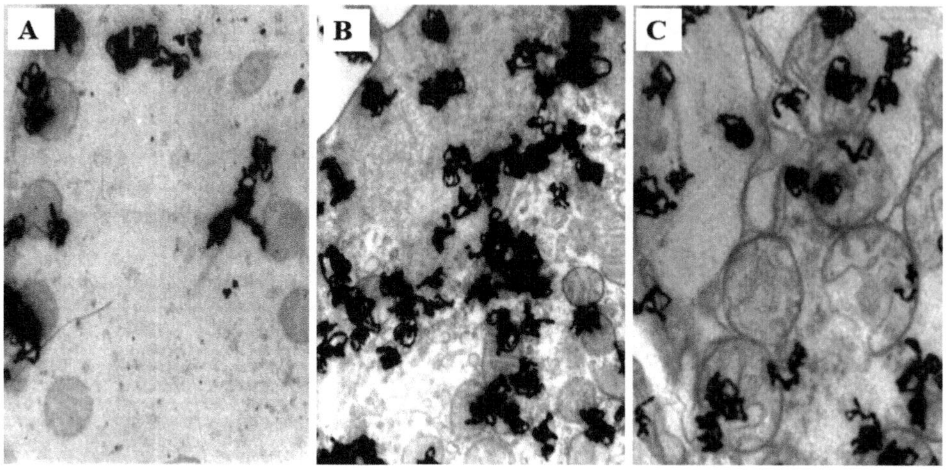

Fig. 7.35 Radioautography was used to demonstrate on ultrathin sections of cochlear hair cells that tritium-labeled kanamycin mainly accumulates in the mitochondria after entering the hair cells. (**A**) 30 min after the cochlear perfusion with tritium-labeled kanamycin, kanamycin accumulated in the mitochondria. (**B**) 60 min after cochlear perfusion with tritium-labeled kanamycin, the black ribbon-like tritium-labeled kanamycin mainly accumulated in the mitochondria, lysosomes, and cuticular plate of the hair cells. (**C**) A magnified image of tritium-labeled kanamycin accumulated in mitochondria. This selective mitochondrial targeting provides direct ultrastructural evidence for the organelle-specific binding of kanamycin, supporting the hypothesis that mitochondria serve as the primary subcellular site for kanamycin's ototoxic action. (Reproduced with permission from Ding et al. [68])

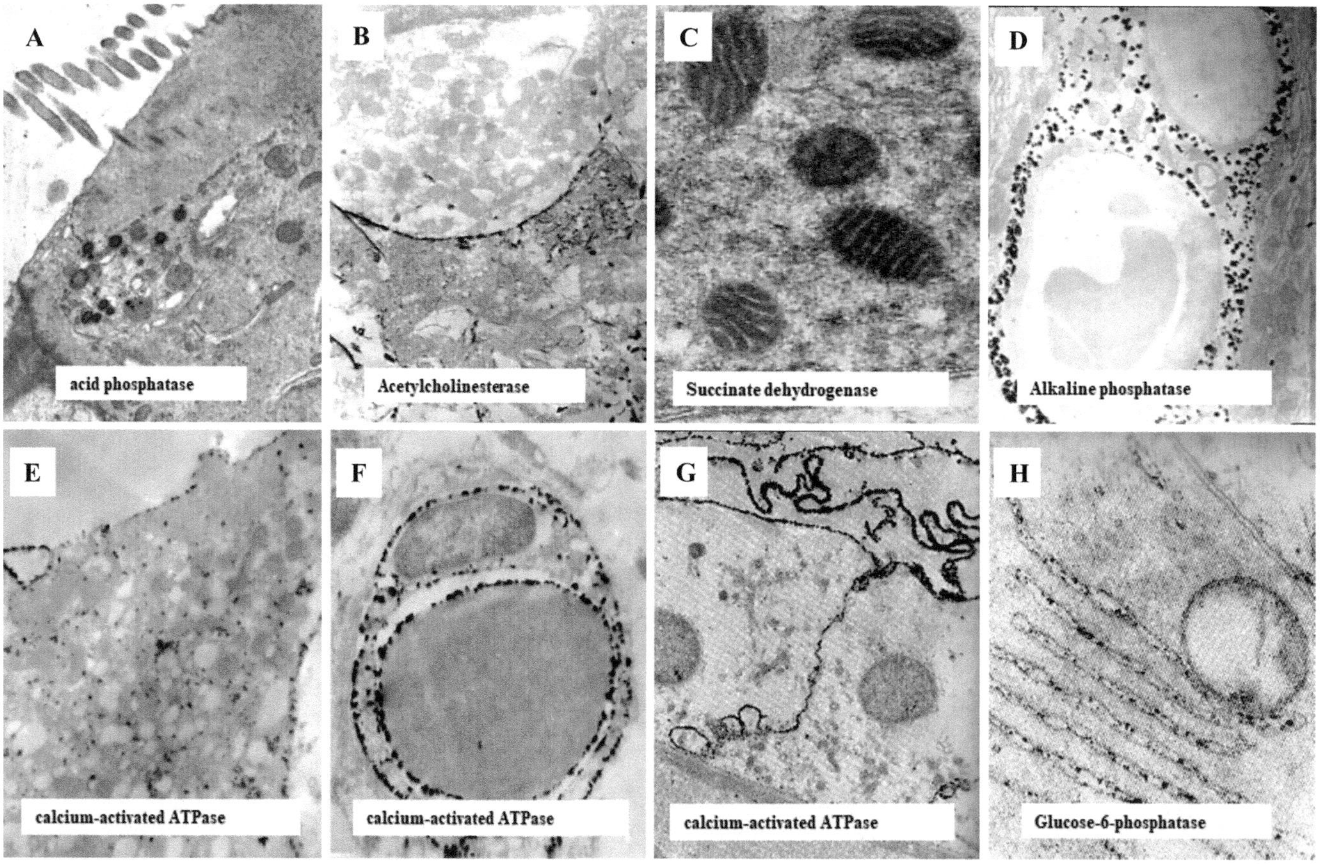

Fig. 7.36 The localization of several enzymes in the cochlea of the normal guinea pig using electron microscopic histochemistry. (**A**) Acid phosphatase activity is specifically confined to primary lysosomes beneath the cuticular plate of cochlear hair cells. (**B**) At the base of the outer hair cells, acetylcholinesterase is specifically expressed on the surface of the efferent synapses that connect to the outer hair cells. (**C**) Succinate dehydrogenase is precisely located on the surface of mitochondrial cristae of hair cells. (**D**) Alkaline phosphatase in the stria vascularis is localized in the capillary wall of the stria vascularis. (**E**) Calcium-activated ATPases in hair cells show dual localization in both plasma membranes and intracellular endomembrane systems. (**F**) Calcium-activated ATPase in the stria vascularis is located in the capillary endothelial cell membrane and erythrocyte membrane. (**G**) Calcium-activated ATPase in Claudius cells is located on their plasma membrane. (**H**) Glucose-6-phosphatase in hair cells is located in their endoplasmic reticulum. These observations establish a comprehensive enzymatic mapping of cochlear ultrastructure, revealing specialized compartmentalization of various enzymes and their ultrastructural localization

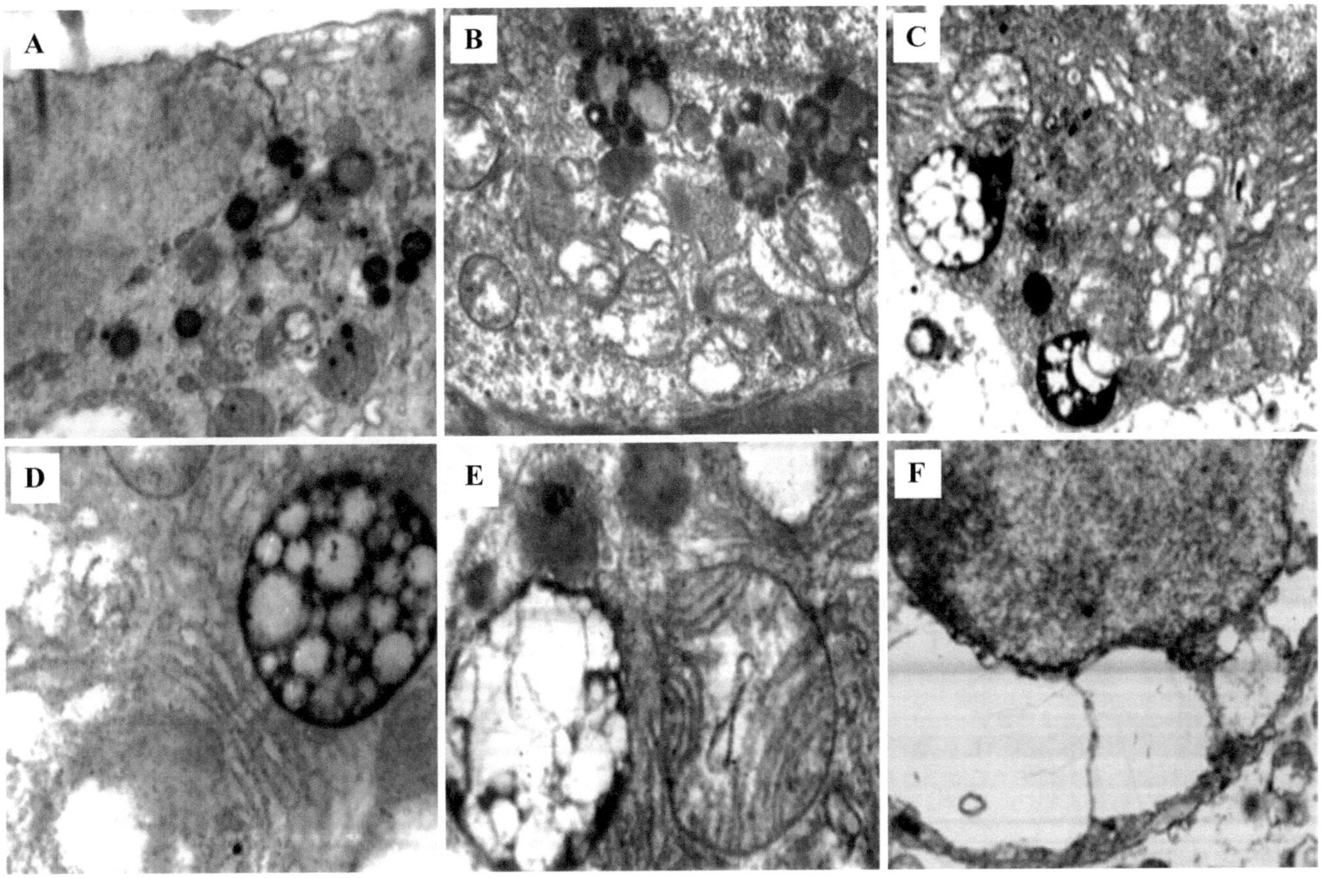

Fig. 7.37 Dynamic ultrastructural alterations of acid phosphatase activity during kanamycin-induced hair cell degeneration. (**A**) In normal hair cells, acid phosphatase serves as a definitive lysosomal marker, localized specifically in primary lysosomes beneath the cuticular plate. (**B**) After seven days of daily kanamycin injections, acid phosphatase-labeled primary lysosomes were relocated from their original location beneath the cuticular plate to around damaged mitochondria beneath the hair cell nuclei. (**C**) Acid phosphatase labeling shows that secondary lysosomes appear as multivesicular bodies after engulfing kanamycin and damaged organelles. The arrow points to a secondary lysosome with a multivesicular morphology that is attempting to engulf neighboring damaged mitochondria. (**D**) Acid phosphatase labeling showed that the secondary lysosomes gradually expanded as they continued to engulf the destroyed mitochondria. (**E**) Progressive lysosomal overload manifests as the fusion of small vacuoles into expanding large vacuolar structures. (**F**) When the membrane of the secondary lysosome ruptures due to overload, the degradative enzymes in the lysosome are released into the cytoplasm, eventually digesting the cytoplasm into large cavities. This sequence records the complete activity trajectory of lysosomes during kanamycin-induced cochlear hair cell destruction, from the initial lysosomal translocation to phagocytosis and finally to cell autolysis, highlighting the core destructive role of lysosomes in the process of aminoglycoside-induced hair cell necrosis

Cryosubstitution is a useful alternative in the analysis of cellular fine structure. Freeze-substitution is a physicochemical process in which biological specimens are immobilized and stabilized for microscopy. In this process, the water within the cells is rapidly replaced by organic solvents under extremely low temperatures, resulting in cells instantly drying. Multiple enzymes and antigenic proteins are best protected and preserved in a low-temperature and dry environment. Therefore, cryosubstitution is an ideal method of fixation to preserve the morphology and activities of cells [77].

Our optimized cryo-substitution protocol for spiral ligament fixation incorporates a novel "sandwich" embedding technique that addresses multiple technical challenges simultaneously. The dissected spiral ligament is carefully positioned between two thin liver tissue slices from the same animal, creating a composite block that is then flash-frozen in dry ice-cooled acetone or liquid nitrogen. This innovative approach provides mechanical support during processing while preventing ice crystal formation, enabling superior preservation of both enzymatic activities and antigenic structures that would otherwise be compromised by aldehyde fixation. The liver-embedded tissue blocks facilitate all subsequent steps from cryo-substitution to cryosectioning, with frozen sections mounted on slides for either enzyme histochemistry or immunohistochemistry. Remarkably, upon immersion in reaction solutions, the preserved biomolecules rapidly regain full activity from their cryopreserved state. For experimental rigor, we embed control and experimental spiral ligament samples within the same liver block, ensuring identical section thickness and identical processing conditions across all samples—a critical design

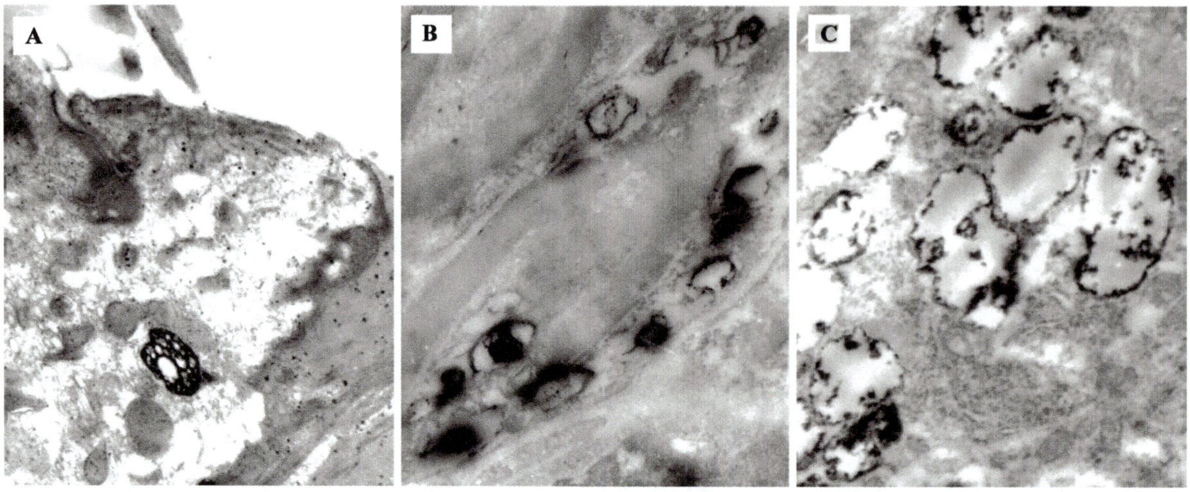

Fig. 7.38 Transmission electron micrographs show the activity changes of calpain in the cochlear inner hair cells, type I afferent nerve fibers, and spiral ganglion neurons after carboplatin injection. (**A**) Calcium-activated protease appears in vacuoles in chinchilla inner hair cells 48 h after carboplatin injection. (**B**) Calcium-activated protease appears in vacuoles within auditory nerve fibers 24 h after carboplatin injection. (**C**) Calcium-activated protease appears in vacuoles in spiral ganglion cells 48 h after carboplatin injection. These results suggest that calpain plays an important role in carboplatin-induced destruction of inner hair cells, type I afferent nerve fibers, and type I spiral ganglion neurons in chinchilla

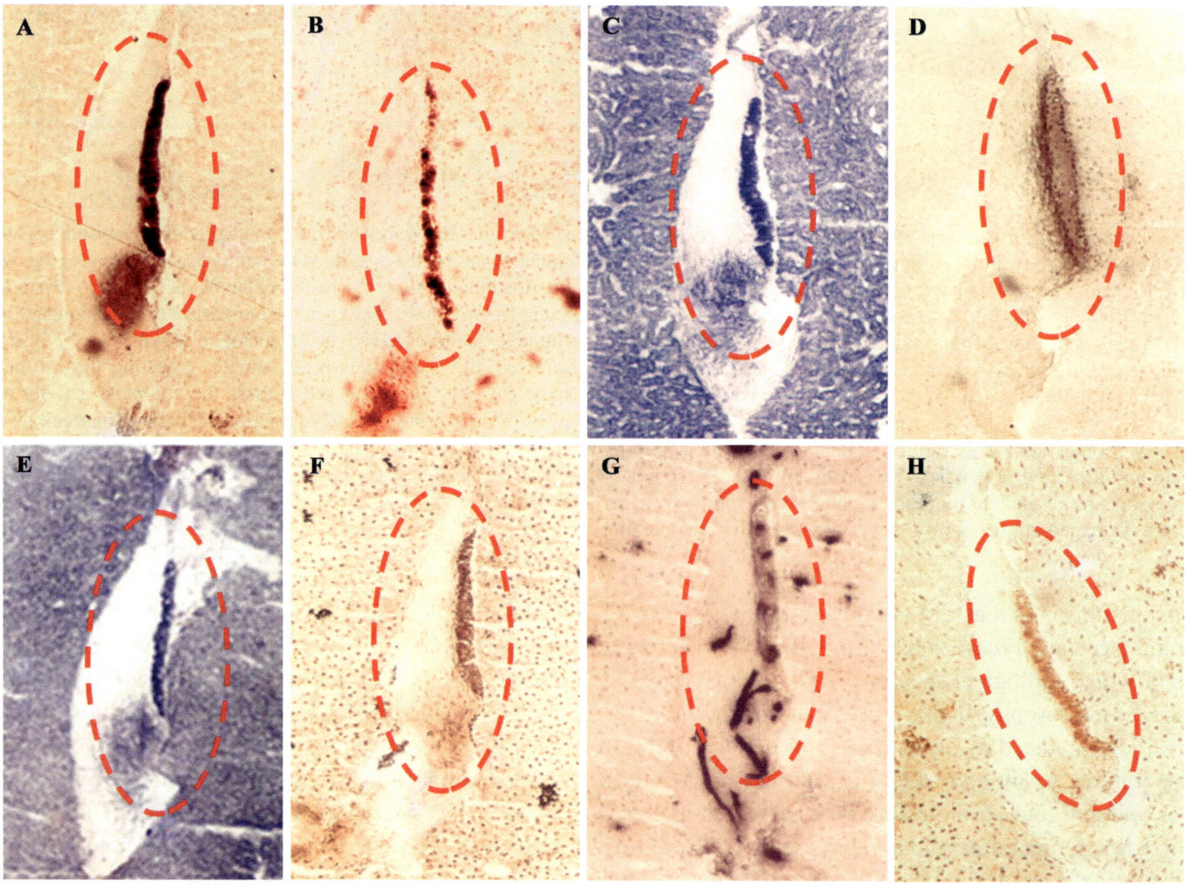

Fig. 7.39 The enzyme histochemical observations of stria vascularis epithelial cells using our optimized liver-embedded cryosection technique. (**A**) Sodium-potassium activated ATPase in the stria vascularis of the normal guinea pig. (**B**) 60 min after intravenous injection of ethacrynic acid, the activity of sodium-potassium activated ATPase in the epithelial cells of stria vascularis was greatly decreased. (**C**) Succinate dehydrogenase in the epithelial cells of stria vascularis. (**D**) 5′ Nucleotidase in the epithelial cells of stria vascularis. (**E**) Lactate dehydrogenase in the epithelial cells of stria vascularis. (**F**) Calcium-activated ATPase in the epithelial cells of stria vascularis. (**G**) Adenylate cyclase in the epithelial cells of stria vascularis. (**H**) Magnesium-activated ATPase in the epithelial cells of stria vascularis. This comprehensive enzymatic profiling of the stria vascularis was enabled by the liver embedding and cryosubstitution technique, which preserves the tissue cellularity while preserving the various enzymatic reactions. This sample preparation procedure uses a consistent technical approach to ensure direct comparability of enzymatic profiles and activities

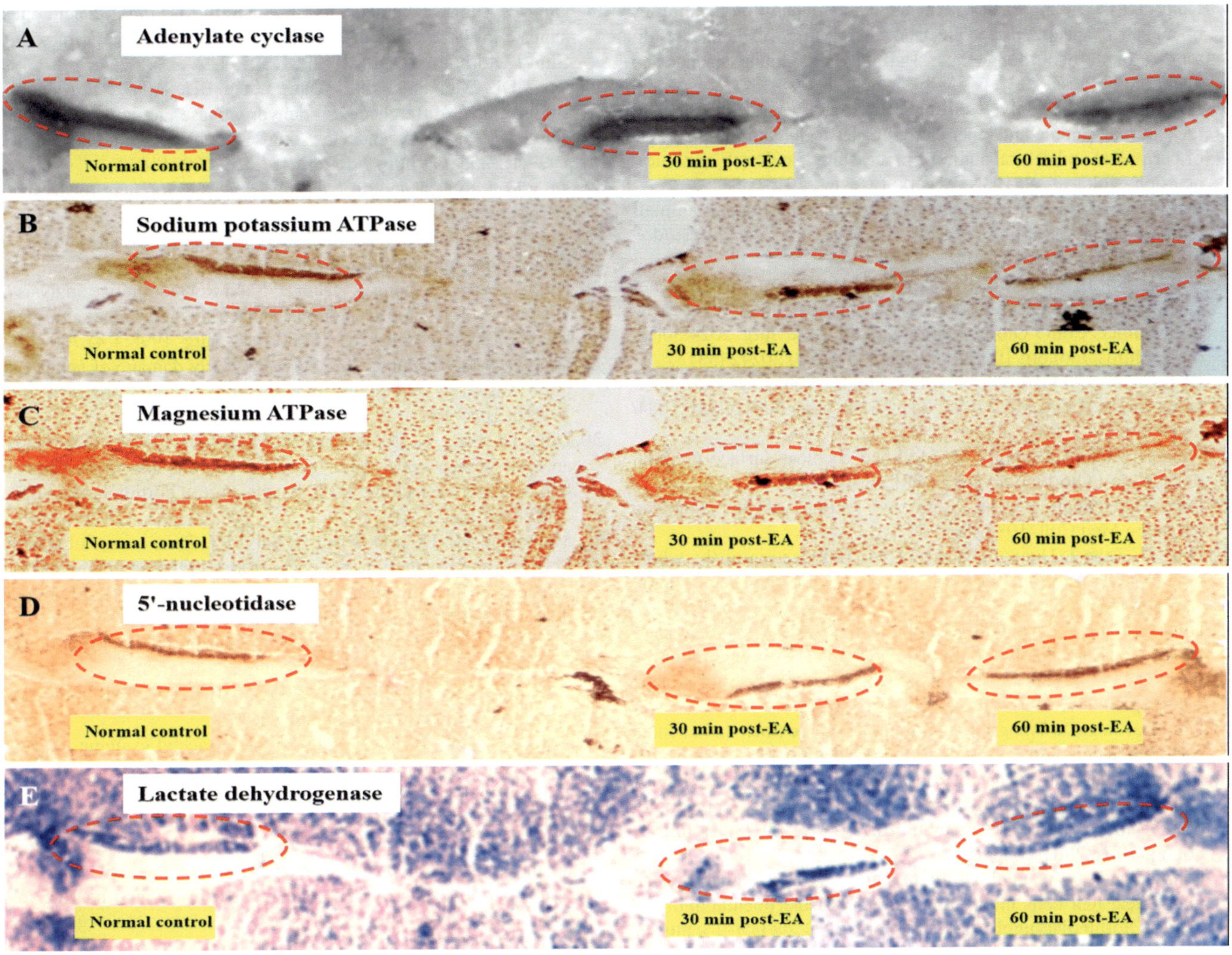

Fig. 7.40 Spiral ligaments under different experimental conditions were embedded in the same piece of liver tissue to obtain frozen sections of the stria vascularis with the same thickness and stained under the same conditions, ensuring the comparability of the results of enzyme histochemical staining under different experimental conditions. (**A**) Adenylate cyclase activity was attenuated 60 min after intravenous injection of ethacrynic acid. (**B**) Sodium-potassium-activated ATPase activity was greatly attenuated 60 min after injection of ethacrynic acid. (**C**) Magnesium-activated ATPase activity was attenuated in epithelial cells of the stria vascularis 60 min after injection of ethacrynic acid. (**D**) There was no change in 5′-nucleotidase activity 60 min after injection of ethacrynic acid. (**E**) There was no change in lactate dehydrogenase activity 60 mi after intravenous injection of ethacrynic acid. These differential responses, reliably documented through our controlled comparative methodology, reveal the specific metabolic pathways most susceptible to ethacrynic acid toxicity. The consistent experimental conditions eliminate technical variables, allowing unambiguous interpretation of the distinct patterns of enzymatic vulnerability in stria vascularis epithelium

that eliminates variability from cutting parameters or incubation conditions. This methodological refinement allows direct comparison of histochemical results between experimental conditions while additionally providing optimal exposure of stria vascularis epithelial proteins to incubation solutions through cross-sectional access, bypassing the diffusion barriers posed by intact marginal cell surfaces [3, 20, 21, 38, 51, 74] (Figs. 7.39 and 7.40). The protocol represents a comprehensive solution that overcomes the major limitations of conventional fixation methods while introducing quality controls for comparative studies of cochlear biochemistry.

References

1. Schuknecht H. 1. Histological method. In: Schuknecht H, editor. Pathology of the ear. 1st ed. Cambridge: Harvard University Press; 1974. pp. 1–20.
2. Ding D, Jiang S. Chapter 7: Slicing techniques of the inner ear. In: Ding D, editor. Manual of anatomical examination of the inner ear of the guinea pig. Shanghai: Xuelin Publishing House; 1989. p. 61–66.
3. Ding D, Li M, Jiang C, Salvi R. Chapter 6: Sectioning of the inner ear. In: Ding D, editor. Morphology of the inner ear. Harbin: Heilongjiang Science and Technology Press; 2001. p. 38–54.

4. Ding D, Li M, Jiang C, Salvi R. Chapter 7: Preparation technology of inner ear specimens for electron microscopy. In: Ding D, editor. Morphology of the inner ear. Harbin: Heilongjiang Science and Technology Press; 2001. p. 55–85.
5. Hayes SH, Ding D, Salvi R, Allman BL. Anatomy and physiology of the external, middle and inner ear. In: Celesia GG, editor. Disorders of peripheral and central auditory processing. Handbook of clinical neurophysiology, vol. 10. New York: Elsevier; 2013. p. 3–23.
6. Ding D, Yu J, Li P, et al. Standardization of experimental animals temporal bone sections. J Otol. 2015;10(2):66–71. https://doi.org/10.1016/j.joto.2015.08.001.
7. Ding D, Shi L, Xing Y, et al. Sagittal sectioning of temporal bones and quantitative measurement of neural densities in the inner ear in normal mice. Chin J Otorhinolaryngol Skull Base Surg. 2024;30(2): 69–75. https://doi.org/10.11798/j.issn.1007-1520.202424331.
8. Bliss CL, Novy FG. Action of formaldehyde on enzymes and on certain proteins. J Exp Med. 1899;4(1):47–80. https://doi.org/10.1084/jem.4.1.47.
9. Ding D, Zhao J, Huangfu M. Modified cochlear surface preparations. Chin J Otorhinolaryngol. 1981;16(4):207–9.
10. Ding D, Huangfu M, Jin X. Frozen sections of the inner ear. J Bengbu Med Coll. 1987;12(3):222.
11. Ding D, Zhao J, Huangfu M, Jin X. Microdissection of the whole membranous labyrinth in guinea pigs. J Clin Otorhinolaryngol. 1987;1(1):9–11.
12. Ding D, Jiang S. Chapter 5: Fixation techniques for inner ear specimens. In: Ding D, editor. Manual of anatomical examination of the inner ear of the guinea pig. Shanghai: Xuelin Publishing House; 1989. pp. 36–48.
13. Ding D, Zheng X, Wang J. [Quantitation of nerve fibers in habenula perforata in chinchilla]. Chin JOtorhinolaryngol. 1998;33(1):30–31.
14. Zhang F, Woods TJ, Zhu L, Rauchfuss TB. Inhibition of [FeFe]-hydrogenase by formaldehyde: proposed mechanism and reactivity of FeFe alkyl complexes. Chem Sci. 2021;12(47):15673–81. https://doi.org/10.1039/d1sc05803g.
15. Ding D, Li P, Qi W, et al. Different patterns of age-related damage to cochlear hair cells in different species of experimental animals. Chin J Otorhinolaryngol Skull Base Surg. 2023;29(1):7–13. https://doi.org/10.11798/j.issn.1007-1520.202323084.
16. Ding D, Manohar S, Kador PF, Salvi R. Multifunctional redox modulator prevents blast-induced loss of cochlear and vestibular hair cells and auditory spiral ganglion neurons. Sci Rep. 2024;14(1):15296. https://doi.org/10.1038/s41598-024-66406-1.
17. Ding D, Shi L, Xing Y, et al. Secondary neural damage in the inner ear induced by intratympanic gentamicin injection. Chin J Otorhinolaryngol Skull Base Surg. 2024;30(1):11–19. https://doi.org/10.11798/i.issn.1007-1520.202424356.
18. Dapson RW. Macromolecular changes caused by formalin fixation and antigen retrieval. Biotech Histochem. 2007;82(3):133–40. https://doi.org/10.1080/10520290701567916.
19. Otali D, Stockard CR, Oelschlager DK, et al. Combined effects of formalin fixation and tissue processing on immunorecognition. Biotech Histochem. 2009;84(5):223–47. https://doi.org/10.3109/10520290903039094.
20. Ding D, Qi W, Yang K, et al. Technical evolution of pathology in the inner ear. Chin J Otorhinolaryngol Skull Base Surg. 2016;22(2):169–78. https://doi.org/10.11798/i.issn.1007-520.201603001.
21. Ding D, Qi W, Qu Y, Salvi R. Chapter 6: Research techniques of the inner ear morphology. In: Ding D, editor. Science of the inner ear. Beijing: China Science and Technology Press; 2010. p. 50–88.
22. Ding D, Jiang H, Salvi R. Cochlear spiral ganglion neuron degeneration following cyclodextrin-induced hearing loss. Hear Res. 2021;400:108125 https://doi.org/10.1016/j.heares.2020.108125.
23. Ding D, Li P, Qi W, et al. Study on delayed secondary lesions in the cochlea triggered by cochlear hair cell death. Chin J Otorhinolaryngol Skull Base Surg. 2022;28(1):1–10. https://doi.org/10.11798/j.issn.1007-1520.2022221001.
24. Ding D, Zhu X, Chen H, Zhao J, Huangfu M. Study on acid phosphatase in the cochlea of guinea pigs with kanamycin ototoxicity. Chin J Otorhinolaryngol. 1986;21(2):121–2.
25. Ding DL, McFadden SL, Wang J, Hu BH, Salvi RJ. Age- and strain-related differences in dehydrogenase activity and glycogen levels in CBA and C57 mouse cochleas. Audiol Neurotol. 1999;4(2):55–63. https://doi.org/10.1159/000013822.
26. Ding D, Luo D, Huangfu M. Embryonic development of the inner ear in guinea pigs. Shanghai Lab Anim Sci. 1991;11(2):45–46.
27. Xia G, Ding D. Pathological changes of suppurative labyrinthitis in guinea pigs. Acta Otorhinolaryngol Sin. 1992;6(2):84–86.
28. Ding D, Wang J, Zhang XY, Sun H, Salvi R. Quantitative analysis of hair cells, spiral ganglion neurons, and nerve fibers in the same cochlea. Chin J Otorhinolaryngol Skull Base Surg. 1998;4(4):200–4.
29. Ding D, Wang J, Zheng XY, Salvi RJ. Early damage of spiral ganglion caused by carboplatin in chinchilla. J Audiol Speech Pathol. 1998;6(2):65–67.
30. Ding D, Jiang H, McFadden SL, Salvi RJ, Li M. Quantitative analysis of hair cells, spiral ganglion neurons and nerve fibers in knock out mice lacking SOD 1 gene. Acta Otorhinolaryngol Sin. 1999;30(6):1693–705.
31. McFadden SL, Ding D, Jiang H, Salvi RJ. Time course of efferent fiber and spiral ganglion cell degeneration following complete hair cell loss in the chinchilla. Brain Res. 2004;997(1):40–51. https://doi.org/10.1016/j.brainres.2003.10.031.
32. Zheng QY, Ding D, Yu H, Salvi RJ, Johnson KR. A locus on distal chromosome 10 (ahl4) affecting age-related hearing loss in A/J mice. Neurobiol Aging. 2009;30(10):1693–705. https://doi.org/10.1016/j.neurobiolaging.2007.12.011.
33. Ding D, Jiang H, Chen GD, et al. N-acetyl-cysteine prevents age-related hearing loss and the progressive loss of inner hair cells in gamma-glutamyl transferase 1 deficient mice. Aging. 2016;8(4):730–750. https://doi.org/10.18632/aging.100927.
34. Ding D, Jiang H, Manohar S, et al. Spatiotemporal developmental upregulation of prestin correlates with the severity and location of cyclodextrin-induced outer hair cell loss and hearing loss. Front Cell Dev Biol. 2021;9:643709 https://doi.org/10.3389/fcell.2021.643709.
35. Fu Y, Ding D, Jiang H, Salvi R. Ouabain-induced cochlear degeneration in rat. Neurotoxic Res. 2012;22(2):158–69. https://doi.org/10.1007/s12640-012-9320-0.
36. Fu Y, Ding D, Wei L, Jiang H, Salvi R. Ouabain-induced apoptosis in cochlear hair cells and spiral ganglion neurons in vitro. BioMed Res Int. 2013;2013:628064 https://doi.org/10.1155/2013/628064.
37. El-Badry MM, Ding DL, McFadden SL, Eddins AC. Physiological effects of auditory nerve myelinopathy in chinchillas. Eur J Neurosci. 2007;25(5):1437–46. https://doi.org/10.1111/j.1460-9568.2007.05401.x.
38. Ding D, Li H, Zhao J, Huangfu M. Enzyme histochemical sectioning technique of the stria vascularis in the inner ear of guinea pigs. J Clin Otorhinolaryngol. 1987;1(4):173–74.
39. Ding D, Jiang H, Wang P, Salvi R. Cell death after co-administration of cisplatin and ethacrynic acid. Hear Res. 2007;226(1–2):129–39. https://doi.org/10.1016/j.heares.2006.07.015.
40. Jamesdaniel S, Ding D, Kermany MH, et al. Analysis of cochlear protein profiles of Wistar, Sprague-Dawley, and Fischer 344 rats with normal hearing function. J Proteome Res. 2009;8(7):3520–8. https://doi.org/10.1021/pr900222c.
41. Zhou Y, Ding D, Kraus KS, et al. Functional and structural changes in the chinchilla cochlea and vestibular system following round window application of carboplatin. Audiol Med. 2009;7(3):189–99. https://doi.org/10.3109/16513860903335795.
42. Ding D, Jiang H, Salvi RJ. Mechanisms of rapid sensory hair-cell death following co-administration of gentamicin and ethacrynic acid. Hear Res. 2010;259(1-2):16–23. https://doi.org/10.1016/j.heares.2009.08.008.

43. Ding D, He J, Allman BL, et al. Cisplatin ototoxicity in rat cochlear organotypic cultures. Hear Res. 2011;282(1-2):196–203. https://doi.org/10.1016/j.heares.2011.08.002.
44. Wu X, Ding D, Jiang H, et al. Transfection using hydroxyapatite nanoparticles in the inner ear via an intact round window membrane in chinchilla. J Nanopart Res. 2012;14(6):708. https://doi.org/10.1007/s11051-011-0708-1.
45. Ding D, Salvi R, Roth JA. Cellular localization and developmental changes of the different isoforms of divalent metal transporter 1 (DMT1) in the inner ear of rats. BioMetals. 2014;27(1):125–34. https://doi.org/10.1007/s10534-013-9692-5.
46. Ding D, Salvi R, Roth JA. Cellular localization and developmental changes of Zip8, Zip14 and transferrin receptor 1 in the inner ear of rats. BioMetals. 2014;27(4):731–44. https://doi.org/10.1007/s10534-014-9765-0.
47. Qi W, Ding D, Zhu H, et al. Efficient siRNA transfection to the inner ear through the intact round window by a novel proteidic delivery technology in the chinchilla. Gene Ther. 2014;21(1):10–18. https://doi.org/10.1038/gt.2013.49.
48. Ding D, Liu H, Qi W, et al. Ototoxic effects and mechanisms of loop diuretics. J Otol. 2016;11(4):145–56. https://doi.org/10.1016/j.joto.2016.10.001.
49. Manohar S, Jamesdaniel S, Ding D, et al. Quantitative PCR analysis and protein distribution of drug transporter genes in the rat cochlea. Hear Res. 2016;332:46–54. https://doi.org/10.1016/j.heares.2015.10.020.
50. Yu J, Ding D, Sun H, Salvi R, Roth JA. Trimethyltin-induced cochlear degeneration in rat. J Otol. 2016;11(3):118–26. https://doi.org/10.1016/j.joto.2016.07.001.
51. Zhao J, Ding D, Huangfu M. Effects of ethacrynic acid on enzyme activities in stria vascularis of guinea pigs. J Clin Otorhinolaryngol. 1988;2(2):65–67.
52. Ding D, Li P, Qi W, et al. Quantitative observation of vestibular sensory hair cells in experimental animals. Chin J Otorhinolaryngol. Skull Base Surg. 2022;28(1):11–18. https://doi.org/10.11798/j.issn.1007-1520.202290001.
53. Ding D, Zhang J, Jiang H, et al. Some ototoxic drugs destroy cochlear support cells before damaging sensory hair cells. Neurotoxic Res. 2020;37(4):743–52. https://doi.org/10.1007/s12640-020-00170-8.
54. Ding D, Zhang J, Yang K, et al. Growth and development process of calcitonin gene-related peptide and aceltylcholinesterase in rat cochlear efferent nervous system. Chin J Otorhinolaryngol Skull Base Surg. 2020;28(6):662–8. https://doi.org/10.3969/j.issn.1006-7299.2020.06.012.
55. Ding D, Jiang S. Chapter 9: Staining techniques of the inner ear specimen. In: Ding D, editor. Manual of anatomical examination of the inner ear of the guinea pig. Shanghai: Xuelin Publishing House; 1989. p. 75–99.
56. Li Y, Ding D, Jiang H, Fu Y, Salvi R. Co-administration of cisplatin and furosemide causes rapid and massive loss of cochlear hair cells in mice. Neurotoxic Res. 2011;20(4):307–19. https://doi.org/10.1007/s12640-011-9244-0.
57. Gao K, Ding D, Sun H, Roth J, Salvi R. Kanamycin damages early postnatal, but not adult spiral ganglion neurons. Neurotoxic Res. 2017;32(4):603–13. https://doi.org/10.1007/s12640-017-9773-2.
58. Ding D, Manohar S, Jiang H, Salvi R. Hydroxypropyl-beta-cyclodextrin causes massive damage to the developing auditory and vestibular system. Hear Res. 2020;396:108073 https://doi.org/10.1016/j.heares.2020.108073.
59. Ding D, Prolla T, Someya S, Manohar S, Salvi R. Roles of Bak and Sirt3 in paraquat-induced cochlear hair cell damage. Neurotox Res. 2021;39(4):1227–37. https://doi.org/10.1007/s12640-021-00366-6.
60. Ding D, Qi W, Jiang H, Salvi R. Excitotoxic damage to auditory nerve afferents and spiral ganglion neurons is correlated with developmental upregulation of AMPA and KA receptors. Hear Res. 2021;411:108358 https://doi.org/10.1016/j.heares.2021.108358.
61. Ding D, Chen GD, Zhang C, et al. Supporting cell involvement in cochlear damage and repair: Novel insights from a quantitative analysis of cyclodextrin-induced ototoxicity in mice. Hear Res. 2025;459:109201 https://doi.org/10.1016/j.heares.2025.109201.
62. Zhang J, Sun H, Salvi R, Ding D. Paraquat initially damages cochlear support cells leading to anoikis-like hair cell death. Hear Res. 2018;364:129–41. https://doi.org/10.1016/j.heares.2018.03.014.
63. Li C, Du B, Ding D, Du B. Development of corti organ in kunming mouse. Progress of anatomical. Sciences. 2008;14(2):148–50.
64. Ding D, Luo D, Huangfu M, Gong Z. Enzyme cytochemistry of the inner ear under electron microscopy. J Clin Otorhinolaryngol. 1989;3(4):183–4.
65. Ding D, Luo D, Guo Y, Huangfu M. Study on the mechanism of ototoxicity of aminoglycoside antibiotics. Chin J Otorhinolaryngol. 1991;26(3):154–55.
66. Ding D, Jin X, Huangfu M, Wu D, Lu X. [Functional and morphological changes of the cochlea in guinea pigs during anoxia]. Chin J Otorhinolaryngol. 1993;28(5):265–7.
67. Ding D, Jin X, Zhang Z, Zhu Q. Study on the different susceptibility between red-eyed and black-eyed guinea pigs to gentamicin. Acta Otolaryngol. 1995;9(2):70–74.
68. Ding D, Jin X, Zhao J. [Accumulation sites of kanamycin in the organ of Corti by microautoradiography]. Chin J Otorhinolaryngol. 1997;32(6):348–49.
69. Ding D, Zheng X, Wang J, et al. Mechanisms of carboplatin ototoxicity suggested by cytochemical analysis. J Audiol Speech Dis. 1999;7(4):200–2.
70. Sun H, Hashino E, Ding DL, Salvi RJ. Reversible and irreversible damage to cochlear afferent neurons by kainic acid excitotoxicity. J Comp Neurol. 2001;430(2):172–81. https://doi.org/10.1002/1096-9861(20010205)430:2<172::aid-cne1023>3.0.co;2-w.
71. Ding D, McFadden SL, Salvi RJ. Calpain immunoreactivity and morphological damage in chinchilla inner ears after carboplatin. J Assoc Res Otolaryngol. 2002;3(1):68–79. https://doi.org/10.1007/s101620020004.
72. Wang J, Ding D, Salvi RJ. Carboplatin-induced early cochlear lesion in chinchillas. Hear Res. 2003;181(1-2):65–72. https://doi.org/10.1016/s0378-5955(03)00176-x.
73. Ye HB, Shi HB, Wang J, et al. Bilirubin induces auditory neuropathy in neonatal guinea pigs via auditory nerve fiber damage. J Neurosci Res. 2012;90(11):2201–13. https://doi.org/10.1002/jnr.23107.
74. Ding D, Jiang S. Chapter 8: Preparation techniques for electron microscopy of inner ear specimen. In: Ding D, editor. Manual of anatomical examination of the inner ear of the guinea pig. Shanghai: Xuelin Publishing House; 1989. p. 67–74.
75. Luo D, Ding D, Huangfu M. [Ultracytochemical observation on lysosome of hair cells in kanamycin ototoxic guinea pigs]. Zhonghua Er Bi Yan Hou Ke Za Zhi. 1990;25(5):281–2.
76. Ding D, Salvi R. Review of cellular changes in the cochlea due to aminoglycoside antibiotics. Volta Rev. 2005;105(3):407–38.
77. von Schack ML, Fakan S, Villiger W, Muller M. Cryofixation and cryosubstitution: a useful alternative in the analyses of cellular fine structure. Eur J Histochem. 1993;37(1):5–18.

8 Technique of Cochlear Micro-Dissections and Surface Preparations

The surface preparation technique of the cochlear basilar membrane was originally developed in 1882 by Retzius, who is universally acknowledged as the pioneering histologist to establish this methodology. On this basis, Kolmer successfully prepared the surface preparations of the cochlear basilar membrane by silver plating in 1927. Regrettably, despite its technical merits, this innovation did not gain immediate widespread recognition during that period. The pivotal turning point came in 1962 when Engstrom reintroduced and vigorously promoted the application of this technique, which was gradually accepted and continuously improved in subsequent practice, which became a turning point [1–10]. The sophisticated technique involves the meticulous dissection of the delicate membranous labyrinth from the surrounding bony labyrinth cavity. The isolated membrane is then carefully mounted on a glass slide, enabling comprehensive microscopic examination of the surface structure of sensory hair cells throughout various regions of the inner ear. In terms of technical classification, the surface preparation of the inner ear methodology encompasses two principal categories: the surface preparations of the vestibular membranous labyrinth and the cochlear membranous labyrinth. The surface preparations of the cochlear membrane labyrinth are further divided into surface preparations of the whole spiral ligament and the whole cochlear basilar membrane. These two surface preparation techniques provide complementary perspectives for investigating the organizational structure and physiological functions of the whole cochlear membranous labyrinth [8, 9, 11–19].

8.1 Surface Preparation Technique of the Entire Cochlear Spiral Ligament

The spiral ligament, forming the lateral wall of the cochlear duct, is of paramount importance in cochlear physiology. The entire spiral ligament was micro-dissected out and placed on a glass slide as flat surface preparations. This technique enables comprehensive examination of both the epithelial architecture covering the stria vascularis and spiral prominence, as well as the intricate microcirculatory network within the stria vascularis capillaries. The detailed preparation protocol initiates with thorough fixation of the temporal bone using 10% formalin solution, ensuring optimal tissue preservation. The fixed specimen is then transferred into a glass container filled with distilled water for subsequent processing (Fig. 8.1A). Under a dissecting microscope, use a separating sharp needle to carefully separate and remove the osseous cochlear wall along the gap between the spiral ligament and the bony cochlear shell to fully expose the entire spiral ligament (Fig. 8.1B). Then use a separating needle to cut off the connection between the spiral ligament and the cochlear basilar membrane along the lateral sulcus and take off the entire spiral ligament (Fig. 8.1C). To facilitate specific research objectives, various histological staining protocols can be performed on the spiral ligament to emphasize particular cellular constituents or functional elements. The spiral ligament is then mounted on a glass slide in glycerin with the stria vascularis surface oriented upwards to ensure optimal optical clarity for examinations under light or fluorescence microscope [11, 14, 15, 17, 19–25] (Figs. 8.2–8.6). Alternatively, for ultrastructural analysis, the spiral ligament can be mounted on a conductive adhesive-coated specimen holder. Following precise gold sputter-coating procedures using high-vacuum systems, the samples are ready for high-resolution imaging under scanning electron microscopy [18, 19, 26–32] (Figs. 8.7 and 8.8).

8.2 Surface Preparation Technique of the Entire Cochlear Basilar Membrane

The cochlear basilar membrane, as the membranous lower boundary of the cochlear duct that separates the scala media from the scala tympani, extends continuously from the basal turn to the apical turn throughout the cochlear cavity.

D. Ding et al., *Histopathological Atlas of the Inner Ear*,
https://doi.org/10.1007/978-981-95-6338-8_8

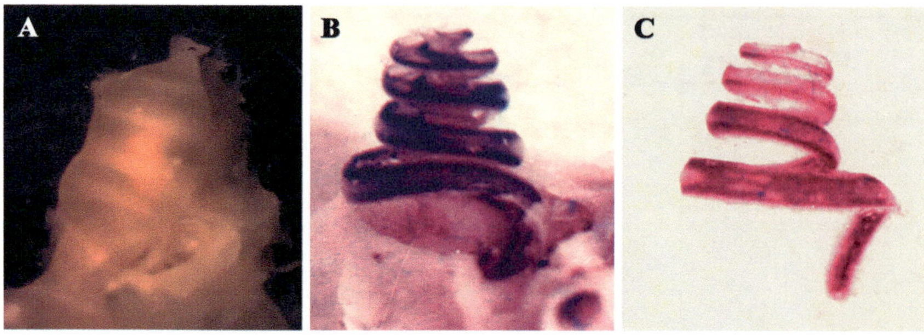

Fig. 8.1 Sampling steps of the cochlear spiral ligament. (**A**) The middle ear cavity is surgically opened to fully expose the bony cochlear structure. (**B**) The cochlear bony wall is carefully stripped away to reveal the spiral ligament. (**C**) Under a dissecting microscope, the entire spiral ligament is precisely separated along the lateral sulcus of the cochlear basilar membrane. This well-established protocol maintains excellent structures of the spiral ligament for various histochemical examinations

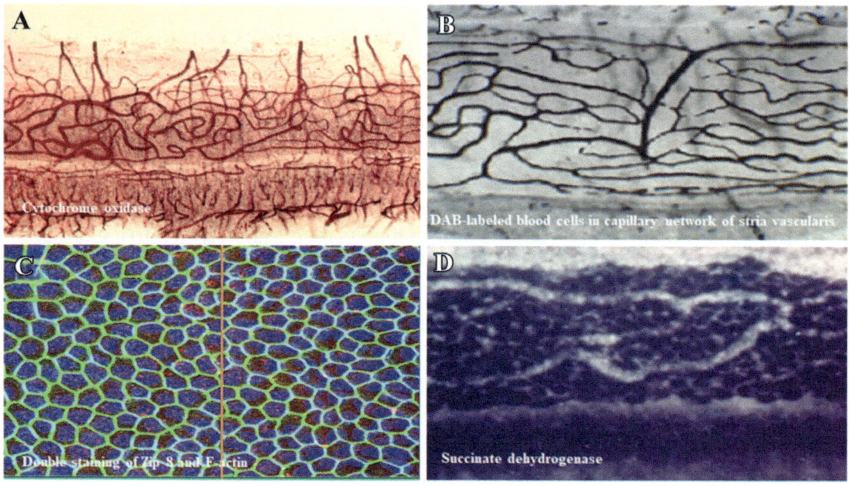

Fig. 8.2 Histochemical staining of surface preparations of stria vascularis. (**A**) Cytochrome oxidase staining clearly labels both the epithelial cells and capillary walls within the stria vascularis. (**B**) 3,3'-diaminobenzidine (DAB) staining effectively highlights red blood cells, providing clear visualization of the capillary network architecture. (**C**) Double immunofluorescence staining demonstrates the localization of the metal transporter Zip8 (red fluorescence) in epithelial cells and F-actin (green fluorescence via phalloidin staining) in tight junctions between marginal cells. (**D**) Intense succinate dehydrogenase staining reveals the abundant mitochondrial content and high metabolic activity in stria vascularis epithelial cells. Collectively, these specialized staining techniques provide comprehensive morphological and functional characterization of this critical cochlear structure

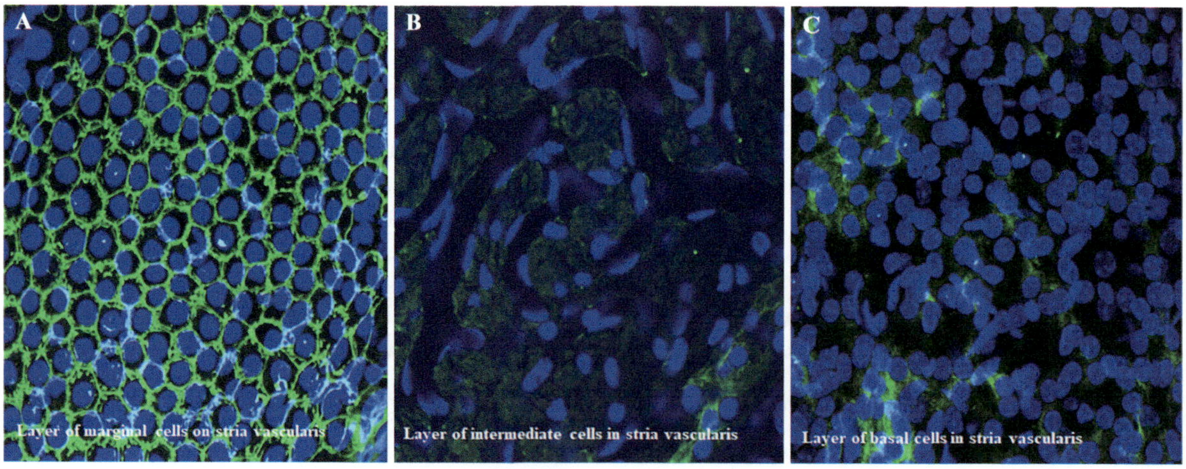

Fig. 8.3 Double staining for phalloidin and ToPro-3 showing the three-layered tissue structure of stria vascularis. (**A**) The marginal cell layer exhibits distinct polygonal morphology with intense F-actin staining delineating cellular boundaries. (**B**) The intermediate cell layer displays an intricate capillary network permeating throughout the cellular interstices. (**C**) The basal cell layer shows densely packed cellular organization, with notably smaller nuclear size compared to marginal cells. This tri-laminar architecture demonstrates the specialized structural organization of stria vascularis, with each layer maintaining unique cellular characteristics that support its vital role in cochlear homeostasis

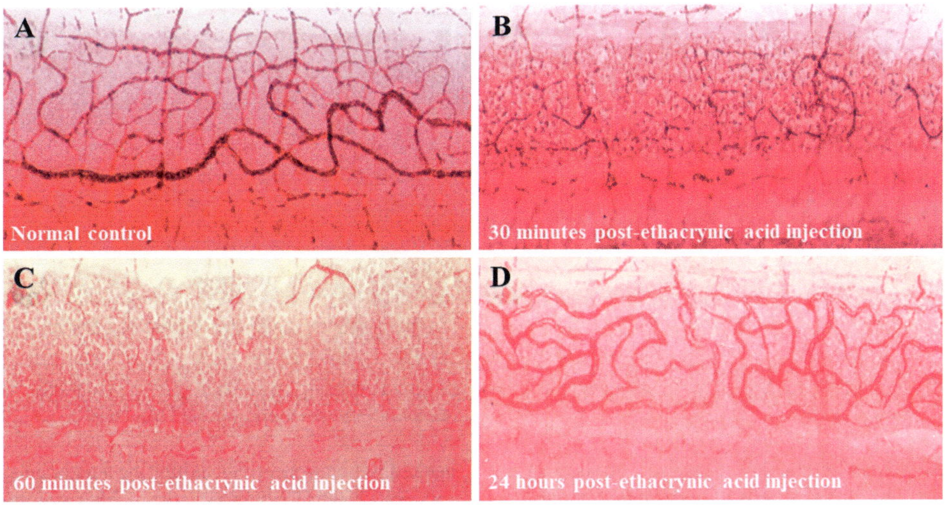

Fig. 8.4 Surface preparation of spiral ligament showing eosin-stained erythrocytes in stria vascularis capillaries. (**A**) Control specimens demonstrate capillaries fully packed with erythrocytes in normal stria vascularis. (**B**) Marked ischemia develops within 30 min post-ethacrynic acid injection, evidenced by dramatic reduction in the number of erythrocytes within the capillaries of the stria vascularis, resulting in empty capillary lumens. (**C**) By 60 min post-injection, ischemic damage progresses to characteristic hypoxic vacuolization in stria vascularis epithelial cells. (**D**) Complete microcirculatory recovery is achieved by 24 h, with full resolution of epithelial cell swelling and regeneration of damaged cellular elements. This temporal series precisely documents the ischemic cascade and subsequent reparative processes following intravenous injection of ethacrynic acid

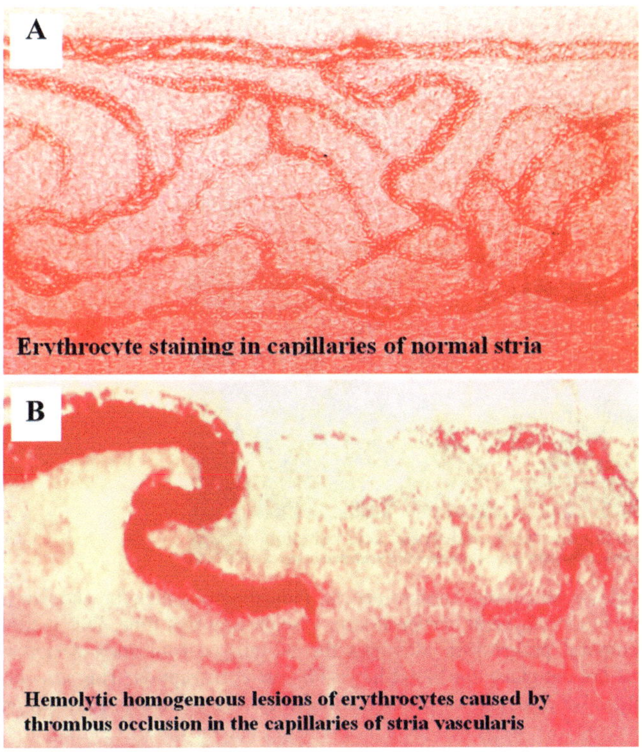

Fig. 8.5 Surface preparations of the spiral ligament with eosin staining demonstrating erythrocyte distribution in the stria vascularis capillaries. (**A**) Capillaries in the normal stria vascularis are filled with erythrocytes. (**B**) Experimental barium sulfate microembolization, by retrograde injection into the axillary artery, revealed embolism-induced erythrolysis at the site of embolization of the stria vascularis capillaries with barium sulfate particles and produced unique homogeneous hemolytic lesions in the affected capillaries, which not only demonstrated the vulnerability of the cochlear microvasculature to embolism but also explained the ensuing ischemic pathological changes

The organ of Corti, the specialized auditory sensory epithelium, is precisely situated upon this basilar membrane. Under the dissecting microscope, the entire cochlear basilar membrane can be carefully separated and mounted on a glass slide as a surface preparation. This method enables detailed microscopic examination along the entire length of the cochlear basilar membrane, including the evaluation of sensory hair cells, supporting cells, as well as the intricate neural elements of nerve fibers and synaptic connections within the organ of Corti.

The detailed protocol for preparing cochlear basilar membrane surface specimens involves the following meticulous steps: Initially, the temporal bone is thoroughly fixed using 10% formalin solution to ensure optimal tissue preservation. The fixed specimen is then carefully transferred into a glass container filled with distilled water for subsequent processing (Fig. 8.9A). Under a high-magnification dissecting microscope, microsurgical instruments are used to peel off the bony cochlear shell. The spiral ligament surrounding the lateral edge of the basilar membrane is separated and removed to fully expose the entire cochlear basilar membrane (Fig. 8.9B). Using a separating needle to separate the entire cochlear basilar membrane from the apical turn to the basal turn along the spiral lamina of modiolus (Fig. 8.9C). Depending on specific research objectives, the isolated basilar membrane can be subjected to various histological staining protocols designed to highlight particular cellular components or pathological features. The cochlear basilar membrane is finally mounted in glycerin on glass slides as surface preparation for examinations under optical microscopy or confocal laser scanning microscopy systems [8, 9, 14–16, 18, 22–24, 32–73] (Figs. 6.10, 6.19,

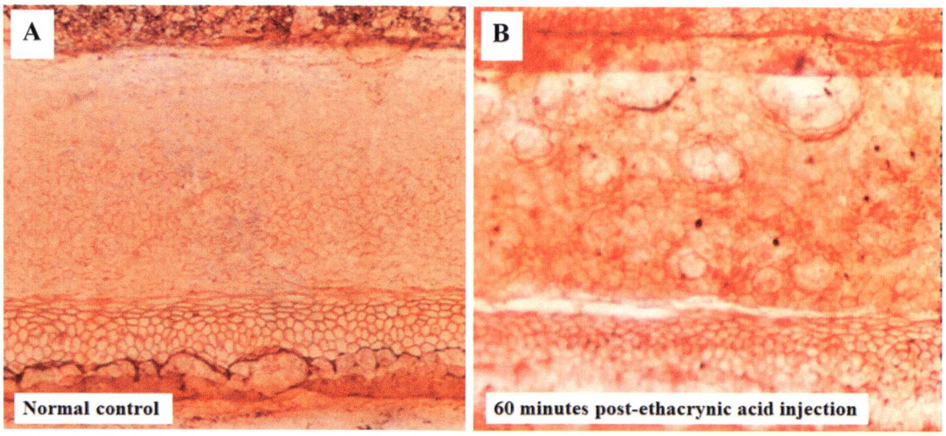

Fig. 8.6 Silver nitrate precipitation staining of stria vascularis marginal cell surface morphology. (**A**) Marginal cells in normal guinea pigs display characteristic flattened morphology with distinct cellular borders. (**B**) Within 60 min post-ethacrynic acid injection, these cells develop marked ischemic swelling, exhibiting a pathognomonic cauliflower-like appearance due to hypoxic stress. This staining technique provides exceptional visualization of both the normal cytoarchitecture and the obvious swelling changes of marginal cells

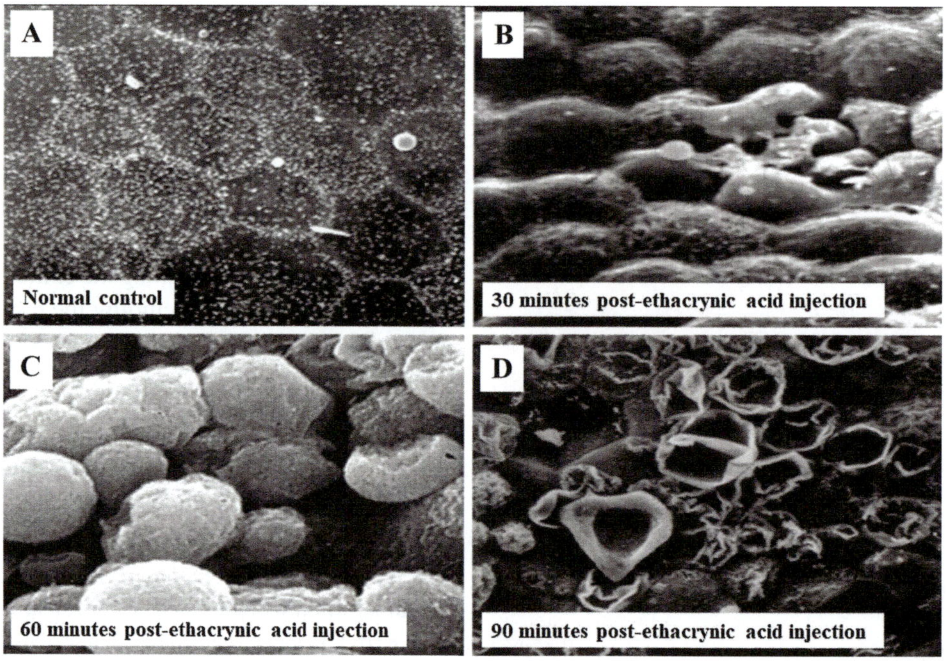

Fig. 8.7 Scanning electron micrographs demonstrating ultrastructural alterations in stria vascularis marginal cells following ethacrynic acid administration. (**A**) Control micrographs exhibit the characteristic polygonal morphology of normal marginal cells with intact surface architecture. (**B**) Within 30 min post-injection, early ischemic changes become evident as cellular swelling due to hypoxia-induced edema. (**C**) By 60 min, cells develop severe swollen into spheres with loss of surface microarchitecture. (**D**) At the 90-min timepoint, widespread cellular rupture occurs, indicating complete breakdown of the blood-labyrinth barrier at stria vascularis at this time. This precise temporal progression identifies the 90-min post-injection period as the critical phase for blood-labyrinth barrier disruption. This provides objective evidence for understanding why ethacrynic acid causes rapid hearing loss, its pathological mechanisms, and the timing of eliminating the blood-cochlear barrier

6.22, and 6.23; Figs. 8.10–8.30). For ultrastructural analysis via scanning electron microscopy, two preparation methods are available: either the entire modiolus with its attached basilar membrane is securely mounted on specimen stubs using conductive adhesive, or the isolated basilar membrane is precisely positioned on double-sided conductive tape. Following standardized gold sputter-coating procedures in high-vacuum systems, these preparations enable nanometer-scale resolution imaging of the organ of Corti's surface architecture [22, 28, 30, 32, 73–80] (Figs. 6.11–6.15; Figs. 8.31–8.38).

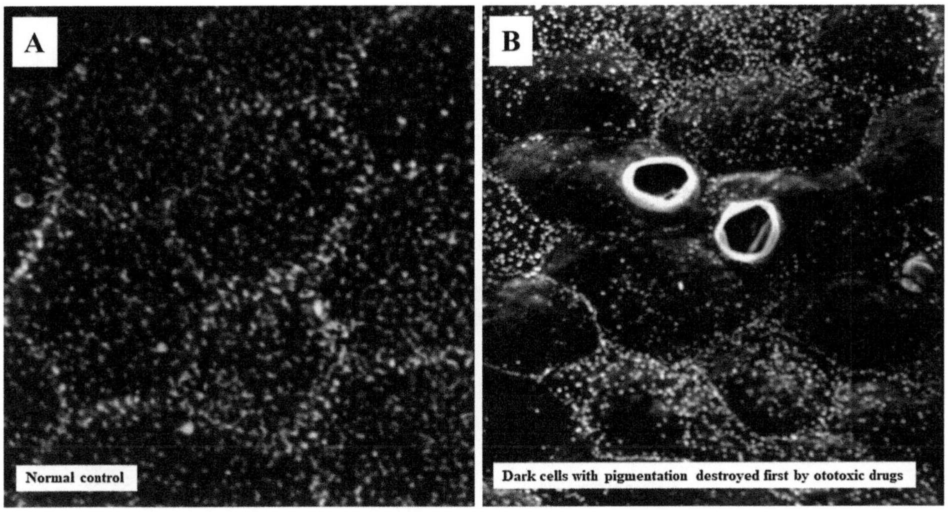

Fig. 8.8 Ultrastructural comparison of the different destructive effects of gentamicin on dark cells containing melanin and dark cells without melanin in the stria vascularis. (**A**) Albino guinea pigs (devoid of melanin production capability) receiving 14 intramuscular gentamicin injections (125 mg/kg per dose at 12-h intervals) demonstrate intact dark cell morphology in stria vascularis. (**B**) Black-eyed pigmented guinea pigs subjected to an identical dosing regimen exhibit significant dark cell destruction. It is known that melanin-rich cells show a special affinity for a variety of chemical agents and can actively take up chemical agents. Therefore, the pigmented dark cells located in the stria vascularis of pigmented guinea pigs can actively take up more gentamicin from the perilymph and endolymph. This uptake mechanism may reduce the accumulation of gentamicin in the cochlear lymph fluid. When the melanin-containing dark cells that have taken up a large amount of drugs are ruptured due to overload, the damaged dark cells may become a pathway for gentamicin to leak from the inner ear fluid, which will also cause a decrease in the concentration of gentamicin in the inner ear fluid. In contrast, the dark cells of albino animals that lack melanin have a relatively weak ability to absorb drugs, resulting in a higher concentration of gentamicin accumulated in the inner ear fluid and thus more severe damage to the cochlear hair cells. Our previous pharmacokinetic studies have confirmed the effect of whether dark cells contain melanin on the concentration of gentamicin in the inner ear fluid and its effect on the degree of damage to the cochlear hair cells [29]

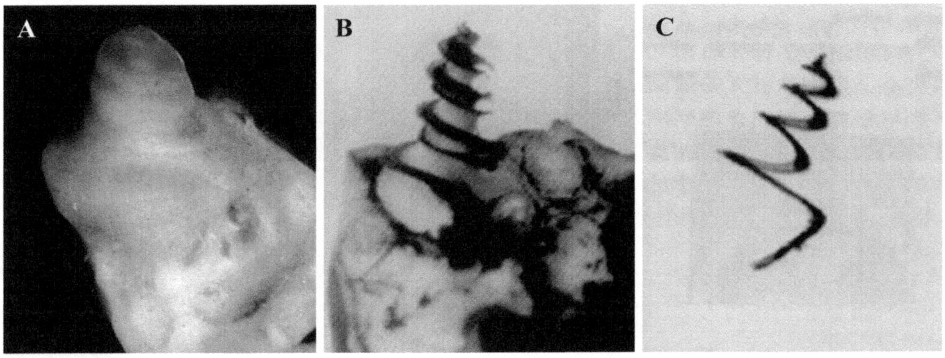

Fig. 8.9 Sampling steps of the cochlear basilar membrane. (**A**) The entire bony labyrinth of the cochlea is exposed by stripping away the surrounding cochlear bony wall. (**B**) The cochlear shell and spiral ligament are removed to fully expose the spiral-shaped cochlear basilar membrane surrounding the modiolus. (**C**) Using a separating needle to separate the entire cochlear basilar membrane from the spiral lamina of the modiolus.(Reproduced with permission from Ding et al. [8])

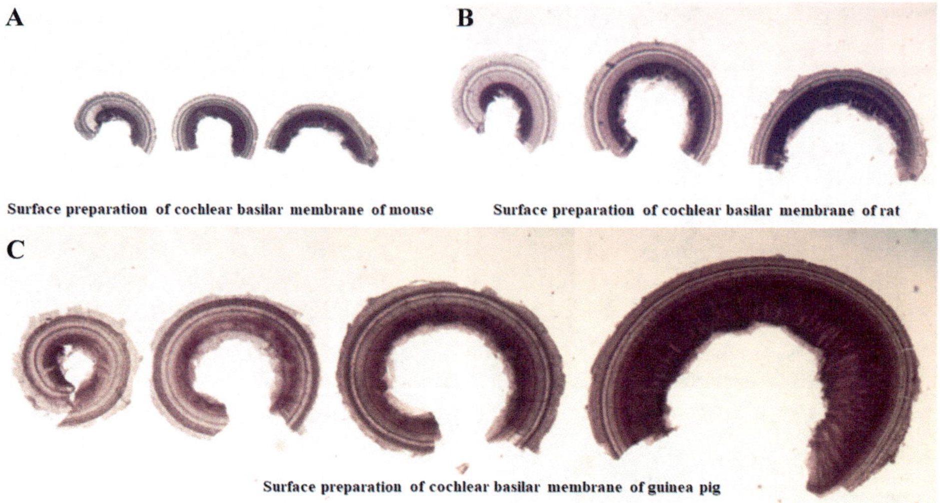

Fig. 8.10 Comparative surface preparations of cochlear basilar membranes from three experimental rodent species. (**A**) Surface preparation of the whole cochlear basilar membrane of the mouse. (**B**) Surface preparation of the whole cochlear basilar membrane of the rat. (**C**) Surface preparation of the whole cochlear basilar membrane of the guinea pig

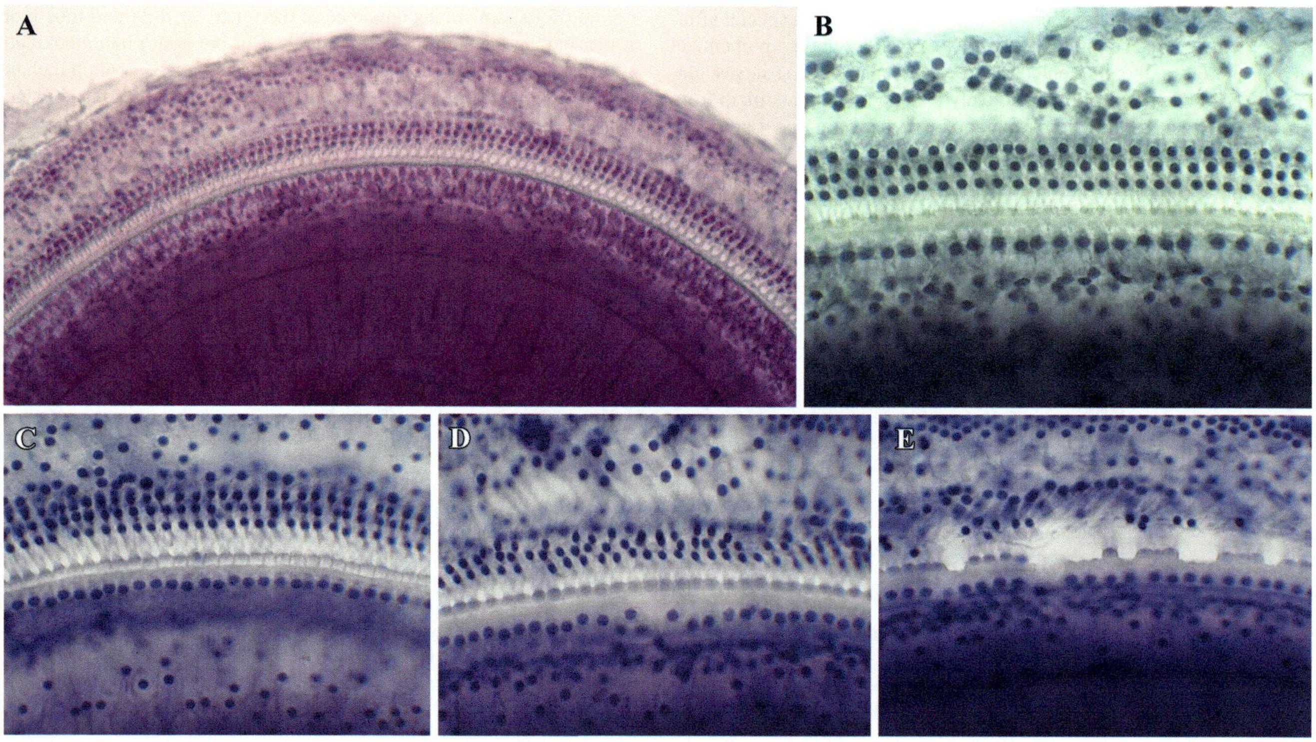

Fig. 8.11 Hematoxylin-stained surface preparations of cochlear basilar membranes under various experimental conditions. (**A**) Surface preparation of the cochlear basilar membrane from a normal mouse shows an orderly arrangement of cochlear hair cells. (**B**) Surface preparation of the cochlear basilar membrane from a normal guinea pig shows neatly arranged inner and outer hair cells. (**C**) Surface preparation of the cochlear basilar membrane in a normal rat. (**D**) Mild ototoxic damage caused by aminoglycoside antibiotics results in loss of only individual outer hair cells. (**E**) Severe ototoxic drug-induced damage was manifested by the loss of a large number of outer hair cells, but most inner hair cells were intact, indicating that outer hair cells are more sensitive to antibiotic-induced damage than inner hair cells

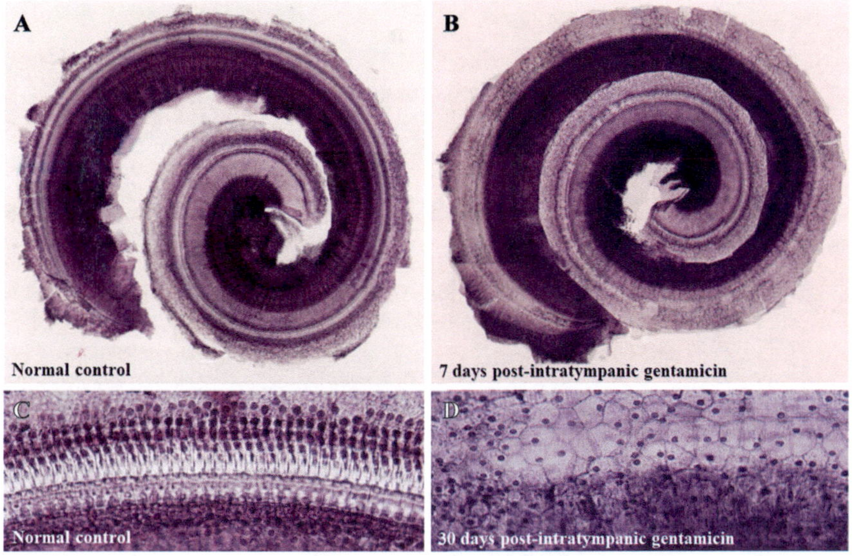

Fig. 8.12 Progressive destruction of cochlear hair cells induced by intratympanic gentamicin administration. (**A**) The inner and outer hair cells in a normal control rat are neatly arranged along the entire length of the cochlear basilar membrane. (**B**) 7 days after gentamicin intratympanic injection, the hair cells in the cochlear basal turn disappeared completely, but the hair cells in the apical turn were basically intact, forming a vulnerability gradient from the basal turn to the apical turn of the cochlea. (**C**) Under high magnification, the inner and outer hair cells of the normal cochlea are arranged in a characteristic geometric pattern. (**D**) 30 days after intratympanic injection of gentamicin, all the original hair cells and supporting cells in the cochlear basal turn have disappeared, replaced by a single layer of squamous epithelial cells. The temporal and spatial patterns of gentamicin-induced cochlear damage described above confirm that aminoglycoside antibiotics cause irreversible and complete destruction of the cochlear sensory epithelium.(Reproduced with permission from Ding et al. [71])

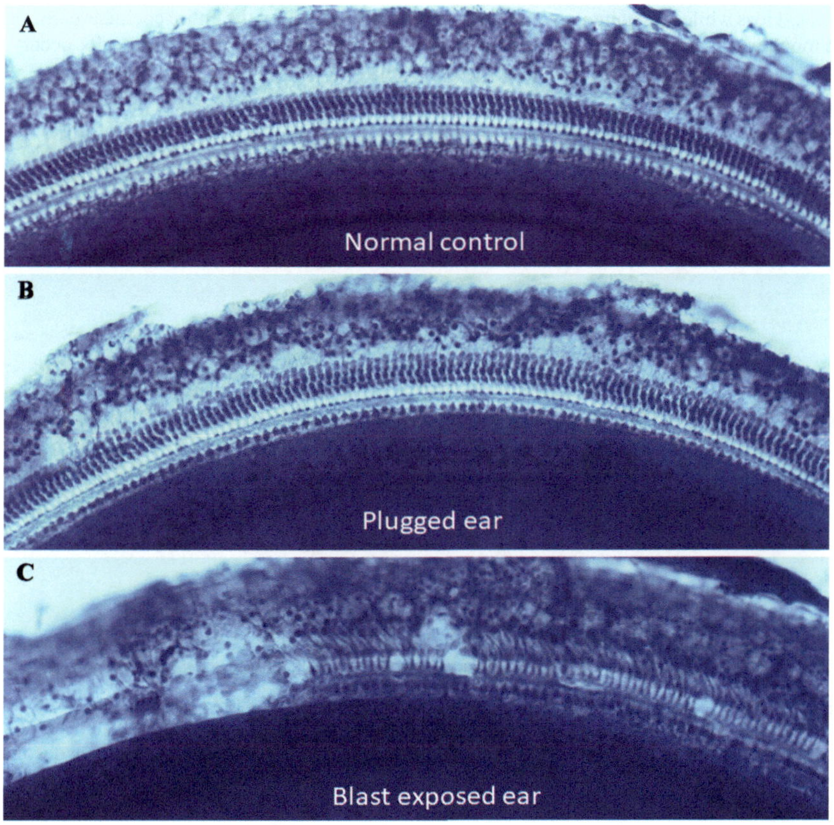

Fig. 8.13 Hematoxylin-stained surface preparation of cochlear basilar membrane confirms the protective effect of blocking the external auditory canal against blast-induced cochlear damage. (**A**) The arrangement of inner and outer hair cells in the normal mouse cochlea presents a characteristic complete array structure. (**B**) The results of the surface preparation of the cochlear basilar membrane in the plugged external auditory canal showed complete preservation of cochlear hair cells after blast exposure. (**C**) In stark contrast, the unoccluded ear displays extensive blast-induced hair cell loss and structural disintegration, illustrating the devastating consequences of unobstructed blast energy propagation into the inner ear. These comparative results provide solid evidence that ear protection devices can effectively protect the cochlear sensory organ from blast-induced mechanical damage

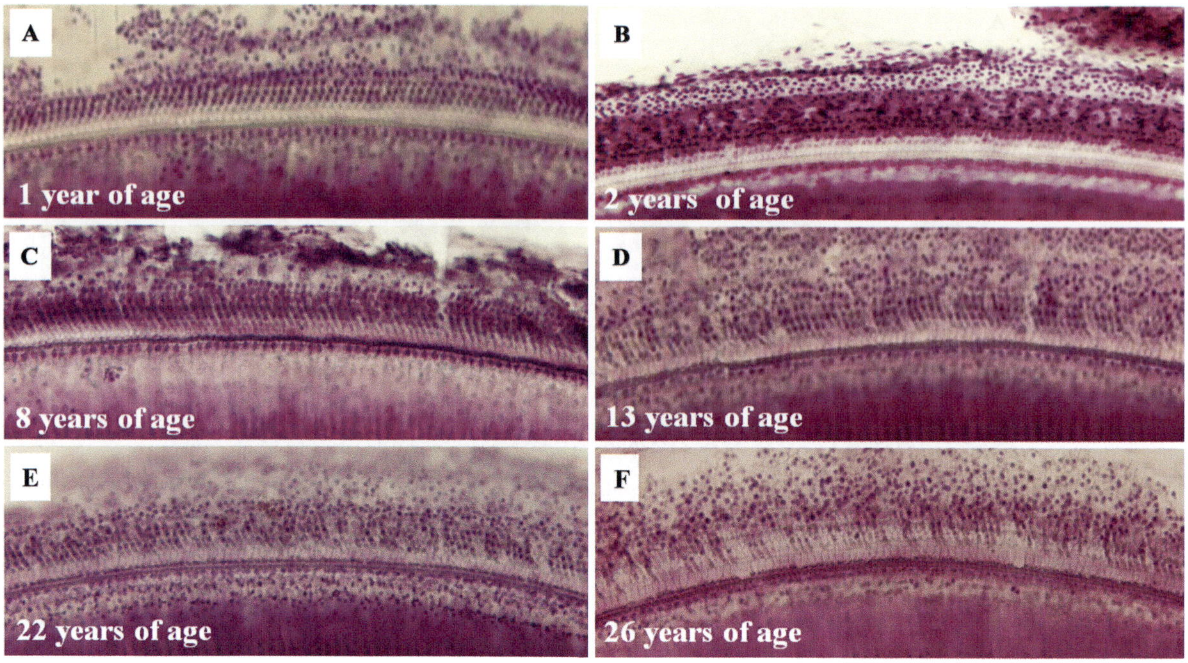

Fig. 8.14 Age-dependent cochlear hair cell degeneration patterns in primate cochlear basilar membrane preparations. (**A–C**) Specimens from juvenile monkeys (<10 years) demonstrate complete preservation of cochlear hair cell populations with intact morphological organization. (**D**) Adult specimens (10–15 years) exhibit initial signs of evenly distributed, sporadic outer hair cell loss while maintaining overall cochlear architecture. (**E–F**) Aged monkeys (>20 years old) showed that the loss of outer hair cells gradually increases, and the sites of hair cell loss were evenly distributed along the entire length of the cochlea, showing no tendency for regional damage. These systematically documented morphological changes establish the characteristic spatiotemporal progression of presbycusis in primate models, confirming that age-related cochlear degeneration in primates occurs as a diffuse, non-traumatic process affecting the entire cochlear partition uniformly, and the age-related destruction of outer hair cells occurs earlier than the inner hair cells

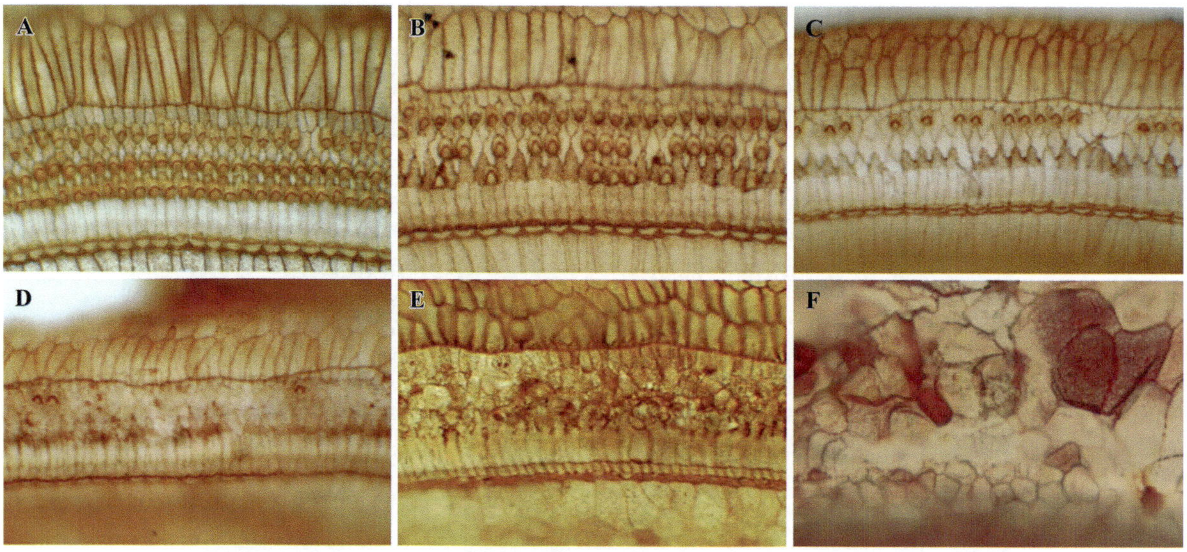

Fig. 8.15 Silver nitrate precipitation staining was used to identify the progressive damage pattern of cochlear hair cells caused by gentamicin. (**A**) In a normal animal, silver staining accurately shows the surface structure of the organ of Corti, clearly outlining the cuticle plates and stereocilia bundles of cochlear hair cells. (**B**) Gentamicin-induced cochlear hair cell loss shows a stereotyped pattern, with hair cell loss always starting in the first row and gradually spreading to the second and third rows. (**C**) As the lesion progresses, the first and second rows of outer hair cells are completely lost, but some outer hair cells in the third row still survive. This once again proves that gentamicin-induced outer hair cell destruction in the same location expands from the first row to the third row. (**D**) The late stage shows that the three rows of outer hair cells are almost completely lost, while the inner hair cells still maintain normal morphology, indicating that the outer hair cells are more sensitive to the damage of aminoglycosides than the inner hair cells. (**E**) Co-administration of ethacrynic acid (40 mg/kg, I.V.) and gentamicin (125 mg/kg, I.M.) potentiates gentamicin ototoxic effects, resulting in the death of all inner and outer hair cells within 24 h. (**F**) Terminal pathology demonstrates complete collapse of the organ of Corti architecture following hair cell loss, including secondary degeneration of supporting cells and basilar membrane structural disintegration. These findings systematically describe the spatiotemporal progression and cellular specificity of gentamicin-induced destruction of cochlear hair cells

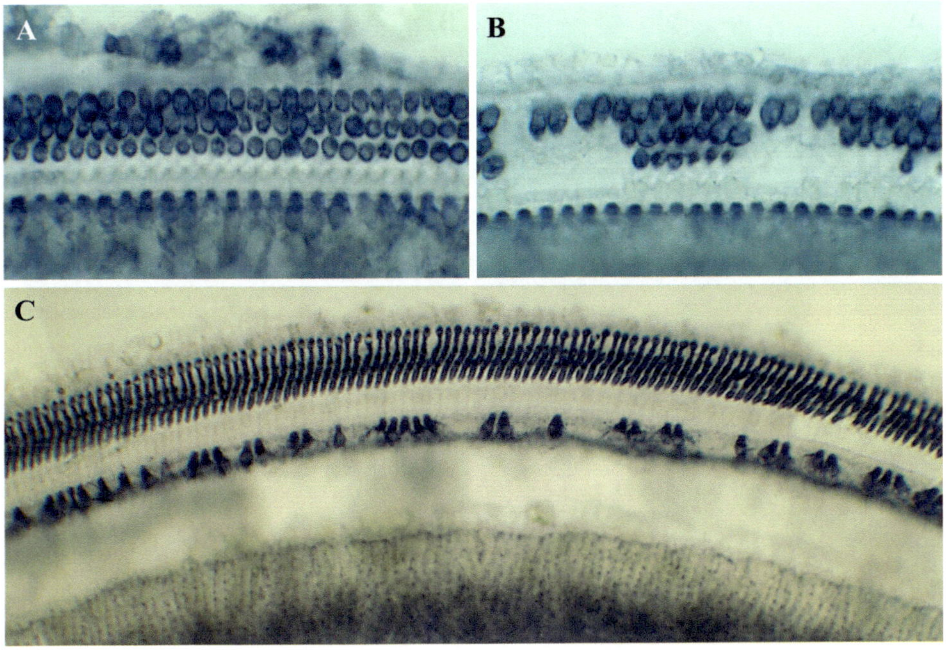

Fig. 8.16 Application of succinate dehydrogenase histochemical staining for cochlear pathological evaluation in chinchilla models. (**A**) As a marker enzyme of mitochondria, succinate dehydrogenase is strongly expressed in normal cochlear hair cells rich in mitochondria, while supporting cells show little staining due to their lack of mitochondria, resulting in a clear contrast between hair cells and supporting cells. (**B**) Surface preparation of cochlear basilar membrane reveals noise-induced outer hair cell loss, with the resultant cellular voids occupied by mitochondria-deficient Deiters cells that remain unstained by succinate dehydrogenase. (**C**) Succinate dehydrogenase staining clearly demonstrates carboplatin-induced selective loss of inner hair cells in chinchillas

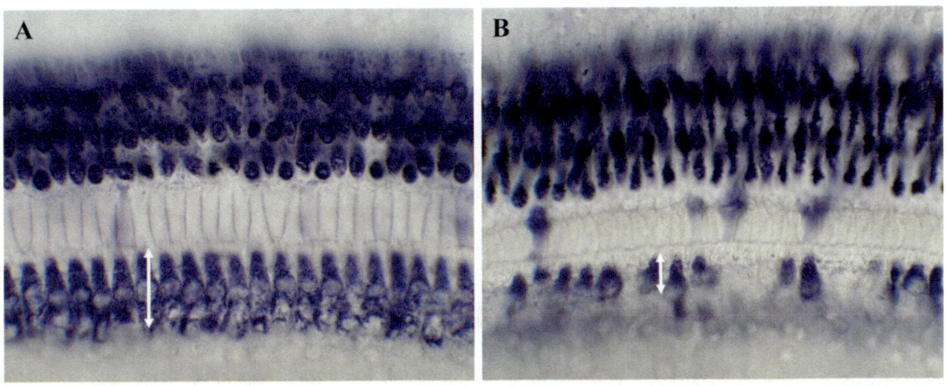

Fig. 8.17 Succinate dehydrogenase-stained cochlear basilar membrane of chinchillas. (**A**) Succinate dehydrogenase is strongly expressed in cochlear hair cells in normal chinchilla. (**B**) 3 days post-carboplatin (100 mg/kg, i. p.), the succinate dehydrogenase in outer hair cells maintains normal, while inner hair cells exhibit scattered loss and significant morphological changes in surviving cells, characterized by apparent shortening. These alterations likely result from swelling of type I afferent nerve terminals beneath inner hair cells, which causes the nuclei of the inner hair cells to be pushed toward the cuticular plate

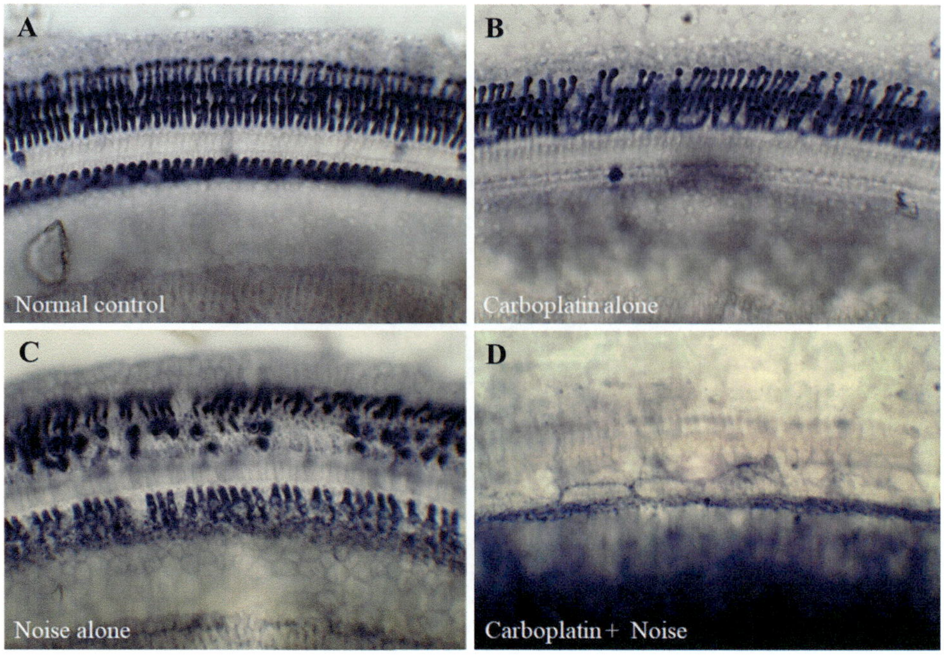

Fig. 8.18 Succinate dehydrogenase-stained cochlear basilar membrane demonstrates exacerbated noise-induced outer hair cell damage following inner hair cell loss. (**A**) Surface preparation of the normal cochlear basilar membrane showing the normal arrangement of inner and outer hair cells. (**B**) Carboplatin administration (100 mg/kg, i.p.) selectively eliminates almost all inner hair cells in chinchilla while preserving outer hair cell integrity. (**C**) Narrowband noise exposure (105 dB SPL at 4 kHz for 5 h) primarily damages the outer hair cells within the frequency-matched region in normal chinchilla, while with minimal inner hair cell loss. (**D**) First, all inner hair cells were eliminated using carboplatin, followed by the same noise exposure, resulting in the destruction of all inner and outer hair cells in the region of the basilar membrane that responds to the 4 kHz frequency. These results indicate that intact inner hair cells are essential for maintaining protective auditory reflexes, including middle ear muscle contractions and efferent-mediated cochlear protections, which collectively mitigate noise-induced cochlear damage. The findings establish the pivotal role of inner hair cells in coordinating physiological defenses against acoustic trauma [40]

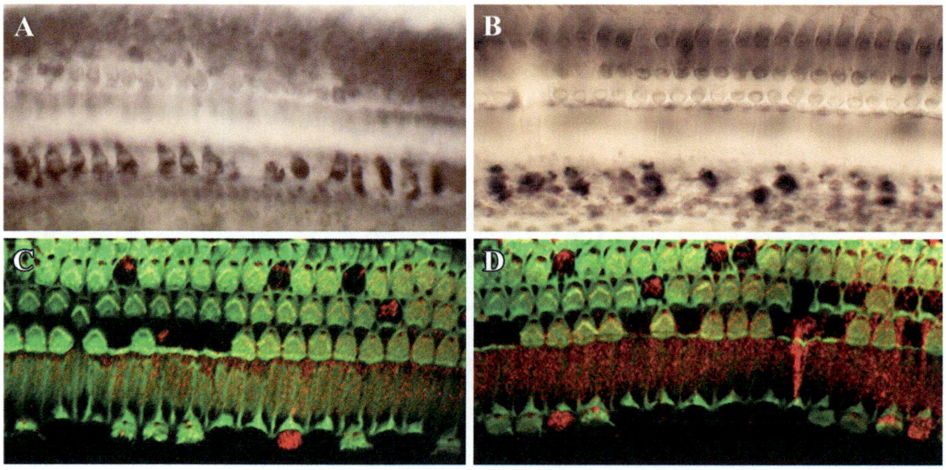

Fig. 8.19 Temporal progression of P53-mediated apoptosis in carboplatin-induced inner hair cell death in chinchilla. (**A**) 48 h after carboplatin injection (100 mg/kg, subcutaneous injection), biotinylation immunostaining showed that in the early apoptosis process, P53-positive brown reaction products were only present in the remaining inner hair cells, while no P53 expression was observed in the outer hair cells. (**B**) 72 h after carboplatin injection, the number of inner hair cells lost increased, and the remaining inner hair cells were all P53 positive, showing typical apoptotic features such as cell deformation and nuclear condensation. (**C–D**) 5 days post-carboplatin, extensive inner hair cell loss and initial outer hair cell loss were detected. P53 fluorescent signals were absent in regions of inner hair cell missing. However, P53-positive immunohistochemical products can still be detected in the fragments of dead outer hair cells. These observations establish P53 as a critical regulator in the apoptotic cascade initiated by carboplatin ototoxicity

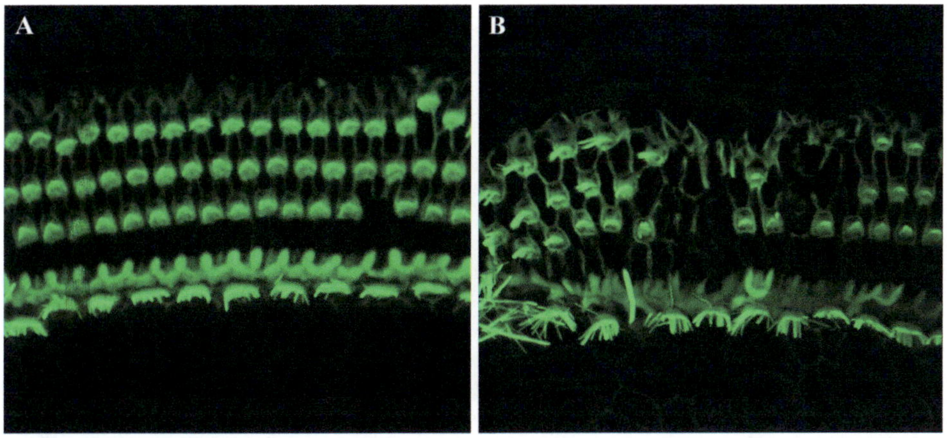

Fig. 8.20 Surface preparation of the cochlear basilar membrane with phalloidin-staining confirmed that blockage of the external auditory canal protected cochlear hair cells from mechanical damage induced by blast wave. (**A**) The plugged right ear maintains intact inner and outer hair cells, indicating effective protection from blast-induced mechanical damage. (**B**) The external auditory canal of the left ear was not blocked; it suffered serious hair cell damage due to the violent explosion of the shock wave, indicating that in the absence of protective measures, the cochlear hair cells would inevitably be damaged by the explosion of the blast wave

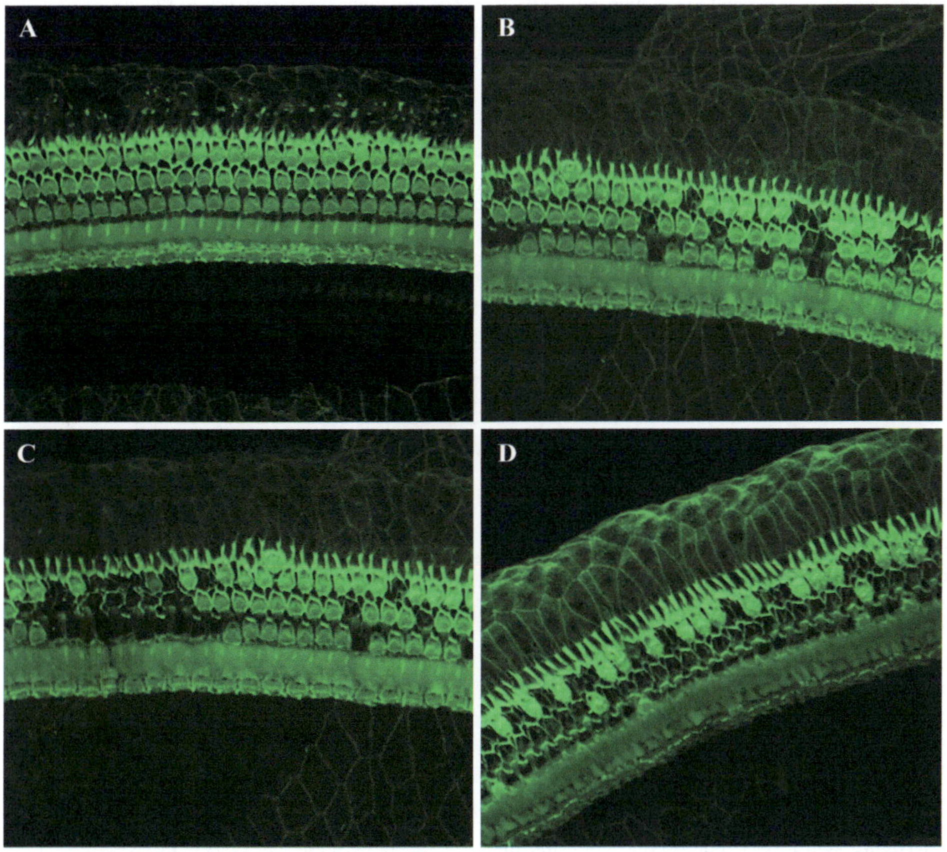

Fig. 8.21 Phalloidin-stained surface morphology of rat cochlear basilar membrane. (**A**) Normal specimens demonstrate the characteristic, organized architecture of sensory hair cells in the organ of Corti. (**B**) 48 h after exposure to narrowband noise (105 dB SPL, center frequency 4 kHz, for 5 h), one rat exhibits scattered loss of outer hair cells in the area on the basilar membrane corresponding to the 4 kHz frequency response. (**C**) Another rat subjected to the same noise conditions showed moderate outer hair cell destruction in the area of the basilar membrane corresponding to the 4 kHz frequency response 48 h after noise exposure. (**D**) 48 h after the same noise exposure, the outer hair cells of the third rat in the 4 kHz frequency corresponding area on the basilar membrane were severely destroyed, with the first and second rows of outer hair cells completely missing, and the third row of outer hair cells lost about 50%. The areas of missing outer hair cells were sealed by the cuticular plate of Deiters cells to form the typical scars. These experimental observations confirm that standardized noise exposure can produce variable degrees of cochlear hair cell damage across individual animals

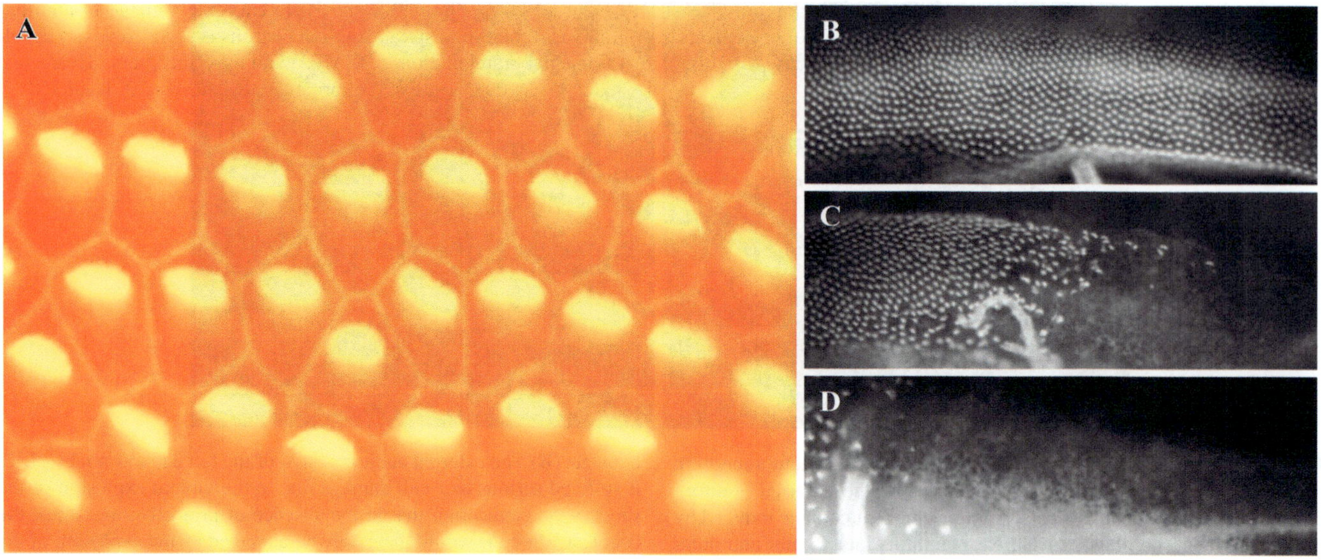

Fig. 8.22 Phalloidin staining of surface preparation of the cochlear basilar membrane in the chicken. (**A**) High-magnification fluorescence microscopy shows the characteristic pentagonal or hexagonal cuticular plates and their ciliary bundles of normal avian hair cells. (**B**) A low-magnification view demonstrates the organized mosaic pattern of hair cells in the normal chicken cochlea. (**C**). On day 2, after 10 days of kanamycin treatment (400 mg/kg/day, IM), hair cell missing started from the basal turn and toward the apical turn. (**D**) On day 4, after 10 days of kanamycin treatment (400 mg/kg/day, IM), the loss of hair cells has extended from the basal to the apical turn. These observations support the normal cellular architecture of the avian auditory epithelium and the basal-to-apical extension of aminoglycoside-induced hair cell loss

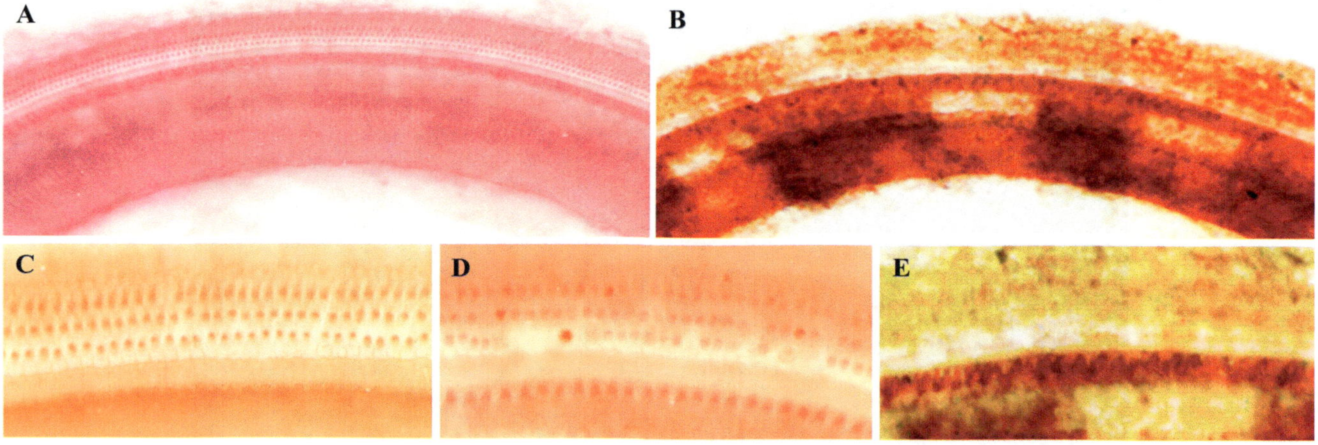

Fig. 8.23 Azo-coupling histochemical demonstration of acid phosphatase activity in guinea pig cochlear hair cells. (**A**) In normal specimens, acid phosphatase appears as red azo-dye deposits within lysosomes beneath the cuticular plates of both inner and outer hair cells. (**B**) 10 days after kanamycin treatment (400 mg/kg/day i.m.), while many hair cells are destroyed, surviving cells exhibit either reduced or enhanced acid phosphatase staining, indicating variable lysosomal activity responses. (**C**) High-magnification microscopy confirms the subcuticular localization of azo-coupled acid phosphatase in normal hair cells. (**D**) On day 1 after 7 days of kanamycin treatment (500 mg/kg/day, IM), scattered loss of first-row outer hair cells occurs. The acid phosphatase staining in the remaining outer hair cells was mostly weakened, but it was enhanced in some individual outer hair cells, reflecting that the lysosomes were in a different state of activity. (E) Daily injections of kanamycin continued until the 10th day, most of the outer hair cells have been destroyed, acid phosphatase activity is no longer seen in those destroyed outer hair cells, but the expression of acid phosphatase in surviving inner hair cells is increased. As a lysosomal marker, these temporary changes in acid phosphatase activity confirmed the involvement of lysosomes in kanamycin-induced hair cell destruction [33]

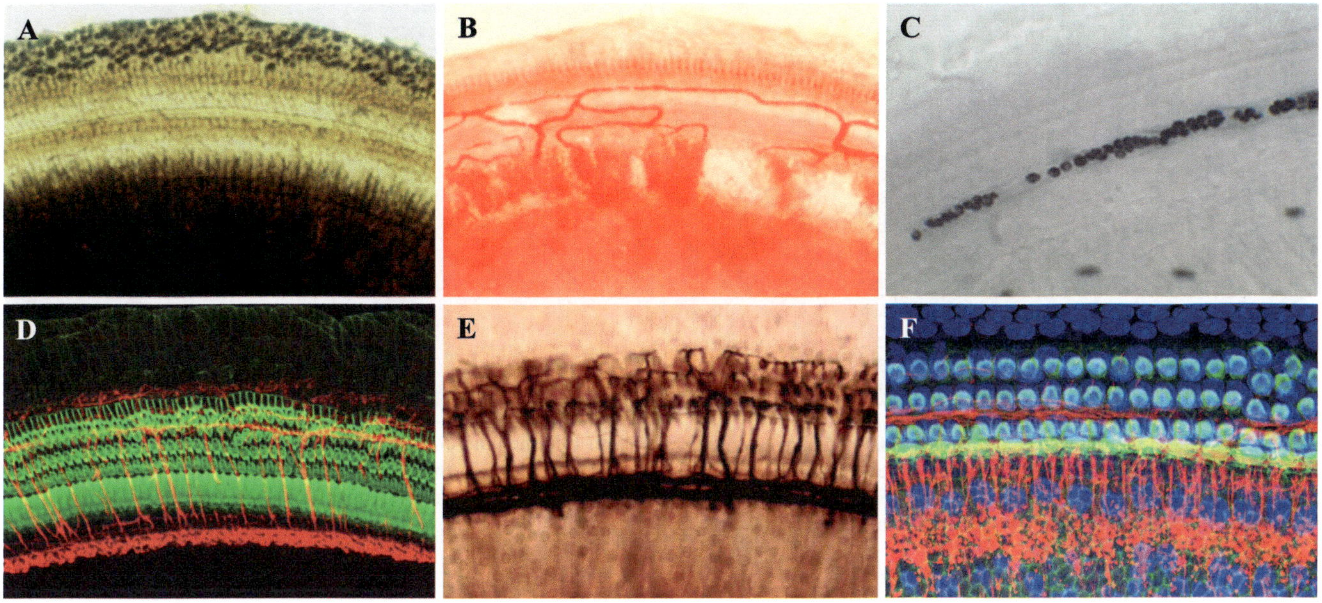

Fig. 8.24 Several histochemical staining methods were used to observe the different components and structures in the cochlear basilar membrane. (**A**) Osmium tetroxide staining marks fat droplets on the surface of Hensen's cells in the apical turn of the guinea pig cochlea and the auditory nerve fibers wrapped by myelin in the habenular perforata. (**B**) Eosin stain shows erythrocytes within spiral capillaries located in the tunnel of Corti. (**C**) Diaminobenzidine staining enhances the contrast of erythrocytes in the spiral capillaries at the bottom of the tunnel of Corti. (**D**) Double fluorescence staining of phalloidin and tubulin shows the surface structure (green) and the nerve fiber distribution (red) in the basilar membrane of the chinchilla cochlea. (**E**) Acetylcholinesterase staining specifically identifies efferent nerve fibers and their synapse in the chinchilla cochlea. (**F**) The cochlear basilar membrane of the rat was triple-stained with anti-tubulin antibody, phalloidin, and Topro-3 to label the nerve fibers in red, stereocilia of the hair cells in green, and cell nuclei in blue, respectively

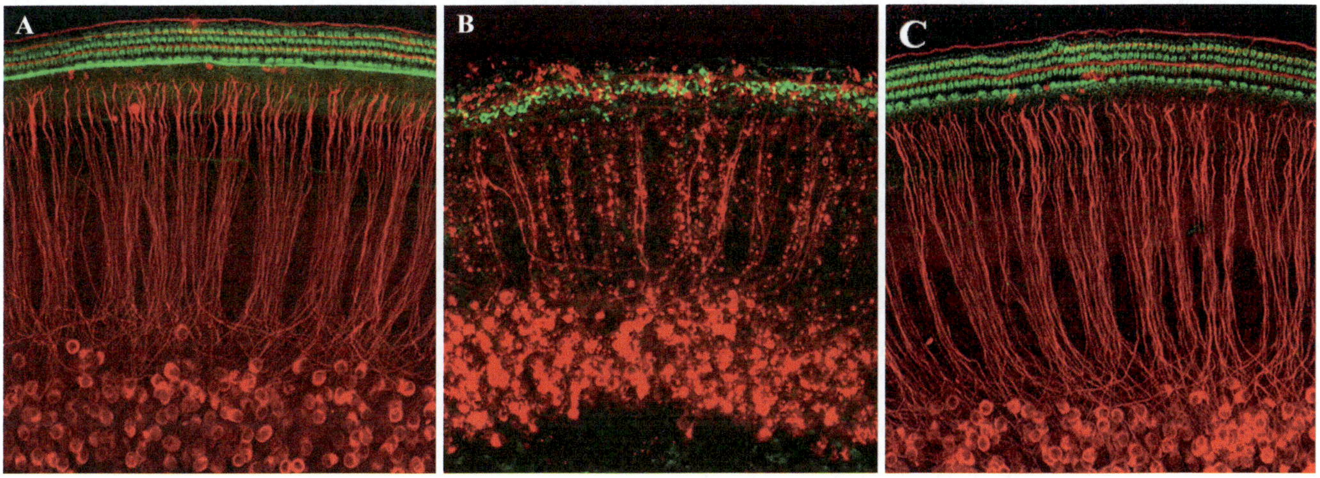

Fig. 8.25 Cochlear explants were stained with neurofilament-200 antibody and phalloidin. (**A**) Normal cochlear explants cultured in standard serum-free medium without cisplatin for 48 h show intact cochlear hair cells, spiral ganglion, and their nerve fibers. (B) Cochlear explants were cultured in serum-free medium containing 50 μM cisplatin for 48 h, and all cochlear hair cells, spiral ganglion neurons, and auditory nerve fibers were completely destroyed. (**C**) The cochlear explants were cultured in serum-free medium containing 100 μM cimetidine (copper transporter blocker) and 50 μM cisplatin for 48 h, and almost all cochlear hair cells, spiral ganglia, and auditory nerve fibers were intact. This indicates that copper transport inhibition prevents cellular uptake of cisplatin through copper transport channels, thereby effectively protecting the cochlear hair cells and the cochlear peripheral nervous system [48, 81]

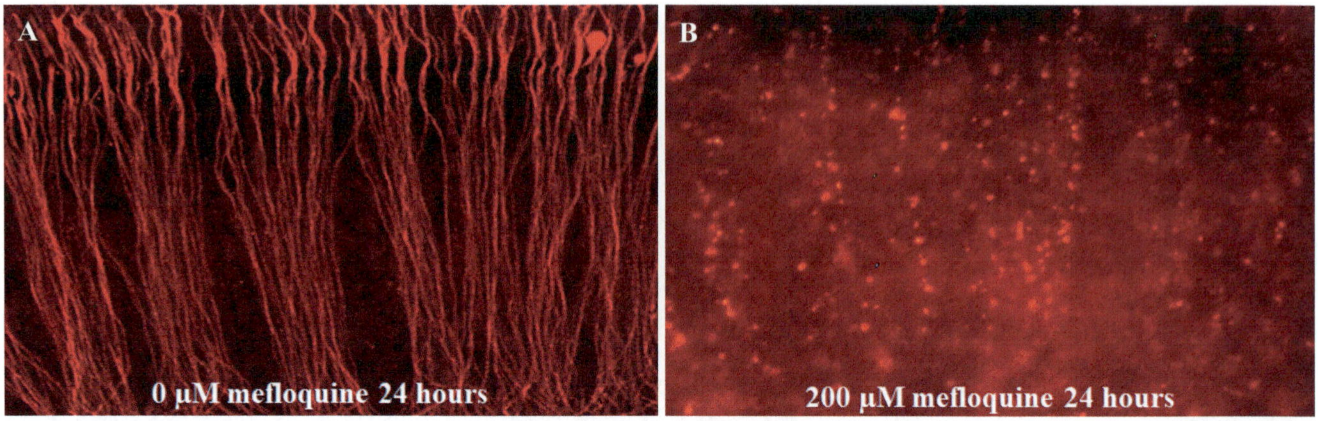

Fig. 8.26 Mefloquine-induced auditory nerve fiber damage in cochlear explants. (**A**) Cochlear explant maintained in mefloquine-free serum-free medium for 24 h shows intact auditory nerve fibers within the cochlear basilar membrane. (**B**) Cochlear explants were cultured in serum-free medium containing 200 µM mefloquine for 24 h; the auditory nerve fibers in the basilar membrane were severely fragmented (Reproduced with permission from Ding et al. [46])

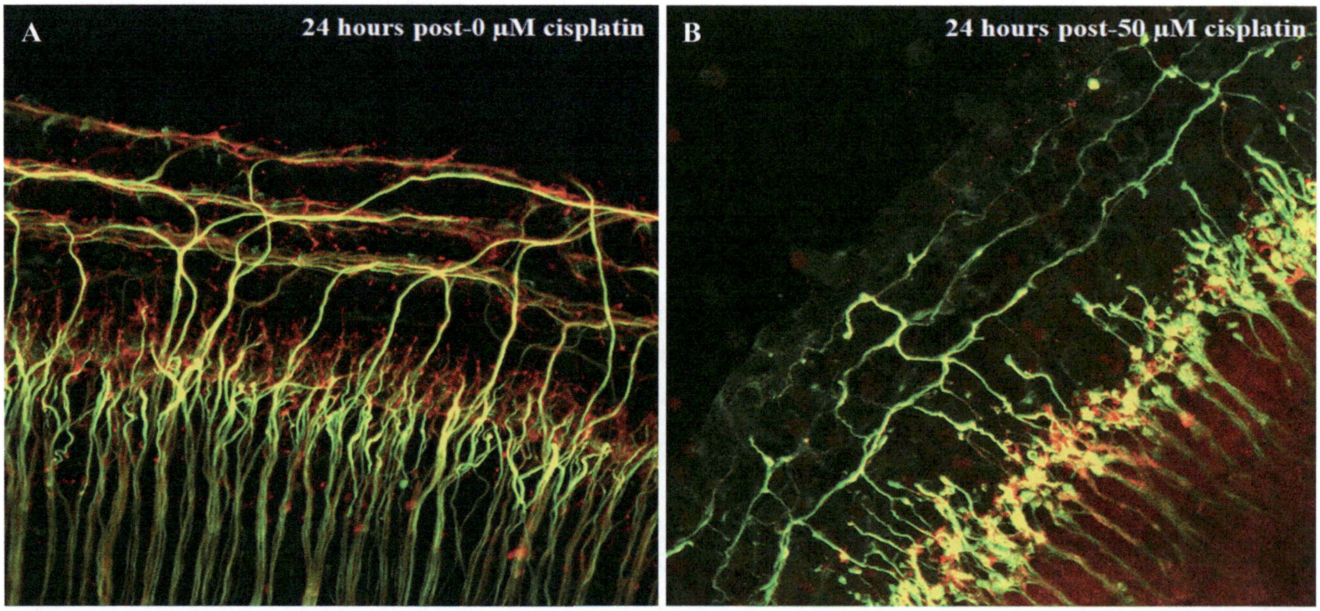

Fig. 8.27 Double staining of neurofilament and synapse in rat cochlear explants. (**A**) A normal control cochlear explant at postnatal day 3 was cultured in serum-free medium without cisplatin for 24 h; the auditory nerve fibers (labeled with anti-neurofilament-200 antibody, green) and synapses (labeled with anti-synapsin antibody, red) in the cochlear basilar membrane were intact. (**B**) Cochlear explant was cultured in serum-free medium containing 50 µM cisplatin for 24 h, the synapses labeled with anti-synapsin antibody at the base of outer hair cells were completely lost, but the nerve fibers labeled with anti-neurofilament-200 antibody remained intact. This indicates that cisplatin-induced synaptic damage preceded the degeneration of nerve fibers

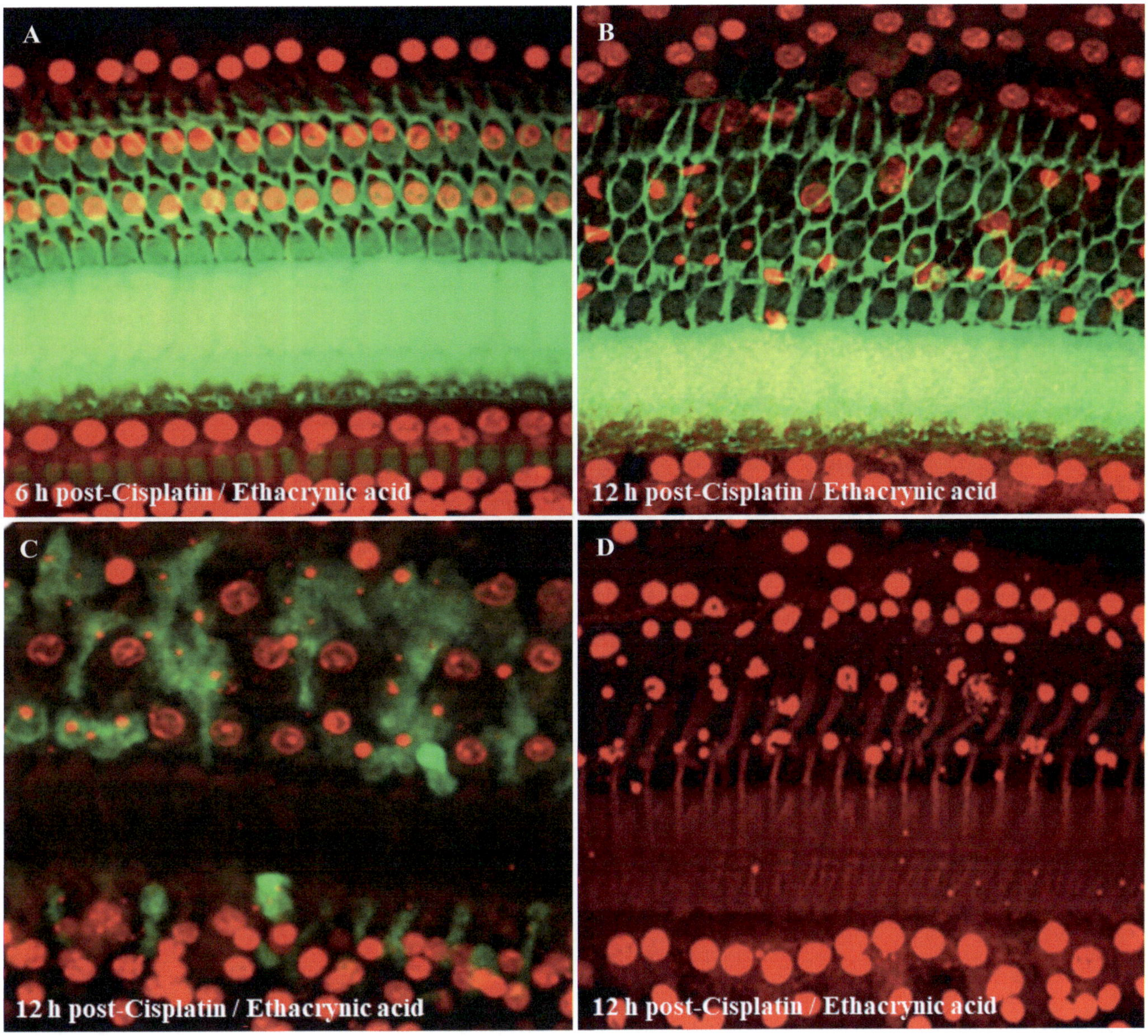

Fig. 8.28 Double staining of surface preparation of chinchilla cochlear basilar membrane to assess cisplatin-induced lesions of hair cell nucleus and surface structures or caspase-mediated apoptotic pathways. (**A**) 6 h after co-administration of cisplatin (0.2 mg/kg) and ethacrynic acid (40 mg/kg), Dual phalloidin and propidium iodide staining reveals both the cuticular plate and the nuclei of hair cells present normally. (B) 12 h after the simultaneous injection of cisplatin and ethacrynic acid, the nuclei in most outer hair cells showed typical apoptotic features such as obvious nuclear condensation or nuclear fragmentation. (**C**) Twelve hours post-cisplatin and ethacrynic acid, caspase-8, one of the initiating caspases that responds exclusively to cell death receptors on the cell membrane, was present in outer hair cells with nuclear condensation. However, the positive labeling of caspase-8 did not appear in the hair cells without nuclear condensation. This suggests that cisplatin-induced hair cell apoptosis may be closely related to the apoptotic signal released by cell death factor receptors on the cell membrane. (**D**) 12 h after the simultaneous injection of cisplatin and ethacrynic acid, although most outer hair cells expressed nuclear shrinkage or nuclear rupture, another initiator caspase, caspase-9, was not activated. Since caspase-9 is only activated by the complex of cytochrome c bound to the cytosolic protein Apaf-1 and dATP in the cytoplasm, cisplatin-induced hair cell apoptosis does not appear to be via the mitochondrial apoptotic pathway. The above characteristics of nuclear lesions in cochlear hair cells indicate that cisplatin-induced hair cell death is through the initiation of programmed cell apoptosis. The differential activation patterns of these initiator caspases demonstrate that cisplatin primarily activates the extrinsic apoptotic pathway rather than the intrinsic apoptotic pathway in cochlear hair cells

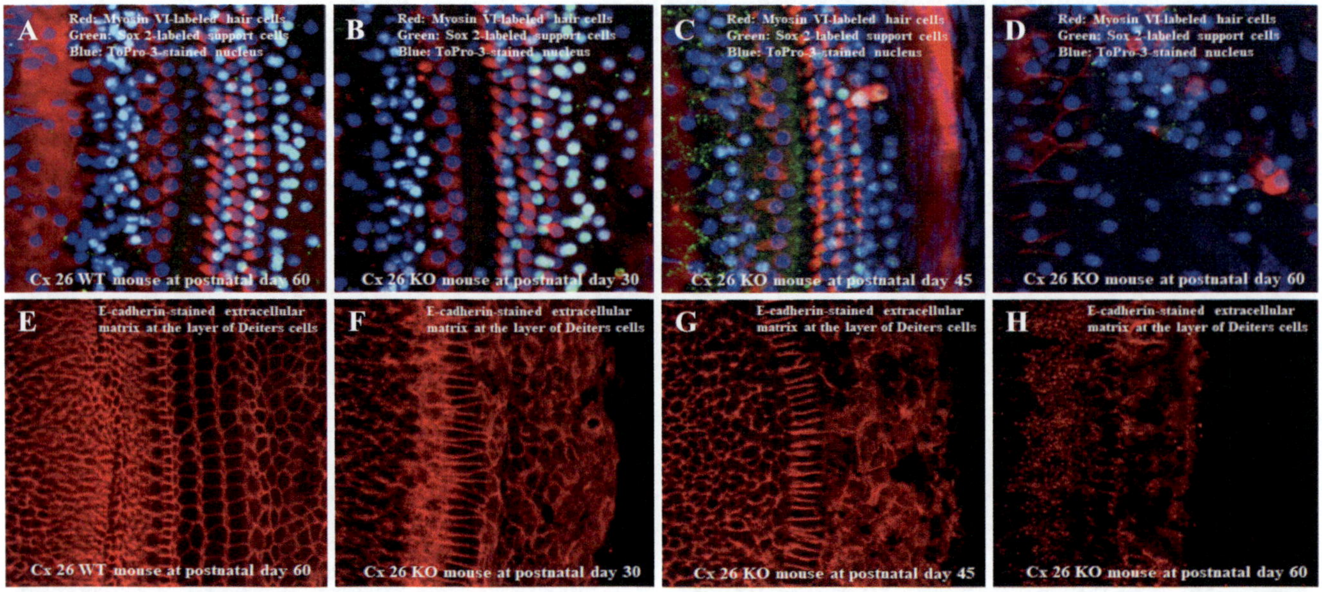

Fig. 8.29 The lesions of the organ of Corti caused by connexin 26 gene deficiency originate from the destruction of the extracellular matrix surrounding the supporting cells beneath the hair cells. (**A**) Triple staining with anti-myosin VI antibody, anti-Sox-2 antibody, and ToPro-3 stains hair cells, supporting cells, and nuclei in red, green, and blue, respectively. 60 days after birth, cochlear hair cells and supporting cells of connexin 26 wild-type mice were intact. (**B**) Connexin 26 knockout mice begin to partially lose supporting cells beneath outer hair cells 30 days after birth. (**C**) Connexin 26 knockout mice showed an obvious decrease in the number of supporting cells beneath the outer hair cells 45 days after birth, but the hair cells were intact. (**D**) All hair cells and supporting cells in the Corti organ of Connexin 26 knockout mice were completely destroyed 60 days after birth. Only a thin layer of flat epithelium remained on the basilar membrane of the cochlea. (**E**) Anti-E-cadherin antibody labeling shows that the extracellular matrix surrounding the Deiters cells maintains intact normal connection patterns 60 days after birth. (**F**) Anti-E-cadherin antibody labeling shows that the extracellular matrix surrounding Deiters cells has begun to be partially destroyed in connexin 26 knockout mice 30 days after birth. (**G**) Anti-E-cadherin antibody labeling shows that the extracellular matrix surrounding the Deiters cells was severely destroyed in connexin 26 knockout mice 45 days after birth. (**H**) Anti-E-cadherin antibody labeling showed that the extracellular matrix surrounding Deiters cells in connexin 26 knockout mice was completely gone at postnatal day 60. The above-mentioned series of pathological processes of the cochlear organ of Corti in Connexin 26 mutant mice indicates that the death of hair cells occurs after the destruction of supporting cells, and the destruction of supporting cells originates from the destruction of the extracellular matrix. Therefore, it is possible that the loss of the Connexin 26 gene causes the loss of intercellular gap junction proteins and the loss of extracellular matrix, which in turn interrupts the connection between cochlear supporting cells, causing anoikis and secondary apoptosis of cochlear hair cells

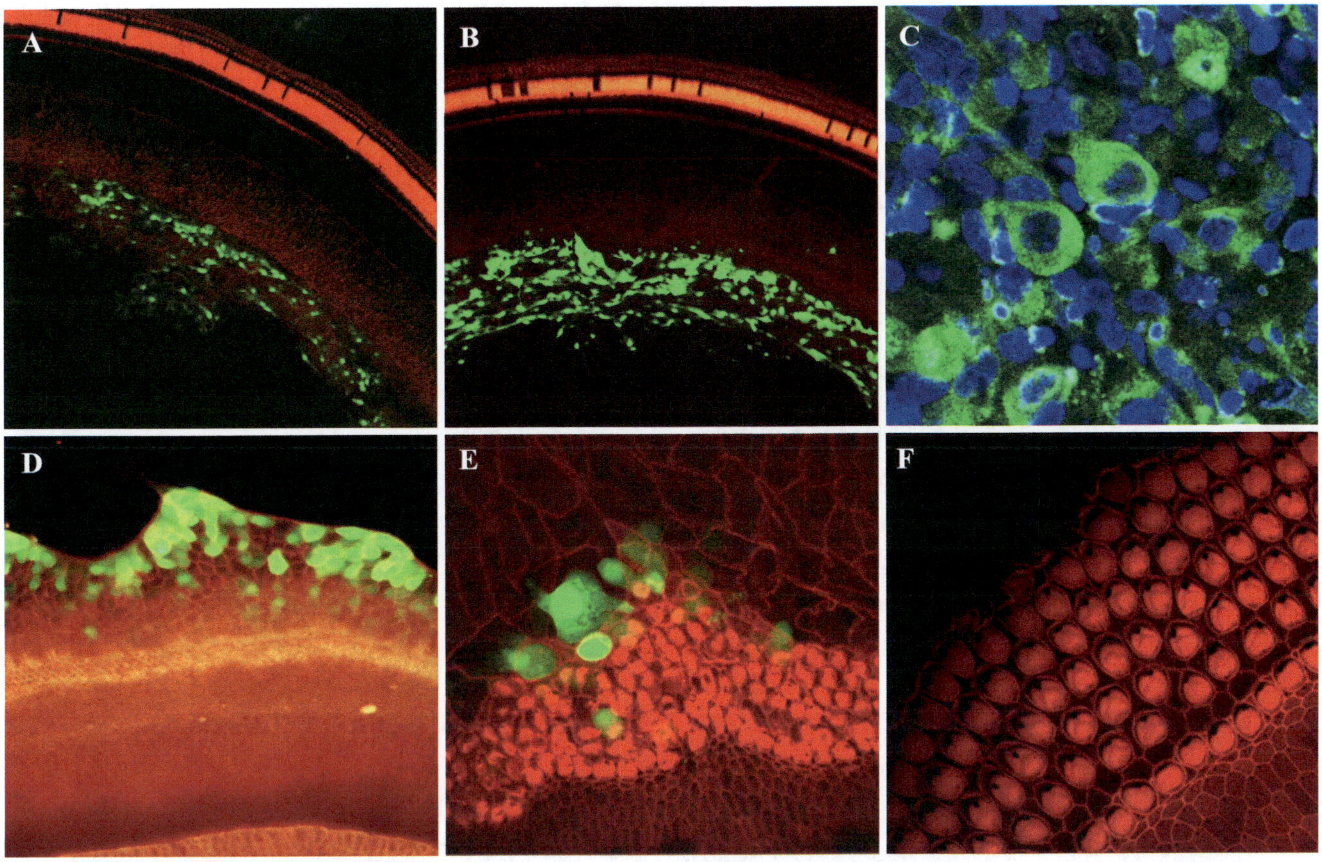

Fig. 8.30 Different transfection tropisms of viral vectors for different cell types in the mammalian cochlea. (**A**) On the second day after the herpes simplex virus (HSV) vector carrying the green fluorescent protein gene entered the perilymph of the scala tympani of the cochlea through the round window membrane, some spiral ganglion neurons began to express green fluorescent protein, but the hair cells and supporting cells on the basilar membrane of the cochlea were not transfected, indicating that the herpes virus tends to transfect neurons. (**B**) On the fifth day after the herpes simplex virus vector carrying the green fluorescent protein gene infiltrated the perilymph of the chinchilla cochlea through the round window membrane, a large amount of green fluorescent protein appeared in the spiral ganglion cells in Rosenthal's canal. This once again proves that herpes simplex virus tends to transduce neurons rather than inner ear epithelial cells. Therefore, herpes simplex virus can be regarded as an ideal neuron-targeted transfection vector. (**C**) In the rat cochlea, it was also observed that the herpes simplex virus vector carrying the green fluorescent protein gene that entered the cochlea through the round window membrane caused many spiral ganglion cells to express green fluorescent protein on the third day after transfection. (**D**) On the third day after the adenovirus vector carrying the green fluorescent protein gene entered the cochlea of the chinchilla through the round window membrane, many supporting cells in the lateral sulcus region of the basilar membrane began to express green fluorescent protein, but no green fluorescent protein was expressed in the cochlear hair cells, suggesting that the adenovirus vector may prefer to transfect the supporting cells of the cochlea. (**E**) On the third day after the adenovirus vector carrying the Math1 gene and the green fluorescent gene was transfected into the cochlea at postnatal day 1, the supporting cells at the lateral sulcus region began to express green fluorescent protein and differentiated into additional hair cell-like cells, suggesting that the Math1 gene may induce the transfected supporting cells to begin to differentiate into hair cell-like cells. (**F**) 1 week after adenovirus vector carrying the Math1 gene transfection to the mouse cochlear explants, multiple rows of cells similar in appearance to outer hair cells were detected outside the third row of outer hair cells. It is speculated that these additional cell populations may be from the supporting cells transfected with adenoviral vectors carrying the Math1 gene. This implies that once the Math1 gene is transfected into supporting cells, it is likely to induce the transfected supporting cells to differentiate into hair cell-like cells

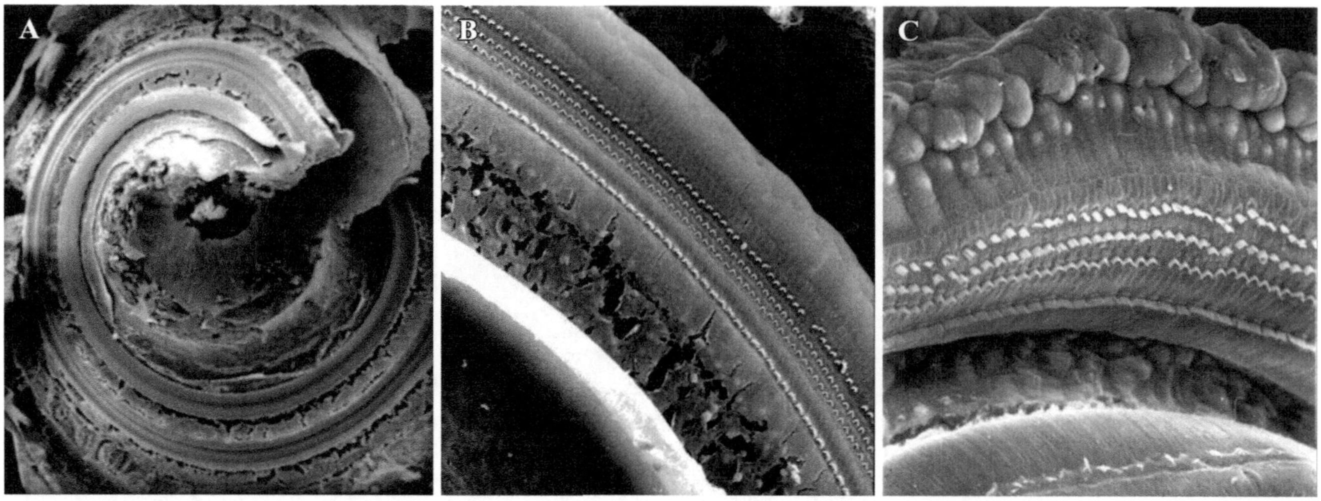

Fig. 8.31 Observation of the ultrastructure on the surface of the cochlear basilar membrane using scanning electron microscopy. (**A**) Low-magnification view of the exposed basilar membrane surface at the second cochlear turn in chinchilla. (**B**) Surface morphology and structure of the organ of Corti in the second turn in the normal chinchilla. (**C**) Surface ultrastructure of the organ of Corti in the third turn in a normal guinea pig

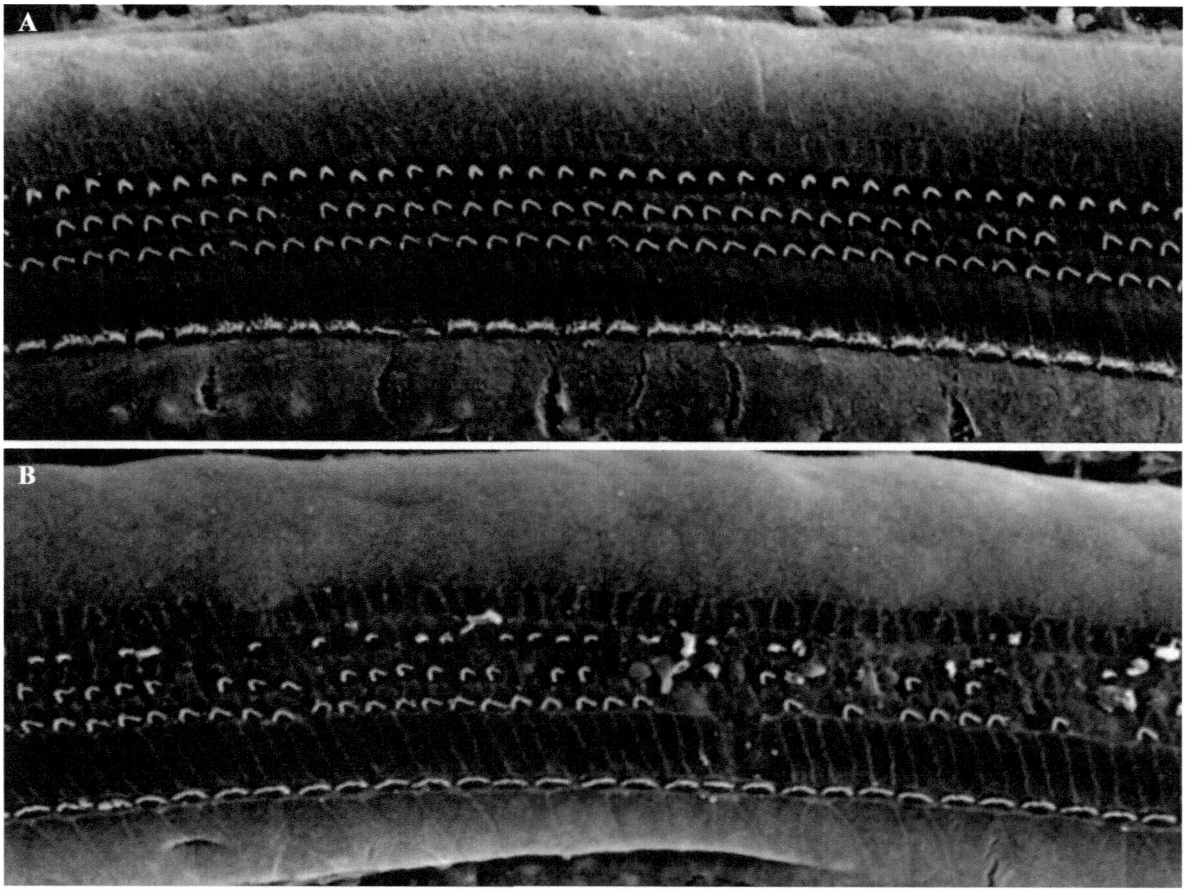

Fig. 8.32 Scanning electron microscopic view of the surface structure on the cochlear basilar membrane of the chinchilla. (**A**) Surface ultrastructure of the organ of Corti in a normal chinchilla, showing the characteristic arrangement of three rows of outer hair cells and one row of inner hair cells. (**B**) Intense noise (105 dB, SPL) exposure resulted in damage to some outer hair cells, while the inner hair cells in the same region were intact. This suggests that outer hair cells are more susceptible to being injured by intense noise than inner hair cells

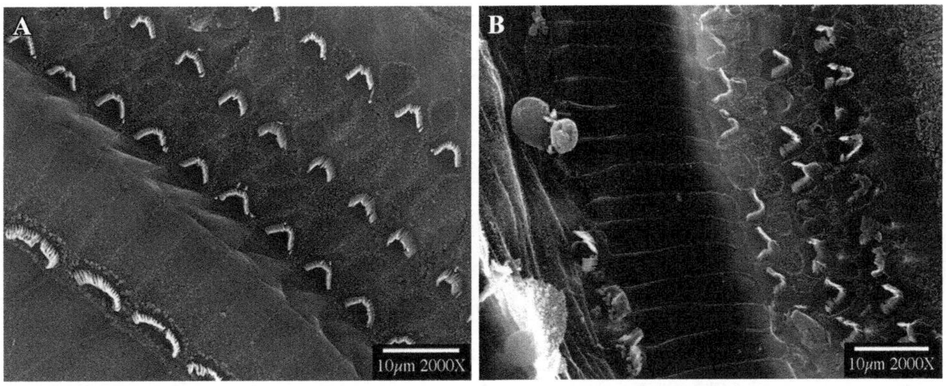

Fig. 8.33 Scanning electron micrograph showing the surface submicroscopic structure of the cochlear organ of Corti. (**A**) Scanning electron micrograph of a normal cochlear basilar membrane showing the orderly arrangement of the submicroscopic structure of the stereocilia and cuticle plate of the inner and outer hair cells. (**B**) When carboplatin was placed in the round window niche, both the inner and outer hair cells of the chinchilla were damaged, but the range and degree of damage to the inner hair cells were more severe than the outer hair cells

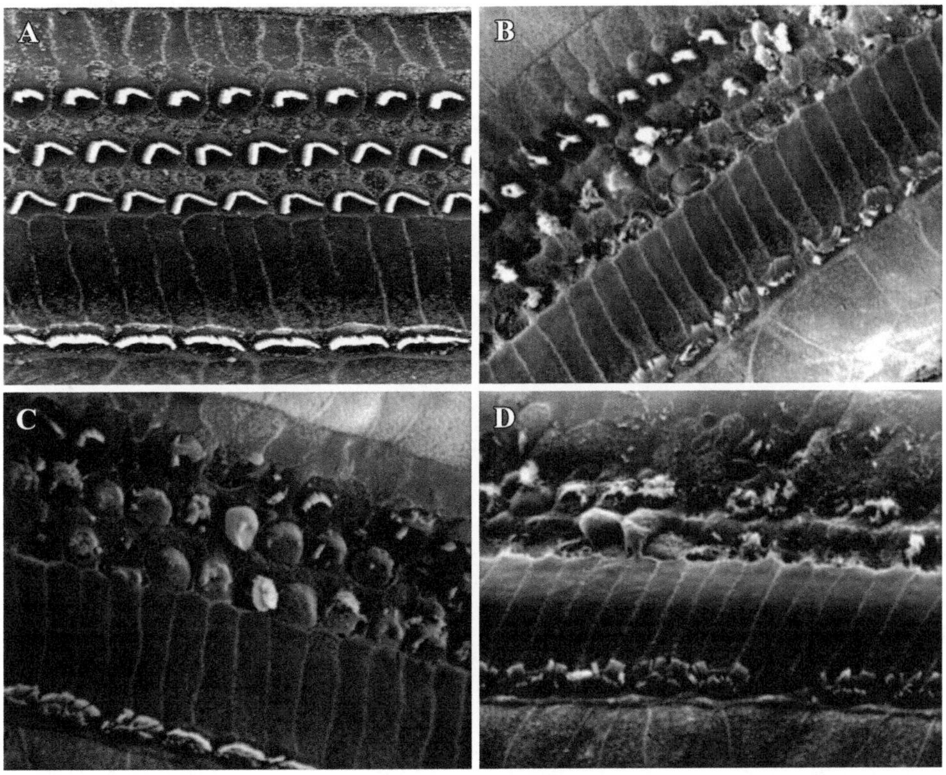

Fig. 8.34 Scanning electron micrographs of the surface structure of the organ of Corti in normal chinchilla and noise-exposed chinchillas. (**A**) The surface ultrastructure of the inner and outer hair cells of the organ of Corti in normal chinchilla shows a neat arrangement order. (**B**) On the second day after exposure to narrowband noise (105 dB SPL octave band noise centered at 4 kHz, 5 h), in the region of cochlear basilar membrane corresponding to the frequency of 4 kHz, the outer hair cells in the first row and second row were completely destroyed, and although the outer hair cells in the third row and the inner hair cells were not absent, but the stereocilia of these hair cells were obviously scattered, lodged, or fused. (**C**) On the third day after exposure to 4 kHz narrowband noise, the three rows of outer hair cells corresponding to the 4 kHz frequency were severely damaged. Although the cuticular plate of most outer hair cells still existed, the stereocilia of these outer hair cells had fallen off, and the cuticle plate also showed swelling and bulges. (**D**) On the fifth day after exposure to 4 kHz narrow-band noise, all three rows of outer hair cells in the region of the cochlear basilar membrane corresponding to the frequency of 4 kHz were completely destroyed, leaving some cellular debris and scar tissue on the surface of the organ of Corti. The inner hair cells in this region also presented obvious dispersion or lodging of stereocilia. The above experimental results show that the outer hair cells located in the area of the maximum vibration amplitude of the basilar membrane corresponding to the center frequency of the noise are most severely destroyed

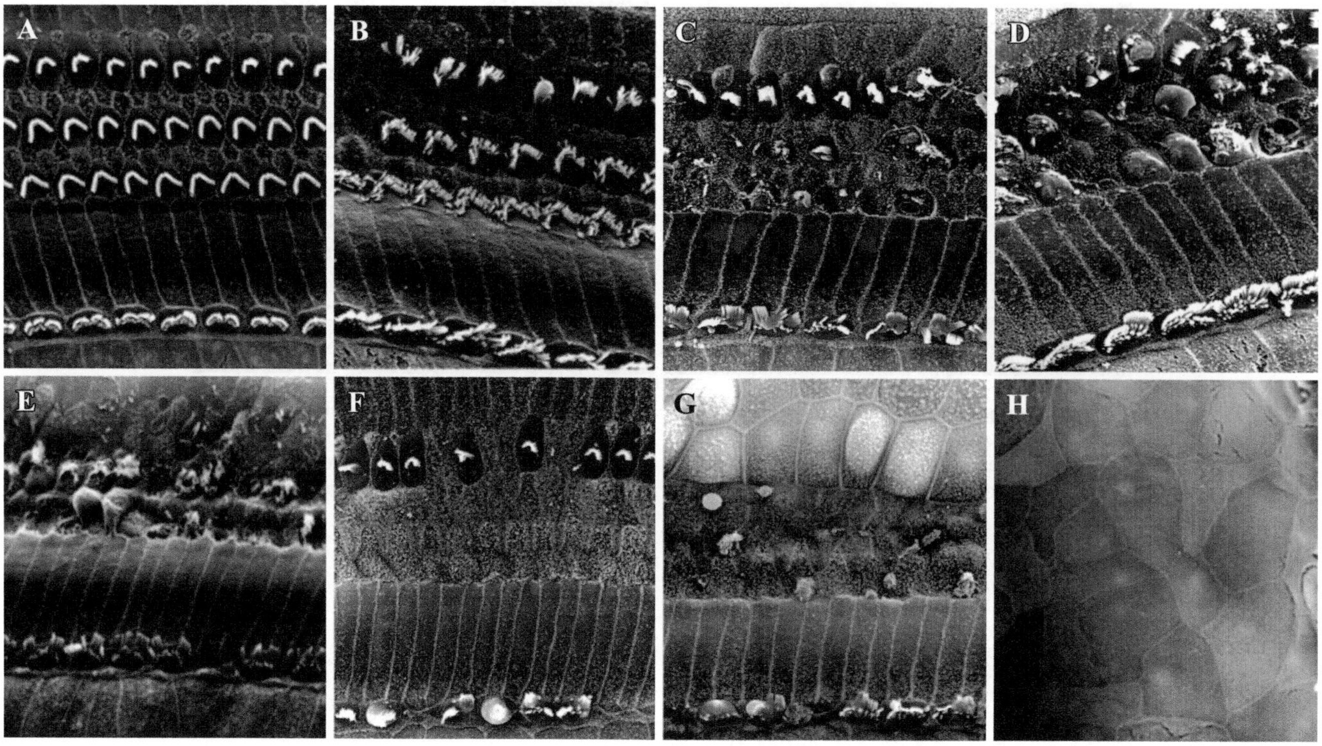

Fig. 8.35 Surface ultrastructure of cochlear hair cells in the chinchilla was observed under a scanning electron microscope. (**A**) The surface ultrastructure of cochlear hair cells on the basilar membrane was arranged in an orderly geometric pattern in normal chinchillas. (**B**) Early damage to cochlear hair cells often manifests as dispersion and prostration of stereocilia. (**C**) Ototoxic chemical-induced damage to the cochlear outer hair cells usually extends from the first row toward the third row, indicating potential differences in vulnerability among outer hair cell populations. (**D**) After the stereocilia of the damaged outer hair cells are shed, the cuticular plate often exhibits prominent bulges, suggesting increased pressure within the organ of Corti. (**E**) Cellular debris or tissue fragments are often seen in the area where the outer hair cells have just been destroyed. (**F**) After hair cells are completely destroyed, the cuticular plate of Deiters cells expands and fuses with each other to form scars, effectively sealing the reticular lamina. (**G**) The scar effectively seals the reticular lamina, preventing the mixing of endolymph and cortilymph. (**H**) Large-scale hair cell death leads to delayed secondary destruction of supporting cells, and ultimately causes the collapse of the entire supporting structure of the Corti organ. After all hair cells and supporting cells die, only a thin layer of flat epithelium remains on the cochlear basilar membrane. It is worth noting that this flat epithelium is different from any of the original supporting cell types on the basilar membrane, so this flat epithelium is speculated to be a new cell involved in basilar membrane repair

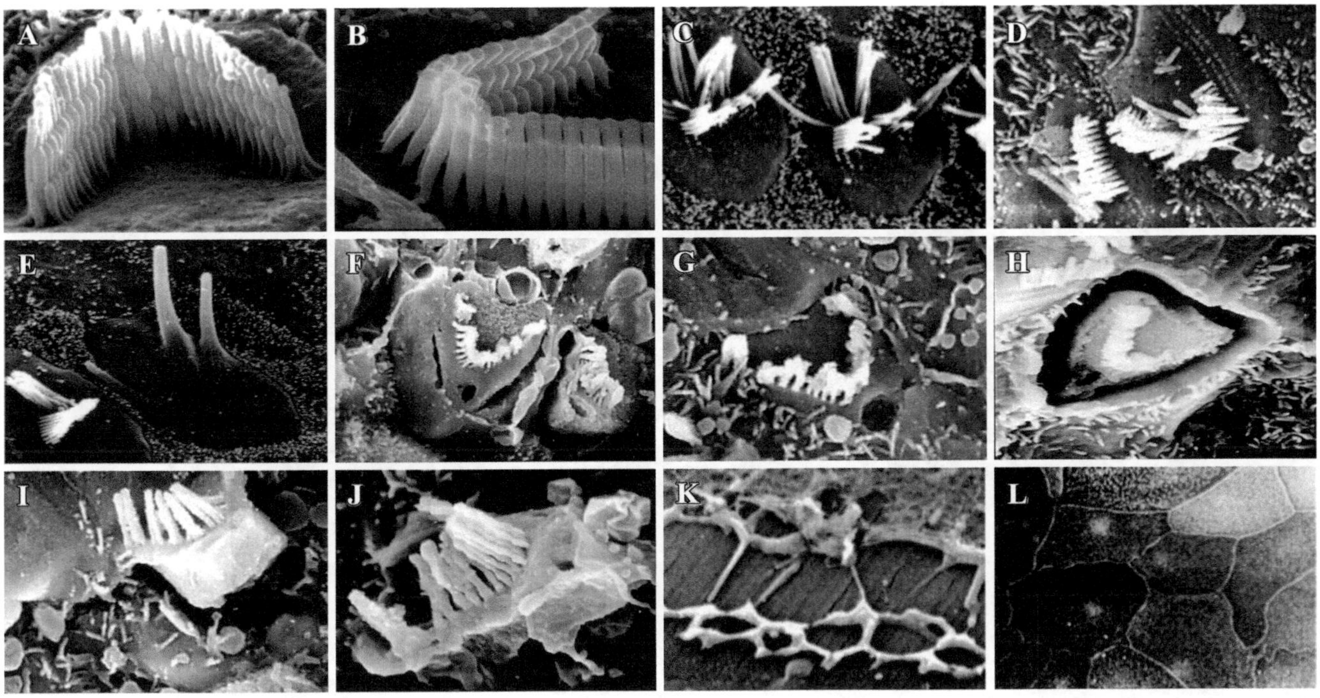

Fig. 8.36 Scanning electron microscopy was used to observe the surface ultrastructure of outer hair cells and the process of pathological changes. (**A**) Normal outer hair cells exhibit the characteristic W-shaped stereocilia bundles on the cuticular plate when viewed from the front. (**B**) The W-shaped stereocilia of outer hair cells have three rows, of which the stereocilia facing the modiolus are the shortest, while the stereocilia adjacent to the Hensen's cells are the longest. (**C**) Disordered arrangement of stereocilia can often be seen as one of the early pathological changes occurring on the surface of cochlear hair cells. (**D**) As the lesion progresses, the stereocilia of the hair cells can be seen falling off, exposing the stereocilia root sockets in the cuticular plate of hair cells. (**E**) Adjacent damaged stereocilia on the injured hair cells can fuse with each other to form an abnormal giant ciliary. (**F**) In the late stage of hair cell damage, perforation of the cuticular plate of hair cells, and cracks or gaps surrounding the cuticular plate of hair cells can be detected. (**G**) The cytoplasm of the damaged hair cell is expelled through the perforation in the cuticular plate, and the hair cell is considered to be dying at this point. (**H**) Before the cuticular plate of the damaged hair cells is expelled into the scala media, a circular fissure appears around the cuticular plate of the damaged hair cell, indicating that the cuticular plate of the damaged hair cells has been completely separated from the cuticle plate of surrounding Deiters cells. (**I**) During the destruction of the hair cells in the organ of Corti and the extreme expansion of Deiters cells, the destroyed cuticular plate of hair cells is expelled through perforations on the reticular membrane onto the surface of the organ of Corti. (**J**) The cuticular plate of destroyed hair cells that were expelled to the surface of the organ of Corti was then progressively broken down. (**K**) Complete destruction of cochlear hair cells leads to subsequent secondary destruction of supporting cells. After engulfing and digesting all tissue cell debris, macrophages are finally exposed on the surface of the basilar membrane. (**L**) The ultimate outcome of the complete destruction of the organ of Corti is the withdrawal of macrophages, with only a thin layer of squamous epithelium remaining on the cochlear basilar membrane. These observations systematically document the complete cytopathological cascade from initial stereociliary disarray to final structural collapse

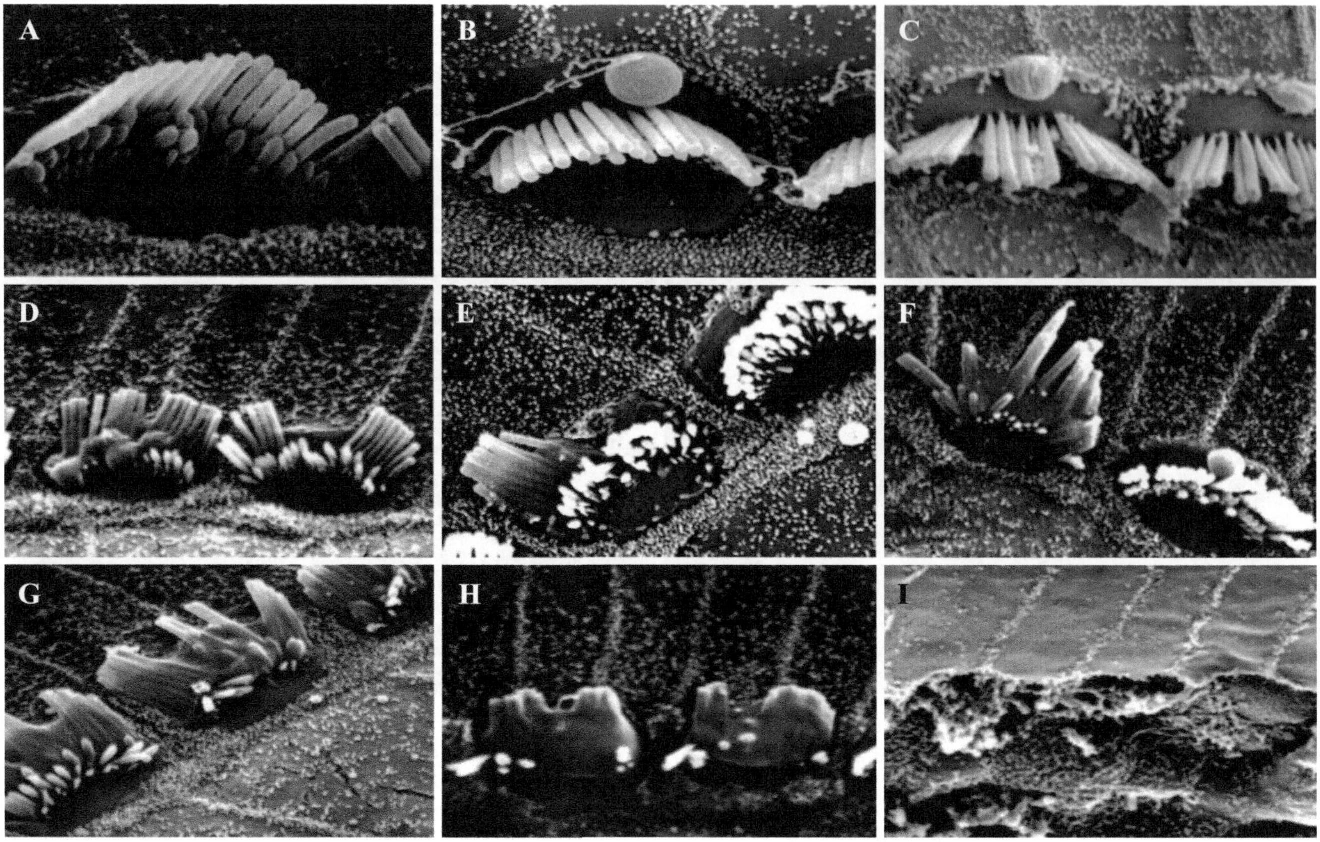

Fig. 8.37 A scanning electron microscope system was used to record the process of carboplatin-induced ultrastructural pathological changes on the surface of inner hair cells in chinchillas. (**A**) In a normal chinchilla, the stereocilia of inner hair cells are arranged in a unique double row on the cuticular plate, with longer stereocilia facing the inner pillar cells and shorter ones facing the inner sulcus. (**B**) 24 h after injection of carboplatin (100 mg/kg), spherical objects appeared on the surface of the epidermal plate of inner hair cells, which may be some kind of cellular contents discharged from the inner hair cells. (**C**) In the early stage of carboplatin ototoxicity, the spherical objects that first appear on the cuticular plate of inner hair cells may be considered as an early pathological sign of inner hair cell damage. (**D**). 48 h post-carboplatin, the long stereocilia of inner hair cells begin to scatter or fall off while the short stereocilia remain intact, suggesting that the long stereocilia of inner hair cells may be more sensitive to the destruction of carboplatin. (**E**) 48 h after carboplatin injection, long stereocilia of many inner hair cells were lost, but the short stereocilia had not yet fallen off. (**F**) 72 h after carboplatin injection, the long stereocilia on the surface of many inner hair cells began to fuse. (**G**) 72 h after carboplatin injection, fusion of long stereocilia on the inner hair cell begins to spread to short stereocilia. (**H**) 5 days post-carboplatin, all stereocilia disappear, and the cuticular plate begins to show lytic lesions. (**I**) 1 week after injection, the inner hair cells completely disappear. The original location of inner hair cells was sealed by the interconnected cuticular plates of inner phalangeal cells and inner pillar cells to form a scar structure. This pathological progression reveals the sequential ultrastructural changes during carboplatin-induced inner hair cell death

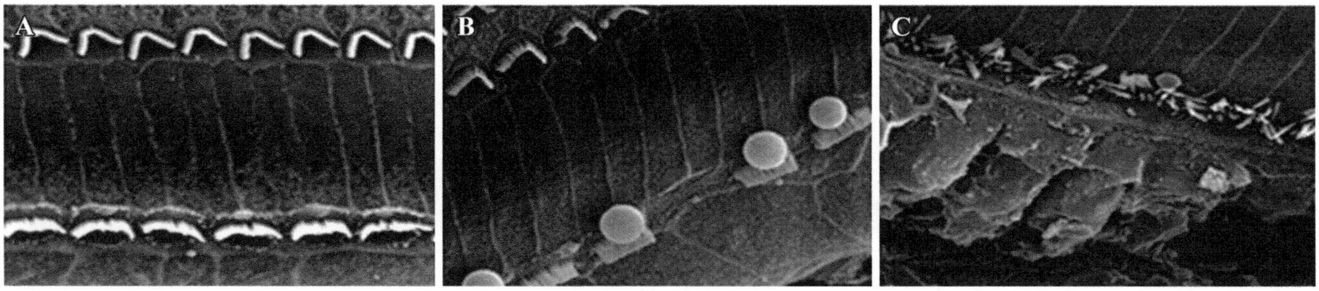

Fig. 8.38 Early ultrastructural pathological changes on the surface of inner hair cells after carboplatin injection in chinchillas. (**A**) The surface ultrastructure of inner hair cells and surrounding supporting cells in the normal chinchilla cochlea shows intact morphology. (**B**) 48 h after carboplatin injection (100 mg/kg), spherical secretions appear along the longer stereocilia of inner hair cells, while the stereociliary bundles maintain the normal morphology, indicating cellular exudation precedes stereocilia damage. (**C**) 72 h post-injection, many stereocilia became scattered or collapsed, accompanied by destruction of adjacent inner border cells and inner phalangeal epithelial cells, suggesting these destroyed supporting cells may be secondary to the destruction of type I afferent nerve terminals beneath the inner hair cells. The submicroscopic structural destruction that occurred successively on the surface of inner hair cells and surrounding supporting cells indicated that the ultrastructural changes on the surface of the organ of Corti might be one of the early pathological sites of carboplatin

References

1. Engström H. Cochlear damage from ototoxic antibiotics. Acta Otolaryngol. 1965;59(2-3):171–8.
2. Engström H. Structural pattern of the organ of Corti. Sweden: Almqvist & Wiksells Boktryckeri AB; 1966.
3. Engström H. The pathological sensory cell in the cochlea. Acta Otolaryngol. 1967;63(Suppl 226):20–26. https://doi.org/10.3109/00016486709128795.
4. Bohne BA. Location of small cochlear lesions by phase contrast microscopy prior to thin sectioning. Laryngoscope. 1972;82(1):1–16. https://doi.org/10.1002/lary.5540820101.
5. Spoendlin H, Brun JP. The block-surface technique for evaluation of cochlear pathology. Arch Otorhinolaryngol. 1974;208(2):137–45. https://doi.org/10.1007/BF00453927.
6. Ylikoski J. Guinea-pig hair cell pathology from ototoxic antibiotics. Acta Otolaryngol Suppl. 1974;326:5–22. https://doi.org/10.3109/00016487409129729.
7. Dai S, Wang C, Ji M. Surface preparation technique of the whole cochlea. Chin J Otorhinolaryngol. 1981;16(2): 72–75.
8. Ding D, Zhao J, Huangfu M. Modified cochlear surface preparations. Chin J Otorhinolaryngol. 1981;16(4):207–9.
9. Ding D, Zhao J, Huangfu M, Jin X. Microdissection of the whole membranous labyrinth in guinea pigs. J Clin Otorhinolaryngol. 1987;1(1):9–11.
10. Spoendlin H, Schrott A. The spiral ganglion and the innervation of the human organ of Corti. Acta Otolaryngol. 1988;105(5-6):403–10. https://doi.org/10.3109/00016488809119493.
11. Ding D, Wang J, He Y. Surface preparation technique of the spiral ligament of the cochlea in guinea pig. Shanghai Med J. 1984;7(11):657–8.
12. Ding D, Luo S, Jin X. Microdissection of the vestibular end-organs in guinea pigs. Shanghai Med J. 1986;9(3):153–4.
13. Ding D, Li H, Zhao J, Huangfu M. Enzyme histochemical sectioning technique of the stria vascularis in the inner ear of guinea pigs. J Clin Otorhinolaryngol. 1987;1(3):173–74.
14. Ding D, Jiang S. Chapter 6: Surface preparation techniques of the inner ear. In: Ding D, editor. Manual of anatomical examination of the inner ear of the guinea pig. Shanghai: Xuelin Publishing House; 1989. pp. 49–60.
15. Ding D, Li M, Jiang C, Salvi R. Chapter 5: Surface preparation techniques of membranous labyrinth. In: Ding D, editor. Morphology of the inner ear. Harbin: Heilongjiang Science and Technology Press; 2001. pp. 24–37.
16. Ding D, McFadden SL, Salvi R. Cochlear hair cell densities and inner-ear staining techniques. In: Willott JF, editor. Handbook of mouse auditory research from behavior to molecular biology. Boca Raton: CRC Press; 2001. p. 189–204.
17. Ding D, McFadden SL, Woo JM, Salvi RJ. Ethacrynic acid rapidly and selectively abolishes blood flow in vessels supplying the lateral wall of the cochlea. Hear Res. 2002;173(1–2):1–9. https://doi.org/10.1016/s0378-5955(02)00585-3.
18. Ding D, Qi W, Qu Y, Salvi R. Chapter 6: Research techniques of the inner ear morphology. In: Ding D, editor. Science of the inner ear. Beijing: China Science and Technology Press; 2010. pp. 50–88.
19. Ding D, Liu H, Qi W, et al. Ototoxic effects and mechanisms of loop diuretics. J Otol. 2016;11(4):145–56. https://doi.org/10.1016/j.joto.2016.10.001.
20. Li Y, Ding D, Jiang H, Fu Y, Salvi R. Co-administration of cisplatin and furosemide causes rapid and massive loss of cochlear hair cells in mice. Neurotox Res. 2011;20(4):307–19. https://doi.org/10.1007/s12640-011-9244-0.
21. Liu H, Ding DL, Jiang HY, et al. Ototoxic destruction by co-administration of kanamycin and ethacrynic acid in rats. J Zhejiang Univ Sci B. 2011;12(10):853–61. https://doi.org/10.1631/jzus.B1100040.
22. Ding D, Jiang H, Fu Y, et al. Ototoxic model of oxaliplatin and protection from nicotinamide adenine dinucleotide. J Otol. 2013;8(2):63–71. https://doi.org/10.1016/s1672-2930(13)50009-2.
23. Ding D, Salvi R, Roth JA. Cellular localization and developmental changes of the different isoforms of divalent metal transporter 1 (DMT1) in the inner ear of rats. BioMetals. 2014;27(1):125–34. https://doi.org/10.1007/s10534-013-9692-5.
24. Ding D, Salvi R, Roth JA. Cellular localization and developmental changes of Zip8, Zip14 and transferrin receptor 1 in the inner ear of rats. BioMetals. 2014;27(4):731–44. https://doi.org/10.1007/s10534-014-9765-0.
25. Manohar S, Jamesdaniel S, Ding D, et al. Quantitative PCR analysis and protein distribution of drug transporter genes in the rat cochlea. Hear Res. 2016;332:46–54. https://doi.org/10.1016/j.heares.2015.10.020.
26. Engström H, Engström B. The inner ear. J Otolaryngol Soc Aust. 1972;3(3):307–16.
27. Engstrom B. Scanning electron microscopy of the inner structure of the organ of Corti and its neural pathways. Acta Otolaryngol Suppl. 1974;319:57–66. https://doi.org/10.1080/16512251.1974.11675752.
28. Ding D, Jiang S. Chapter 8: Preparation techniques for electron microscopy of inner ear specimen. In: Ding D, editor. Manual of anatomical examination of the inner ear of the guinea pig. Shanghai: Xuelin Publishing House; 1989. pp. 67–74.
29. Ding D, Jin X, Zhang Z, Zhu Q. Study on the different susceptibility between red-eyed and black-eyed guinea pigs to gentamicin. Acta Otorhinolaryngol. 1995;9(2):70–74.
30. Ding D, Li M, Jiang C, Salvi R. Chapter 7: Preparation technology of inner ear specimens for electron microscopy. In: Ding D, editor. Morphology of the inner ear. Harbin: Heilongjiang Science and Technology Press; 2001. p. 55–85.
31. Ding D, Li M, Jiang S, Salvi R. Chapter 9: Electron microscopic cytochemical techniques of inner ear cells. In: Ding D, editor. Morphology of the inner ear. Harbin: Heilongjiang Science and Technology Press; 2001. pp. 125–7.
32. Ding D, Salvi R. Review of cellular changes in the cochlea due to aminoglycoside antibiotics. Volta Rev. 2005;105(3): 407–38.
33. Ding D, Zhu X, Chen H, Zhao J, Huangfu M. Study on acid phosphatase in the cochlea of guinea pigs with kanamycin ototoxicity. Chin J Otorhinolaryngol. 1986;21(2):121–2.
34. Willott JF, Turner JG, Carlson S, et al. The BALB/c mouse as an animal model for progressive sensorineural hearing loss. Hear Res. 1998;115(1-2):162–74. https://doi.org/10.1016/s0378-5955(97)00189-5.
35. Ding D, Jiang H, McFadden SL, Salvi RJ, Li M. Quantitative analysis of hair cells, spiral ganglion neurons and nerve fibers in knock out mice lacking SOD 1 gene. Acta Otorhinolaryngol Sin. 1999;30(3):1693–705.
36. McFadden SL, Ding D, Reaume AG, Flood DG, Salvi RJ. Age-related cochlear hair cell loss is enhanced in mice lacking copper/zinc superoxide dismutase. Neurobiol Aging. 1999;20(1):1–8. https://doi.org/10.1016/s0197-4580(99)00018-4.
37. McFadden SL, Ding D, Jiang H, Woo JM, Salvi RJ. Chinchilla models of selective cochlear hair cell loss. Hear Res. 2002;174(1-2):230–8. https://doi.org/10.1016/s0378-5955(02)00697-4.
38. Ding D, Stracher A, Salvi RJ. Leupeptin protects cochlear and vestibular hair cells from gentamicin ototoxicity. Hear Res. 2002;164(1-2):115–26. https://doi.org/10.1016/s0378-5955(01)00417-8.
39. Ding D, McFadden SL, Browne RW, Salvi RJ. Late dosing with ethacrynic acid can reduce gentamicin concentration in perilymph and protect cochlear hair cells. Hear Res. 2003;185(1-2):90–96. https://doi.org/10.1016/s0378-5955(03)00258-2.

40. Ding D, Jiang H, Wang J, et al. Inner hair cell missing potentiates noise induced outer hair cell lesion. J Audiol Speech Pathol. 2004;12(6):413–5.
41. Ding D, Seigel GM, Salvi RJ. Migration of R28 retinal precursor cells into cochlear and vestibular organs. J Otol. 2006;1(1):51–56. https://doi.org/10.13489/j.cnki.11-4883/r.2006.01.009.
42. Willott JF, Bosch JV, Shimizu T, Ding DL. Effects of exposing DBA/2J mice to a high-frequency augmented acoustic environment on the cochlea and anteroventral cochlear nucleus. Hear Res. 2006;216–217:138–45. https://doi.org/10.1016/j.heares.2006.01.010.
43. Ding D, Jiang H, Wang P, Salvi R. Cell death after co-administration of cisplatin and ethacrynic acid. Hear Res. 2007;226(1–2):129–39. https://doi.org/10.1016/j.heares.2006.07.015.
44. Qi W, Ding D, Jiang H, Salvi R. Quantified analytic system for cochlear hair cells. J Audiol Speech Pathol. 2007;15(2):158–60.
45. Qi W, Ding D, Salvi RJ. Cytotoxic effects of dimethyl sulphoxide (DMSO) on cochlear organotypic cultures. Hear Res. 2008;236(1–2):52–60. https://doi.org/10.1016/j.heares.2007.12.002.
46. Ding D, Qi W, Yu D, Jiang H, Salvi R. Ototoxic effects of mefloquine in cochlear organotypic cultures. J Otol. 2009;4(2):76–85. https://doi.org/10.13489/j.cnki.11-4883/r.2009.02.008.
47. Ding D, Jiang H, Salvi RJ. Mechanisms of rapid sensory hair-cell death following co-administration of gentamicin and ethacrynic acid. Hear Res. 2010;259(1–2):16–23. https://doi.org/10.1016/j.heares.2009.08.008.
48. Ding D, He J, Allman BL, et al. Cisplatin ototoxicity in rat cochlear organotypic cultures. Hear Res. 2011;282(1–2):196–203. https://doi.org/10.1016/j.heares.2011.08.002.
49. Ding D, Roth J, Salvi R. Manganese is toxic to spiral ganglion neurons and hair cells in vitro. Neurotoxicology. 2011;32(2):233–41. https://doi.org/10.1016/j.neuro.2010.12.003.
50. Ding D, Allman BL, Salvi R. Review: ototoxic characteristics of platinum antitumor drugs. Anat Rec (Hoboken). 2012;295(11):1851–67. https://doi.org/10.1002/ar.22577.
51. Ding D, Jiang H, Fu Y, et al. Ototoxic effects of carboplatin in organotypic cultures in chinchillas and rats. J Otol. 2012;7(2):92–101. https://doi.org/10.1016/S1672-2930(12)50023-1.
52. Ye HB, Shi HB, Wang J, et al. Bilirubin induces auditory neuropathy in neonatal guinea pigs via auditory nerve fiber damage. J Neurosci Res. 2012;90(11):2201–13. https://doi.org/10.1002/jnr.23107.
53. Ding D, Qi W, Yu D, et al. Addition of exogenous NAD+ prevents mefloquine-induced neuroaxonal and hair cell degeneration through reduction of caspase-3-mediated apoptosis in cochlear organotypic cultures. PLoS One. 2013;8(11):e79817 https://doi.org/10.1371/journal.pone.0079817.
54. Hayes SH, Ding D, Salvi R, Allman BL. Anatomy and physiology of the external, middle and inner ear. In: Celesia GG, editor. Disorders of peripheral and central auditory processing. Handbook of clinical neurophysiology, vol. 10. New York: Elsevier; 2013. p. 3–23.
55. Qi W, Ding D, Zhu H, et al. Efficient siRNA transfection to the inner ear through the intact round window by a novel proteidic delivery technology in the chinchilla. Gene Ther. 2014;21(1):10–18. https://doi.org/10.1038/gt.2013.49.
56. Wang L, Ding D, Salvi R, Roth JA. Nicotinamide adenine dinucleotide prevents neuroaxonal degeneration induced by manganese in cochlear organotypic cultures. Neurotoxicology. 2014;40:65–74. https://doi.org/10.1016/j.neuro.2013.11.007.
57. Ding D, Jiang H, Chen GD, et al. N-acetyl-cysteine prevents age-related hearing loss and the progressive loss of inner hair cells in gamma-glutamyl transferase 1 deficient mice. Aging. 2016;8(4):730–50. https://doi.org/10.18632/aging.100927.
58. Salvi R, Sun W, Ding D, et al. Inner hair cell loss disrupts hearing and cochlear function leading to sensory deprivation and enhanced central auditory gain. Front Neurosci. 2016;10:621 https://doi.org/10.3389/fnins.2016.00621.
59. Ye H, Xing Y, Zhang L, et al. Bilirubin-induced neurotoxic and ototoxic effects in rat cochlear and vestibular organotypic cultures. Neurotoxicology. 2019;71:75–86. https://doi.org/10.1016/j.neuro.2018.12.004.
60. Ding D, Manohar S, Jiang H, Salvi R. Hydroxypropyl-beta-cyclodextrin causes massive damage to the developing auditory and vestibular system. Hear Res. 2020;396:108073 https://doi.org/10.1016/j.heares.2020.108073.
61. Ding D, Zhang J, Jiang H, et al. Some ototoxic drugs destroy cochlear support cells before damaging sensory hair cells. Neurotox Res. 2020;37(4):743–52. https://doi.org/10.1007/s12640-020-00170-8.
62. Ding D, Zhang J, Liu F, et al. Antioxidative stress-induced damage in cochlear explants. J Otol. 2020;15(1):36–40. https://doi.org/10.1016/j.joto.2019.11.005.
63. Yuan F, Ding DL, Wang J, et al. [Inner hair cells loss by carboplatin and the changes of cochlear compound action potential in chinchillas]. Zhonghua Er Bi Yan Hou Tou Jing Wai Ke Za Zhi. 2020;55(6):506–13. https://doi.org/10.3760/cma.j.cn.115330-20200426-00332.
64. Ding D, Jiang H, Manohar S, et al. Spatiotemporal developmental upregulation of prestin correlates with the severity and location of cyclodextrin-induced outer hair cell loss and hearing loss. Front Cell Dev Biol. 2021;9:643709 https://doi.org/10.3389/fcell.2021.643709.
65. Ding D, Jiang H, Salvi R. Cochlear spiral ganglion neuron degeneration following cyclodextrin-induced hearing loss. Hear Res. 2021;400:108125 https://doi.org/10.1016/j.heares.2020.108125.
66. Ding D, Qi W, Jiang H, Salvi R. Excitotoxic damage to auditory nerve afferents and spiral ganglion neurons is correlated with developmental upregulation of AMPA and KA receptors. Hear Res. 2021;411:108358 https://doi.org/10.1016/j.heares.2021.108358.
67. Zhang L, Ye H, Xing Y, Ding D, Shi H. Experimental study on the effect of psalmotoxin-1 in bilirubin-induced ototoxicity. Chin Arch Otolaryngol-Head Neck Surg. 2021;28(1):26–30. https://doi.org/10.16066/j.1672-7002.2021.01.007.
68. Ding D, Li P, Qi W, et al. Study on delayed secondary lesions in the cochlea triggered by cochlear hair cell death. Chin J Otorhinolaryngol Skull Base Surg. 2022;28(1):1–10. https://doi.org/10.11798/j.issn.1007-1520.2022221001.
69. Ding D, Li P, Qi W, Zhang J. Different patterns of age-related damage to cochlear hair cells in different species of experimental animals. Chin J Otorhinolaryngol Skull Base Surg. 2023;29(1):7–13. https://doi.org/10.11798/j.issn.1007-1520.202323084.
70. Ding D, Manohar S, Kador PF, Salvi R. Multifunctional redox modulator prevents blast-induced loss of cochlear and vestibular hair cells and auditory spiral ganglion neurons. Sci Rep. 2024;14:15296. https://doi.org/10.1038/s41598-024-66406-1.
71. Ding D, Shi L, Xing Y, et al. Secondary neural damage in the inner ear induced by intratympanic gentamicin injection. Chin J Otorhinolaryngol Skull Base Surg. 2024;30(6):11–19. https://doi.org/10.11798/j.issn.1007-1520.202424356.
72. Li L, Chen D, Lin X, et al. Antioxidative stress-induced destruction to cochlear cells caused by blind antioxidant therapy. Chin Arch Otolaryngol Head Neck Surg. 2024;170(5):1421–9. https://doi.org/10.1002/ohn.659.
73. Ding D, Chen GD, Zhang C, et al. Supporting cell involvement in cochlear damage and repair: novel insights from a quantitative analysis of cyclodextrin-induced ototoxicity in mice. Hear Res. 2025;459:109201 https://doi.org/10.1016/j.heares.2025.109201.
74. Gao WY, Ding DL, Zheng XY, Ruan FM. Changes in the stereocilia and non-monotonic pattern of threshold shift after exposure to impulse noise. Hear Res. 1991;54(2):296–304. https://doi.org/10.1016/0378-5955(91)90123-q.

75. Ding D, Fan J, Gong Z, Huangfu M. Combined observation of guinea pig cochlea by scanning electron microscopy and transmission electron microscopy. J Clin Otorhinolaryngol. 1992;6(1):8–10.
76. Gao WY, Ding DL, Zheng XY, Ruan FM, Liu YJ. A comparison of changes in the stereocilia between temporary and permanent hearing losses in acoustic trauma. Hear Res. 1992;62(1):27–41. https://doi.org/10.1016/0378-5955(92)90200-7.
77. Ding D, Zhao J. Combined observation of the cuticular plate of auditory hair cells by light and electron microscopy. J Audiol Speech Pathol. 1994;2(1):28–31.
78. Zhang S, Ding D. An investigation on the lesions of reticular laminae of cochlear hair cells. Chin Arch Otolaryngol Head Neck Surg. 1995;2(4):242–5. https://doi.org/10.16066/j.1672-7002.1995.04.028.
79. Ma J, Ding D, Zheng M, et al. Scanning electron microscopic analyses of inner hair cell damage in chinchilla caused by carboplatin. Otorhinolaryngol J Integr Traditional Western Med China. 1998;6(1):58–60.
80. McFadden SL, Woo JM, Michalak N, Ding D. Dietary vitamin C supplementation reduces noise-induced hearing loss in guinea pigs. Hear Res. 2005;202(1–2):200–8. https://doi.org/10.1016/j.heares.2004.10.011.
81. He J, Ding D, Yu D, et al. Modulation of copper transporters in protection against cisplatin-induced cochlear hair cell damage. J Otol. 2011;6(2):53–61. https://doi.org/10.13489/j.cnki.11-4883/r.2011.02.007.

9 Technique of Cochlear Cultures

The study of the cochlear auditory peripheral system can be performed using in vivo and in vitro experimental techniques. The in vitro methods are further divided into cochlear cell line culture, cochlear primary cell culture, and cochlear organotypic culture. Each method has its own advantages for studying cochlear physiology and pathology at the cellular and tissue levels.

9.1 Cochlear Cell Line Cultures

Cochlear cell line cultures are derived from a single cell type originating in the cochlea and maintained in culture dishes with growth medium, where they can proliferate indefinitely under appropriate conditions. However, only a limited number of cochlear cells can be genetically modified to undergo complete dedifferentiation and transform into conditionally immortalized cell lines capable of continuous division. During this dedifferentiation process, these cells lose their original highly specialized functions and morphological characteristics and transition into proliferative but undifferentiated states. Consequently, experimental data obtained from such cell lines primarily reflect the behavior of dedifferentiated proliferating cells rather than native, fully differentiated cochlear hair cells, as the dedifferentiation process fundamentally alters their biological identity and functional properties [1].

In adult mammals, cochlear cells typically cease proliferating shortly after birth; however, when the cochlear basilar membrane is isolated and cultured in vitro, the lateral edge rapidly generates new proliferating cells, demonstrating that these cells can undergo dedifferentiation and re-enter the cell cycle within a short timeframe. While those highly differentiated cells such as hair cells fail to achieve complete dedifferentiation eventually die in an in vitro culture environment. Although this phenomenon suggests that cell lines could theoretically be derived from these dividing lateral edge cells [2] (Figs. 9.1–9.4), significant questions remain regarding their biological relevance. Specifically, whether fully dedifferentiated cochlear-derived cell lines can accurately represent native, highly specialized cochlear cells is debatable, as the dedifferentiation process likely alters their original characteristics. If experimentally modified cell lines with fundamentally changed properties were considered valid proxies for mature cochlear hair cells, then by extension, even a fertilized egg or morula-stage embryonic cell could theoretically represent any somatic cell—an obviously flawed premise. Following this logic, prokaryotic cells, as evolutionary precursors to eukaryotes, would paradoxically qualify as models for all eukaryotic cell types. These conceptual inconsistencies have led to growing skepticism about whether in vitro cell line behavior can reliably reflect in vivo physiological processes in terminally differentiated cells [3].

D. Ding et al., *Histopathological Atlas of the Inner Ear*,
https://doi.org/10.1007/978-981-95-6338-8_9

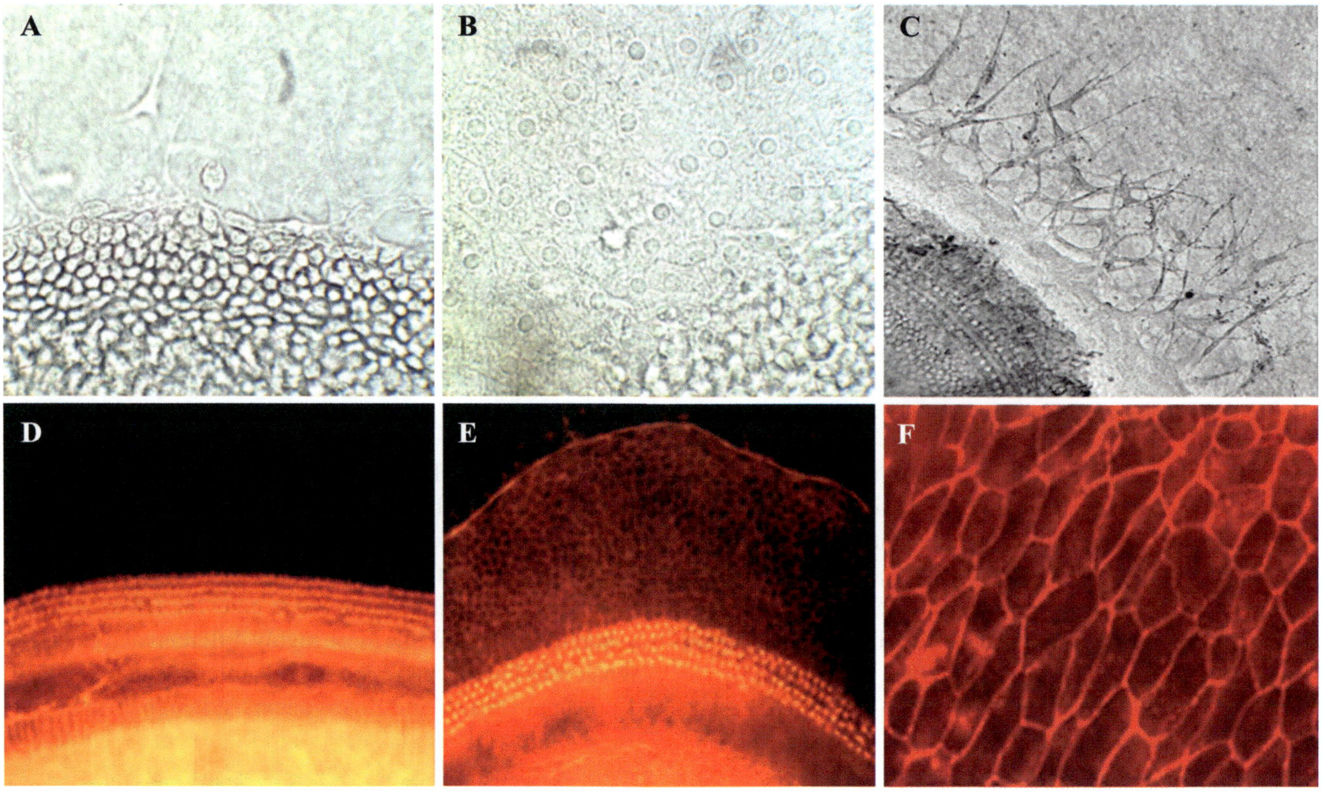

Fig. 9.1 The dedifferentiation and proliferation of supporting cells in postnatal day 1 mouse cochlear explants under organotypic culture conditions. (**A**) 12 h after culture in serum-free culture, cells at the peripheral edge of the cochlear basilar membrane initiate division and proliferation. (**B**) 24 h after culturing in serum-free medium, the range of proliferating dividing cells at the lateral edge of the cochlear basilar membrane gradually expanded to the periphery. (**C**) When the cochlear explants were cultured in DMEM/F-12 medium with 10% serum for 24 h, the proliferating cells at the lateral edge of the cochlear basilar membrane presented the fibroblast-like morphology, which is completely different in cellular morphology from the proliferating pattern observed in serum-free conditions. It is suggested that different culture medium conditions may result in the production of different types of dividing cells. (**D**) No proliferating cells were observed in freshly dissected cochlear explants cultured in serum-free medium. (**E**) When the cochlear explants were cultured in serum-free medium for 72 h, the proliferating cells at the lateral edge of the basilar membrane gradually expanded outward. (**F**) Higher magnification reveals detailed morphological characteristics of these proliferating edge cells. (Reproduced with permission from Ding et al. [2])

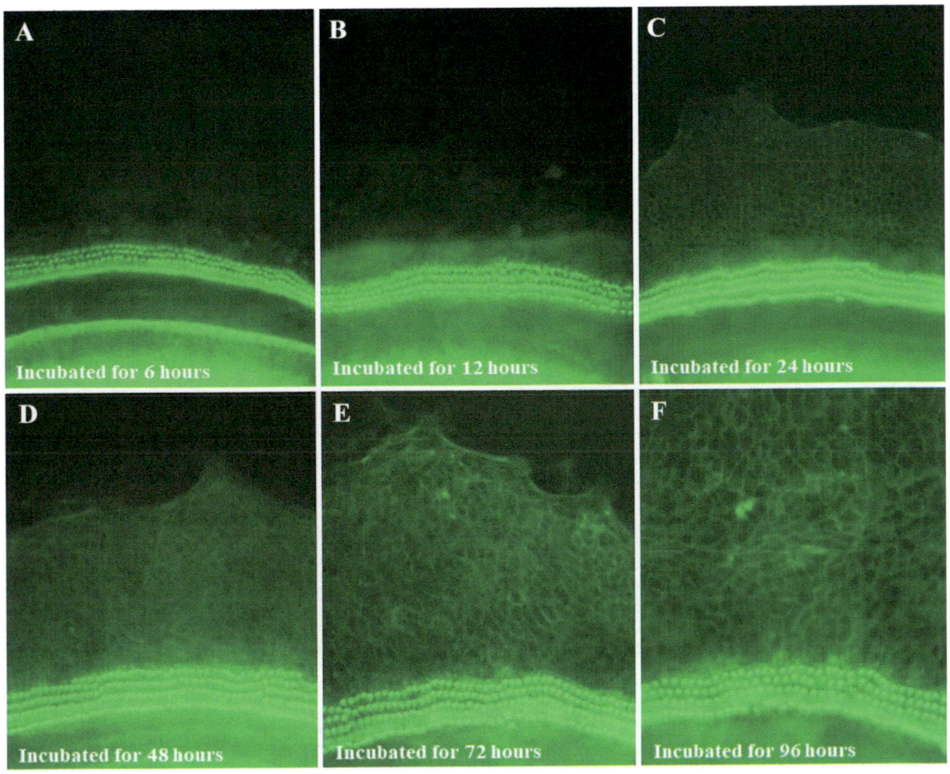

Fig. 9.2 The temporal progression of cellular dedifferentiation and proliferation at the outer edge of the cochlear basilar membrane from mice at postnatal day 5. (**A**) Initial proliferation is observed 6 h post-culture in serum-free medium, with a small cluster of dividing cells emerging at the lateral edge. (**B**) By 12 h, the proliferative zone begins expanding radially from the lateral edge of the basilar membrane. (**C**) At 24 h, the cell population exhibits a marked numerical increase while maintaining distinct spatial organization. (**D**) After 48 h, proliferating cells demonstrate continued quantitative expansion with preserved edge-localized distribution. (**E**) The 72-h timepoint reveals sustained proliferative activity with progressive population growth. (**F**) By day 4, the proliferating cell mass shows both numerical increase and spatial expansion across the lateral edge of the cochlear basilar membrane. (Reproduced with permission from Ding et al. [2])

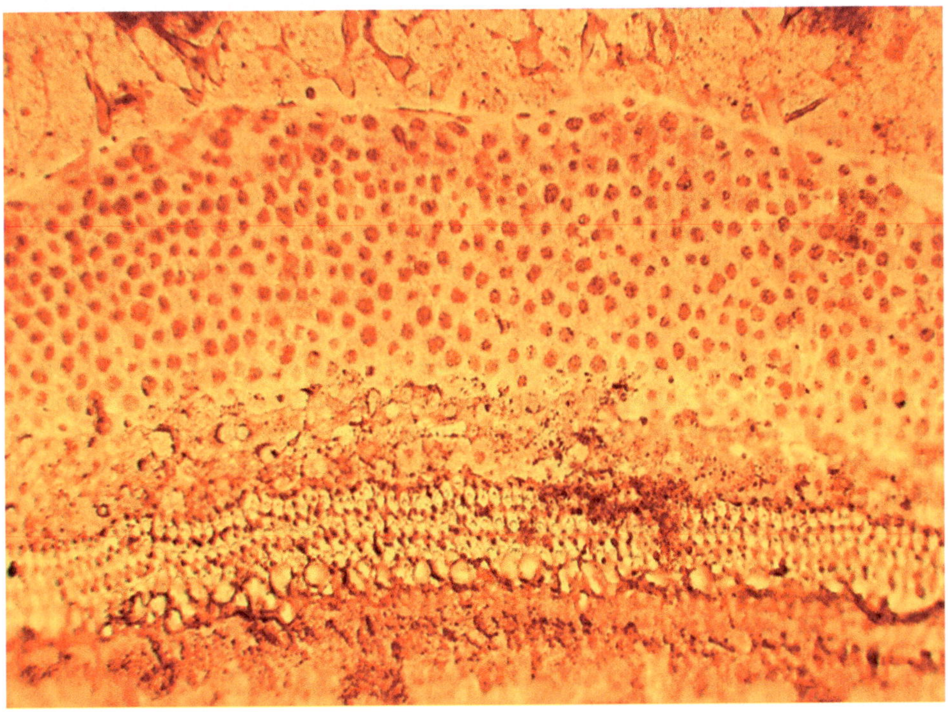

Fig. 9.3 Bromodeoxyuridine (BrdU) immunolabeling in a cochlear explant cultured for 3 days in serum-free medium from a mouse at postnatal day 5. Nuclear BrdU incorporation was consistently observed in all newly proliferated cells at the lateral edge of the cochlear basilar membrane, providing definitive evidence that these cells originated through mitotic division rather than cellular migration or other mechanisms. The uniform BrdU positivity across the proliferative zone confirms active DNA replication and validates the mitotic nature of this edge cell population. (Reproduced with permission from Ding et al. [2])

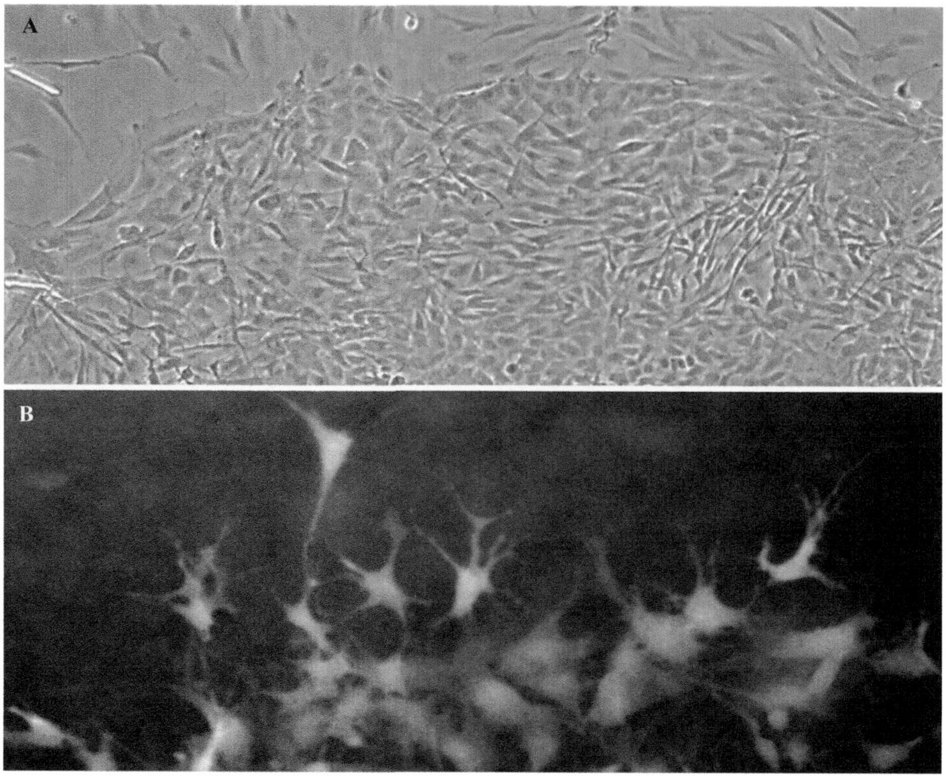

Fig. 9.4 The morphological characteristics of proliferating cells in serum-supplemented culture conditions. (**A**) Within 24 h of culture in DMEM/F-12 medium containing 10% serum, extensive cellular proliferation is observed at the lateral edge of the cochlear basilar membrane. (**B**) Higher magnification reveals that these newly proliferated cells exhibit an irregular, flattened morphology distinct from the original supporting cells in the lateral sulcus region, raising important questions about whether such dedifferentiated cell lines can accurately represent native cochlear auditory cells—a matter requiring further scientific investigation. (Reproduced with permission from Ding et al. [2])

9.2 Cochlear Primary Cell Cultures

The technique of cochlear primary cell culture refers to the technology that quickly completes some targeted experimental research after taking out the isolated cells from the inner ear. To utilize the cells of the inner ear for specific experimental studies in vitro, primary cochlear cell culture involves two steps: cell isolation and cell culture. This technique preserves the original diploid state and highly differentiated characteristics of the cells, making it particularly valuable for studies involving cell transplantation, transfection, and chemical toxicity assessments. For instance, when spiral ganglion neurons are isolated from Rosenthal's canal through enzymatic and mechanical dissociation, they initially appear as rounded cell bodies after losing their nerve fibers. However, under the culture condition, these isolated neurons demonstrate a remarkable ability to regenerate nerve fibers, extending new neurites and forming synaptic connections with neighboring ganglion cells (Fig. 9.5). While primary cultures maintain many intrinsic cellular properties, the absence of normal tissue interactions limits their ability to fully replicate cochlear physiology, particularly regarding intercellular communication mechanisms. In serum-containing co-culture experiments with retinal precursor cell lines, spiral ganglion neurons reestablished neural networks while the retinal precursors continued proliferating and did not stop proliferating (Fig. 9.6). Interestingly, when the isolated cells were cultured in serum-free medium, the same co-culture system produced markedly different results: retinal precursors ceased proliferation and, when influenced by adjacent spiral ganglion neurons, adopted neuronal-like morphologies resembling spiral ganglion cells [4] (Fig. 9.7). These findings highlight both the utility and limitations of primary cochlear cell cultures in auditory research.

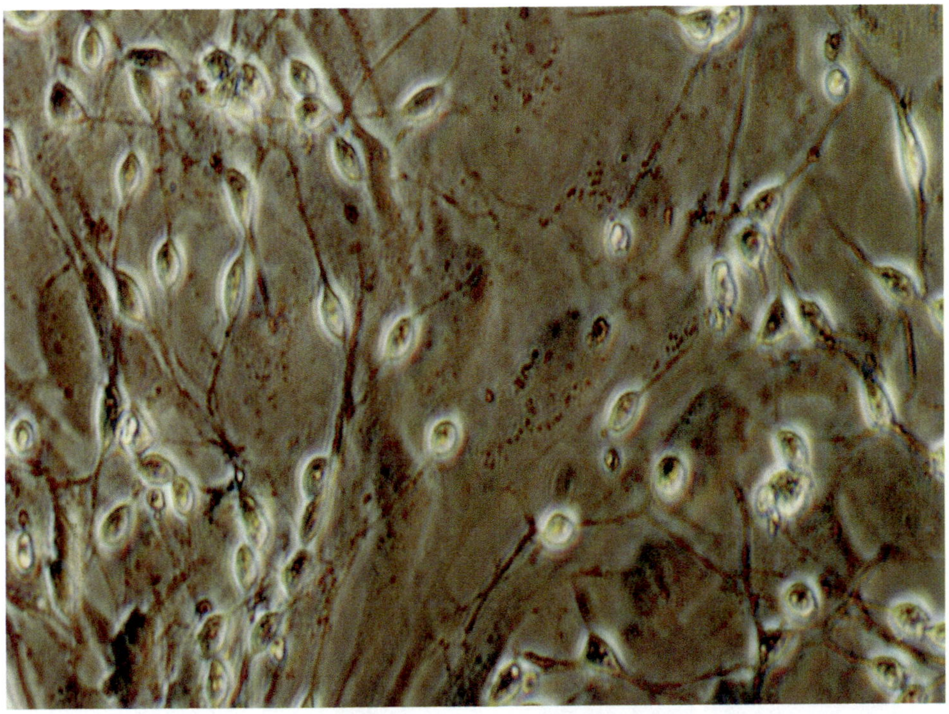

Fig. 9.5 Regeneration of nerve fibers from dissociated, isolated cochlear spiral ganglion neurons in vitro. By day 3 of culture, bipolar neurons extend regenerated neurites from both poles, exhibiting robust axonal outgrowth characteristic of their native morphology. These extending processes establish new synaptic connections between neighboring neurons, recapitulating key aspects of their neural network formation capacity in vivo, despite the absence of their original peripheral and central targets. This regenerative process highlights the intrinsic growth potential of spiral ganglion neurons when maintained in appropriate culture conditions

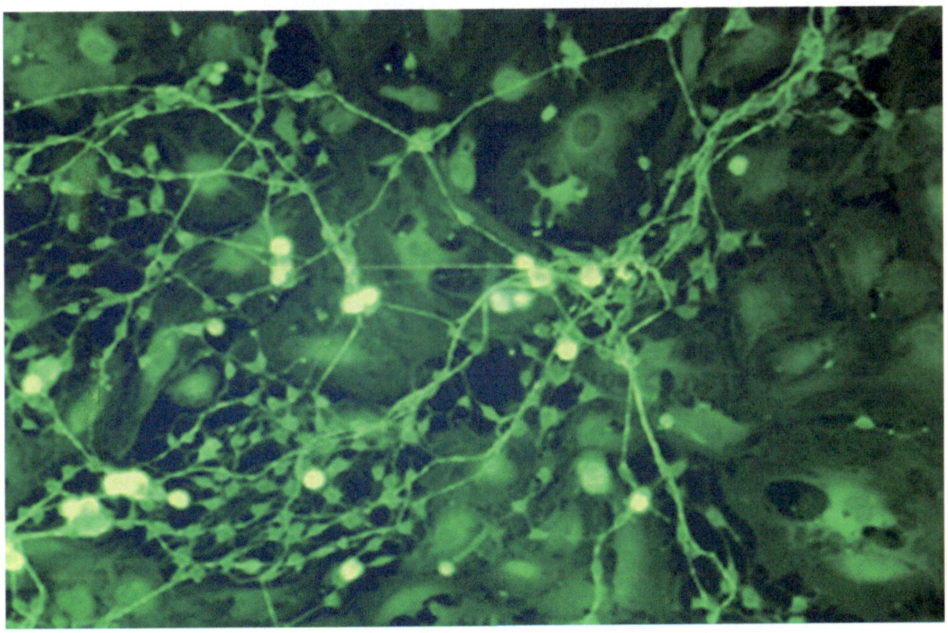

Fig. 9.6 The differential cellular responses in a co-culture system of retinal precursors (R28 cells) and spiral ganglion neurons under serum-supplemented conditions. After 3 days in DMEM-F12 medium containing 10% calf serum, spiral ganglion neurons and their neurites exhibit strong neurofilament-200 immunoreactivity with distinct FITC fluorescence labeling, while R28 cells show comparatively weaker neurofilament expression. The R28 cells maintain their undifferentiated state, continuing to proliferate and form a monolayer beneath the neuronal network, demonstrating that serum-containing medium supports their proliferation while inhibiting differentiation. (Reproduced with permission from Ding et al. [2])

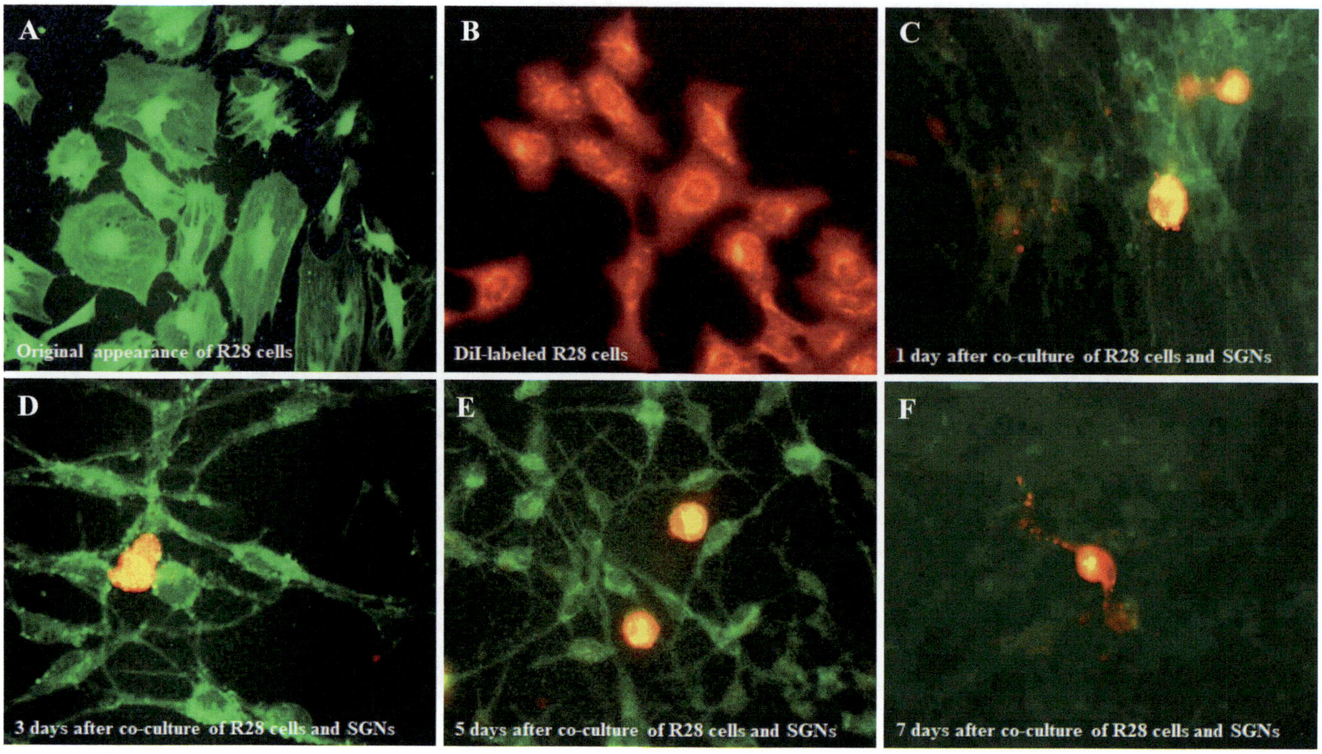

Fig. 9.7 DiI-labeled R28 retinal progenitor cells exhibit significant differentiation potential when co-cultured with spiral ganglion neurons in serum-free medium. (**A**) In serum-containing medium, R28 cells maintain an undifferentiated state, adhering to the culture dish with characteristic flat, irregular morphology. (**B**) DiI labeling confirms cellular identity through distinct cytoplasmic red fluorescence. (**C**) Within 24 h of serum-free co-culture, DiI-positive R28 cells migrate into spiral ganglion neuron regions. (**D**) By day 3, R28 cells undergo morphological changes, transitioning from flat to rounded shapes similar to adjacent neurons. (**E**) After 5 days, the cellular transformation progresses further, with R28 cells adopting spherical morphologies nearly identical to mature spiral ganglion neurons. (**F**) By day 7, differentiated R28 cells exhibit bipolar neuronal morphology, extending neurite-like processes in opposite directions, demonstrating complete phenotypic conversion under the inductive influence of spiral ganglion neuron-derived signals. (Reproduced with permission from Ding et al. [2])

9.3 Technique of Cochlear Organotypic Culture

Cochlear organotypic culture involves maintaining whole or partial cochlear structures in vitro while preserving their native tissue architecture and cellular interactions. This technique offers significant advantages as the cultured organ of Corti retains both the original intercellular connections and highly differentiated cellular morphology, allowing for more physiologically relevant investigation of cochlear responses to experimental manipulations. The thin, multilayered structure of the cochlear basilar membrane facilitates optimal nutrient exchange and waste removal between cells and culture medium. Importantly, this method maintains functional synaptic connections between sensory hair cells and spiral ganglion neurons, preserving critical intercellular communication pathways and creating a more representative microenvironment for both hair cells and ganglion neurons compared to dissociated culture systems. The preserved tissue integrity in organotypic cultures enables more accurate assessment of cellular responses while maintaining the complex interactions found in vivo. Cochlear organotypic culture represents the most physiologically relevant in vitro model for cochlear research, as it maintains cellular organization and function closest to native in vivo conditions. This technique has been extensively validated through numerous studies [5–28], demonstrating its superior ability to evaluate experimental effects on cochlear cells compared to either cell line or primary culture systems. The method's unique advantage lies in preserving the intricate cellular interactions and microenvironment of the organ of Corti, enabling more accurate assessment of pharmacological, genetic, or environmental impacts on cochlear physiology. Given this methodological superiority in maintaining tissue integrity and cellular responses that closely mirror in vivo conditions, cochlear organotypic culture has become the gold standard for in vitro cochlear research, warranting detailed discussion of its technical implementation in this chapter.

The cochlear dissection procedure begins with surface sterilization using 75% alcohol, followed by decapitation of the experimental animal. After opening the parietal bone and removing brain tissue to expose the skull base (Figs. 9.8A, B and 9.9A), the temporal bone is carefully separated from the sphenoid bone using a dissection needle and completely excised (Figs. 9.8C, D and 9.9B). The isolated temporal bone is immediately transferred to Hank's balanced salt solution for microdissection, where the bony cochlear capsule is removed under stereomicroscopic visualization to expose the membranous labyrinth (Figs. 9.8E and 9.9C).

The cochlear modiolus with attached membranous labyrinth is then extracted, followed by careful separation of the cochlear basilar membrane from the modiolus along the bony spiral lamina, and final isolation of the basilar membrane from the spiral ligament along the lateral sulcus (Figs. 9.8F–H and 9.9D–G), completing preparation of the intact cochlear sensory epithelium for organotypic culture.

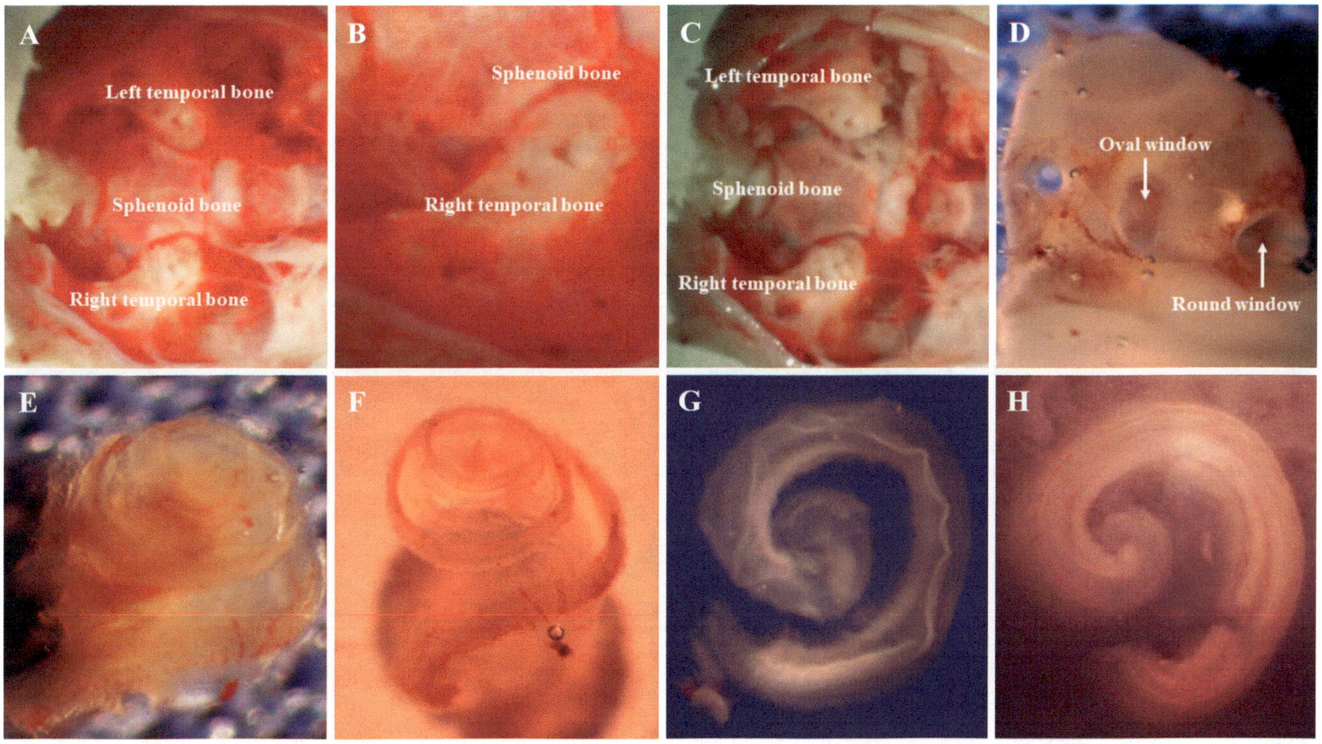

Fig. 9.8 The sequential microdissection procedure for isolating the cochlear basilar membrane from rats at postnatal day 3. (**A**) Following skull opening and brain removal, the bilateral temporal bones become visible at the skull base. (**B**) Higher magnification reveals anatomical details of the right temporal bone at the skull base. (**C**) Precise separation of the temporal bone is achieved by tracing its natural junction with the sphenoid bone using fine dissection tools. (**D**) The intact bony cochlea is carefully liberated from surrounding bony structures. (**E**) Removal of the osseous cochlear shell exposes the delicate membranous labyrinth. (**F**) The complete cochlear membranous structure is then detached from the modiolus. (**G**) Final separation of the spiral ligament yields an intact basilar membrane preparation. (**H**) For optimal preservation, the isolated basilar membrane is mounted on rat tail collagen gel as a surface preparation

The collagen gel matrix was prepared by combining type I rat tail collagen (Collaborative Biomedical Products #40236), 10× Basal Medium Eagle (Sigma B9638), and 2% sodium carbonate (Sigma S-2127) in a 9:1:1 ratio with thorough mixing. For culture preparation, 10 μL aliquots of this collagen mixture were pipetted onto the center of 35 mm culture dishes (Falcon 1008) and allowed to polymerize for 15 min at room temperature. Following gelation, 1300 μL of serum-free culture medium was carefully added to create a liquid layer flush with the gel surface. The serum-free culture medium formulation consisted of 2 g bovine serum albumin (BSA, Sigma A-4919), 2 mL serum-free supplement (Sigma I-1884), 4.8 mL 20% glucose (Sigma G-2020), 0.4 mL penicillin G (Sigma P-3414), 2 mL of 200 mM glutamine (Sigma G-6392), and 190.8 mL of 1× BME (Sigma B-1522), providing optimal nutritional support while maintaining the differentiated state of cochlear explants.

For cochlear organotypic culture, the intact basilar membrane or spiral ligament was carefully positioned as a surface preparation on the polymerized collagen gel matrix in serum-free medium (Figs. 9.8H and 9.9 H). Following a 60-min incubation period (Forma Scientific 3029, 37°C, 5% CO_2) to allow tissue adherence, an additional 700 μL of serum-free medium was added to completely submerge the explants. After overnight culture, experimental compounds were introduced according to study protocols, with cultures maintained until predetermined endpoints. Termination involved careful medium aspiration followed by fixation with 10% neutral buffered formalin. The fixed explants were then processed for various histological and immunohistochemical analyses to evaluate specific cochlear structures and cellular components (Figs. 9.9J–L, 9.10–9.14), enabling comprehensive morphological and molecular assessment of treatment effects on the organotypic cultures.

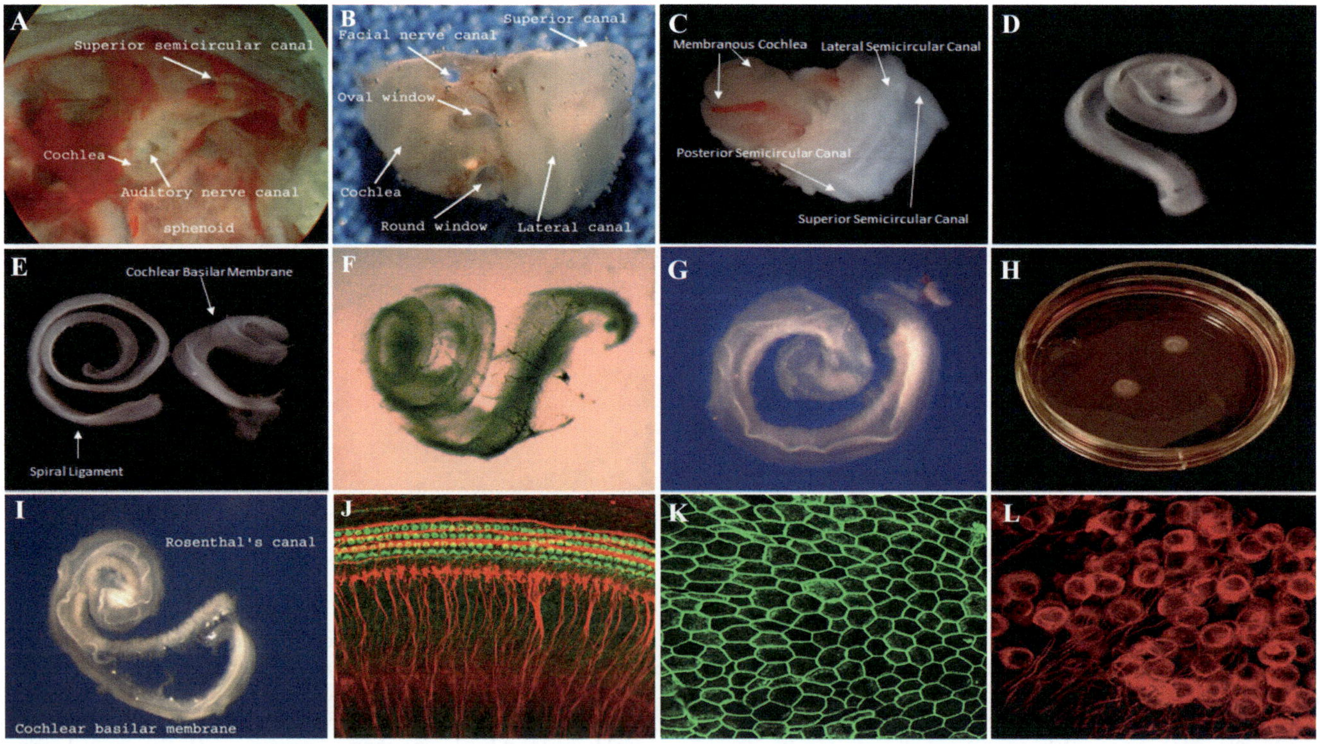

Fig. 9.9 The detailed microdissection process for preparing cochlear explants from rats on postnatal day 3. (**A**) Initial exposure of the temporal bone following brain removal reveals the anatomical landmarks at the skull base. (**B**) The intact temporal bone is carefully isolated while preserving its structural integrity. (**C**) Delicate removal of the osseous cochlear shell exposes the underlying membranous labyrinth. (**D**) The complete cochlear membranous structure is meticulously separated from surrounding tissues. (**E**) Precise dissection along the lateral sulcus allows separation of the basilar membrane from the spiral ligament. (**F**) The spiral ligament is isolated as a distinct structural component. (**G**) Final isolation yields an intact cochlear basilar membrane preparation. (**H**) For optimal culture conditions, the basilar membrane is placed on rat tail collagen gel in serum-free medium. (**I**) Selective microdissection separates Rosenthal's canal, containing spiral ganglion neurons, from the epithelial cell-rich basilar membrane. (**J**) Immunofluorescence double labeling simultaneously visualizes auditory nerve fibers (neurofilament, red) and the stereocilia of hair cells (phalloidin, green). (**K**) Phalloidin staining highlights the distinctive surface morphology of the marginal cells on the surface of stria vascularis. (**L**) Spiral ganglion neurons are specifically identified by neurofilament-200 immunoreactivity

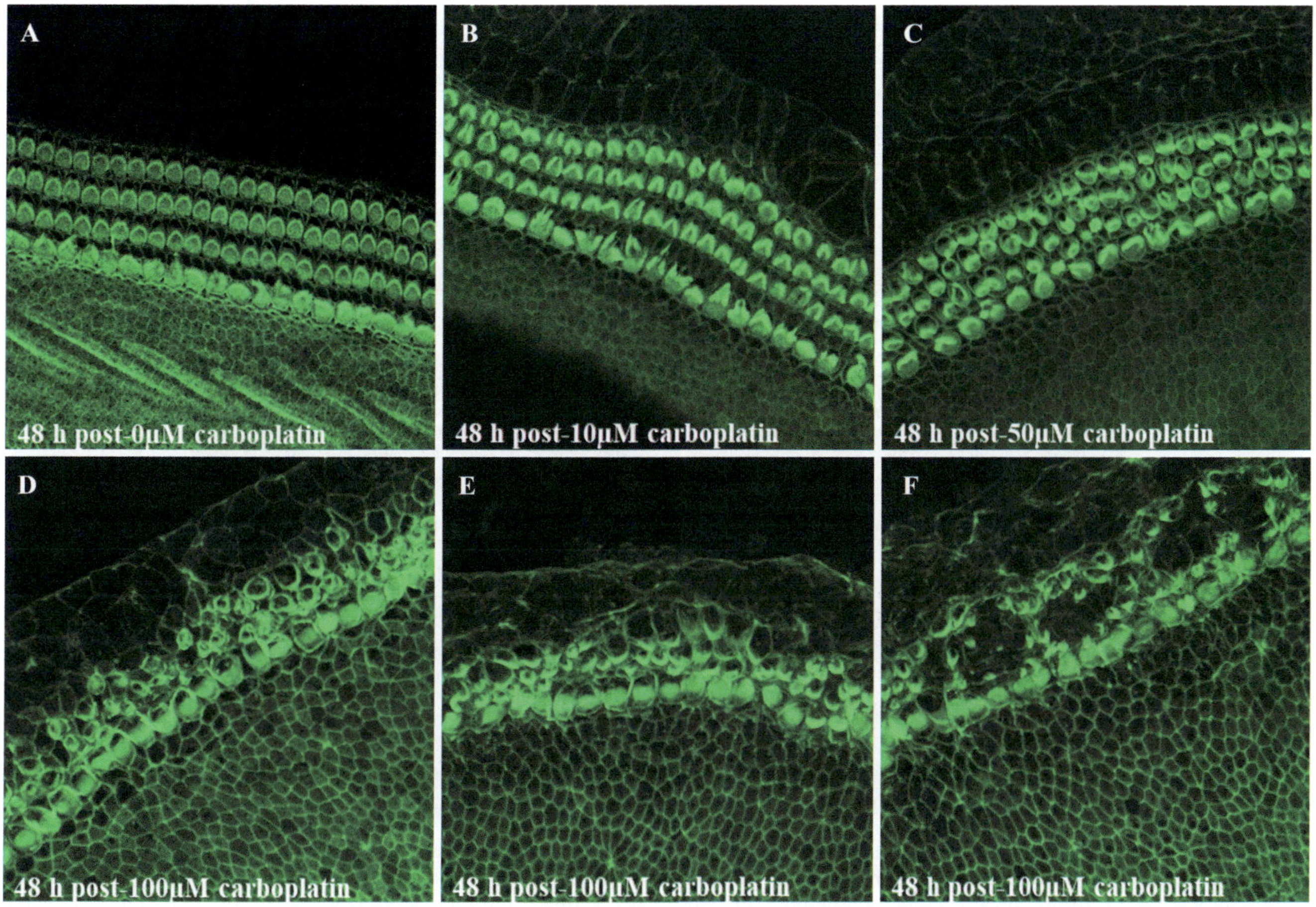

Fig. 9.10 The dose-dependent ototoxic effects of carboplatin on cochlear explants of adult rats. (**A**) Control cultures maintained in serum-free medium for 48 h preserve normal hair cell morphology with intact stereociliary bundles. (**B**) Exposure to 10 μM carboplatin for 48 h induces initial stereociliary disorganization while maintaining overall cellular architecture. (**C**) At 50 μM concentration, carboplatin causes stereociliary shrinkage and deformation in select outer hair cells, marking the onset of cellular damage. (**D**) With 100 μM treatment for 48 h, progressive outer hair cell degeneration manifests through complete stereociliary loss in affected cells. (**E**) 48 h post-100 μM carboplatin, the cuticular plate of outer and inner hair cells was swollen. (**F**) 48 h after 100 μM carboplatin treatment, advanced toxicity results in complete destruction of outer hair cells, while inner hair cells show relative resistance, retaining their cuticular plates despite stereociliary loss. These findings collectively establish the selective vulnerability of outer hair cells to carboplatin-induced damage in the organotypic culture model. (Reproduced with permission from Ding et al. [13])

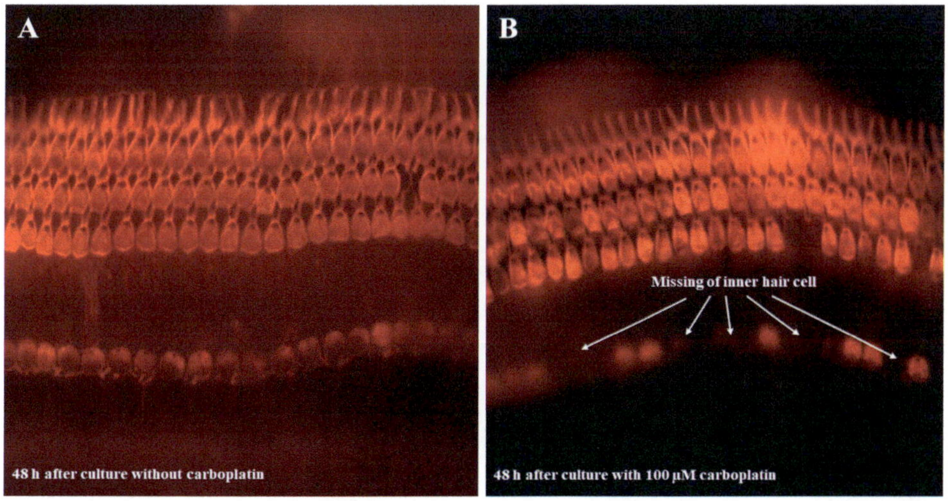

Fig. 9.11 The species-specific ototoxic effects of carboplatin in chinchilla cochlear explants. (**A**) Control cultures maintained for 48 h in serum-free medium demonstrate preserved cytoarchitecture of both inner and outer hair cell populations. (**B**) Following 48 h of 100 μM carboplatin exposure, histological analysis shows selective degeneration of inner hair cells while maintaining normal outer hair cell morphology, establishing a distinct contrast to the outer hair cell vulnerability observed in rat models. (Reproduced with permission from Ding et al. [13])

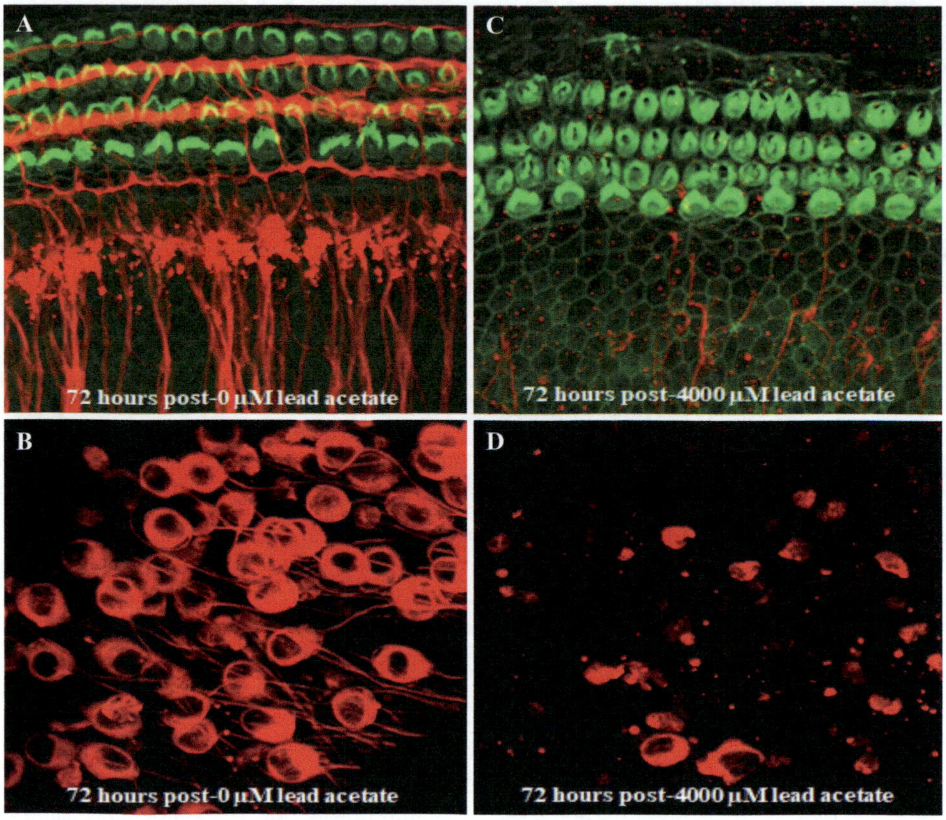

Fig. 9.12 The neurotoxic effects of lead acetate on cochlear neural elements in organotypic culture. (**A**) In control cochlear explants cultured in lead-free medium for 3 days, the morphology of inner and outer hair cells, as well as their auditory nerve fibers and synapses remained intact. (**B**) 3 days after culturing in lead acetate-free medium, the soma of spiral ganglion neurons in the cochlear explant also maintained their normal structure. (**C**) After three days of culture in serum-free medium containing 4 mM lead acetate, although the stereocilia and their surface structures of the hair cells appeared abnormal, no hair cell loss was observed. Notably, the afferent nerve fibers and their terminals beneath the hair cells completely degenerated. (**D**) 3 days after being cultured in medium containing 4 mM lead acetate, all spiral ganglion neurons were destroyed completely. These results indicate a distinct pattern of primary neural toxicity preceding potential sensory hair cell damage in heavy metal-induced neuron destruction

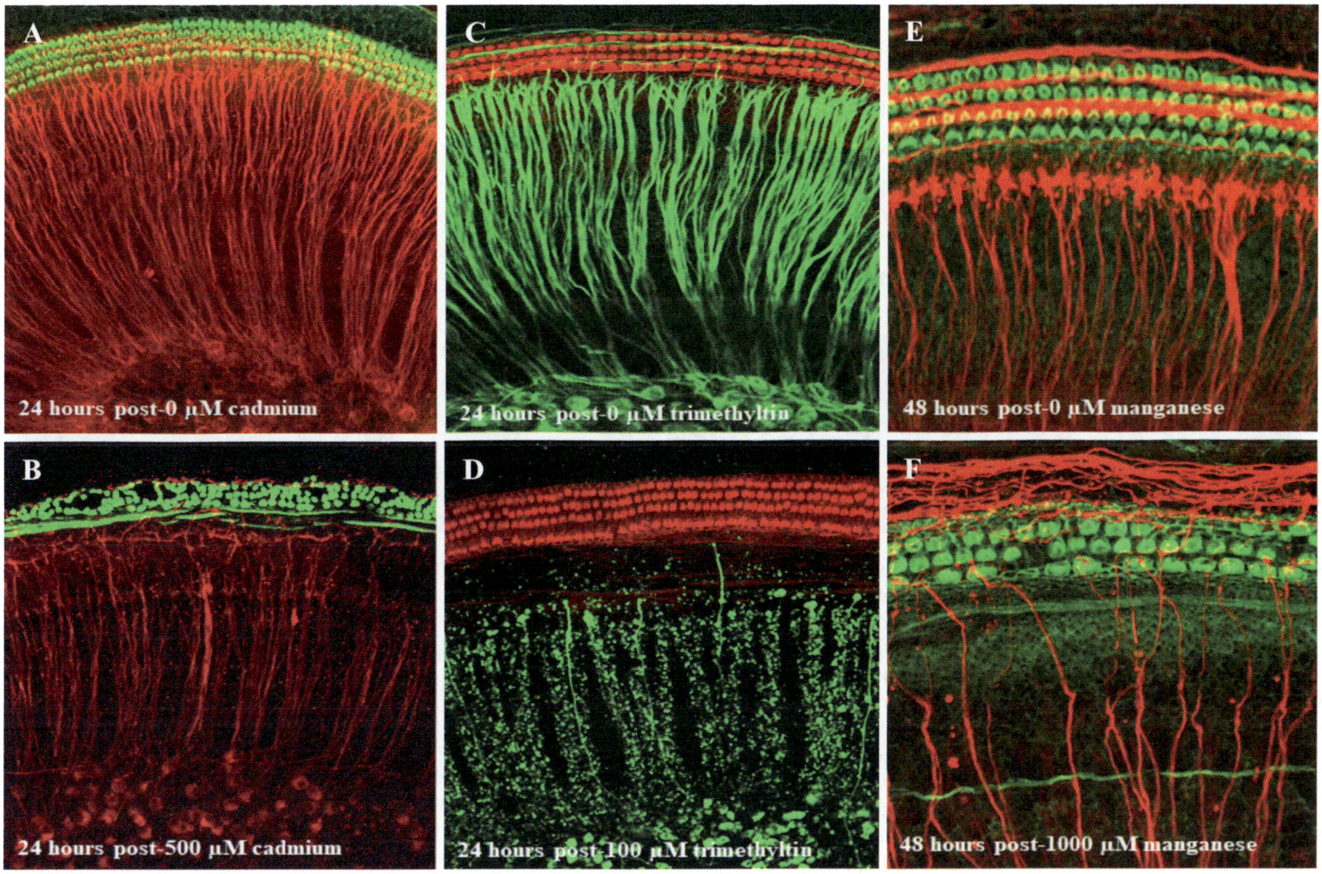

Fig. 9.13 The preferential neurotoxicity of heavy metals in cochlear explants. (**A**) Control cultures after 24 h in cadmium chloride-free medium maintain intact hair cells and auditory nerve fibers. (**B**) Exposure to 500 μM cadmium chloride for 24 h induces mild deletion of hair cells, while accompanied by significant nerve fiber degeneration. (**C**) Trimethyltin-free controls preserve the normal cytoarchitecture of both sensory and neural elements. (**D**) Treatment with 100 μM trimethyltin for 24 h severely damages the auditory nerve fibers while sparing the hair cells. (**E**) After 48 h in manganese chloride-free conditions, all cochlear structures remain unaffected. (**F**) Exposure to 500 μ M manganese chloride for 48 h causes disintegration of type II afferent fiber bundles connecting outer hair cells and complete synaptic loss of type I afferent nerve fibers connecting inner hair cells, and preceding sporadic hair cell degeneration, collectively demonstrating that heavy metal toxicity primarily targets cochlear neural elements before affecting sensory cells

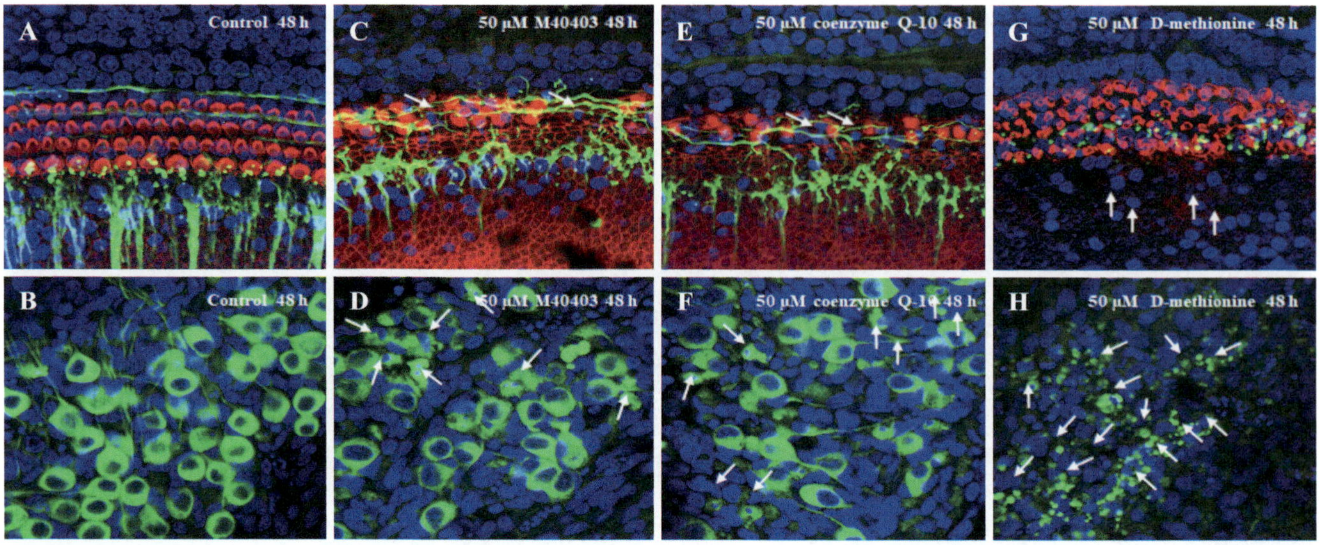

Fig. 9.14 The paradoxical ototoxicity of various antioxidants in cochlear organotypic cultures. (**A**) Control explants maintained for 48 h in an antioxidant-free medium preserve the normal morphology of both hair cells and auditory nerve fibers. (**B**) Spiral ganglion neurons in control conditions similarly demonstrate intact cytoarchitecture. (**C**) Treatment with 50 μM M40403 (a superoxide dismutase mimetic) causes severe hair cell damage with mildly affecting nerve fibers. (**D**) Corresponding spiral ganglion neurons show remarkable resistance to M40403-induced toxicity. It is suggested that excess M40403 first causes the destruction of cochlear hair cells. (**E**) Coenzyme Q-10 exposure (50 μM) disrupts most hair cells and eliminates auditory nerve synapses. (**F**) In the same coenzyme Q-10-treated cochlear explant, most spiral ganglion neurons were basically normal, but only a few neurons were shrunken. It is suggested that excess coenzyme Q-10 will first damage the cochlear hair cells and the auditory synapse. (**G**) The cochlear explant was cultured for 48 h with serum-free medium containing an antioxidant of 50 μM D-methionine although the reduction in the number of hair cells has not yet occurred, the morphology of all hair cells is already in a state of pathological changes. Remarkably, the auditory nerve fibers and their synapse were completely disappeared. (**H**) In the same 50 μM D-methionine-treated cochlear explant, all spiral ganglion neurons were destroyed completely. It is suggested that excessive 50 μM D-methionine has stronger destructive effects on spiral ganglia than hair cells. The above experimental results demonstrated that blind or excessive antioxidant treatment can cause serious damage to the cochlea, which challenges the presumed universal protective role of antioxidants. (Reproduced with permission from Ding et al. [26])

References

1. Li L, Chen D, Lin X, et al. Antioxidative stress-induced destruction to cochlear cells caused by blind antioxidant therapy. Otolaryngol Head Neck Surg. 2024;170(5):1421–9. https://doi.org/10.1002/ohn.659.
2. Ding D, Wang J, Yu Z, et al. Spontaneous proliferation in organotypic cultures of mouse cochleae. J Otol. 2008;3(2):76–83. https://doi.org/10.1016/S1672-2930(08)50018-3.
3. Kalinec G, Thein P, Park C, Kalinec F. HEI-OC1 cells as a model for investigating drug cytotoxicity. Hear Res. 2016;335:105–17. https://doi.org/10.1016/j.heares.2016.02.019.
4. Ding D, Seigel GM, Salvi RJ. Migration of R28 retinal precursor cells into cochlear and vestibular organs. J Otol. 2006;1(1):51–56. https://doi.org/10.1016/S1672-2930(06)50009-1.
5. Ding D, Stracher A, Salvi RJ. Leupeptin protects cochlear and vestibular hair cells from gentamicin ototoxicity. Hear Res. 2002;164(1-2):115–26. https://doi.org/10.1016/s0378-5955(01)00417-8.
6. McFadden SL, Ding D, Salvemini D, Salvi RJ. M40403, a superoxide dismutase mimetic, protects cochlear hair cells from gentamicin, but not cisplatin toxicity. Toxicol Appl Pharmacol. 2003;186(1):46–54. https://doi.org/10.1016/s0041-008x(02)00017-0.
7. Hou Q, Ding D, Jiang H, Salvi R, Yin S. Gentamicin ototoxic model in mouse cochlear organotypic cultures. Chin J Otol. 2005;3(3):191–3. https://doi.org/10.1007/s11655-010-0258-x.
8. Qi W, Ding D, Salvi RJ. Cytotoxic effects of dimethyl sulphoxide (DMSO) on cochlear organotypic cultures. Hear Res. 2008;236(1-2):52–60. https://doi.org/10.1016/j.heares.2007.12.002.
9. Ding D, Qi W, Yu D, Jiang H, Salvi R. Ototoxic effects of mefloquine in cochlear organotypic cultures. J Otol. 2009;4(2):76–85. https://doi.org/10.1016/S1672-2930(09)50018-9.
10. Ding D, He J, Allman BL, et al. Cisplatin ototoxicity in rat cochlear organotypic cultures. Hear Res. 2011;282(1-2):196–203. https://doi.org/10.1016/j.heares.2011.08.002.
11. Ding D, Roth J, Salvi R. Manganese is toxic to spiral ganglion neurons and hair cells in vitro. Neurotoxicology. 2011;32(2):233–41. https://doi.org/10.1016/j.neuro.2010.12.003.
12. Wu X, Ding D, Sun H, et al. Lead neurotoxicity in rat cochlear organotypic cultures. J Otol. 2011;6(2):45–52. https://doi.org/10.1016/S1672-2930(11)50021-2.
13. Ding D, Jiang H, Fu Y, et al. Ototoxic effects of carboplatin in organotypic cultures in chinchillas and rats. J Otol. 2012;7(2):92–101. https://doi.org/10.1016/S1672-2930(12)50023-1.
14. Deng L, Ding D, Su J, Manohar S, Salvi R. Salicylate selectively kills cochlear spiral ganglion neurons by paradoxically up-regulating superoxide. Neurotox Res. 2013;24(3):307–19. https://doi.org/10.1007/s12640-013-9384-5.
15. Ding D, Qi W, Yu D, et al. Addition of exogenous NAD+ prevents mefloquine-induced neuroaxonal and hair cell degeneration through reduction of caspase-3-mediated apoptosis in cochlear organotypic cultures. PLoS One. 2013;8(11):e79817. https://doi.org/10.1371/journal.pone.0079817.
16. Fu Y, Ding D, Wei L, Jiang H, Salvi R. Ouabain-induced apoptosis in cochlear hair cells and spiral ganglion neurons in vitro. BioMed Res Int. 2013;2013:628064. https://doi.org/10.1155/2013/628064.

17. Liu H, Ding D, Sun H, et al. Cadmium-induced ototoxicity in rat cochlear organotypic cultures. Neurotox Res. 2014;26(2):179–89. https://doi.org/10.1007/s12640-014-9461-4.
18. Wang L, Ding D, Salvi R, Roth JA. Nicotinamide adenine dinucleotide prevents neuroaxonal degeneration induced by manganese in cochlear organotypic cultures. Neurotoxicology. 2014;40:65–74. https://doi.org/10.1016/j.neuro.2013.11.007.
19. Li P, Ding D, Salvi R, Roth JA. Cobalt-induced ototoxicity in rat postnatal cochlear organotypic cultures. Neurotox Res. 2015;28(3):209–21. https://doi.org/10.1007/s12640-015-9538-8.
20. Yu J, Ding D, Sun H, Salvi R, Roth JA. Neurotoxicity of trimethyltin in rat cochlear organotypic cultures. Neurotox Res. 2015;28(1):43–54. https://doi.org/10.1007/s12640-015-9531-2.
21. Ding D, Liu H, Qi W, et al. Ototoxic effects and mechanisms of loop diuretics. J Otol. 2016;11(4):145–56. https://doi.org/10.1016/j.joto.2016.10.001.
22. Gao K, Ding D, Sun H, Roth J, Salvi R. Kanamycin damages early postnatal, but not adult spiral ganglion neurons. Neurotox Res. 2017;32(4):603–13. https://doi.org/10.1007/s12640-017-9773-2.
23. Zhang J, Sun H, Salvi R, Ding D. Paraquat initially damages cochlear support cells leading to anoikis-like hair cell death. Hear Res. 2018;364:129–41. https://doi.org/10.1016/j.heares.2018.03.014.
24. Ye H, Xing Y, Zhang L, et al. Bilirubin-induced neurotoxic and ototoxic effects in rat cochlear and vestibular organotypic cultures. Neurotoxicology. 2019;71:75–86. https://doi.org/10.1016/j.neuro.2018.12.004.
25. Ding D, Manohar S, Jiang H, Salvi R. Hydroxypropyl-beta-cyclodextrin causes massive damage to the developing auditory and vestibular system. Hear Res. 2020;396:108073. https://doi.org/10.1016/j.heares.2020.108073.
26. Ding D, Zhang J, Liu F, et al. Antioxidative stress-induced damage in cochlear explants. J Otol. 2020;15(1):36–40. https://doi.org/10.1016/j.joto.2019.11.005.
27. Ding D, Zhang J, Jiang H, et al. Some ototoxic drugs destroy cochlear support cells before damaging sensory hair cells. Neurotox Res. 2020;37(3):743–52. https://doi.org/10.1007/s12640-020-00170-8.
28. Ding D, Qi W, Jiang H, Salvi R. Excitotoxic damage to auditory nerve afferents and spiral ganglion neurons is correlated with developmental upregulation of AMPA and KA receptors. Hear Res. 2021;411:108358. https://doi.org/10.1016/j.heares.2021.108358.

Quantitative Analysis of Cochlear Hair Cells

10

Cochlear hair cells, situated on the cochlear basilar membrane, serve as the primary sensory receptors in the auditory peripheral system. These cells are regularly arranged into one row of inner hair cells and three rows of outer hair cells, which align along both sides of the tunnel of Corti, extending from the cochlear base around the modiolus to its apex. The spatial arrangement of hair cells on the basilar membrane is critical, as their resonance and sensory responses to sound stimuli vary according to their specific location and the corresponding frequency. High-frequency sounds predominantly activate hair cells in the basal turn, mid-frequency sounds target those in the middle turn, and low-frequency sounds are detected by hair cells in the apical turn. Consequently, the density of cochlear hair cells at distinct locations reflects the population of cells responsive to the frequency range associated with that region. This spatial-frequency relationship underscores the necessity of precise localization in quantitative analyses of cochlear hair cells, as emphasized in previous studies [1–7].

Quantitative assessment of cochlear hair cells can be achieved through two primary methodologies: serial section analysis or surface preparation analysis of the entire cochlear basilar membrane. The serial section approach involves meticulously counting hair cells on individual cochlear slices and subsequently integrating these data into a three-dimensional reconstruction of the cochlear architecture, as demonstrated in earlier studies [8–10]. Alternatively, the surface preparation technique entails systematically enumerating hair cells across successive microscopic fields along the entire length of the basilar membrane, progressing from the apical to the basal region. This data is then computationally processed to generate a quantitative profile of hair cell distribution, comparing experimental results with normative control values to calculate percentage hair cell loss relative to position along the cochlear length. Advanced cochlear mapping software facilitates the automated generation of comprehensive hair cell distribution maps, enabling precise spatial analysis of hair cell populations. This methodological framework has been extensively validated and refined through numerous investigations [4, 6, 11–34], establishing it as a robust and reliable technique for cochlear hair cell quantification.

10.1 Hair Cell Counting from Serial Slices of Cochlea and Cochlear Graphic Reconstruction

In the early stages of inner ear pathology research, technological limitations restricted hair cell analysis to semi-quantitative observations on cochlear slices. Initial quantification methods involved counting hair cells in discrete regions of the cochlea, with a typical focus on the upper half-turn and basal half-turn segments. However, this localized sampling approach failed to provide comprehensive data on the extent and distribution of hair cell loss across the entire cochlear basilar membrane, significantly limiting its clinical and research utility. In 1921, Guild introduced an improved technique involving cochlear slice tracing and reconstruction [8], marking a methodological advancement. Nevertheless, this approach remained constrained by its two-dimensional representation of the spiral cochlear structure, which inherently could not accurately capture the three-dimensional spatial distribution of hair cell pathology along the entire basilar membrane. Consequently, despite its innovative nature, Guild's method saw limited adoption among researchers due to these fundamental limitations in representing the true spatial organization of cochlear hair cell lesions.

10.1.1 Observation of Serial Sections of the Cochlea

Quantitative analysis of cochlear hair cells through serial sectioning employs a cutting plane parallel to the modiolar axis, revealing the spiral architecture of the basilar membrane, where

D. Ding et al., *Histopathological Atlas of the Inner Ear*,
https://doi.org/10.1007/978-981-95-6338-8_10

the basal turn exhibits the largest diameter and the apical turn the smallest. Initial sections typically penetrate the cochlear duct of the basal turn first, establishing this as the reference point for subsequent hair cell tracing and three-dimensional reconstruction. As sectioning progresses sequentially, the knife traverses through Claudius cells in the lateral sulcus before encountering the organ of Corti's cellular components: Hensen's cells, Deiters' cells, outer hair cells, pillar cells (both outer and inner), inner hair cells, and inner phalangeal cells. Further advancement reveals internal sulcus cells, habenula perforata in the osseous spiral lamina's tympanic lip, and spiral ganglion neurons within Rosenthal's canal. Notably, when sectioning reaches the basal turn's spiral lamina, the second cochlear turn's duct becomes exposed, with continued sectioning progressively revealing the third turn until reaching the modiolar mid-axis plane, where true axial sections perpendicular to the organ of Corti are obtained. Importantly, all sections acquired before or after this mid-axis plane present oblique cuts through cellular structures, significantly complicating accurate hair cell identification and quantification [9, 35–38] (Fig. 10.1). This technical challenge underscores the complexity of obtaining reliable quantitative data from serial cochlear sections.

10.1.2 Tracing and Reconstructing from Cochlear Slices

In guinea pig cochlear reconstruction using 20 μm serial sections, key anatomical landmarks are systematically identified for spatial mapping: point "a" marks the junction of inner and outer pillar cells in the basal turn, with corresponding junctions in subsequent turns designated as points "b" (second turn), "c" (third turn), and "d" (fourth turn). Following sectioning through the modiolar central axis, contralateral pillar cell junctions are sequentially labeled as "e" (fourth turn), "f" (third turn), "g" (second turn), and "h" (basal turn). The reconstruction process involves connecting specific point pairs (a-h, a-g, b-g, b-f, c-f, c-e, and e-d) to form a spiral plane, with each segment's length calculated using circular geometry formulas. The sum of these interconnected segments yields the total length of the pillar cell junction line, which functionally represents the cochlear basilar membrane's complete extension (Fig. 10.2). Spatial data from each section are plotted on a spiral coordinate system where the vertical axis indicates slice sequence numbers and the horizontal axis shows measurement scales. While this tracing method enables basilar membrane length measurement from serial sections, it presents significant challenges for precise whole-cochlea hair cell localization and quantification due to inherent spatial reconstruction limitations [10].

10.2 Hair Cell Count and Cochleogram from Surface Preparations of the Cochlear Basilar Membrane

The introduction of cochlear surface preparation techniques by Engström in 1960 revolutionized inner ear pathology research by overcoming the limitations of traditional temporal bone sectioning methods. This innovative approach provides optimal visualization for precise localization and quantitative assessment of cochlear hair cells through direct en face examination. The technique involves microdissection of the intact basilar membrane from the osseous spiral lamina under

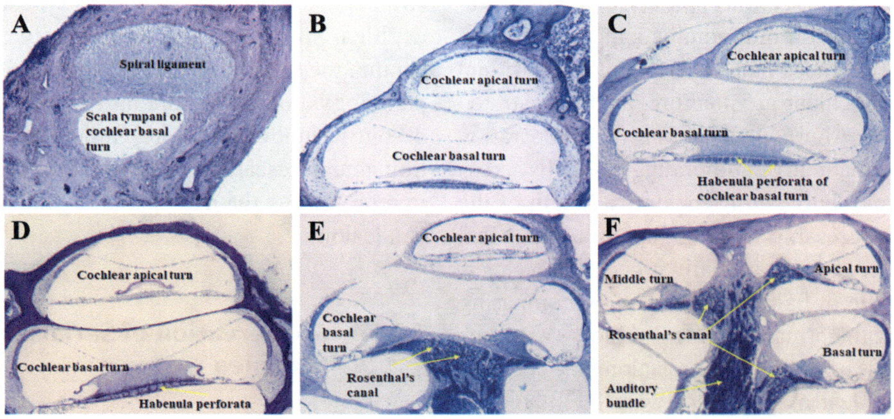

Fig. 10.1 Sequential semi-thin sections through the mouse cochlea demonstrating progressive anatomical planes from lateral to medial structures. (**A**) Initial section plane revealing the scala tympani and spiral ligament in the cochlear basal turn. (**B**) Advancement to the osseous spiral lamina (basal turn) and lateral sulcus (apical turn). (**C**) Section plane reaching the habenula perforata in the basal turn. (**D**) Subsequent plane intersecting both the osseous spiral lamina (basal turn) and the medial sulcus (apical turn). (**E**) Section plane encompassing Rosenthal's canal (basal turn) and medial sulcus (apical turn). (**F**) Final section reaching the central modiolar axis, representing the most medial plane of sectioning. This series demonstrates the three-dimensional relationships of cochlear structures across different sectional planes

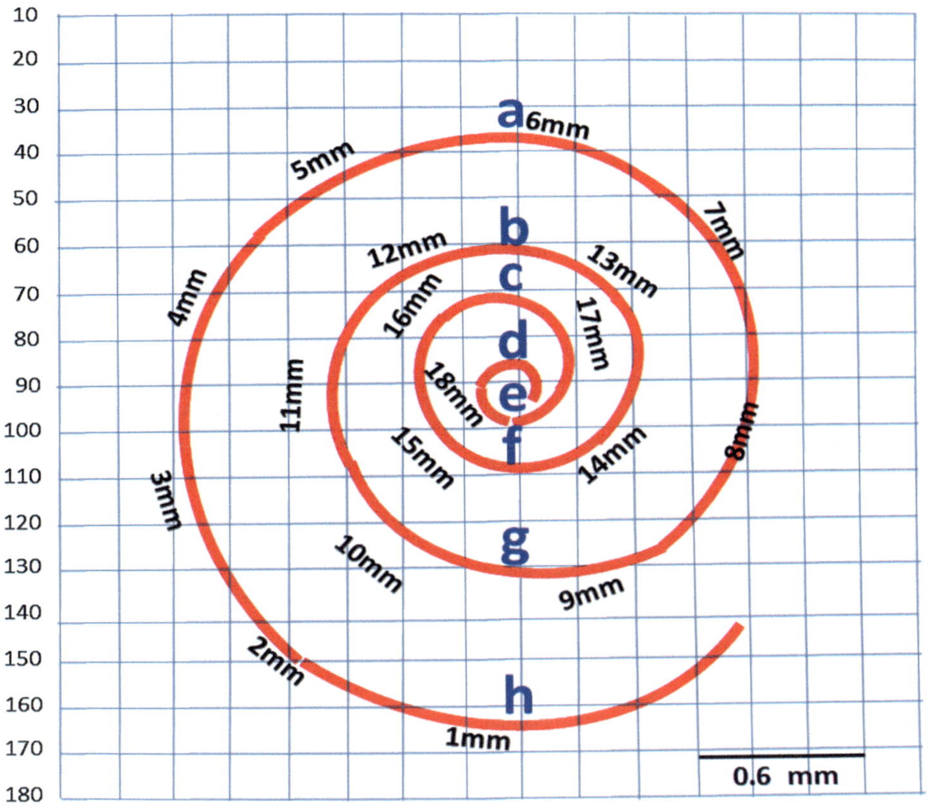

Fig. 10.2 The spiral reconstruction method for guinea pig cochlear serial sections. In the coordinate system, the ordinate represents the slice serial number, and the abscissa represents the measurement scale. The reconstruction algorithm constructs successive semicircular segments using specific diameter parameters: segment ah forms the basal turn's first semicircle, ag completes the basal turn's remaining portion, while diameters bg, bf, cf, ce, and de generate subsequent turns, collectively forming a continuous spiral representation of the cochlear architecture. Each semicircular segment's basilar membrane length is calculated using the formula $L = 1/2\pi \times$ slice thickness (20 μm) × number of slices, with the summation of all segments yielding the cochlear basilar membrane's total length. This geometric reconstruction approach provides a method for dimensional analysis of the spiral cochlear structure from serial sectional data

stereomicroscopic guidance, followed by flat-mounting in glycerol on glass slides. This preparation enables comprehensive topographic mapping and accurate enumeration of every hair cell along the entire cochlear spiral with superior spatial resolution [4, 5, 12–15, 21, 25, 28, 29, 39–44]. The methodological superiority of this approach is demonstrated in multiple figures throughout the literature (Figs. 8.10–8.16 and 8.22; Figs. 10.3 and 10.4), establishing it as the gold standard for quantitative cochleogram analysis in modern auditory research.

10.2.1 Method of Hair Cell Count on Surface Preparations of the Cochlear Basilar Membrane

The dissected cochlear basilar membrane segments are systematically mounted on glass slides in anatomical sequence from basal to apical turns using glycerol as mounting medium and covered with coverslips [45] (Fig. 10.3A). Quantitative analysis is performed at 400× magnification using a calibrated eyepiece micrometer (0.24 mm scale length) as the standardized measurement reference (Fig. 10.4A). Hair cell counts were performed scale-by-scale, field of view from apex to base, with separate counts recorded for the single row of inner hair cells and three rows of outer hair cells within each scale unit (Fig. 10.4B). Data entry into specialized cochleogram software follows standardized protocols: pressing Enter indicates no hair cell loss within the measured segment, negative values (e.g., −5) denote specific numbers of missing hair cells, while positive numbers (e.g., 5) indicate surviving hair cell counts in severely degenerated regions (Fig. 10.5). This standardized quantification protocol significantly enhances the efficiency and reliability of cochlear hair cell analysis [4].

10.2.2 Preparation of Cochleogram using DOS Software

The quantitative hair cell data input into the computer undergoes automated comparison with species-specific normative values through the DOS cochleogram software (Fig. 10.5), which systematically generates cochleograms depicting the

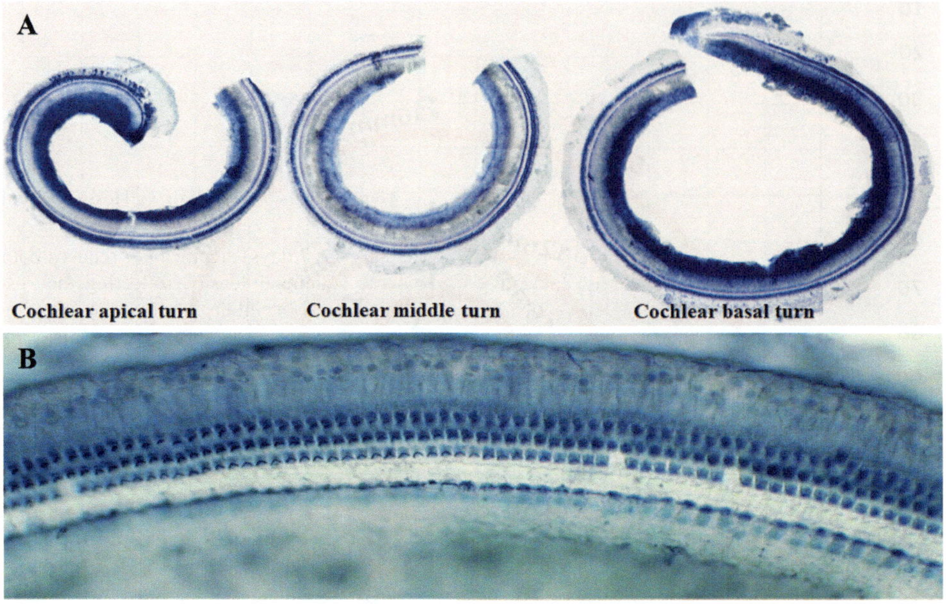

Fig. 10.3 Surface preparation of the cochlear basilar membrane using different histological techniques. (**A**) Surface preparation of the entire chinchilla cochlear basilar membrane stained with succinate dehydrogenase, revealing metabolic activity patterns across the entire cochlear spiral. (**B**) Surface preparation of rat cochlear basilar membrane stained with hematoxylin, with microscopic focus on the surface structure of the organ of Corti, showing detailed cellular architecture (**A**: Reproduced with permission from Yuan et al. [42]). These preparations exemplify the two principal staining approaches for cochlear surface observations—enzymatic activity visualization and structural cytological demonstration

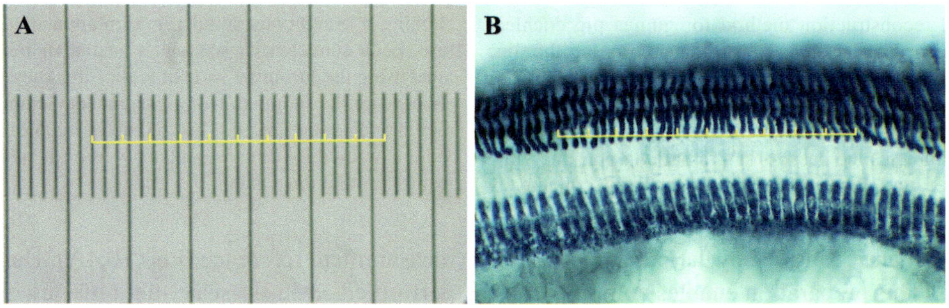

Fig. 10.4 The methodology for precise morphometric analysis of cochlear structures. (**A**) Calibration of the microscopic measurement system showing the yellow micrometer ruler within the eyepiece at 400× magnification, with scale verification confirming 0.24 mm actual length per graduated unit. (**B**) Systematic quantification protocol demonstrating sequential measurement of the cochlear basilar membrane's length using the calibrated micrometer scale, accompanied by simultaneous enumeration of both inner and outer hair cells within each standardized measurement segment, ensuring accurate spatial correlation between anatomical dimensions and cellular distributions

percentage loss of inner and outer hair cells at 10% intervals along the cochlear length from apex to base (Fig. 10.6). This specialized software incorporates advanced functionality for creating composite cochleograms by averaging data across experimental groups. Subsequent data processing through integrated analysis with GraphPad Prism version 5.0 enables precise spatial quantification of hair cell loss patterns at defined cochlear locations, facilitating statistically robust topographic assessment of cochlear pathology [4, 12, 13, 21, 25, 28, 33, 37, 39–43]. This integrated analytical approach is visually demonstrated in Figs. 10.7 and 10.8, showcasing the system's capability for detailed spatial mapping and statistical evaluation of cochlear hair cell distributions.

The cochleogram employs a dual-axis quantitative representation. The vertical axis of the cochleogram marks the percentage of hair cell loss, and the horizontal axis of the cochleogram marks the location of resonant response of the cochlear basilar membrane to different frequency sound stimuli (Figs. 10.6, 10.7, and 10.8). The cochleogram not only accurately reflects the loss of hair cells in various locations of the cochlea, but also comprehensively analyzes the relation between the hair cell loss and the threshold shift of specific auditory frequencies. This is termed a quantitative analysis map of cochlear hair cells corresponding to frequency positions [6, 12, 13, 21, 25, 28, 33, 37, 41]. Referred to as the cochlear frequency-position analysis map, this standardized visualization

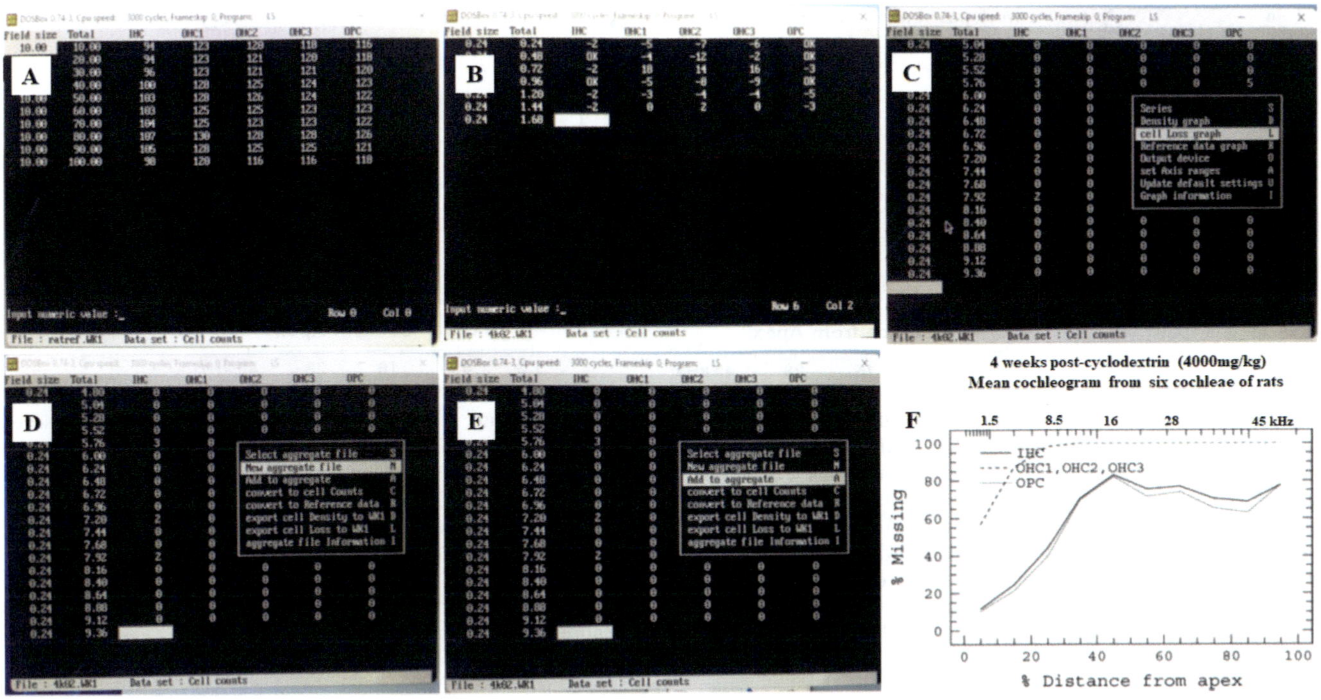

Fig. 10.5 The comprehensive workflow for generating an averaged cochleogram from experimental data. (**A**) Normal rat cochlear hair cell density values (cells/mm) serve as baseline reference data for the cochleogram software. (**B**) Quantitative hair cell analysis involves sequential entry of cell counts per 0.24 mm segment, where "OK" indicates intact cell populations, negative values denote missing cells relative to normal density, and positive numbers represent absolute counts in degenerated regions. (**C**) Completed cochlear analyses are stored as WK1 format files. (**D**) For group analysis, individual WK1 files are converted to the Aggregate format. (**E**) Aggregate files from all specimens are compiled into a master group file. (**F**) The final Aggregate file undergoes format conversion to Postscript for visualization in graphic software, displaying group-averaged cochleograms with percentage hair cell loss (vertical axis) versus cochlear location (lower horizontal axis) and corresponding frequency positions (upper horizontal axis). The representative cochleogram demonstrates complete outer hair cell loss (20%–100% cochlear length) and >70% inner hair cell loss (40%–100% length) four weeks post-cyclodextrin injection, with inner hair cell degeneration patterns mirroring outer pillar cell loss, suggesting secondary degeneration due to supporting structure collapse. This standardized analytical pipeline enables precise spatial mapping of cochlear pathology patterns

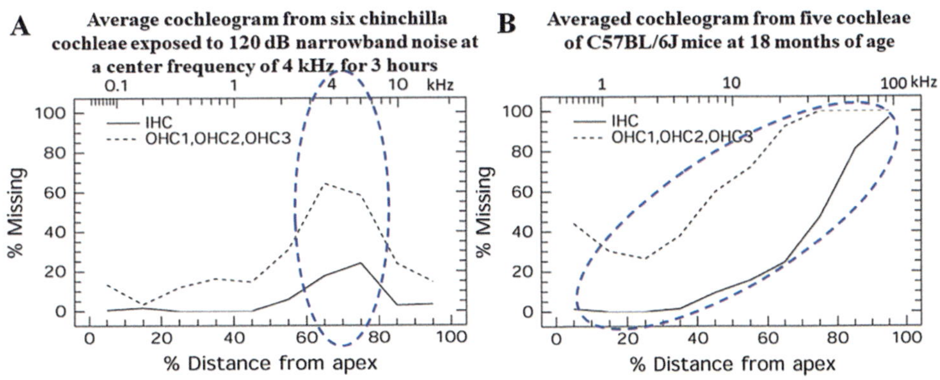

Fig. 10.6 Two different averaged cochleograms reveal distinct patterns of hair cell loss across the cochlear basilar membrane in two different experimental models. (**A**) Mean cochleogram from six chinchilla cochleae reveals targeted hair cell damage in the 4 kHz frequency responding region of the cochlear basilar membrane following acoustic trauma (120 dB narrow-band noise centered at 4 kHz for 3 h), with maximal lesion severity corresponding to the tonotopic representation of the traumatic stimulus. (**B**) Mean cochleogram from five cochleae of eighteen-month-old C57BL/6J mice ($n = 5$ cochleae) exhibits that the cochlear hair cell loss in the cochlea occurs in a stereotypic pattern, with the hair cell missing beginning at the base of the cochlea and progressing toward the apex. These representative cochleograms illustrate the system's capacity to identify both noise-induced and genetic defect-related hair cell loss patterns through quantitative spatial analysis

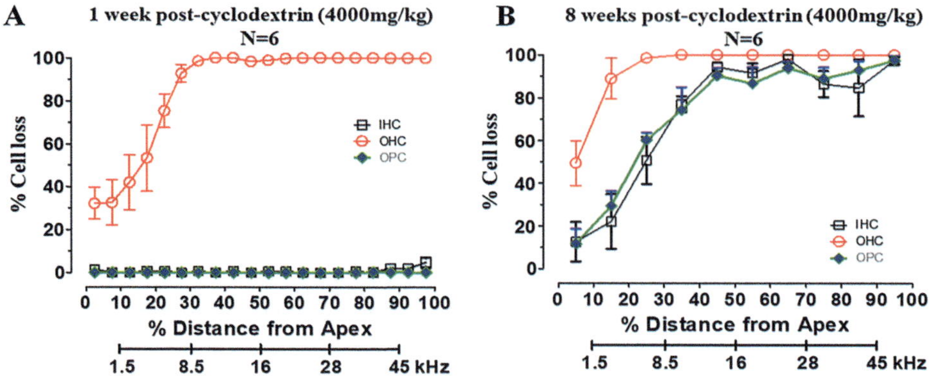

Fig. 10.7 Averaged rat cochleograms plotted using GraphPad Prism version 5.0 software illustrate delayed destruction of inner hair cells and supporting structures caused by specific outer hair cell destruction. (**A**) Pathological changes in early-stage (1 week after cyclodextrin administration with a dose of 4000 mg/kg) reveal selective outer hair cell destruction in basal and second turns with complete preservation of inner hair cells throughout the cochlea, demonstrating that the compound's primary ototoxic target is outer hair cells. (**B**) Eight weeks after cyclodextrin (4000 mg/kg) injection, following the secondary destruction of outer pillar cells and collapse of the Corti tunnel, severe destruction of inner hair cells also occurred. This mean cochleogram shows that the percentage of inner hair cell missing is exactly the same as that of outer pillar cells, suggesting that the delayed death of inner hair cells is entirely secondary to the collapse of the supporting structures of the organ of Corti. These temporal and spatial patterns of cochlear damage elucidate the mechanistic progression from primary outer hair cell toxicity to subsequent structural and functional compromise of the entire organ of Corti

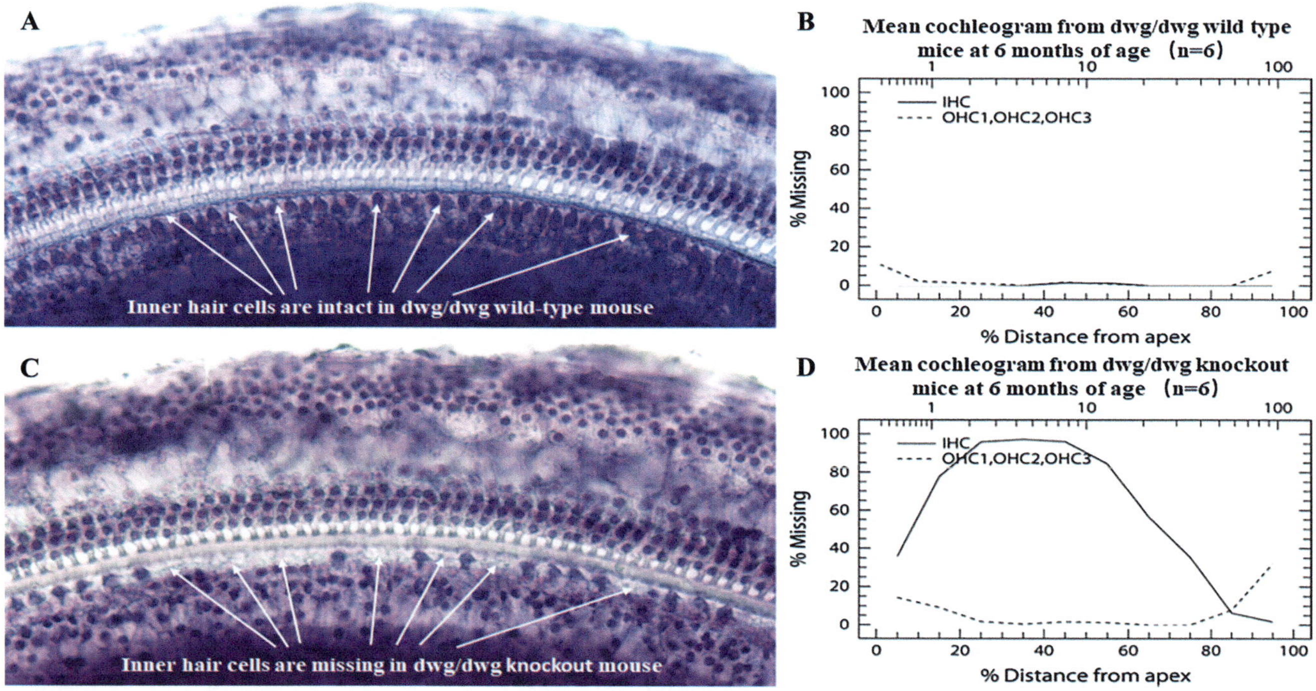

Fig. 10.8 As an enzyme that catalyzes the conversion of γ-glutamyl, the deficiency of γ-glutamyl transferase often results in Ggt1 dwg/dwg homozygous mutations of Dwarf gray mice are unable to synthesize glutathione due to the γ-glutamyltransferase 1 gene. Unexpectedly, Ggt1 dwg/dwg homozygous mice lacking the γ-glutamyltransferase 1 gene not only developed synthesis impairment to glutathione synthesis but also exhibited selective inner hair cell loss. (**A**) Cochlear surface preparations from 6-month-old wild-type mice demonstrate normal morphological organization of both inner and outer hair cell arrays. (**B**) An averaged cochleogram from six age-matched wild-type animals confirms the complete preservation of hair cell populations throughout the entire length of the cochlear basilar membrane in genetically intact mice. (**C**) Striking pathological findings in Ggt1 dwg/dwg mutants reveal selective loss of inner hair cells despite preserved outer hair cell architecture at 6 months of age. (**D**) Averaged cochleogram from six Ggt1 dwg/dwg gene mutant mice documents near-total (100%) inner hair cell loss in mid-cochlear regions with minimal (<5%) outer hair cell involvement, establishing a novel pattern of preferential inner hair cell vulnerability associated with glutathione metabolism disruption. These findings suggest that the γ-glutamyltransferase plays an unexpectedly important role in maintaining the survival of inner hair cells but does not appear to affect the lifespan of outer hair cells

method has been extensively validated for its accuracy in reflecting structure-function relationships in cochlear auditory pathology research, as demonstrated in Figs. 10.6, 10.7, and 10.8. The methodology's strength lies in its ability to simultaneously represent both cochlear hair cell loss and functional consequences through this integrated coordinate system.

The tonotopic organization of the cochlea dictates that specific basilar membrane locations respond to distinct frequency ranges, yet absolute position varies significantly between specimens due to natural variations in basilar membrane length, with equivalent frequency representations potentially differing by half an octave or more in their physical distance from the apex. This anatomical variability necessitates normalization of measurements, as direct comparison using absolute lengths would artifactually superimpose different frequency representations. The established solution involves converting physical distances to percentage positions along the basilar membrane's total length, enabling accurate comparison of equivalent tonotopic regions across specimens. By standardizing hair cell counts against species-specific normative values at matched percentage locations, this methodology effectively eliminates technical artifacts arising from dimensional variations while preserving the critical frequency-position relationships essential for meaningful cochleogram interpretation [12, 13, 21, 25, 28, 29, 33, 37, 41]. This normalization process represents a fundamental principle in quantitative cochlear histopathology, ensuring reliable correlation between structural damage and functional auditory deficits.

10.3 A Windows-Compatible System for Quantitative Analysis of Cochlear Hair Cell Localization

Our comprehensive database system incorporates cochlear hair cell reference values derived from surface preparation analyses across multiple experimental species, including BALB/C mice, CBA/Ca mice, C57BL/6J mice, C57BL/10J mice, DBA/2J mice, Kunming mice, Sprague Dawley rats, Wistar rats, gerbils, guinea pigs, chinchillas, New Zealand white rabbits, and African vervet monkeys, with data acquisition through systematic microscopic photography. These standardized reference values form the foundation for quantitative cochlear hair cell assessment. The software platform, developed for Windows operating systems (Win10 compatible) with Excel 2003+ integration, utilizes Visual Basic.Net 2015 programming language with an English interface. Designed with dual user/developer modules, the system not only provides preloaded normative data but also enables customization of laboratory-specific reference databases. This versatile tool has received formal certification from China's National Copyright Administration (Certificate No. 3064966, Registration No. 2018SR735871;

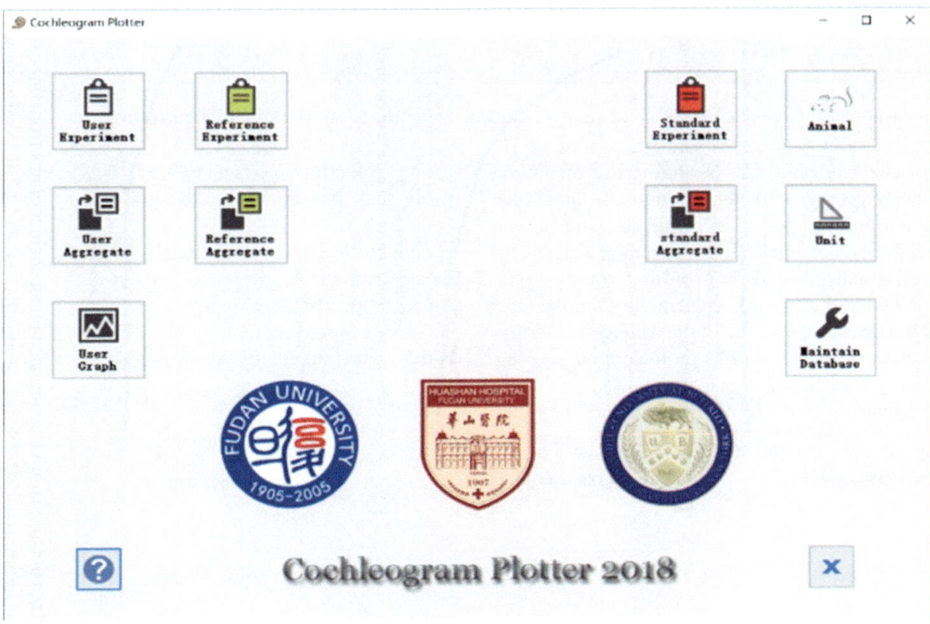

Fig. 10.9 Interface of Windows-compatible software for quantitative analysis of cochlear hair cells

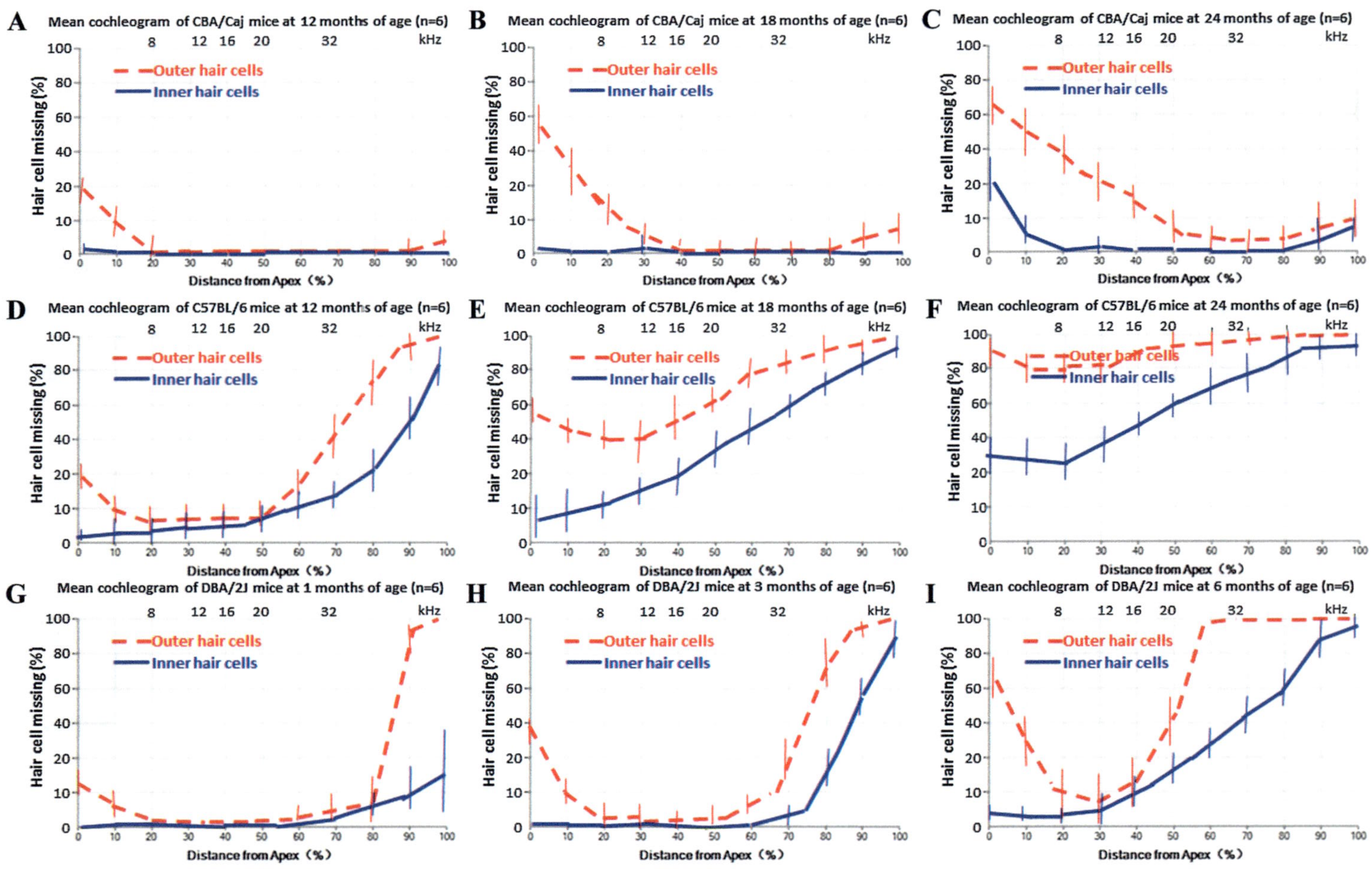

Fig. 10.10 Comparative age-related mean cochleograms from three mouse strains demonstrating distinct patterns of progressive hair cell loss. (**A–C**) CBA/Caj mice exhibit apical-to-basal outer hair cell degeneration at 12, 18, and 24 months. (**D–F**) C57BL/6 mice show basal-to-apical progression of hair cell loss across 12, 18, and 24 months of age. G-I. DBA/2J mice display unique dual-origin pathology by 1, 3, and 6 months of age, with inner hair cell loss beginning from the basal turn toward the apical turn, while outer hair cell loss initiates simultaneously at both cochlear extremities before converging centrally. The above results indicate that the patterns of cochlear hair cell loss differ between mice without and with deafness-associated gene defects (Reproduced with permission from Ding et al. [43]). These strain-specific trajectories illustrate how genetic background determines both spatial patterns and temporal progression of age-related cochlear degeneration

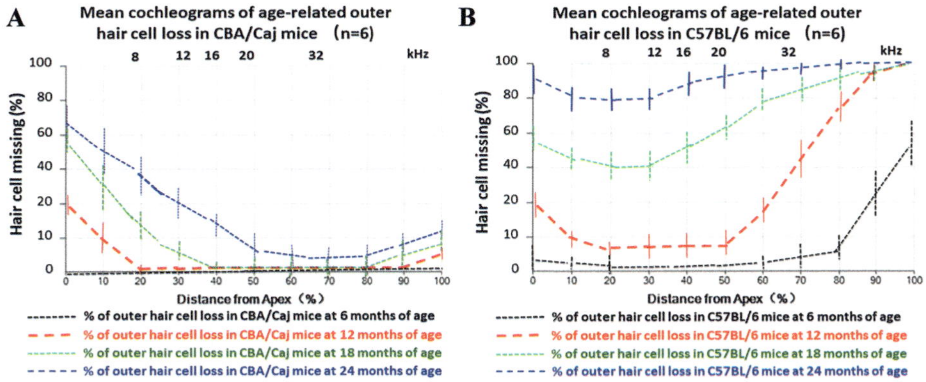

Fig. 10.11 Different patterns of outer hair cell loss among mice with different strains and ages. (**A**) CBA/Caj mice exhibit progressive outer hair cell loss from the apical turn to the basal turn, with degeneration initiating in the low-frequency responding region at the apical turn and gradually extending toward the high-frequency responding region at the basal turn over time. (**B**) The outer hair cell loss in C57BL/6 mice displays an inverse basal-to-apical progression pattern, where the outer hair cell loss begins in the high-frequency responding region at the basal turn and advances toward the low-frequency responding region at the apical turn with age. These contrasting trajectories highlight fundamental differences in the spatial and temporal progression of presbycusis between mouse strains, reflecting distinct underlying mechanisms of age-related cochlear degeneration

Development team: Weidong Qi, Dalian Ding, Xiaoguang Sun, Fang Yuan), with technical specifications detailed in peer-reviewed publications [40, 42, 46] as illustrated in Fig. 10.9.

The quantitative analysis of cochlear hair cells begins with high-resolution microscopic imaging (100–400× magnification) of stained basilar membrane surface preparations, systematically documenting the entire cochlear length from apex to basal hook region. This standardized imaging protocol employs flexible measurement units (100 μm, 200 μm, etc.) within microscope software to establish consistent observation parameters. Manual enumeration proceeds tonotopically, counting all inner and outer hair cell rows sequentially from apical to basal regions, with data entered into specialized cochleogram software using a standardized coding system: "OK" indicates intact populations, "-X" denotes missing cells, "+X" represents surviving cells in degenerated regions, and "bad" flags mechanical artifacts that the software automatically excludes from analysis. The system performs critical data transformations, converting absolute lengths to percentage positions and raw cell counts to percentage loss values relative to species-specific normative databases. Advanced analytical features include: (1) Flexible output of cochleograms at user-defined resolution (1%, 5%, 10% intervals); (2) Generation of group-averaged cochleograms with incorporated variability metrics (standard deviation/error); (3) Comparative analysis between experimental groups; and (4) Customizable visualization formats. This integrated methodology, validated through extensive research applications [25, 28, 33, 40, 42, 44, 46], significantly enhances the efficiency and reliability of cochlear histopathological assessment while maintaining flexibility for diverse research applications. The system's capacity for both detailed individual analysis and robust group comparisons is illustrated in Figs. 10.10 and 10.11, demonstrating its comprehensive analytical capabilities.

References

1. Schuknecht H. 1. Histological method. In: Pathology of the ear. 1st ed. Cambridge: Harvard University Press; 1974. p. 1–20.
2. Muller M. Frequency representation in the rat cochlea. Hear Res. 1991;51(2):247–54. https://doi.org/10.1016/0378-5955(91)90041-7.
3. Ding D, Li M, Jiang C, Salvi R. Chapter 3: Anatomy of the temporal bone and inner ear. In: Morphology of the inner ear. Harbin: Heilongjiang Science and Technology Press; 2001. p. 10–17.
4. Ding D, McFadden SL, Salvi R. Cochlear hair cell densities and inner-ear staining techniques. In: Willott JF, editor. Handbook of mouse auditory research from behavior to molecular biology. Boca Raton: CRC Press; 2001. p. 189–204.
5. Viberg A, Canlon B. The guide to plotting a cochleogram. Hear Res. 2004;197(1-2):1–10. https://doi.org/10.1016/j.heares.2004.04.016.
6. Ding D, Jiang H, Wang P, Salvi R. Cell death after co-administration of cisplatin and ethacrynic acid. Hear Res. 2007;226(1–2):129–39. https://doi.org/10.1016/j.heares.2006.07.015.
7. Ding D, Qi W, Qu Y, Salvi R. Chapter 6: Research techniques of the inner ear morphology. In: Science of the inner ear. Beijing: China Science and Technology Press; 2010. p. 50–88.
8. Guild SR. A graphic reconstruction method for the study of the organ of Corti. Anat Rec. 1921;20(2):140–57. https://doi.org/10.1002/ar.1090220205.
9. Schuknecht HF. Techniques for study of cochlear function and pathology in experimental animals; development of the anatomical frequency scale for the cat. AMA Arch

Otolaryngol. 1953;58(4):377–97. https://doi.org/10.1001/archotol.1953.00710040399001.
10. Zeng Y, Yin J, Wang Y, et al. Tracing and remaking of cochlear sections of guinea pig. Zhonghua Er Bi Yan Hou Ke Za Zhi. 1964;10:299–303.
11. McFadden SL, Ding D, Jiang H, Woo JM, Salvi RJ. Chinchilla models of selective cochlear hair cell loss. Hear Res. 2002; 174(1–2):230–38. https://doi.org/10.1016/s0378-5955(02)00697-4.
12. Ding D, McFadden SL, Browne RW, Salvi RJ. Late dosing with ethacrynic acid can reduce gentamicin concentration in perilymph and protect cochlear hair cells. Hear Res. 2003;185(1–2):90–96. https://doi.org/10.1016/s0378-5955(03)00258-2.
13. Ding D, Jiang H, Wang J, et al. Inner hair cell missing potentiates noise induced outer hair cell lesion. J Audiol Speech Pathol. 2004;12(6):413–15.
14. Qi W, Ding D, Jiang H, Salvi R. Quantified analytic system for cochlear hair cells. J Audiol Speech Pathol. 2007;15(2):158–60.
15. Ding D, Qi W, Yu D, Jiang H, Salvi R. Ototoxic effects of mefloquine in cochlear organotypic cultures. J Otol. 2009;4(2):76–85. https://doi.org/10.13489/j.cnki.11-4883/r.2009.02.008.
16. He J, Yin S, Wang J, Ding D, Jiang H. Effectiveness of different approaches for establishing cisplatin-induced cochlear lesions in mice. Acta Otolaryngol. 2009;129(12):1359–67. https://doi.org/10.3109/00016480902856604.
17. Ding D, He J, Allman B, et al. Cisplatin ototoxicity in rat cochlear organotypic cultures. Hear Res. 2011;282(1–2):196–203. https://doi.org/10.1016/j.heares.2011.08.002.
18. He J, Ding D, Yu D, et al. Modulation of copper transporters in protection against cisplatin-induced cochlear hair cell damage. J Otol. 2011;6(2):53–61. https://doi.org/10.13489/j.cnki.11-4883/r.2011.02.007.
19. Li Y, Ding D, Jiang H, Fu Y, Salvi R. Co-administration of cisplatin and furosemide causes rapid and massive loss of cochlear hair cells in mice. Neurotox Res. 2011;20(4):307–19. https://doi.org/10.1007/s12640-011-9244-0.
20. Deng L, Ding D, Su J, Manohar S, Salvi R. Salicylate selectively kills cochlear spiral ganglion neurons by paradoxically up-regulating superoxide. Neurotox Res. 2013;24(3):307–19. https://doi.org/10.1007/s12640-013-9384-5.
21. Ding D, Qi W, Yu D, et al. Addition of exogenous NAD+ prevents mefloquine-induced neuroaxonal and hair cell degeneration through reduction of caspase-3-mediated apoptosis in cochlear organotypic cultures. PLoS One. 2013;8(11):e79817. https://doi.org/10.1371/journal.pone.0079817.
22. Dong Y, Ding D, Jiang H, et al. Ototoxicity of paclitaxel in rat cochlear organotypic cultures. Toxicol Appl Pharmacol. 2014;280(3):526–33. https://doi.org/10.1016/j.taap.2014.08.022.
23. Liu H, Ding D, Sun H, et al. Cadmium-induced ototoxicity in rat cochlear organotypic cultures. Neurotox Res. 2014;26(2):179–89. https://doi.org/10.1007/s12640-014-9461-4.
24. Li P, Ding D, Salvi R, Roth JA. Cobalt-induced ototoxicity in rat postnatal cochlear organotypic cultures. Neurotox Res. 2015;28(3):209–21. https://doi.org/10.1007/s12640-015-9538-8.
25. Ding D, Jiang H, Chen GD, et al. N-acetyl-cysteine prevents age-related hearing loss and the progressive loss of inner hair cells in gamma-glutamyl transferase 1 deficient mice. Aging (Albany NY). 2016;8(4):730–50. https://doi.org/10.18632/aging.100927.
26. Zhang J, Sun H, Salvi R, Ding D. Paraquat initially damages cochlear support cells leading to anoikis-like hair cell death. Hear Res. 2018;364:129–41. https://doi.org/10.1016/j.heares.2018.03.014.
27. Liu X, Ding D, Chen GD, et al. 2-hydroxypropyl-beta-cyclodextrin ototoxicity in adult rats: rapid onset and massive destruction of both inner and outer hair cells above a critical dose. Neurotox Res. 2020;38(3):808–23. https://doi.org/10.1007/s12640-020-00252-7.
28. Ding D, Jiang H, Manohar S, et al. Spatiotemporal developmental upregulation of prestin correlates with the severity and location of cyclodextrin-induced outer hair cell loss and hearing loss. Front Cell Dev Biol. 2021;9:643709. https://doi.org/10.3389/fcell.2021.643709.
29. Ding D, Jiang H, Salvi R. Cochlear spiral ganglion neuron degeneration following cyclodextrin-induced hearing loss. Hear Res. 2021;400:108125. https://doi.org/10.1016/j.heares.2020.108125.
30. Ding D, Prolla T, Someya S, Manohar S, Salvi R. Roles of Bak and Sirt3 in paraquat-induced cochlear hair cell damage. Neurotox Res. 2021;39(4):1227–37. https://doi.org/10.1007/s12640-021-00366-6.
31. Ding D, Li P, Qi W, et al. Study on delayed secondary lesions in the cochlea triggered by cochlear hair cell death. Chin J Otorhinolaryngol Skull Base Surg. 2022;28(6):1–10.
32. Manohar S, Ding D, Jiang H, et al. Combined antioxidants and anti-inflammatory therapies fail to attenuate the early and late phases of cyclodextrin-induced cochlear damage and hearing loss. Hear Res. 2022;414:108409. https://doi.org/10.1016/j.heares.2021.108409.
33. Ding D, Manohar S, Kador PF, Salvi R. Multifunctional redox modulator prevents blast-induced loss of cochlear and vestibular hair cells and auditory spiral ganglion neurons. Sci Rep. 2024;14(1):15296. https://doi.org/10.1038/s41598-024-66406-1.
34. Ding D, Shi L, Xing Y, et al. Sagittal sectioning of temporal bones and quantitative measurement of neural densities in the inner ear in normal mice. Chin J Otorhinolaryngol Skull Base Surg. 2024;30(6): 69–75. https://doi.org/10.11798/j.issn.1007-1520.202424331.
35. Schuknecht H. 2. Anatomy. In: Pathology of the ear. 1st ed. Cambridge: Harvard University Press; 1974. p. 40–96.
36. Ding D, Yu J, Li P, et al. Standardization of experimental animals temporal bone sections. J Otol. 2015;10(2):66–71. https://doi.org/10.1016/j.joto.2015.08.001.
37. Ding D, Shi L, Xing Y, et al. Secondary neural damage in the inner ear induced by intratympanic gentamicin injection. Chin J Otorhinolaryngol Skull Base Surg. 2024;30(6):11–19. https://doi.org/10.1798/j.issn.1007-1520.202424356.
38. Ding D, Qi W, Qu Y, Salvi R Chapter 1: Anatomy of the inner ear. In: Science of the inner ear. Beijing: China Science and Technology Press; 2010. p. 1–8.
39. Ding D, Qi W, Yang K, et al. Technical evolution of pathology in the inner ear. Chin J Otorhinolaryngol Skull Base Surg. 2016;22(3):169–78. https://doi.org/10.1798/j.issn.1007-1520.201603001.
40. Yuan F, Qi W. Progress in plotting and application of cochleogram. Chin J Otorhinolaryngol-Skull Base Surg. 2018;24(6):592–96. https://doi.org/10.11798/j.issn.1007-520.201806023.
41. Ding D, Manohar S, Jiang H, Salvi R. Hydroxypropyl-beta-cyclodextrin causes massive damage to the developing auditory and vestibular system. Hear Res. 2020;396:108073. https://doi.org/10.1016/j.heares.2020.108073.
42. Yuan F, Ding DL, Wang J, et al. [Inner hair cells loss by carboplatin and the changes of cochlear compound action potential in chinchillas]. Zhonghua Er Bi Yan Hou Tou Jing Wai Ke Za Zhi. 2020;55(5):506–13. https://doi.org/10.3760/cma.j.cn.115330-20200426-00332.
43. Ding D, Li P, Qi W, Zhang J. Different patterns of age-related damage to cochlear hair cells in different species of experimental animals. Chin J Otorhinolaryngol. Skull Base Surg. 2023;29(4):7–13.
44. Ding D, Chen GD, Zhang C, et al. Supporting cell involvement in cochlear damage and repair: novel insights from a quantitative analysis of cyclodextrin-induced ototoxicity in mice. Hear Res. 2025;459:109201. https://doi.org/10.1016/j.heares.2025.109201.
45. Ding D, Zhao J, Huangfu M. Modified cochlear surface preparations. Zhonghua Er Bi Yan Hou Ke Za Zhi. 1981;16(4):207–09.
46. Yuan F, Ding D, Cao Y, Qi W. Cochlear hair cell densities in the rabbit. Anat Sci Int. 2019;94(1):144–49. https://doi.org/10.1007/s12565-018-0461-y.

11 Quantitative Observation of Cochlear Auditory Nerve Fibers and Cochlear Spiral Ganglion Neurons

11.1 Quantification of Peripheral Auditory Nerve Fibers in Habenula Perforata

Quantification of auditory nerve fibers in the habenula perforata provides crucial insights into peripheral auditory pathway integrity, as this specialized channel serves as the exclusive conduit connecting spiral ganglion neurons in Rosenthal's canal with cochlear hair cells in the organ of Corti, enabling transmission of auditory impulses signals released from cochlear hair cells to the spiral ganglions within Rosenthal's canal and the signals continue to the central auditory system through the auditory nerve tract. Precise enumeration of nerve fibers traversing individual habenula perforata openings enables detection of spatial variations in neural innervation density along the cochlear spiral and provides data for evaluating the quantitative relationship between spiral ganglion neurons and their target hair cells, a parameter with significant diagnostic and research implications for auditory pathology [1–12]. This quantitative analysis of peripheral auditory nerve fibers can systematically assess potential neurodegenerative patterns by comparing the number of auditory nerve fibers within the habenula perforata and establishing important structure-function correlations between normal and pathological conditions.

The reduction of auditory nerve fibers in the habenula perforata primarily stems from two distinct pathological mechanisms. The first involves ototoxic agents or acoustic trauma initially destroying cochlear hair cells, subsequently leading to a secondary degeneration of peripheral auditory nerve fibers through a secondary delayed destruction mechanism—while central projections may persist temporarily, the permanent loss of hair cells and their synaptic connections ultimately results in irreversible hearing impairment. Alternatively, neurotoxic compounds, heavy metals, or mechanical damage may directly induce spiral ganglion neuron apoptosis, causing simultaneous degeneration of both peripheral and central axonal processes in a retrograde manner. In this scenario, despite preserved hair cell viability and receptor potentials, the interruption of neural transmission pathways prevents signal propagation to the central auditory system, similarly culminating in permanent deafness [13, 14]. These dual mechanisms highlight the critical importance of both sensory and neural elements in maintaining auditory function.

Horizontal cross-sections through the osseous lamina of the cochlear modiolus reveal a distinctive row of neuropores (habenula perforata), which serve as critical conduits for peripheral auditory nerve fibers to traverse the bony structure and establish synaptic connections with cochlear hair cells via specialized afferent terminals [1–3, 6, 8–12]. This anatomical arrangement facilitates the precise topographic organization of spiral ganglion neuron projections, enabling efficient transmission of auditory signals from hair cells to the central nervous system while maintaining the cochlea's tonotopic mapping (Figs. 6.20, and 7.5–7.7; Figs. 11.1 and 11.2). The structural integrity of habenula perforata is essential for preserving both the quantitative and qualitative aspects of auditory neural transmission throughout the cochlear spiral.

Quantitative analysis of habenula perforata innervation patterns reveals significant species-specific and tonotopic variations in auditory nerve fiber distribution. In chinchillas, fiber counts demonstrate a characteristic cochlear gradient, ranging from 93.7 ± 12.2 fibers per habenula perforata in the basal hook region to 181.5 ± 30.4 at the basal-apical transition zone, with intermediate densities of 129.7 ± 27.8 in the second turn and 75.8 ± 13.2 in the apical turn [1–3, 15, 16]. Similarly, rat specimens exhibit comparable tonotopic organization but with reduced absolute fiber numbers: 45.18 ± 9.31 per habenula perforata in the basal hook, 124.53 ± 19.37 at the basal-middle turn, and 84.21 ± 16.62 in the mid-middle turn region [8–10, 16]. The habenular perforations of mice had similar distribution patterns of sound-localizing fibers, but the number of nerve fibers per perforation was even smaller, measuring 25.18 ± 7.24 in the basal hook region, 58.23 ± 10.31 in the basal-median junction, and 42.64 ± 9.33 in the

D. Ding et al., *Histopathological Atlas of the Inner Ear*,
https://doi.org/10.1007/978-981-95-6338-8_11

middle of the second turn [6, 7, 11, 12, 17]. These comparative anatomical studies demonstrate significant interspecies variability in habenula perforata innervation density, with smaller species generally showing fewer nerve fibers per neuropore. Importantly, substantial intraspecies regional differences exist along the cochlear spiral, necessitating standardized sampling protocols that account for both longitudinal (turn-specific) and radial (modiolus-to-cochlear lateral wall) positions when quantifying auditory nerve fibers. Such methodological rigor ensures valid comparisons within and between experimental groups while controlling for the cochlea's inherent structural heterogeneity.

The habenula perforata mainly contains three functionally distinct nerve fiber populations: type I afferents (comprising approximately 85.7% of total fibers), type II afferents, and cochlear efferents, which collectively account for the remaining 14.3% of fibers. This disproportionate distribution establishes type I afferent fibers as the dominant neural component within each neuropore, reflecting their primary role in transmitting auditory signals from inner hair cells to the central nervous system [2, 3, 18]. The numerical predominance of type I fibers correlates with their functional specialization for high-fidelity sound encoding, while the sparse type II and efferent fibers likely serve more modulatory functions in auditory processing.

11.2 Quantitative Observation of Afferent Nerve Synapse Beneath the Cochlear Inner Hair Cells

The primary afferent pathway of the auditory system is dominated by type I spiral ganglion neurons, which constitute over 95% of cochlear peripheral neurons and form specialized synaptic connections with inner hair cells, establishing this neural population as the principal conduit for acoustic signal transmission to the central nervous system. This overwhelming numerical predominance of type I neurons, coupled with the fact that they directly receive nerve impulse signals from inner hair cells, underscores their critical role in encoding and relaying precise auditory information, while the sparse type II afferent system appears to serve more ancillary functions in cochlear signaling.

The afferent synapse between inner hair cells and type I spiral ganglion neurons constitutes a specialized neuroepithelial junction where mechano-electrical transduction occurs. This synaptic complex comprises three key elements: the presynaptic membrane of inner hair cells containing neurotransmitter vesicles, the postsynaptic membrane of spiral ganglion neuron terminals, and the intervening synaptic cleft. As the primary auditory receptors, inner hair cells transform mechanical sound vibrations into electrochemical signals through glutamate release from presynaptic ribbons (Fig. 11.2), with synaptic transmission involving precisely coordinated vesicle production, mobilization, and calcium-triggered exocytosis at active zones. The presynaptic machinery's exquisite organization enables temporally precise neurotransmitter release essential for sound encoding fidelity.

Glutamate released from inner hair cells binds to AMPA receptors on type I spiral ganglion neuron terminals, inducing cation influx (primarily $Na+$ and $K+$) that generates excitatory postsynaptic potentials through localized membrane depolarization. This synaptic transmission is tightly regulated by glutamate recycling via high-affinity transporters (EAAT1/5) and enzymatic breakdown, maintaining optimal cleft concentrations. However, pathological glutamate accumulation triggers excitotoxicity through a well-characterized cascade: initial postsynaptic edema progresses to dendritic retraction and ultimately spiral ganglion neuron apoptosis via retrograde degeneration. Remarkably, when neuronal somata remain viable, robust synaptic regeneration occurs within 3–7 days through neurite sprouting and ribbon synapse reformation, enabling full functional recovery of auditory thresholds [19–21]. This intrinsic repair capacity highlights the plasticity of cochlear afferent synapses while underscoring the critical window for therapeutic intervention before irreversible neuronal loss occurs.

Irreversible loss of type I spiral ganglion neurons leads to permanent reductions in postsynaptic densities beneath inner hair cells, often accompanied by secondary presynaptic remodeling through retrograde trophic effects [13, 22]. Notably, inner hair cells exhibit intrinsic resistance to glutamate excitotoxicity despite being the primary source of afferent neurotransmitter production and release. This is due to the lack of functional glutamate receptors within their bodies—suggesting that glutamate excitotoxic damage specifically targets postsynaptic elements bearing ionotropic glutamate receptors, rather than the inner hair cells that produce glutamate transmitters [23] (Fig. 7.15; Fig. 11.3). The consequent degeneration of supporting cells and feedback reduction of presynaptic ribbon in the inner hair cells likely represent downstream effects rather than primary insults, highlighting the selective vulnerability of the afferent neural components in cochlear glutamatergic neurotransmission (Fig. 11.4).

11.3 Quantitative Observation of the Spiral Ganglion Neurons in Rosenthal's Canal

The spiral ganglion neurons within Rosenthal's canal serve as the exclusive first-order afferent neurons of the auditory pathway, forming critical neural connections between cochlear hair cells and the central auditory system. These bipolar neurons extend peripheral processes through the habenula perforata to synapse with both inner and outer hair cells, while their central axons traverse modiolar bony channels to coalesce into the auditory nerve bundle projecting to cochlear nuclei in the brainstem. This precise neural architecture facilitates

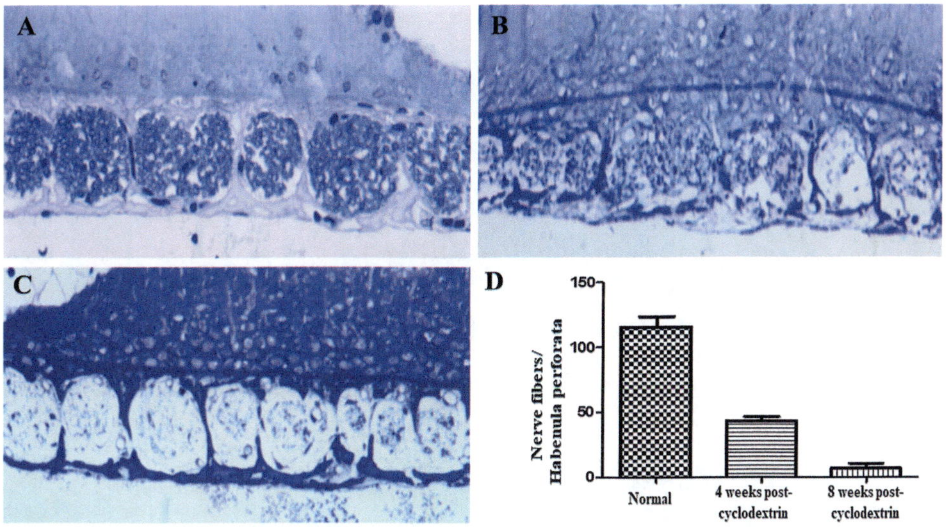

Fig. 11.1 Progressive degeneration of auditory nerve fibers in the habenula perforata following cyclodextrin administration. (**A**) Control specimens show that the intact myelinated nerve fibers are densely packed within the habenula perforata. (**B**) Four weeks post-treatment (4000 mg/kg cyclodextrin), significant fiber demyelination and approximately 60% reduction in fiber density become evident. (**C**) By 8 weeks, near-complete (>90%) loss of auditory nerve fibers is observed, leaving the habenula perforata largely empty. (**D**) Quantitative analysis confirms the time-dependent neurodegeneration within habenula perforata, with progressive fiber loss reaching over 90% at the 8-week endpoint, illustrating that the peripheral auditory nerve system of the cochlea undergoes severe secondary delayed damage after the complete destruction of hair cells

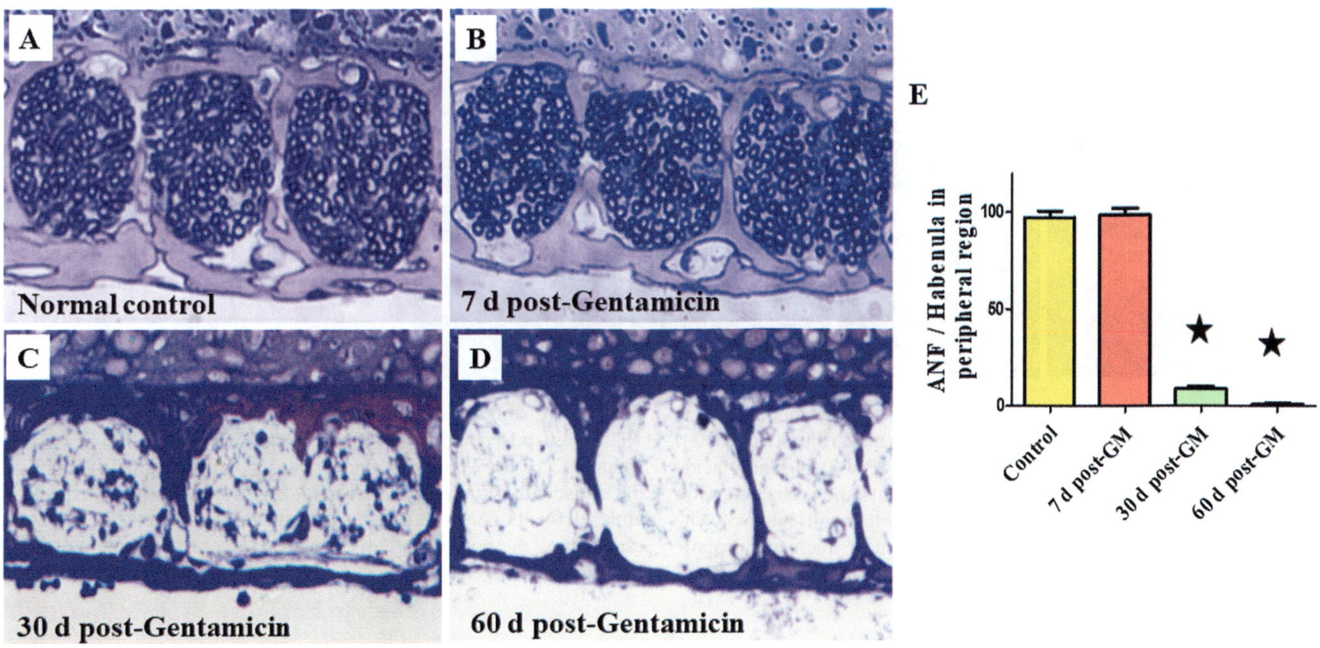

Fig. 11.2 Sagittal section of the habenula perforata of the rat shows delayed secondary destruction of peripheral auditory nerve fibers induced by intratympanic injection of gentamicin. (**A**) The cochlear peripheral nerve fibers in a control rat are present normally. (**B**). Seven days after intratympanic injection of gentamicin, the auditory peripheral nerve fibers were intact. (**C**) Thirty days after intratympanic injection of gentamicin, most auditory peripheral nerve fibers in the habenula perforata were missing. (**D**) Sixty days after intratympanic injection of gentamicin, the auditory peripheral nerve fibers were completely destroyed. (**E**) Quantitative analysis of the density of the auditory peripheral nerve fibers showed that delayed secondary destruction of the auditory peripheral nerve fibers occurs 30 days after intratympanic injection of gentamicin to destroy the cochlear hair cells (Reproduced with permission from Ding et al. [11, 12]). This indicates that the auditory peripheral nerve fibers develop secondary lesions within 30 days after the complete destruction of cochlear hair cells

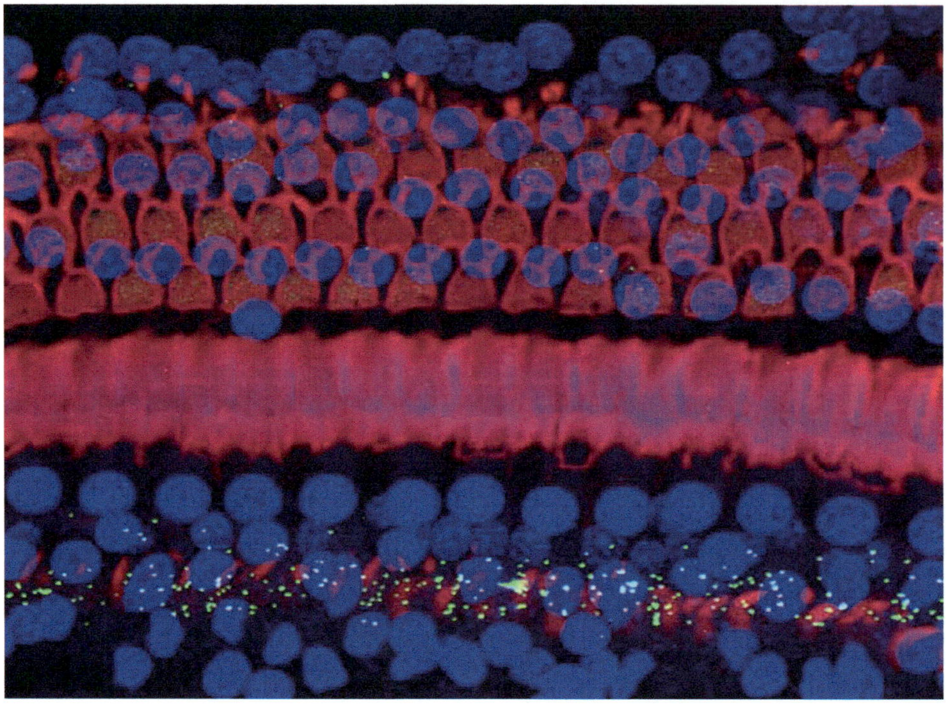

Fig. 11.3 The precise localization of presynaptic ribbons in rat inner hair cells using CtBP2 immunolabeling. The characteristic dense arrangement of these synaptic structures (green fluorescence) facilitates vesicular glutamate release into the synaptic cleft of type I afferent nerve terminals. The distinctive punctate staining pattern reveals highly organized presynaptic active zones, which are crucial for phase-locked neurotransmitter release during auditory transmission

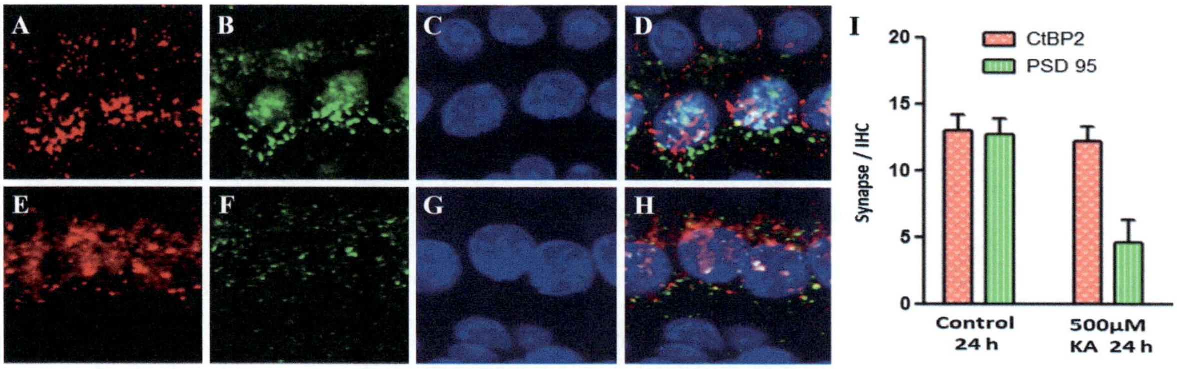

Fig. 11.4 The selective vulnerability of postsynaptic elements to excitotoxic damage using triple-labeling of presynaptic ribbons (CtBP2), postsynaptic densities (PSD-95), and nuclei (ToPro-3) in kainic acid-treated cochlear explants. (**A–D**) Control explants show characteristic paired presynaptic (13.78 ± 1.64 spots per inner hair cell) and postsynaptic (13.8 ± 1.87 spots) organizations with intact nuclear morphology. (**E–H**) Following 500 μM kainic acid exposure for 24 h, while presynaptic ribbons show intact, non-significant reduction (12.15 ± 1.25 spots), postsynaptic densities undergo severe depletion (4.7 ± 2.23 spots; $F(2,15) = 78.37$, $p < 0.001$). (**I**) Quantitative analysis confirms the statistically significant preferential loss of PSD-95-positive postsynaptic elements compared to CtBP2-labeled presynaptic components, establishing the postsynaptic membrane as the primary target of glutamate-mediated excitotoxicity in cochlear afferent synapses

the transmission of auditory signals through a well-defined ascending pathway: from cochlear nuclei to superior olivary complex, through lateral lemniscus to inferior colliculus, then to medial geniculate body of thalamus, and ultimately to auditory cortex—constituting the complete neural circuit for sound perception and processing [4, 24–26]. The strategic position of spiral ganglion neurons as the gateway between peripheral transduction and central auditory processing underscores their fundamental role in hearing function.

Quantitative assessment of spiral ganglion neuron populations has evolved through several methodological refinements to improve accuracy in evaluating cochlear nerve integrity. Initial approaches involving exhaustive cell counts across complete serial sections proved impractical due to technical challenges, including sectioning artifacts and counting errors from overlapping profiles in adjacent slices. While subsequent interval sampling methods offered improved efficiency, they introduced significant measurement variability and failed to capture tonotopic variations along the cochlear spiral. Current best practices employ turn-specific density measurements, which provide both regional resolution and statistical reliability by analyzing defined segments of Rosenthal's canal [1, 8–12, 27, 28]. This standardized approach enables precise characterization of neurodegeneration patterns while accounting for the cochlea's anatomical gradients, representing a significant advancement in quantitative auditory histopathology.

11.4 Quantitative Observation of Cochlear Efferent Nerve Fibers in the Tunnel of Corti

The cochlear efferent system originates from distinct neuronal populations within the superior olivary complex, with the lateral olivocochlear neurons primarily projecting ipsilaterally and the medial olivocochlear neurons predominantly innervating the contralateral cochlea. These descending cochlear efferent nerve fibers travel intracranially with the inferior vestibular nerve bundle, pass through the cochlear neuroforamen and enter the modiolus of the cochlea where they bifurcate into two distinct pathways: one pathway is the inner spiral bundle fibers, which synapse with type I afferent dendrites beneath the inner hair cells, and the other pathway traverses the tunnel of Corti to form the tunneled radial fibers that innervate the outer hair cells. The anatomical organization of these pathways reflects their functional specialization—while lateral system fibers form compact bundles that challenge individual fiber resolution, medial system fibers display characteristic radial dispersion through the tunnel of Corti, which enables precise quantification of these cholinergic efferent nerve fibers [2, 3, 29]. This dichotomous innervation pattern underlies the differential modulation of inner versus outer hair cell function in auditory processing.

The acetylcholinesterase histochemical staining technique enables selective visualization of olivocochlear efferent pathways due to the enzyme's exclusive presence in efferent neurons and their processes. This method distinctly labels both the compact internal spiral bundle fibers synapsing with type I afferents and the dispersed tunnel-crossing fibers innervating outer hair cells [2, 3, 15, 29–31] (Figs. 6.23 and 8.21; Fig. 11.5). Quantitative analysis combines

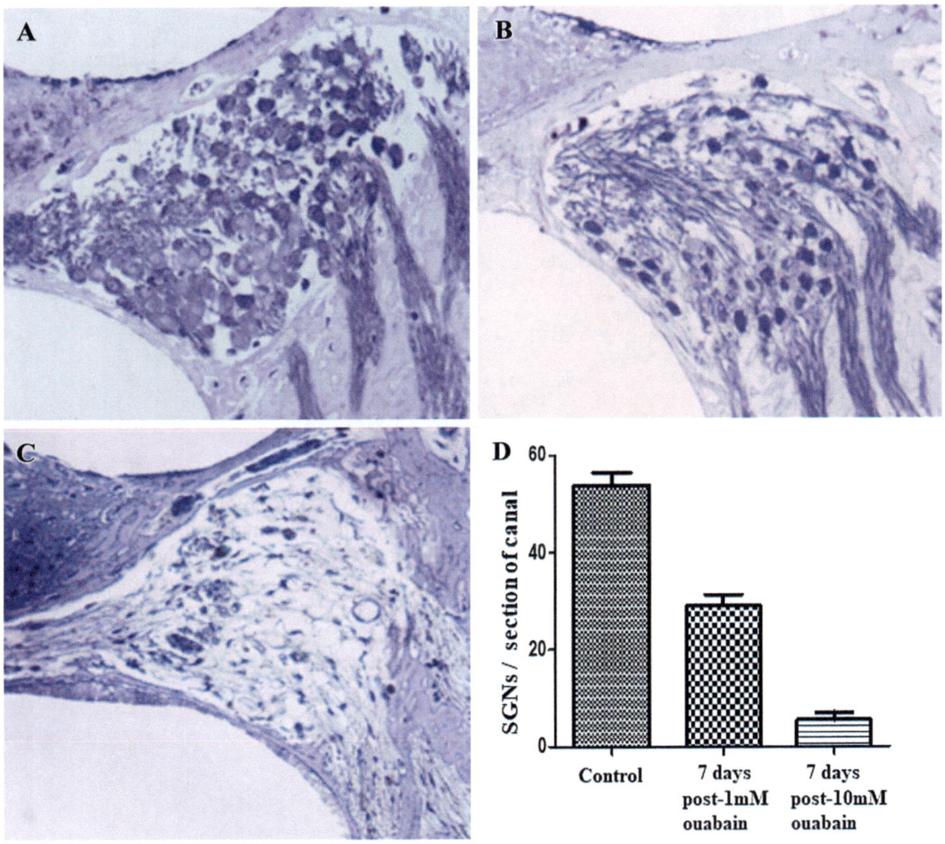

Fig. 11.5 Dose-dependent neurotoxic effects of ouabain on rat spiral ganglion neurons by semi-thin slices. (**A**) Control specimens show normal ganglion cell density (56.17 ± 5.09 cells/section) in Rosenthal's canal at the cochlear basal turn. (**B**) Significant spiral ganglion cell loss was noted one week after application of 1 mM ouabain in the round window niche (31.03 ± 6.34 cells/section). (**C**) One week of application of 10 mM ouabain to the round window niche resulted in near-total ganglion cell depletion (6.12 ± 3.21 cells/section). (**D**) Quantitative analysis confirms the progressive neurodegeneration, establishing ouabain's potency as a selective spiral ganglion toxin when applied locally to the round window niche. This experimental model provides precise control over the degree of primary auditory neuropathy while preserving cochlear hair cells

the succinate dehydrogenase staining to label the hair cells and the acetylcholinesterase staining to label the cochlear efferent nerve fibers and terminals, and employs standardized counting protocols at 400× magnification using a calibrated eyepiece micrometer (0.24-mm scale length) to systematically assess cellular and neural integrity along the entire cochlear spiral. The chinchilla cochleogram software processes these raw counts to generate comprehensive lesion profiles, automatically calculating percentage losses for both sensory cells and efferent fibers while producing group-averaged cochleograms that statistically summarize pathological changes [2, 3, 29, 31] (Fig. 11.6). Combining this double staining labeling method with cochleogram observation and production technology can simultaneously perform quantitative assessment of the entire cochlear hair cells and cochlear efferent nervous system.

11.5 Quantitative Observation of Central Auditory Nerve Fibers in the Cochlear Neuroforamen

The cochlear neuroforamen serves as the exclusive conduit for both the ascending cochlear afferent system and the descending olivocochlear efferent system, with temporal bone sagittal sections providing optimal anatomical visualization [11, 12] (Fig. 11.7). This orthogonal plane permits simultaneous assessment of total fiber counts at low magnification and detailed density measurements at high resolution, enabling comprehensive evaluation of auditory nerve integrity. Advanced immunohistochemical techniques further enhance diagnostic specificity by differentially labeling type I (calretinin-positive) and type II (peripherin-positive) afferent fibers alongside

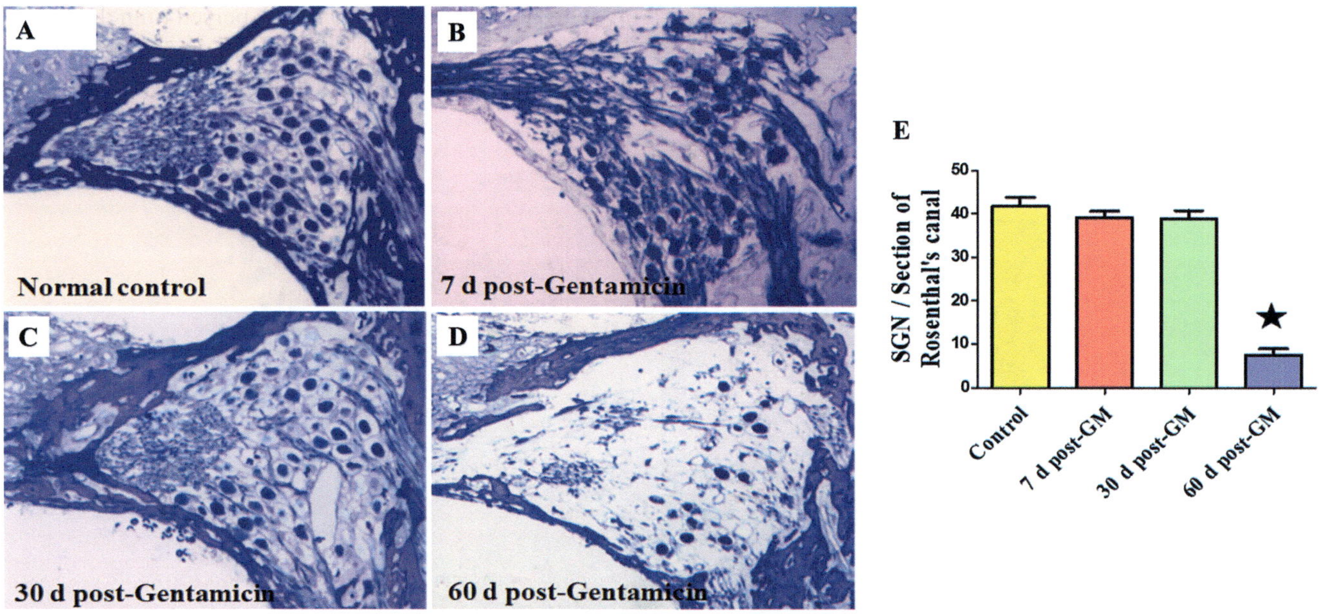

Fig. 11.6 Sagittal section of Rosenthal's canal of the rat shows delayed secondary destruction of spiral ganglion neurons induced by intratympanic injection of gentamicin. (**A**) The spiral ganglion neurons in Rosenthal's canal in a control rat are present normally. (**B**) Seven days after intratympanic injection of gentamicin, the spiral ganglion neurons in Rosenthal's canal were intact. (**C**) Thirty days after intratympanic injection of gentamicin, the spiral ganglion within Rosenthal's canal began to develop pathological swelling. (**D**) Sixty days after intratympanic injection of gentamicin, a large number of spiral ganglion cells are completely destroyed and missing. (**E**) Quantitative analysis of the density of the spiral ganglion neurons in Rosenthal's canal showed that delayed secondary destruction of the spiral ganglion neurons occurs 60 days after intratympanic injection of gentamicin to destroy the cochlear hair cells (Reproduced with permission from Ding et al. [11, 12])

cholinergic efferent projections. This multimodal approach facilitates precise quantification of discrete neural populations while maintaining topological relationships within the nerve bundle, offering superior pathological detection sensitivity compared to conventional histological methods. The sagittal section of the temporal bone is a unique anatomical orientation, therefore, it represents a standard for assessing both quantitative and qualitative changes in the composition of the nerve fibers leading from the cochlea to the intracranial auditory center (Figs. 11.8, 11.9, and 11.10).

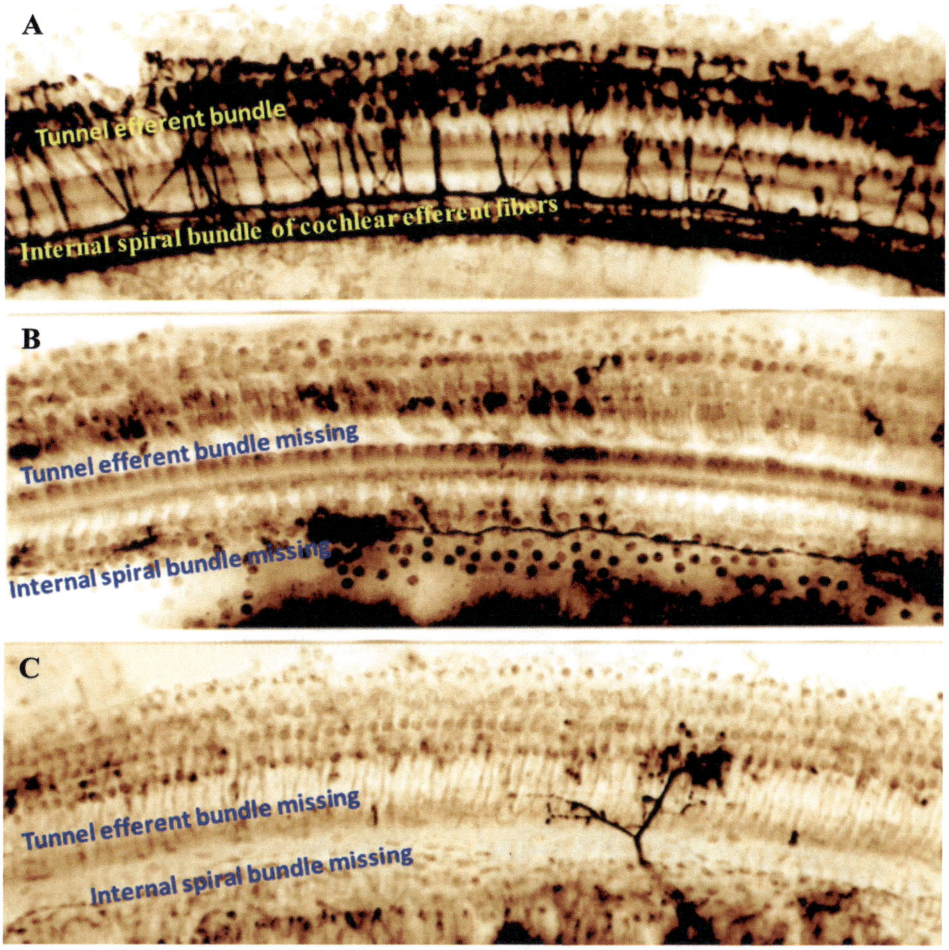

Fig. 11.7 Acetylcholinesterase histochemical staining was used to demonstrate the surgical efficacy of cochlear efferent nerve transection. (**A**) Control specimens show the characteristic organization of both efferent systems: the dense internal spiral bundle innervates type I afferent nerve fibers beneath the inner hair cells, whereas dispersed tunneled radial fibers pass through the tunnel of Corti to innervate the outer hair cells. (**B**) Two weeks after the surgical cutting off the cochlear efferent nerve bundle at the cochlear neuroforamen, the tunnel efferent fibers passing through the tunnel of Corti disappeared completely, but a very few residual cochlear efferent fibers in the internal spiral bundle were occasionally seen in the basilar membrane, suggesting that the medial olivocochlear efferent system may be more severely damaged than the lateral olivocochlear efferent system. (**C**) Two weeks after de-efferent severing, the cochlear efferent nerve fibers in the internal spiral bundle were completely missing. Occasionally, a few remaining efferent nerve fibers passing through the tunnel of Corti can be seen in the basilar membrane

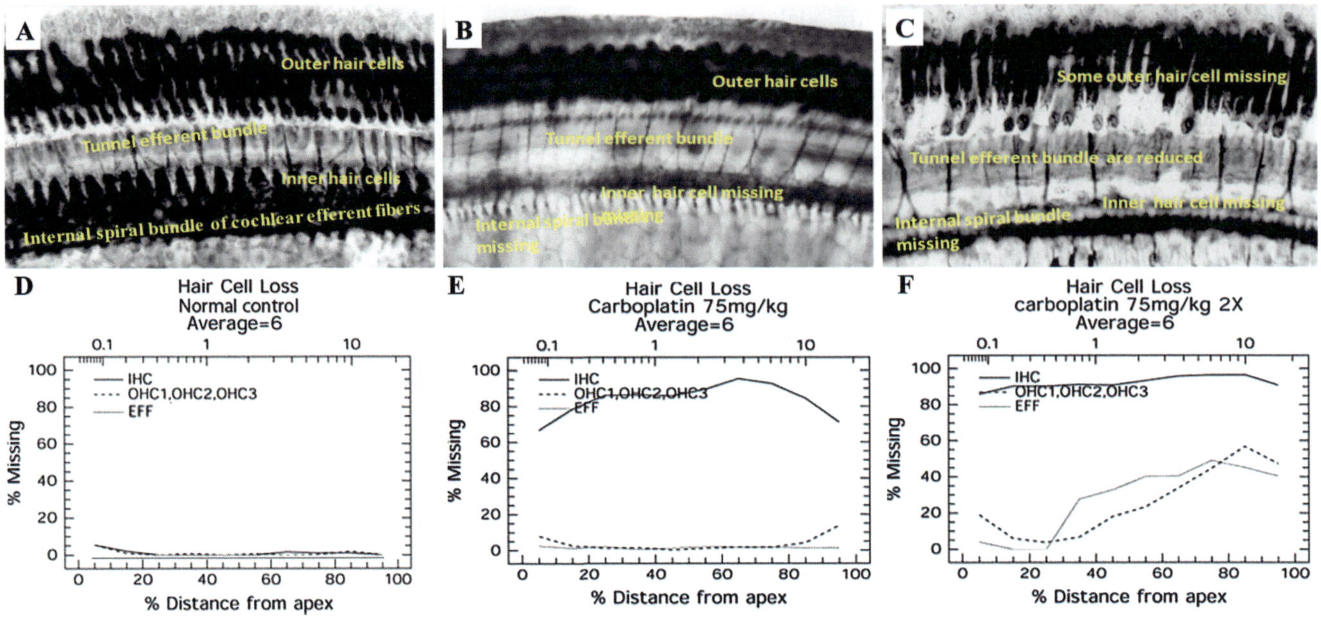

Fig. 11.8 The differential effects of carboplatin toxicity on cochlear hair cells and their associated efferent innervation through histochemical double-labeling. (**A**) Control preparations demonstrate intact succinate dehydrogenase-positive hair cells and acetylcholinesterase-stained efferent fibers in both internal spiral and tunnel radial bundles. (**B**) Single-dose carboplatin (75 mg/kg) selectively eliminates >80% of inner hair cells while sparing outer hair cells, with corresponding loss of internal spiral bundle efferents but preserved tunnel-crossing fibers. (**C**) Double-dose treatment (75 mg/kg×2) produces near-total inner hair cell destruction and 40% outer hair cell loss in the basal turn, accompanied by proportional reduction (40%) of tunnel radial efferent nerve fibers. (**D–F**). Cochleogram analyses quantify these dose-dependent patterns: selective inner hair cell damage affects only the internal spiral efferent bundle, while additional outer hair cell loss correlates with tunnel radial fiber depletion. These findings suggest that the efferent nerve damage after carboplatin treatment represents secondary degeneration rather than primary neurotoxicity, as efferent fiber loss precisely mirrors their target hair cell pathology without evidence of independent neural damage. This hierarchical vulnerability demonstrates the tight trophic coupling and interdependence between hair cells and their efferent innervation

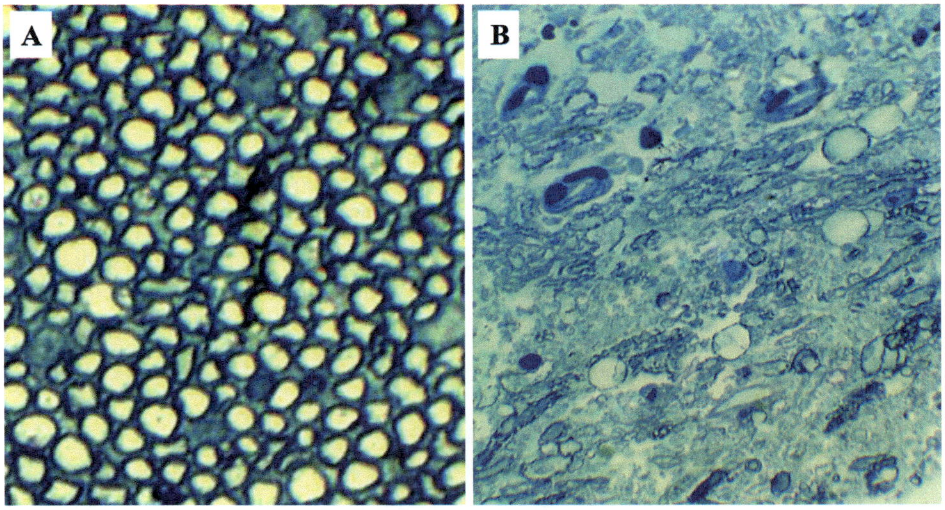

Fig. 11.9 The profound demyelinating effects of doxorubicin on auditory nerve fibers in sagittal temporal bone sections. (**A**) Control specimens show the characteristic organization of myelinated axons within the cochlear neuroforamen, with intact myelin sheaths surrounding densely packed nerve fibers. (**B**) One week after doxorubicin injection into the cochlear neuroforamen, specimens reveal extensive myelin disruption, with complete loss of normal axonal architecture, the Schwann cells, and the glial cells integrity, illustrating the potent neurotoxic effects of doxorubicin on peripheral auditory pathways. This model provides a robust platform for studying drug-induced auditory neuropathy and demyelination mechanisms

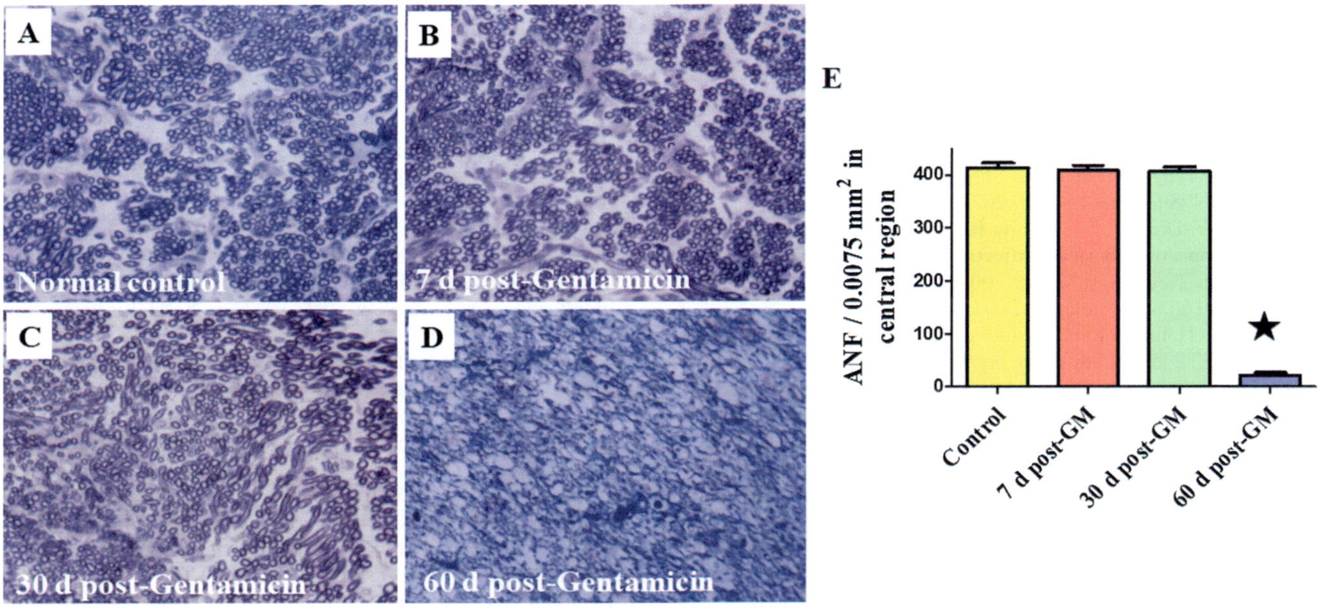

Fig. 11.10 Sagittal section through the cochlear neuroforamen of the rat shows the delayed secondary lesions in auditory fibers leading to the central cochlear nucleus caused by intratympanic injection of gentamicin. (**A**) The auditory nerve fibers leading to the cochlear nucleus in a control rat appear normal. (**B**) Seven days after intratympanic injection of gentamicin, the central end of the auditory nerve fibers leading to the central auditory nervous system expressed normal structure. (**C**) Thirty days after intratympanic injection of gentamicin, the central end of the auditory nerve fibers leading to the cochlear nucleus maintained its intact morphology. (**D**) Sixty days after intratympanic injection of gentamicin, massive destruction of auditory nerve fibers leading to the central auditory nervous system was detected. (**E**) Quantitative analysis of the density of auditory nerve fibers leading to the central auditory nervous system showed that about 60 days after the intratympanic injection of gentamicin to destroy the cochlear hair cells, the auditory nerve fibers leading to the central end of the auditory system were severely demyelinated (Reproduced with permission from Ding et al. [11, 12]). A comprehensive analysis of the experimental results from Figs. 11.2, 11.6, and the present figure shows that after complete destruction of cochlear hair cells, the delayed secondary damage to peripheral auditory nerve fibers occurred earlier than the secondary damage to the ganglion and the central end of auditory nerve fibers. This suggests that the delayed secondary damage to the auditory nervous system caused by cochlear hair cell destruction spreads gradually from the periphery to the central nervous system

References

1. Ding D, Wang J, Zhang XY, Sun H, Salvi R. Quantitative analysis of hair cells, spiral ganglion neurons, and nerve fibers in the same cochlea. Chin J Otorhinolaryngol Skull Base Surg. 1998;4(4):200–4.
2. Ding D, Zheng X, Wang J. [Quantitation of nerve fibers in habenula perforata in chinchilla]. Zhonghua Er Bi Yan Hou Ke Za Zhi. 1998;33(1):30–31.
3. Ding D, Zheng XY, Hu BH, Henderson D, Richard S. Quantitative analysis of cochlear efferent fibers in the tunnel of Corti. Acta Otolaryngol. 1998;12(2):65–68.
4. Ding D, Qi W, Qu Y, Salvi R. Chapter 1: Anatomy of the inner ear. In: Ding D, editor. Science of the inner ear. China Science and Technology Press; 2010. p. 1–8.
5. Ding D, Qi W, Qu Y, Salvi R. Chapter 6: Research techniques of the inner ear morphology. In: Ding D, editor. Science of the inner ear. China Science and Technology Press; 2010. p. 50–88.
6. Ding D, Yu J, Li P, et al. Standardization of experimental animals temporal bone sections. J Otol.. 2015;10(2):66–71. https://doi.org/10.1016/j.joto.2015.08.001.
7. Ding D, Jiang H, Chen GD, et al. N-acetyl-cysteine prevents age-related hearing loss and the progressive loss of inner hair cells in gamma-glutamyl transferase 1 deficient mice. Aging (Albany NY). 2016;8(4):730–50. https://doi.org/10.18632/aging.100927.
8. Ding D, Jiang H, Manohar S, et al. Spatiotemporal developmental upregulation of prestin correlates with the severity and location of cyclodextrin-induced outer hair cell loss and hearing loss. Front Cell Dev Biol. 2021;9:643709. https://doi.org/10.3389/fcell.2021.643709.
9. Ding D, Jiang H, Salvi R. Cochlear spiral ganglion neuron degeneration following cyclodextrin-induced hearing loss. Hear Res. 2021;400:108125. https://doi.org/10.1016/j.heares.2020.108125.
10. Ding D, Manohar S, Kador PF, Salvi R. Multifunctional redox modulator prevents blast-induced loss of cochlear and vestibular hair cells and auditory spiral ganglion neurons. Sci Rep. 2024;14(1):15296. https://doi.org/10.1038/s41598-024-66406-1.
11. Ding D, Shi L, Xing Y, et al. Sagittal sectioning of temporal bones and quantitative measurement of neural densities in the inner ear in normal mice. Chin J Otorhinolaryngol. Skull Base Surg. 2024;30(6):69–75. https://doi.org/10.11798/j.issn.1007-1520.202424331.
12. Ding D, Shi L, Xing Y, et al. Secondary neural damage in the inner ear induced by intratympanic gentamicin injection. Chin J Otorhinolaryngol. Skull Base Surg. 2024;30(6):11–19. https://doi.org/10.11798/j.issn.1007-1520.202424356.
13. Fu Y, Ding D, Jiang H, Salvi R. Ouabain-induced cochlear degeneration in rat. Neurotox Res. 2012;22(2):158–69. https://doi.org/10.1007/s12640-012-9320-0.
14. Yu J, Ding D, Sun H, Salvi R, Roth JA. Trimethyltin-induced cochlear degeneration in rat. J Otol. 2016;11(3):118–26. https://doi.org/10.1016/j.joto.2016.07.001.

15. McFadden SL, Ding D, Jiang H, Salvi RJ. Time course of efferent fiber and spiral ganglion cell degeneration following complete hair cell loss in the chinchilla. Brain Res. 2004;997(1):40–51. https://doi.org/10.1016/j.brainres.2003.10.031.
16. Ding D, Li P, Qi W, et al. Study on delayed secondary lesions in the cochlea triggered by cochlear hair cell death. Chin J Otorhinolaryngol. Skull Base Surg. 2022;28(6):1–10. https://doi.org/10.11798/j.issn.1007-1520.2022221001.
17. Zheng QY, Ding D, Yu H, Salvi RJ, Johnson KR. A locus on distal chromosome 10 (ahl4) affecting age-related hearing loss in A/J mice. Neurobiol Aging. 2009;30(10):1693–705. https://doi.org/10.1016/j.neurobiolaging.2007.12.011.
18. Spoendlin H. Innervation densities of the cochlea. Acta Otolaryngol. 1972;73(2):235–48. https://doi.org/10.3109/00016487209138937.
19. Puel JL, Ruel J, Gervais d'Aldin C, Pujol R. Excitotoxicity and repair of cochlear synapses after noise-trauma induced hearing loss. Neuroreport. 1998;9(9):2109–14. https://doi.org/10.1097/00001756-199806220-00037.
20. Pujol R, Puel JL. Excitotoxicity, synaptic repair, and functional recovery in the mammalian cochlea: a review of recent findings. Ann N Y Acad Sci. 1999;884:249–54. https://doi.org/10.1111/j.1749-6632.1999.tb08646.x.
21. Zheng XY, Salvi RJ, McFadden SL, Ding DL, Henderson D. Recovery of kainic acid excitotoxicity in chinchilla cochlea. Ann N Y Acad Sci. 1999;884:255–69. https://doi.org/10.1111/j.1749-6632.1999.tb08647.x.
22. Sun H, Hashino E, Ding DL, Salvi RJ. Reversible and irreversible damage to cochlear afferent neurons by kainic acid excitotoxicity. J Comp Neurol. 2001;430(2):172–81. https://doi.org/10.1002/1096-9861(20010205)430:2<172::aid-cne1023>3.0.co;2-w.
23. Ding D, Qi W, Jiang H, Salvi R. Excitotoxic damage to auditory nerve afferents and spiral ganglion neurons is correlated with developmental upregulation of AMPA and KA receptors. Hear Res. 2021;411:108358. https://doi.org/10.1016/j.heares.2021.108358.
24. Schuknecht H. Anatomy. In: Schuknecht H, editor. Pathology of the ear. 1st ed. Cambridge: Harvard University Press; 1974. p. 40–96.
25. Ding D, Li M, Jiang C, Salvi R. Chapter 3: Anatomy of the temporal bone and inner ear. In: Ding D, editor. Morphology of the inner ear. Heilongjiang Science and Technology Press; 2001. p. 10–17.
26. Hayes SH, Ding D, Salvi R, Allman BL. Anatomy and physiology of the external, middle and inner ear. In: Celesia GG, editor. Disorders of peripheral and central auditory processing. Handbook of clinical neurophysiology, vol. 10. New York: Elsevier; 2013. p. 3–23.
27. Spoendlin H, Brun JP. The block-surface technique for evaluation of cochlear pathology. Arch Otorhinolaryngol. 1974;208(2):137–45. https://doi.org/10.1007/BF00453927.
28. Keithley EM, Feldman ML. The spiral ganglion and hair cells of Bronx waltzer mice. Hear Res. 1983;12(3):381–91. https://doi.org/10.1016/0378-5955(83)90007-2.
29. Ding D, Li M, Zheng XY, Wang J, Salvi R. Cochleogram for assessing hair cells and efferent fibers in carboplatin-treated ear. J Clin Otorhinolaryngol. 1999;13(11):510–12.
30. Zheng XY, Henderson D, McFadden SL, Ding DL, Salvi RJ. Auditory nerve fiber responses following chronic cochlear de-efferentation. J Comp Neurol. 1999;406(1):72–86. https://doi.org/10.1002/(sici)1096-9861(19990329)406:1<72::aid-cne5>3.3.co;2-1.
31. Ding D, Zhang J, Yang K, et al. Growth and development process of calcitonin gene-related peptide and acetylcholinesterase in rat cochlear efferent nervous system. Chin J Otorhinolaryngol Skull Base Surg. 2020;26(6):662–8. https://doi.org/10.3969/j.issn.1006-7299.2020.06.012.

12 Several Histochemical Staining Techniques Commonly Used to Assess the Pathological Lesions of the Inner Ear

Histochemical staining techniques have emerged as essential methodological tools in life sciences and medical research, offering precise qualitative and quantitative approaches for identifying cellular components, including specific proteins, organelles, and microstructures, while correlating morphological features with functional states. These techniques now represent indispensable scientific methodologies for both research applications and pathological diagnostics. The current discussion focuses specifically on selected staining protocols most frequently employed in evaluating pathological alterations within the cochlear and vestibular systems, providing fundamental technical references for pathology investigations of the inner ear.

12.1 Specific Markers of Hair Cells and Supporting Cells

The membranous labyrinth comprises two principal cell populations—sensory hair cells and supporting cells—whose accurate identification through specific markers is essential for inner ear research. Multiple established techniques exist for selective hair cell labeling, including immunostaining with anti-Myosin VI, anti-Myo7a antibodies, and AM1-43 fluorescence labeling for hair cells, and anti-Prestin antibody for outer hair cells. Similarly, various markers reliably identify supporting cell subtypes: anti-KHRI-1 antibody and anti-galectin-3 antibody for Hensen cells, anti-KHRI-2 antibody for multiple epithelial populations, including border and Hensen cells, anti-KHRI-3 antibody and anti-IFIT3 antibody for Deiters and outer pillar cells, and anti-SOX2 for phalangeal and Deiters' cells, among others [1–7]. As a representative protocol, the dual-labeling technique combining anti-Myo7a (hair cell-specific) and anti-SOX2 (supporting cell-specific) antibodies provides a robust method for simultaneous visualization of both cell populations, with the staining procedure detailed in subsequent sections.

The cochlear basilar membrane was fixed in 10% formalin prior to microdissection and subsequent immunostaining. Specimens were incubated overnight at 4°C in a primary antibody solution containing rabbit anti-Myosin VI antibody (1:100) and goat anti-SOX2 antibody (1:100) diluted in 0.1 M PBS with 1% Triton X-100 and 5% donkey serum. Following PBS washes, tissues were incubated for 2 h with secondary antibodies: TRITC-conjugated donkey anti-rabbit IgG (1:200) and Alexa Fluor 488-conjugated donkey anti-goat IgG (1:200). Nuclear counterstaining was performed using ToPro-3 for 40 min before mounting. Confocal microscopy with appropriate filter sets revealed distinct cellular labeling: Myosin VI-positive hair cells (red), SOX2-positive supporting cells (green), and ToPro-3-stained nuclei (blue) (Figs. 7.24A, 7.25, and 8.28; Fig. 12.1). This protocol enables simultaneous visualization of both major cell populations (hair cells and support cells) in the cochlear and vestibular tissue.

12.2 Staining Methods of Cell Nuclei Commonly Used in the Study of Inner Ear Pathology

The nucleus represents the central regulatory hub of eukaryotic cells, containing essential structural domains—the nuclear envelope, chromatin, nucleolus, nuclear matrix, and nuclear pores—that collectively orchestrate genetic information storage, processing, and cellular metabolism. During pathological cell death, nuclear morphology undergoes characteristic changes: necrosis induces progressive nuclear swelling and dissolution alongside plasma membrane disintegration, whereas apoptosis triggers chromatin condensation and nuclear fragmentation with concomitant cell shrinkage. These distinct nuclear phenotypes serve as fundamental histological markers for discriminating cell death pathways. Investigative applications utilize diverse nuclear staining methodologies ranging from conventional histological dyes (hematoxylin, carmine) to advanced fluorescent probes (DAPI, Hoechst, propidium iodide) and viability indicators (acridine orange, ethidium bromide), and more [8–16], providing researchers

D. Ding et al., *Histopathological Atlas of the Inner Ear*,
https://doi.org/10.1007/978-981-95-6338-8_12

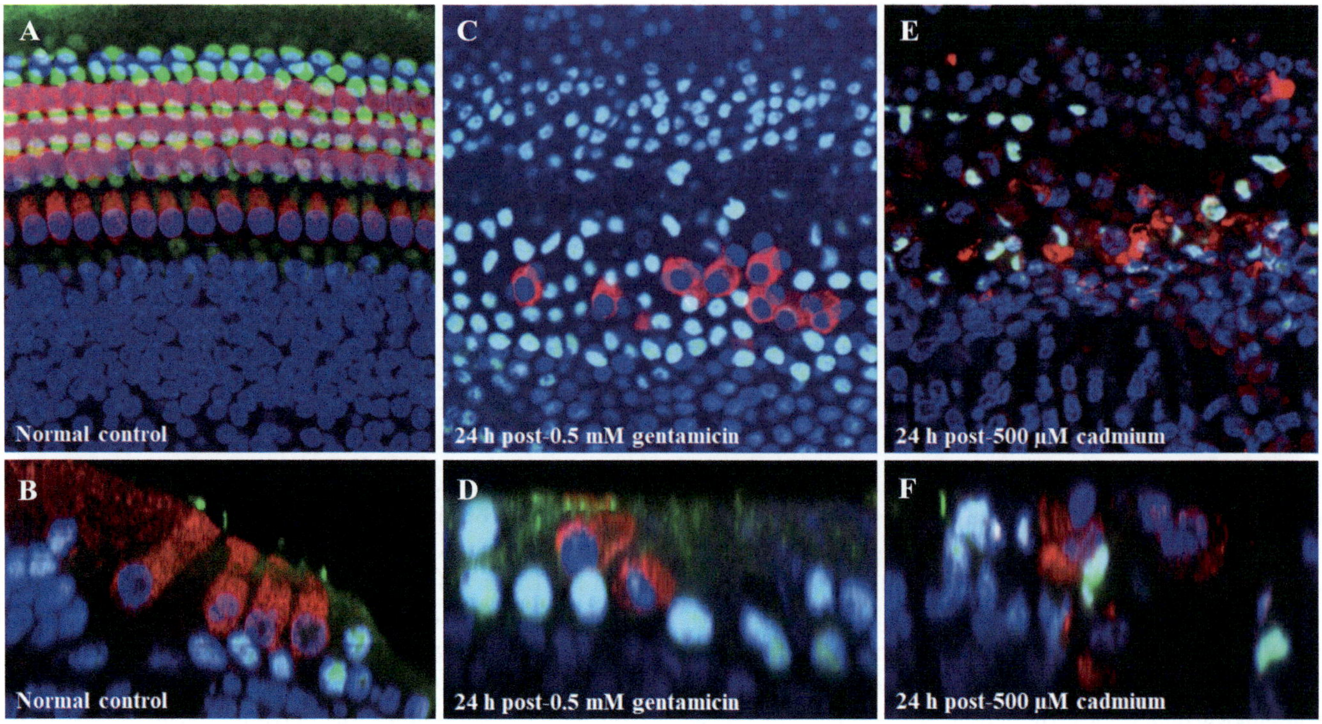

Fig. 12.1 The utility of triple fluorescence labeling for evaluating cochlear pathological changes in rat cochlear explants. (**A**) Surface preparation in a normal cochlear explant reveals characteristic Myosin VI expression (red) in hair cells, SOX2 (green) in supporting cells, and ToPro-3 (blue) in nuclei, establishing baseline cellular architecture. (**B**) A cross-sectional view of the basilar membrane of a normal control cochlear explant showing the spatial relationship between triple-fluorescent labeled cells. (**C**) Triple fluorescent staining of a rat cochlear explant cultured with 0.5 mM gentamicin sulfate for 24 h shows that anti-Myosin VI-antibody labeled hair cells had a large number of absences, but the supporting cells labeled with anti-SOX2-antibody beneath the sensory hair cells are intact. (**D**) A cross-sectional view of the basilar membrane from a cochlear explant treated with 0.5 mM gentamicin for 24 h validates that gentamicin selectively destroys cochlear hair cells without initially destroying supporting cells. (**E**) The surface preparation of cochlear basilar membrane with the triple staining from a rat cochlear explant incubated with 500 μM cadmium chloride for 24 h indicates that all hair cells and supporting cells developed obvious nuclear condensation or nuclear fragmentation, which exhibits typical features of apoptosis. (**F**) A cross-sectional view of the basilar membrane from a cochlear explant treated with 500 μM cadmium chloride for 24 h demonstrates that all hair cells and supporting cells exhibited typical apoptotic features of nuclear condensation or fragmentation. These comparative results highlight differential vulnerability patterns to ototoxic agents through simultaneous visualization of hair cells, supporting cells, and nuclear morphology

with powerful tools to elucidate cellular responses to various toxicological insults.

Common nuclear staining techniques employ diverse chemical classes of dyes including traditional histological stains (hematoxylin, carmine, safranin O, methyl green, crystal violet, Bismarck brown Y, toluidine blue), fluorescent nucleic acid intercalators (acridine orange, ethidium bromide, propidium iodide), and modern fluorescent probes (DAPI, Hoechst dyes, EthD-III, 7-AAD, RedDot1, SYTOX dyes, TO-PRO-3). These reagents provide researchers with multiple options for nuclear visualization and analysis across various experimental applications and imaging modalities.

12.2.1 Hematoxylin Staining Method to Reveal the Nuclei

Hematoxylin is one of the most commonly used nuclear stains in inner ear histological studies due to its low cost, ease of use, and excellent staining durability. The hematoxylin staining technique has low equipment requirements and stable performance, making it easy to use even in laboratories with limited infrastructure while maintaining the diagnostic accuracy of sensory epithelium analysis.

Hematoxylin functions as a cationic nuclear dye through electrostatic interactions between its positively charged molecules and negatively charged nucleic acids, forming stable ionic or hydrogen bonds that enable specific nuclear staining. The standard staining protocol requires only a brief staining of isolated cochlear and vestibular tissues in Harris hematoxylin solution for 5 min, followed by a 15-min tap water rinse that converts the initial red coloration to the characteristic blue-violet nuclear stain. After mounting in glycerol, specimens are ready for light microscopic examination [1, 8, 14–18] (Fig. 3.18B, 5.5–5.7, 5.9, 5.10B, D, 5.11A–C, 5.12A, C, D, 8.10–8.13, and 10.8A, C; Figs. 12.2A, B and 12.3A, B). This straightforward yet reliable technique provides excellent nuclear contrast for morphological analysis of inner ear sensory epithelia.

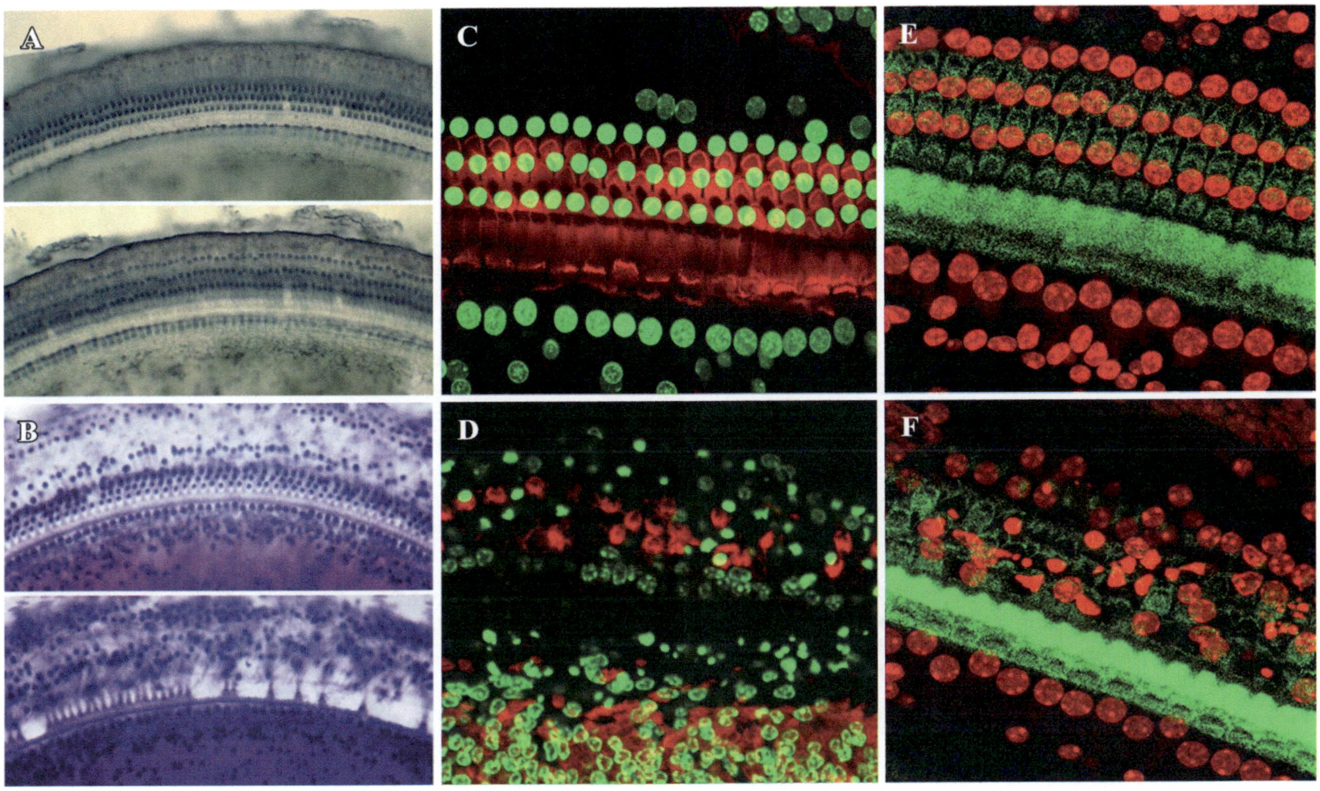

Fig. 12.2 Nuclear staining applications in cochlear pathology assessment using three different dyes. (**A**) Hematoxylin staining enables dual-focus visualization of rat cochlear preparations, with surface focus revealing stereocilia and cuticular plates while the nuclear plane shows hair cell nuclei. (**B**) Comparative hematoxylin staining demonstrates normal cochlear architecture versus blast wave-induced outer hair cell loss, highlighting the technique's diagnostic utility. (**C**) ToPro-3 staining showing the nuclei of inner and outer hair cells in a normal rat cochlear basilar membrane flat mount. (**D**) ToPro-3 staining showing the characteristic apoptotic nuclear shrinkage and fragmentation of the cochlear hair cells after cisplatin treatment. (**E**) Propidium iodide staining showing the nuclei of inner and outer hair cells in the cochlear basilar membrane of a normal chinchilla. (**F**) Several hours after intracochlear electrode implantation, propidium iodide staining revealed that outer hair cells near the implanted electrode began to undergo significant nuclear condensation, suggesting that cochlear electrode implantation may induce programmed apoptosis in surrounding hair cells. These examples illustrate how nuclear staining techniques can discriminate between normal and pathological states while providing insights into underlying cell death mechanisms

12.2.2 TO-PRO®-3 Staining Method to Reveal the Nuclei

TO-PRO®-3 serves as an excellent nuclear counterstain due to its high-affinity binding to dsDNA, enabling precise nuclear visualization in both surface preparations and tissue sections of cochlear and vestibular end-organs. The staining protocol involves fixing cochlear and vestibular tissues, followed by thorough PBS rinsing and incubation in 1:1000 dilution of TO-PRO®-3 solution for 60 min. After mounting in glycerol, specimens are examined using confocal microscopy, with acquired z-stacks images processed through specialized software for enhanced three-dimensional reconstruction [2–4, 11, 19–30] (Figs. 1.27C, 1.29, 1.30, 2.13–2.15, 3.5C, 3.9B, 3.13, 3.18C, 3.20, 4.6, 5.3, 5.8, 5.15B, 6.22B, 6.23B, 7.24, 7.25, 8.3, 8.28A–D, 8.29C, 9.14, 11.2, and 11.3; Figs. 12.1, 12.2C, D, and 12.3C, D). This methodology provides reliable nuclear labeling complementary to other fluorescent markers in pathological research of the inner ear.

12.2.3 Propidium Iodide Staining Method to Reveal the Nuclei

Propidium iodide (PI) represents a photostable red-fluorescent nucleic acid stain with excitation/emission maxima at 530/615 nm, exhibiting high specificity for both DNA and RNA while maintaining excellent staining permanence. For experimental use, PI stock solutions are prepared at 10 mg/mL concentration in deionized water and stored at sub-zero temperatures to ensure long-term stability. This fluorescent probe provides reliable nuclear labeling for various histological applications due to its stable spectral properties and nucleic acid binding characteristics.

For optimal PI staining results, inner ear tissues are first perfused with 10% phosphate-buffered formalin and fixed for 2 h. Following microdissection in PBS, specimens undergo RNase treatment (10 U/mL, 30 min) to minimize cytoplasmic fluorescence background. The staining protocol involves diluting PI stock solution a 1:1000 dilution and incubating

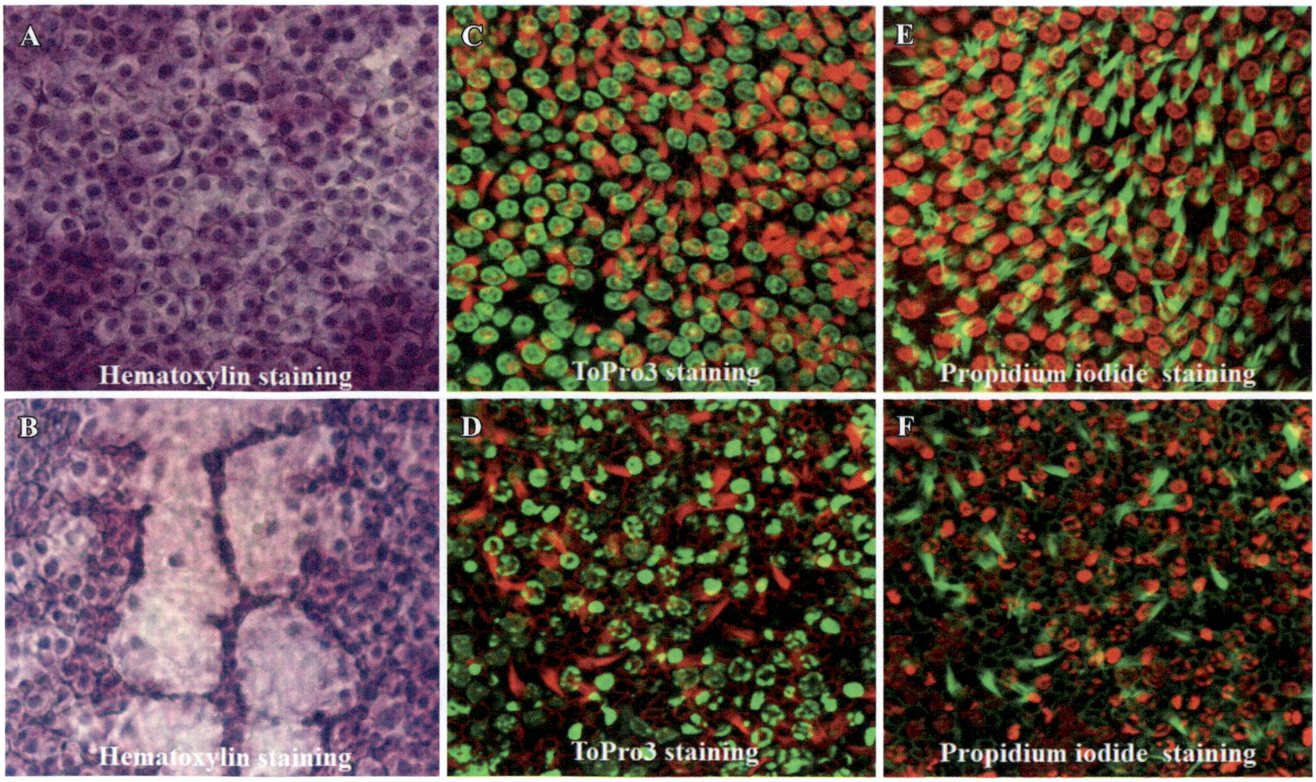

Fig. 12.3 Nuclear staining applications in vestibular pathology assessment using three different dyes. (**A**) Hematoxylin staining shows the nuclei (purple) of vestibular hair cells from the surface preparation of the macula of the utricle in a normal rat. (**B**) Hematoxylin staining shows blast wave-induced missing nuclei of vestibular hair cells in the striola region. (**C**) ToPro-3 staining shows uniform nuclear staining and normal hair cell density in the macula of the utricle of a normal rat. (**D**) ToPro-3 staining shows the characteristic apoptotic nuclear shrinkage and fragmentation of the vestibular hair cells in the macula of the utricle after cisplatin treatment. (**E**) Propidium iodide staining shows the intact nuclei of vestibular hair cells in the macula of the utricle in a normal rat. (**F**) Propidium iodide staining showing the condensed nuclei of vestibular hair cells in the macula of the utricle 24 h after bilirubin treatment. These comparative analyses validate nuclear staining as a sensitive approach for evaluating vestibular hair cell pathology and discriminating mechanisms of cellular injury

tissues for 20 min before mounting in glycerol for fluorescence microscopy. This method ensures specific nuclear labeling with minimal nonspecific staining, providing reliable visualization of cellular morphology [9, 10] (Fig. 8.27; Figs. 12.2E, F and 12.3E, F). The described technique maintains structural integrity while achieving high-contrast nuclear fluorescence for precise pathological evaluation.

12.3 Staining Methods of Ciliary Bundle Commonly Used in the Study of Inner Ear Pathology

The structural and functional differences between cochlear and vestibular hair cells are defined by their distinct ciliary architectures. While mammalian cochlear hair cells lose their kinocilium during late embryonic development, retaining only stereocilia that embed into the tectorial membrane, vestibular hair cells maintain a complete ciliary bundle comprising one kinocilium and multiple stereocilia throughout adulthood. These vestibular bundles project into either the otolithic membrane (in the macula of the saccule and utricle) or the cupula (in the ampullary cristae). Mechanotransduction occurs differently in these systems: cochlear hair cells are stimulated by relative motion between stereocilia and the tectorial membrane during basilar membrane vibration, whereas vestibular hair cells respond to changes in head position, which cause displacement of the otolithic membrane or copula caused by endolymphatic fluid flow, leading to deflection of the hair cell ciliary bundles embedded in the otolithic membrane or copula. Importantly, hair cells that lose their ciliary bundles—though potentially viable—become functionally incompetent, unable to transduce mechanical stimuli or release neurotransmitters. Consequently, evaluation of ciliary bundle integrity or mechanotransduction channel status at stereocilia tips serves as a critical indicator of sensory cell functionality in both auditory and vestibular systems [2, 3]. These structural–functional relationships underscore the importance of ciliary morphology in assessing inner ear sensory cell viability.

Multiple molecular probes are available for analyzing hair cell ciliary bundles, including phalloidin (F-actin staining), anti-Clarin-1 antibody, anti-2A7 antibody, and anti-cadherin 23

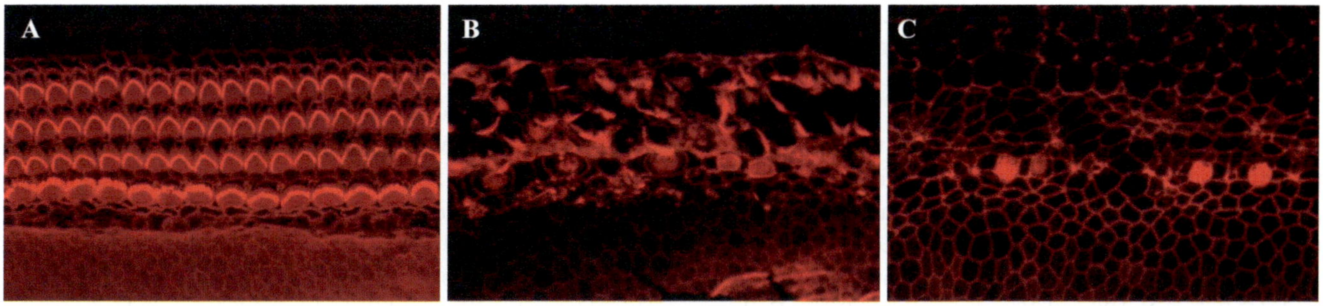

Fig. 12.4 Phalloidin-labeled cochlear pathology in rat cochlear explants under various ototoxic conditions. (**A**) Control specimens exhibit characteristic F-actin organization in stereocilia bundles and the cuticular plate of both inner and outer hair cells. (**B**) Cisplatin exposure (50 µM, 48 h) induces widespread hair cell loss with complete stereocilia degeneration. (**C**) Cadmium treatment (100 µM, 24 h) produces rapid, near-total hair cell destruction, revealing differential vulnerability patterns to these ototoxic agents through distinct temporal progression of ciliary bundle degeneration

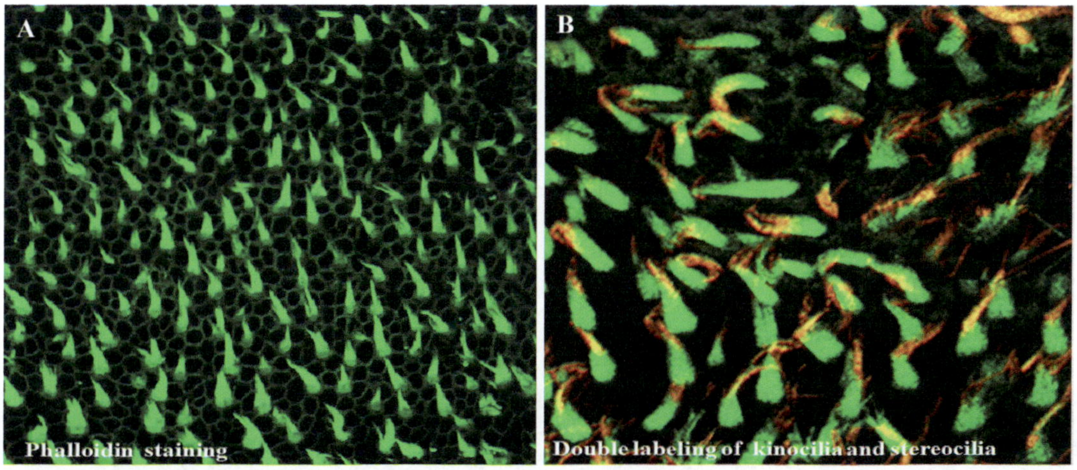

Fig. 12.5 The ciliary bundle staining of vestibular hair cells on the macula of the utricle. (**A**) Phalloidin staining reveals the complete F-actin organization within vestibular hair cell bundles, demonstrating their characteristic structural arrangement. (**B**) Double staining with anti-acetylated tubulin antibody (red) and phalloidin (green) differentially highlights the kinocilium and stereocilia components, respectively, providing clear visualization of the distinct kinocilium and stereocilia microfilament elements that comprise the mechanosensory apparatus of vestibular hair cells. These techniques enable comprehensive morphological assessment of vestibular hair cell bundles at both structural and molecular levels

antibody, along with various cytoskeletal markers for tubulin and actin. In inner ear research, phalloidin remains the most widely used probe for visualizing ciliary bundle morphology, while FM1-43 and AM1-43 fluorescent dyes serve as functional indicators of mechanotransduction channel activity at stereocilia tips. These complementary tools enable comprehensive evaluation of both structural integrity and functional capacity in cochlear and vestibular hair cells during pathological investigations.

12.3.1 Phalloidin Staining Method to Reveal the Ciliary Bundles of the Hair Cells

Phalloidin, a lethal bicyclic heptapeptide from Amanita phalloides mushrooms, serves as an exceptional F-actin probe due to its high binding affinity, making it ideal for visualizing actin-rich ciliary bundles in inner ear hair cells. The standard staining protocol involves fixing tissues in 4% formaldehyde for several hours, PBS rinsing, followed by 40-min incubation in 1:100 dilution of fluorescent phalloidin. After glycerol mounting, specimens are examined using fluorescence or confocal microscopy to reveal detailed ciliary bundle morphology [1–4, 9, 11, 19, 20, 22–26, 28, 30–36] (Figs. 1.23B, C, 1.27B, C, 2.13, 3.4, 3.5A, D, 3.9, 3.10, 3.12, 3.18C, 3.20, 3.21, 4.2D, 4.3C, D, 4.4–4.6, 5.15B, 6.10D–F, 8.2C, 8.3A, 8.18C, D, 8.19, 8.20, 8.23D, F, 8.24, 8.27A, B, 8.29D–F, 9.1D–F, 9.2, 9.9 J, K, 9.10, 9.11, 9.12A, C, 9.13, 9.14A, C, E, G, and 11.2; Figs. 12.3C–F, 12.4, and 12.5).This robust technique provides consistent, high-resolution labeling of hair cell stereocilia for structural and pathological assessments.

12.3.2 Immunolabeling of Kinocilia by Anti-Acetylated Tubulin Antibody

The position of the kinocilium defines vestibular hair cell polarity, necessitating specific labeling techniques for morphological studies. The standard protocol using anti-acetylated tubulin antibody involves incubating fixed vestibular tissues overnight at 4°C in primary antibody solution (1:100 dilution with 1% Triton X-100 and 3% goat serum in PBS). Following PBS washes, specimens are incubated for 2 h with Alexa Fluor 555-conjugated secondary antibody, then counterstained with Alexa 488-phalloidin for 40 min to simultaneously visualize both kinocilia (red) and stereocilia (green) under confocal microscopy (Fig. 12.5B). This dual-labeling approach enables precise determination of hair cell orientation while maintaining the structural context of the entire ciliary bundle.

12.3.3 AM1-43 Labeling of the Mechanotransduction Channel on the Cilia Bundles

AM1-43 serves as a vital functional probe for assessing hair cell viability through its unique uptake mechanism. This membrane-permeant fluorescent dye selectively enters viable hair cells through functional mechanotransduction channels at stereocilia tips, producing characteristic cytoplasmic fluorescence. The dye's inability to label cells with damaged ciliary bundles or nonfunctional transduction channels makes it an essential tool for evaluating both structural integrity and physiological activity of cochlear and vestibular hair cells. This property allows researchers to discriminate between intact, functional hair cells and those with compromised mechanoelectrical transduction capabilities, providing crucial information about hair cell functional status beyond mere morphological preservation.

The AM1-43 labeling protocol varies between in vivo and in vitro applications while maintaining consistent functional evaluation principles. For live animal studies, anesthetized subjects receive direct perfusion of the inner ear cavities with 30 μg/mL AM1-43 solution for 30 min. In vitro preparations involve incubating tissues in culture medium containing the same final AM1-43 concentration for an equivalent duration. Following thorough rinsing with PBS or culture medium, specimens are fixed in 10% phosphate-buffered formalin before surface preparation and confocal microscopy. Successful AM1-43 uptake, evidenced by cytoplasmic fluorescence, confirms functional mechanotransduction channels at stereocilia tips, while absent labeling indicates channel dysfunction or ciliary

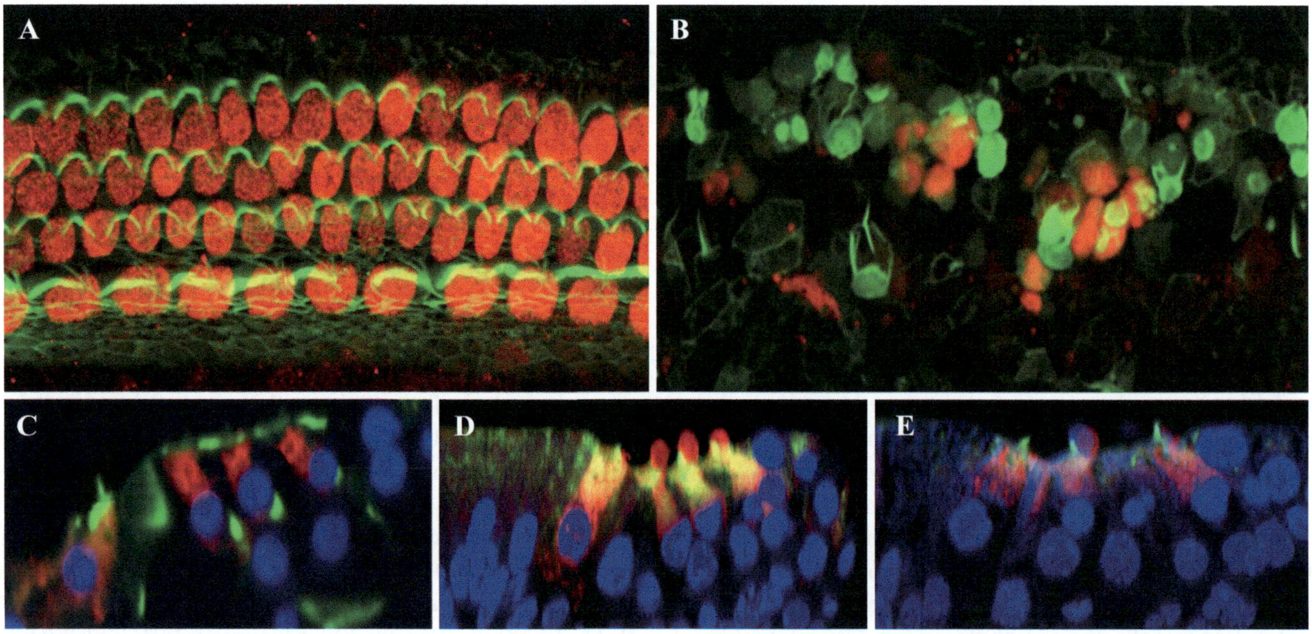

Fig. 12.6 AM1-43 uptake patterns in cochlear hair cells under various experimental conditions using multiplex fluorescence labeling. (**A**) Normal rat cochleae show robust AM1-43 incorporation (red) in all hair cells, this red signal of AM1-43 in the cytoplasm of hair cells is convincingly matches the phalloidin-labeled stereocilia (green), confirming intact mechanotransduction channel function. (**B**) Cisplatin treatment (50 μM, 48 h) severely diminishes AM1-43 uptake due to stereocilia damage, revealing the disruptive effects of cisplatin on mechanoelectrical transduction. (**C**) Cross-sectional views validate cytoplasmic AM1-43 distribution in healthy hair cells. (**D**) The enhanced vesicular release on the cuticular plate of outer hair cells was detected in cyclodextrin-treated rats, representing early pathological changes. (**E**) Complete absence of AM1-43 signals in damaged hair cells demonstrates the critical dependence of dye uptake on stereocilia integrity and channel functionality. These findings establish AM1-43 as a sensitive indicator of both structural and functional hair cell status

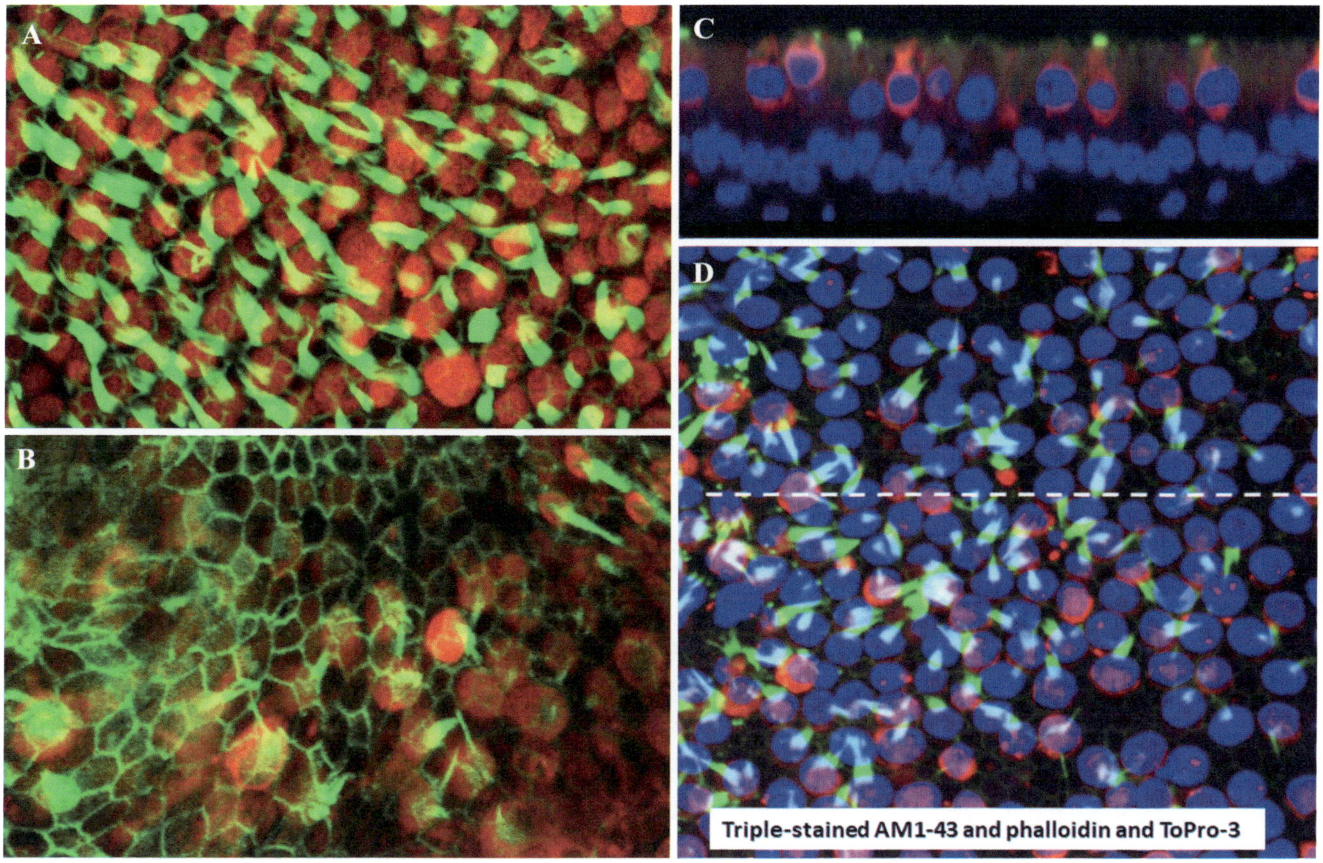

Fig. 12.7 AM1-43 uptake dynamics in vestibular hair cells through multiplex fluorescence imaging. (**A**) Double staining in the normal rat cochlea shows robust AM1-43 incorporation (red) in the cytoplasm of hair cells, and the phalloidin staining in the ciliary bundle of hair cells (green), confirming that functional mechanotransduction of hair cells requires the intact ciliary bundle structure. (**B**) Cisplatin treatment (50 μM, 48 h) significantly reduces AM1-43 uptake due to ciliary bundle damage, demonstrating the vestibulotoxicity of cisplatin. (**C**) Z-stack reconstructions reveal selective AM1-43 labeling in hair cells with preserved ciliary architecture, while those with ciliary bundle damage show no uptake. (**D**) Surface preparations exhibit mosaic AM1-43 uptake patterns, with positive labeling restricted to hair cells maintaining intact mechanotransduction channels at stereocilia tips. These observations confirm AM1-43's strict dependence on functional ciliary bundles for cellular entry, making it a reliable indicator of vestibular hair cell functional status beyond mere morphological preservation. The differential labeling patterns provide clear evidence of both focal and widespread vestibular hair cell dysfunction

damage [2, 3] ((Fig. 5.3; Figs. 12.6 and 12.7). This technique provides a critical functional assessment complementary to structural analyses of hair cell viability.

12.4 Method for Displaying the Outline of the Cuticular Plate of Sensory Hair Cells

The disappearance of circular cuticular plates following hair cell degeneration and their replacement by irregular supporting cell scars provides a reliable morphological marker for quantitative assessment of sensory cell density. This structural transformation allows researchers to accurately determine surviving hair cell populations by counting persistent circular cuticular plates within cochlear and vestibular epithelia, as each plate represents one functional hair cell unit. The method offers a straightforward yet precise approach for evaluating hair cell loss patterns and regeneration potential in inner ear pathology studies.

12.4.1 Silver Precipitation Method to Reveal the Cuticular Plate Outline of Hair Cells

The silver nitrate-negative infiltration technique represents the optimal approach for light microscopic visualization of cuticular plate morphology in inner ear sensory epithelia. This method relies on physical precipitation principles rather than true histochemical reactions, producing silver deposits or silver halide precipitates on tissue surfaces that delineate cellular boundaries with exceptional clarity. The resulting high-contrast images reveal fine structural details of both hair cell and supporting cell cuticular plates, making it particularly valuable for detailed morphological analysis of the surface architecture of cochlear and vestibular sensory hair cells.

The silver nitrate infiltration technique requires surgical preparation beginning with cochlear apex fenestration and stapes footplate removal to access both cochlear and vestibular compartments. Following surgical removal or

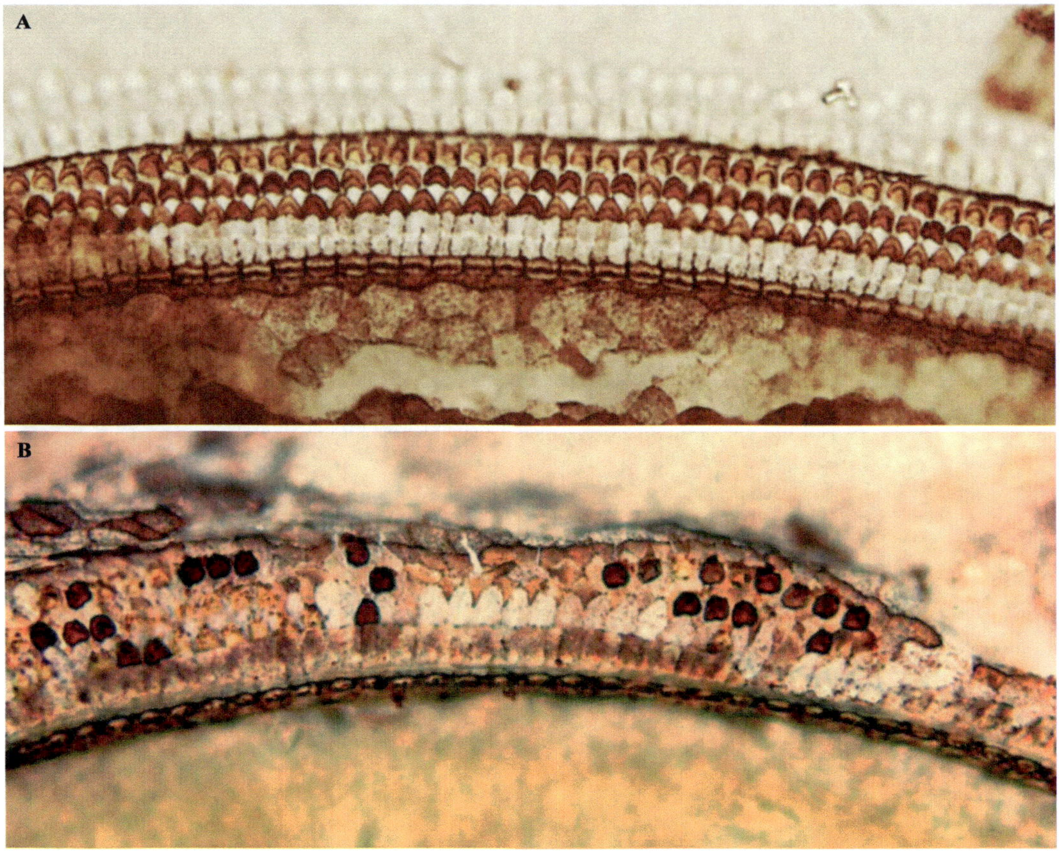

Fig. 12.8 The utility of silver nitrate precipitation for visualizing cochlear hair cell morphology. (**A**) Surface preparation of the cochlear basilar membrane from a normal rat reveals characteristic organization of stereocilia bundles on the inner and outer hair cells and cuticular plates with exceptional clarity. (**B**) Cyclodextrin treatment (4000 mg/kg, 7 days) induces selective outer hair cell degeneration while preserving inner hair cell architecture, highlighting the differential vulnerability of cochlear hair cell populations to cyclodextrin insult. The silver deposition technique provides high-contrast imaging of these pathological changes at the cellular level

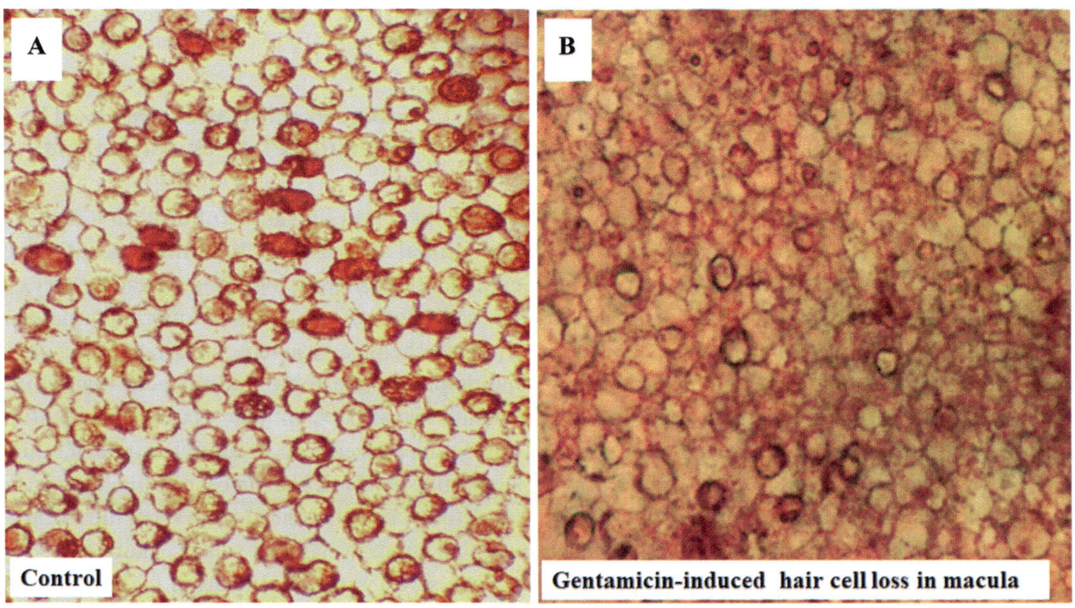

Fig. 12.9 The utility of silver nitrate precipitation for visualizing vestibular hair cell morphology. (**A**) Control specimens demonstrate uniform organization of the cuticular plate of vestibular hair cells across the macula of the utricle in guinea pigs. (**B**) Chronic gentamicin administration (125 mg/kg twice daily for 7 days) produces significant hair cell loss, evidenced by reduced density of cuticular plate of hair cells, confirming the vestibular toxicity of systemic medication of gentamicin. The silver precipitation method enables a precise quantitative assessment of both normal hair cell distribution and drug-induced pathological changes on vestibular epithelia

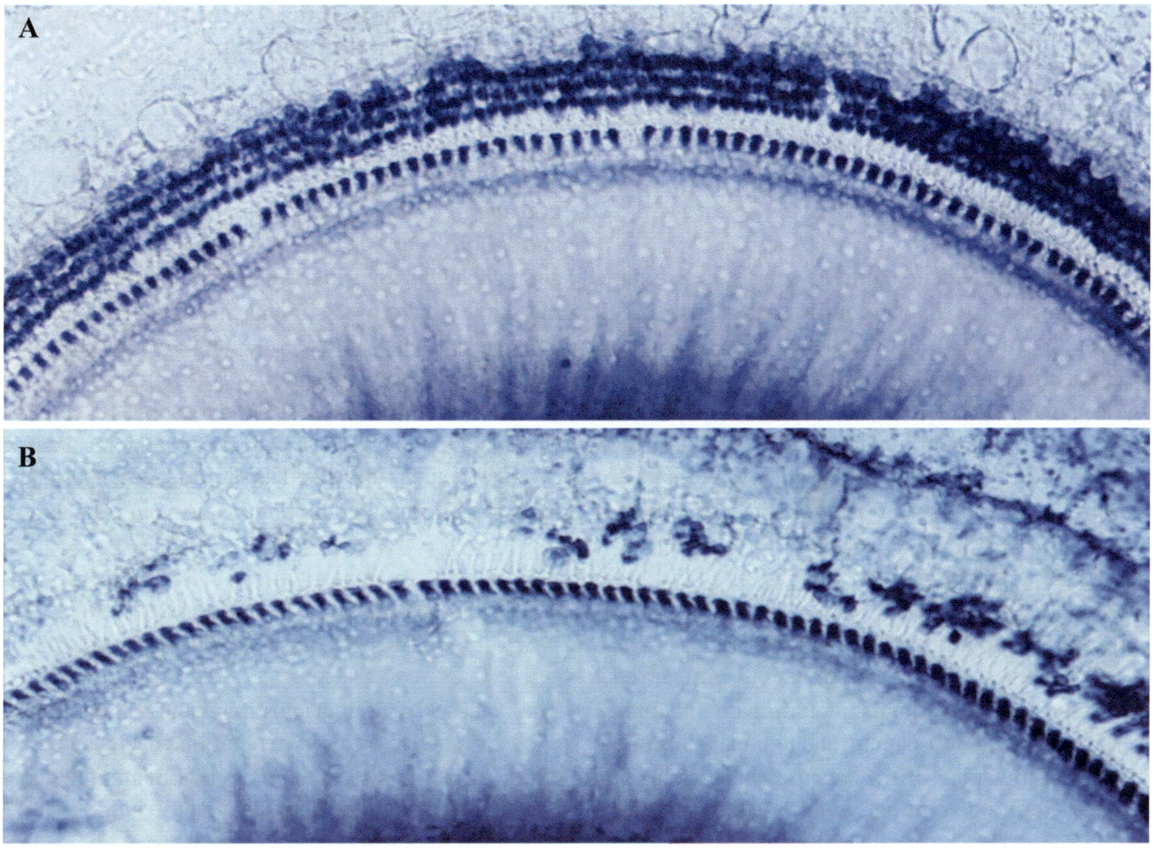

Fig. 12.10 Differential vulnerability of cochlear hair cells through succinate dehydrogenase histochemistry. (**A**) Control specimens exhibit characteristic blue-stained inner and outer hair cell arrays with preserved mitochondrial enzyme activity and normal cellular organization. (**B**) Cyclodextrin administration (4000 mg/kg, subcutaneous injection) induces selective outer hair cell degeneration by day 3 while maintaining inner hair cell integrity, revealing the distinct metabolic susceptibility patterns between cochlear hair cell populations during acute ototoxic injury. This enzymatic staining method effectively highlights both normal mitochondrial distribution and pathological changes in cochlear sensory epithelia

PBS irrigation to clear otolithic membranes from maculae of saccule and utricle and cupula on the ampullary cristae, 0.5% silver nitrate solution is perfused through the cochlear apex (draining through oval and round windows) and individually into each vestibular end-organ. Immediate post-perfusion fixation in 10% formalin overnight precedes microdissection of intact basilar membrane and vestibular end-organs. Mounted specimens undergo 1-h sunlight exposure to develop characteristic tan-colored silver precipitates that delineate cuticular plate contours and cellular junctions with exceptional clarity [1, 37–41] (Figs. 1.24A, 3.11, 3.18A, 3.19, 5.10C, 8.6, and 8.14; Figs. 12.8 and 12.9). This physical deposition method provides unparalleled resolution of inner ear epithelial surface architecture under light microscopy.

12.5 Mitochondrial Staining of Sensory Hair Cell

on of carbohydrates, lipids, and proteins via the tricarboxylic acid cycle and oxidative phosphorylation pathways. These biochemical processes convert metabolic fuels into ATP, establishing mitochondria as the cell's power plants. Mitochondrial dysfunction disrupts this energy production cascade, leading to cellular energy deficits that impair critical ATP-dependent processes and ultimately compromise cell viability. The organelle's central role in bioenergetics makes it particularly vulnerable to various pathological insults with far-reaching consequences for cellular function.

Mitochondrial visualization in inner ear research employs diverse techniques, including fluorescent probes (MitoLite Blue FX490, CytoFixTM Red, JC-10TM ΔΨm indicators, etc.) and histochemical methods targeting respiratory chain enzymes (isocitrate dehydrogenase, succinate dehydrogenase, malate dehydrogenase, cytochrome oxidase, etc.). The membranous labyrinth's cellular composition shows striking metabolic specialization: sensory hair cells exhibit mitochondrial abundance supporting their high energy demands, while supporting cells contain sparse mitochondria. This differential mitochondrial distribution enables selective hair cell identification through mitochondrial labeling approaches, providing important tools for investigating cochlear and vestibular pathophysiology. The techniques' specificity for metabolically active cells makes them particularly useful for assessing hair cell viability and functional status in experimental studies.

12.5.1 Tetrazolium Salt Staining to Reveal the Succinate Dehydrogenase in Mitochondria

Succinate dehydrogenase histochemistry serves as a reliable mitochondrial marker for discriminating between sensory hair cells and supporting cells in the inner ear. This enzymatic staining method, utilizing tetrazolium salt reduction to demonstrate dehydrogenase activity, provides both morphological identification of hair cells and functional assessment of their oxidative metabolic capacity. The technique's specificity for mitochondrial-rich hair cells makes it particularly valuable for evaluating cellular energy metabolism and viability in auditory and vestibular research applications.

The succinate dehydrogenase staining protocol requires vital staining prior to fixation due to the enzyme's sensitivity to aldehyde fixatives. The procedure begins with surgical preparation of anesthetized animals, including cochlear apex fenestration and oval window opening, and removal of otolithic membranes on the maculae of the saccule and utricle. The freshly prepared staining solution containing 0.2 M sodium succinate, 0.2 M phosphate buffer (pH 7.6), and 0.1% nitroblue tetrazolium in a ratio of 1:1:2 is perfused into the inner ear cavities and incubated at 37°C for 60 min. Immediate fixation with 10% formalin, with subsequent 12-h immersion fixation ensuring tissue preservation. Microdissected specimens reveal intense blue formazan deposits in mitochondria-rich hair cells, while supporting cells remain unstained, enabling clear cellular discrimination [1, 10, 38, 42–44] (Figs. 1.17B, 1.18A, 1.19B, 1.24B, 3.17E, 5.13, 5.14A–C, 8.15–8.17, 10.3A, and10.4B; Figs. 12.10 and 12.11). This method provides both morphological identification and functional assessment of hair cell metabolic activity.

12.5.2 MitoTracker Green Staining to Reveal the Mitochondria

The MitoTracker Green protocol involves brief fixation (10% formalin in Hank's balanced salt solution, 15 min at 37°C) followed by acetone permeabilization for mitochondrial labeling in cochlear tissues. Microdissected organs of Corti are incubated in 0.5 μM MitoTracker Green FM for 45 min, then counterstained with TRITC-phalloidin for simultaneous visualization of mitochondria (green) and F-actin structures (red) using confocal microscopy [35] (Fig. 12.12A). This dual-labeling approach enables correlated assessment of mitochondrial distribution and cytoskeletal organization in cochlear hair cells.

12.5.3 Cytochrome c Immunostaining to Reveal the Mitochondria

The cytochrome c immunohistochemistry protocol begins with cochlear fixation (10% formalin, 4 h) followed by microdissection and blocking (Casein solution, 60 min). After PBS rinsing and Triton X-100 permeabilization (0.2%, 30 min), specimens are incubated with primary anti-cytochrome c antibody (2.5 μg/mL, 1 h) followed by Cy2-conjugated secondary antibody (1:200, 1 h). TRITC-phalloidin counterstaining enables simultaneous visualization of cytochrome c distribution (green) and F-actin structures (red) using confocal microscopy [10] (Fig. 12.13B, C). This method can provide the precise cellular localization of mitochondrial cytochrome c and its positional changes in the pathway and process of mitochondrial apoptosis in cochlear hair cells.

12.6 Neural and Synaptic Staining in the Cochlear and Vestibular System

The synapses of afferent and efferent nerve fibers in the inner ear are distributed to the bottom or around each hair cell. The afferent nerve terminals in the inner ear transmit the nerve impulse signals from the inner ear to the central auditory and vestibular system in the brainstem. The efferent system transmits the nerve impulse signals from the central nervous system in the brainstem to both inner ears through crossing and non-crossing efferent nerve fibers, respectively. Although it is theoretically possible to distinguish the transmission direction of nerve signals according to the connection of afferent nerve endings with receptors and the connection of efferent nerve endings with effectors, it is not easy to distinguish the transmission direction of nerve impulse signals in practice, because each hair cell is both a receptor of afferent nerves and an effector of efferent nerve endings. Since both afferent nerve endings and efferent nerve terminals actually have direct or indirect synaptic connections with sensory hair cells, how to judge whether the synapse connected to hair cells is an afferent nerve ending or an efferent nerve ending? The following aspects may be helpful to distinguish whether a synapse is an afferent nerve terminal or an efferent nerve terminal. (1) The nerve terminals containing glutamate receptors, such as α-amino-3-hydroxy-5-methyl-4-isoxazole propionic acid receptors, N-methyl-D-aspartate receptors, or kainic acid receptors, are afferent synapses. (2) The nerve fibers and their synapses containing acetylcholinesterase are efferent nerves. (3) The synaptic vesicles at afferent terminals are located within the hair cells, while the synaptic vesicles at efferent terminals are located within synapses. (4) The CtBP2 immunohistochemical reaction product representing the presynaptic membrane is specifically expressed in the synaptic ribbons of afferent nerve terminals within hair cells. (5) Acetylcholinesterase and calcitonin gene-related peptides and all immunohistochemical reaction

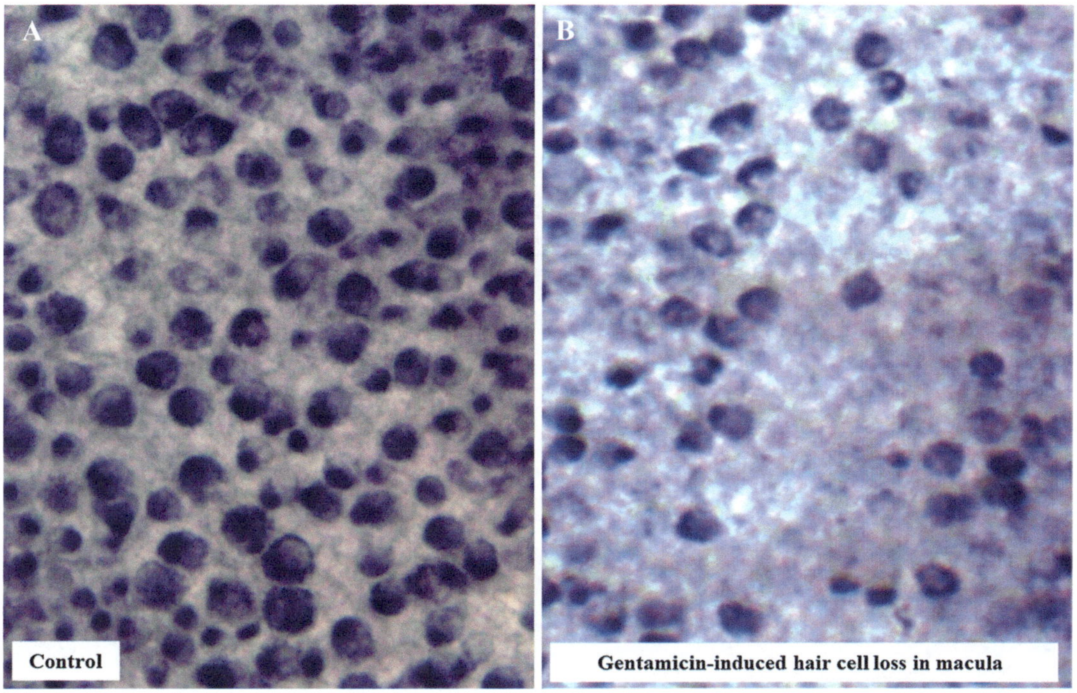

Fig. 12.11 Succinate dehydrogenase staining on the surface preparations of the macula of the saccule in the guinea pig clearly shows the products of the dehydrogenation within the vestibular hair cell. (**A**) Control specimens demonstrate uniform mitochondrial enzyme activity (blue staining) across all vestibular hair cells, confirming normal metabolic function. (**B**) Chronic gentamicin treatment (125 mg/kg twice daily for 7 days) significantly reduces both hair cell density and enzymatic staining intensity, reflecting the vestibulotoxic effects of gentamicin on both cellular survival and mitochondrial integrity. These findings correlate morphological hair cell loss with functional metabolic impairment in gentamicin-induced vestibular damage

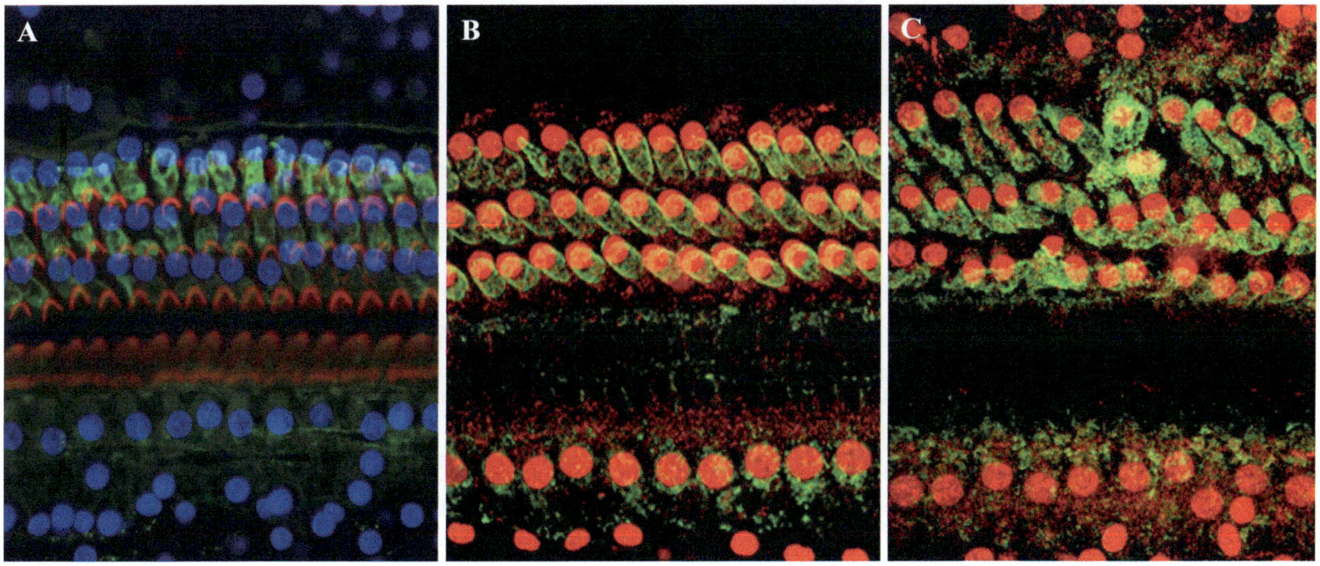

Fig. 12.12 Mitochondrial dynamics during hair cell apoptosis using complementary labeling techniques. (**A**) Triple staining with MitoTracker Green (mitochondria, green), phalloidin (stereocilia, red), and ToPro-3 (nuclei, blue) reveals normal cellular architecture in control rat cochlear hair cells. (**B**) Dual labeling of anti-cytochrome c antibody (green) and propidium iodide (nuclei, red) shows the localization of cytochrome c in mitochondria beneath the plasma membrane of outer hair cells and within the mitochondria of the subnuclear region of inner hair cells. (**C**) Four hours after ethacrynic acid/gentamicin co-administration, the early apoptotic changes are characterized by the dispersion of cytochrome c into cytoplasm from mitochondria, accompanied by nuclear condensation, demonstrating the initiating role of mitochondrial membrane permeabilization in gentamicin-induced hair cell apoptosis. These techniques collectively track the transition from normal mitochondrial distribution to pathological cytochrome c release during ototoxic injury

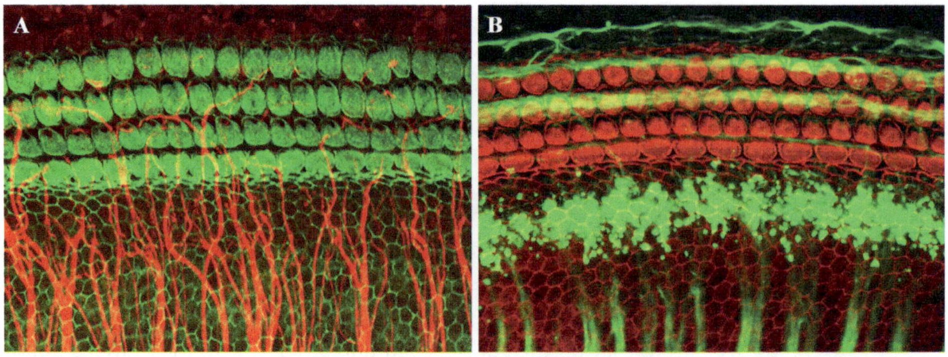

Fig. 12.13 Differential patterns of neural element labeling in mouse cochlear preparations. (**A**) Anti-neurofilament antibody immunohistochemistry selectively highlights auditory nerve fibers, revealing their trajectories through the basilar membrane. However, it is not expressed in the synapse. (**B**) Anti-β-tubulin antibody staining provides more comprehensive neural visualization, labeling both nerve fibers and their terminal arborizations, enabling complete mapping of cochlear innervation patterns. These complementary techniques allow researchers to selectively examine either axonal integrity and/or complete neural architecture, including synaptic terminals

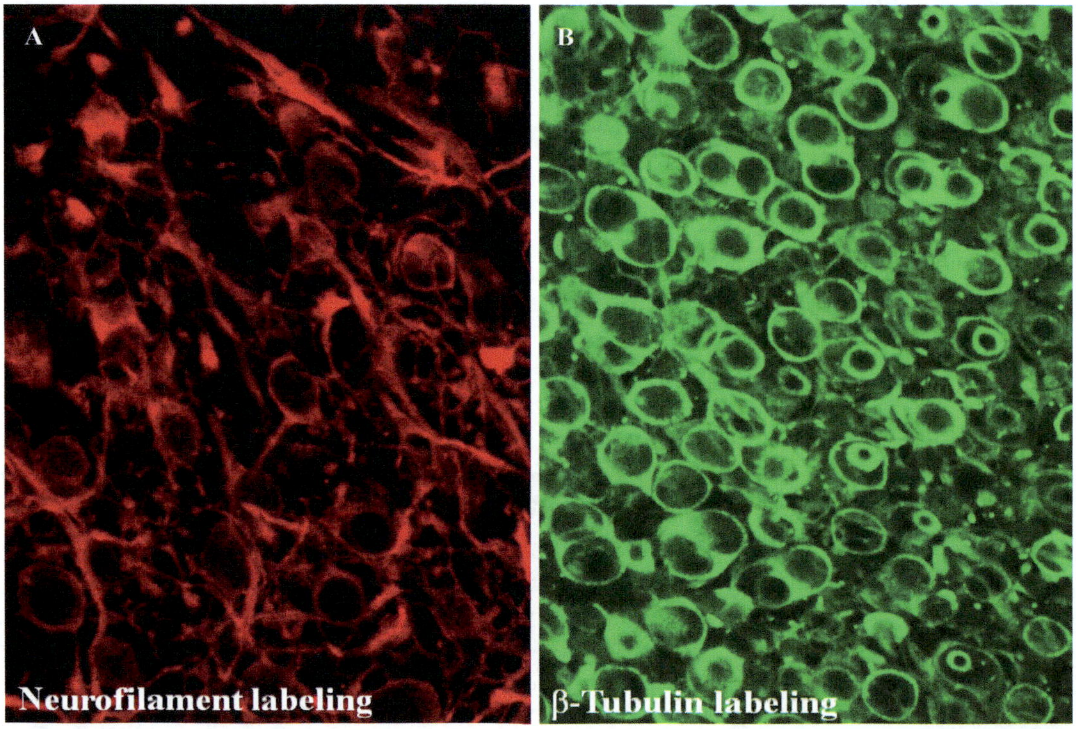

Fig. 12.14 Complementary neural labeling patterns in the macula of the utricle of the rat using distinct immunohistochemical markers. (**A**) Anti-neurofilament-200 antibody immunoreactivity selectively outlines vestibular nerve fiber pathways, demonstrating their projection patterns through vestibular sensory epithelia. (**B**) Anti-β-tubulin antibody staining extends beyond fibers to clearly delineate nerve terminals, revealing complete synaptic architecture beneath the vestibular hair cells. These differential staining profiles enable targeted analysis of either axonal projections or synaptic connectivity within the same vestibular region, providing versatile tools for neural investigation

products of postsynaptic membranes were specifically labeled on the fibers or terminals of efferent nerves.

12.6.1 Immunohistochemical Staining of Neurofilaments and β-Tubulin

Immunohistochemical analysis of inner ear neural elements employs distinct markers with differential specificity: anti-neurofilament-200 antibodies selectively label nerve fibers, making them ideal for assessing axonal pathology, while anti-β -tubulin III antibodies provide more comprehensive neural visualization by staining both fibers and their terminal arborizations. This complementary labeling capacity allows researchers to selectively evaluate either axonal integrity (using neurofilament markers) or complete neural architecture, including synaptic terminals (using tubulin markers), depending on experimental objectives [2, 3, 5, 22, 26, 27, 31, 34, 35]. The choice between

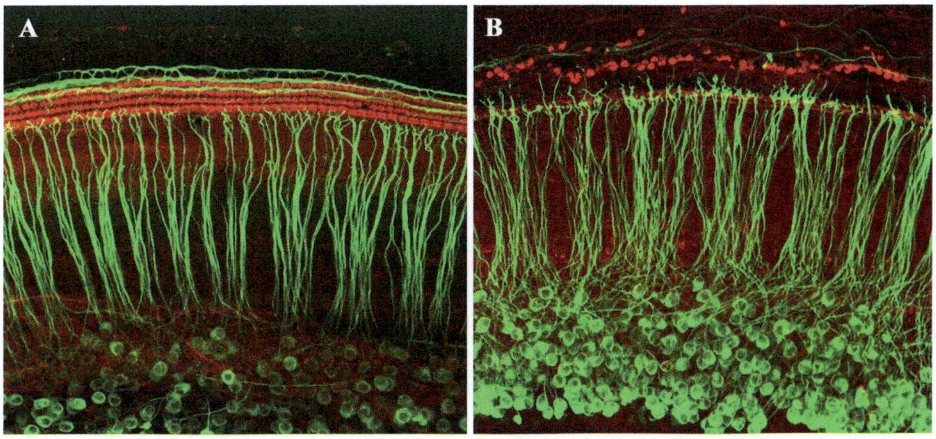

Fig. 12.15 Double-labeling of anti-Tubulin antibody (green) and Phalloidin (red) in the surface preparations of the cochlear basilar membrane in rats. (**A**) Control specimens reveal normal organization of tubulin-positive neural elements (green) connecting phalloidin-labeled hair cells (red), showing intact cochlear innervation patterns. (**B**) Gentamicin-treated cochleae exhibit preserved tubulin-stained spiral ganglion neurons and their processes despite extensive hair cell loss, confirming the primary target of gentamicin is the sensory hair cells rather than neural elements during early ototoxic injury. This differential vulnerability pattern highlights the specific mechanosensory toxicity of gentamicin while sparing cochlear innervation architecture in the early stage of damage

these markers is therefore guided by whether the study requires focused assessment of nerve fiber integrity or more comprehensive evaluation of neural connectivity, including synaptic endings.

The immunohistochemical protocol for neural element visualization begins with 3-h fixation of temporal bones in phosphate-buffered formalin, followed by microdissection of cochlear and vestibular tissues. Specimens undergo overnight incubation at 4°C with primary antibodies (anti-neurofilament-200 antibody or anti-β-tubulin III antibody at 1:100 dilution in PBS containing 1% Triton X-100 and 3% serum). After PBS rinsing, tissues are incubated for 2 h with fluorescent secondary antibodies (1:200 in similar buffer) before surface preparation and confocal microscopy [12, 22, 26, 28, 29, 31, 45–48] (Figs. 1.26C, 1.27C, 1.30, 3.5B, D, 3.10, 6.22, 8.24–8.26, and 9.12–9.14; Figs. 12.13, 12.14, 12.15, and 12.16). This standardized approach enables reliable comparison of neural integrity across studies while accommodating either selective fiber labeling or comprehensive neural visualization, including terminals.

12.6.2 Immunohistochemical Staining to Reveal the Afferent Nerve Fibers

The peripherin immunohistochemical technique offers selective labeling of type II afferent fibers innervating cochlear outer hair cells and vestibular type II hair cells, while excluding both type I afferents and efferent fibers. When combined with anti-β-tubulin antibody immunostaining in dual-labeling experiments, this approach enables differential visualization of specific neural populations, facilitating precise assessment of selective neural vulnerability patterns in inner ear pathology [27]. This immunohistochemical staining method, specific for type II afferents, provides a valuable tool for investigating differential neuropathy mechanisms affecting distinct neural pathways within the auditory and vestibular systems.

The anti-peripherin antibody immunohistochemistry protocol involves microdissection of fixed cochlear and vestibular tissue followed by overnight incubation at 4°C with primary antibody (1:100 dilution in PBS containing 1% Triton X-100 and 3% serum). After thorough PBS rinsing, specimens are incubated for 2 h with fluorescent secondary antibody (1:200 in the same buffer) before glycerol mounting and confocal microscopy (Figs. 1.29B and 6.22; Figs. 12.17, 12.18, and 12.19). This standardized method reliably labels type II afferent fibers while maintaining tissue morphology for precise neural pathway analysis in cochlear and vestibular sensory epithelia.

While no single antibody specifically labels type I afferent fibers, combined peripherin and β-tubulin immunohistochemistry effectively discriminates between afferent subtypes through differential labeling patterns. Peripherin selectively marks type II afferents, including their synapses with outer hair cells in the cochlea and granular terminals contacting vestibular type II hair cells, while β-tubulin labels all neural elements, including type I afferents with their characteristic calyx endings surrounding vestibular type I hair cells [27] (Fig. 6.22; Figs. 12.17, 12.18, and 12.19). This dual-labeling approach enables clear morphological distinction between the fine type II fibers (peripherin-positive only) and thicker type I pathways (β-tubulin-positive) in both auditory and vestibular systems, providing a reliable method for studying the inner ear afferent nerve tissue and its pathological changes.

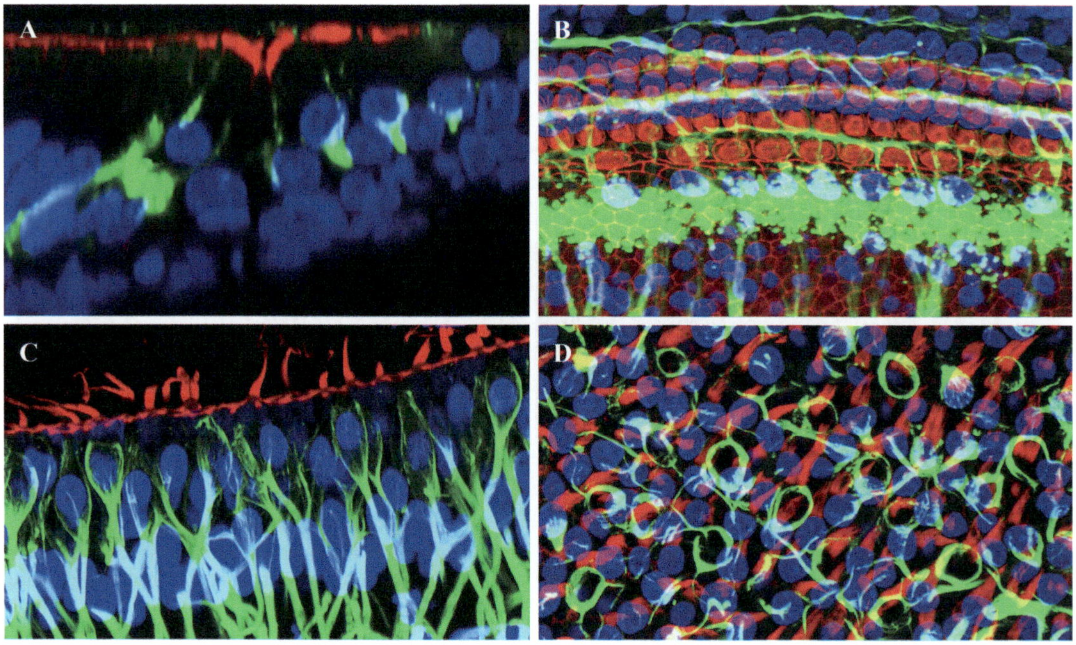

Fig. 12.16 Triple staining shows that the anti-Tubulin antibody labeled nerve fibers and synapses (green) and the phalloidin stains the cilia bundle and cuticular plate (red) of sensory hair cells, and the ToPro-3-stained nuclei in the cochlear and vestibular sensory organs of rats. (**A**) Z-plane reconstruction of the organ of Corti reveals spatial relationships between tubulin-labeled neural synapses (green), phalloidin-stained hair cell structures (red), and ToPro-3-highlighted nuclei (blue). (**B**) View from the surface preparation of the cochlear basilar membrane demonstrates the planar organization of these elements. (**C**) Z-plane reconstructions of the macula of utricle reveal the spatial relationships between tubulin-labeled neural synapses (green), phalloidin-stained hair cell structures (red), and nuclei highlighted by ToPro-3 (blue). (**D**) Surface preparation of the utricular macula shows planar organization of neural-sensory correlations in the macula

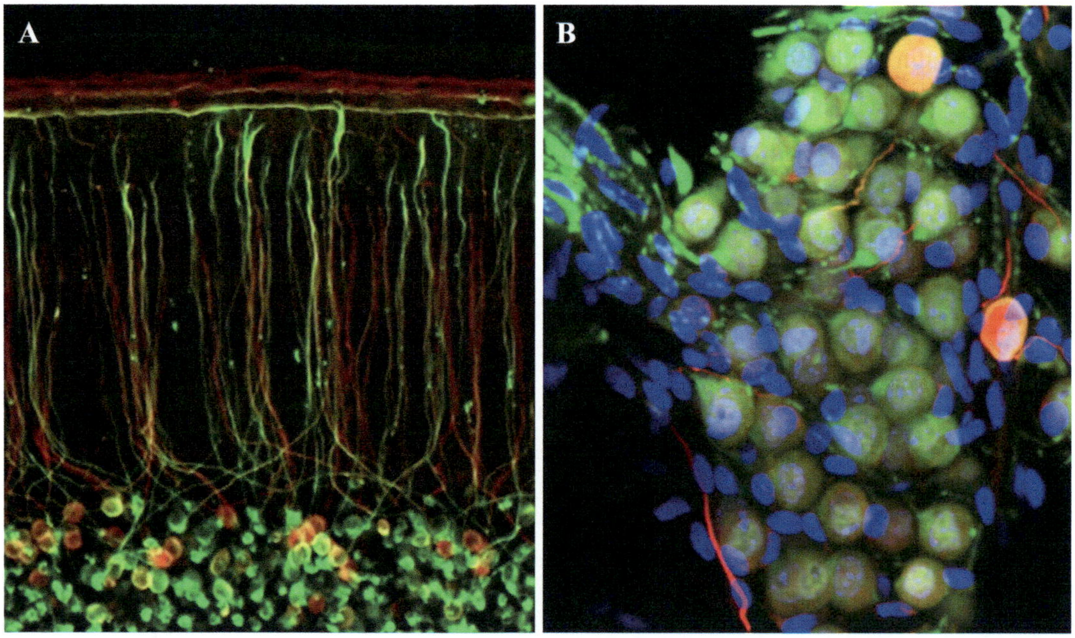

Fig. 12.17 Double immunohistochemical staining with anti-peripherin antibody (red) and anti-neurofilament-200 antibody (green) shows the distribution of type I and type II auditory afferent nervous system in the cochlea. (**A**) In cochlear explants cultured in serum-free medium containing 1 mM kanamycin for 24 h, massive hair cell destruction occurred. Anti-peripherin antibody showed destruction of type II afferent fibers beneath the outer hair cells, but the type II spiral ganglion neurons within Rosenthal's canal remained normal. It may indicate that in the early stage of the lesion, kanamycin destroys the type II afferent fibers while destroying the outer hair cells, but the lesion has not yet spread to the soma of type II spiral ganglion neurons in Rosenthal's canal. Interestingly, while type I afferent nerve fibers labeled with anti-neurofilament-200 antibodies remained intact, the cell bodies of type I spiral ganglia had begun to shrink, which may indicate that kanamycin also destroys the soma of type I spiral ganglion neurons in the early stage, while the lesions had not yet spread to the type I afferent nerve fibers near the synapse beneath the inner hair cells. (**B**) In normal cochlear explants at postnatal day 3, the type I afferent spiral ganglion neurons were stained in green by anti-neurofilament-200 antibody, while the type II afferent spiral ganglion neurons were stained in red by anti-peripherin antibody

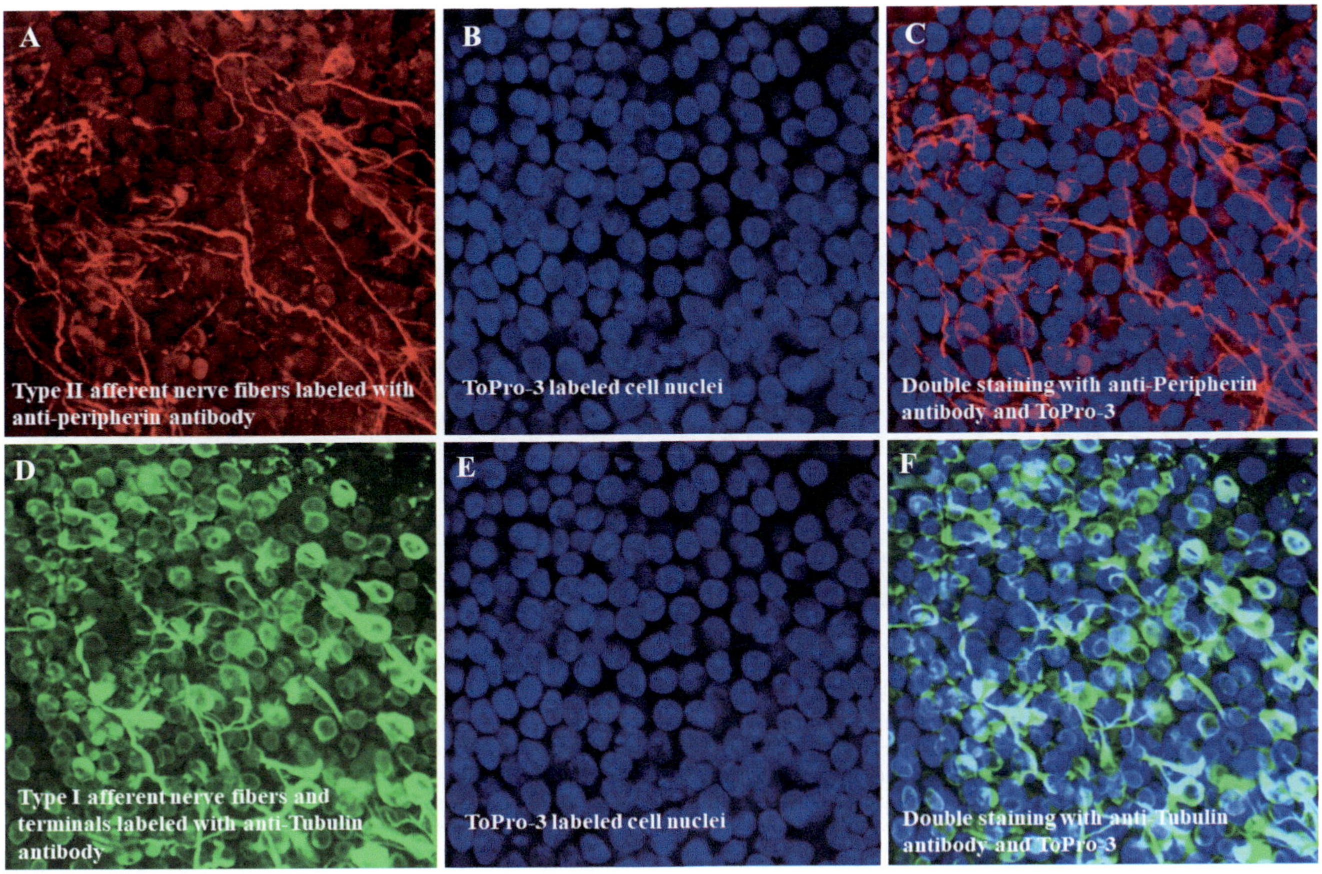

Fig. 12.18 Different distribution of anti-Peripherin antibody-labeled type II afferent nervous system and anti-Tubulin antibody-labeled type I afferent nervous system in the same region of the macula of the utricle. (**A**) On the surface preparation of the macula of the utricle, type II afferent nerve fibers and synapses were labeled in red by anti-Peripherin antibody immunostaining. (**B**) The nuclei of vestibular hair cells in the same region were stained in blue by ToPro-3 staining. (**C**) Merged image of type II afferent nerve fibers and their terminals labeled with anti-Peripherin antibody from image A and ToPro-3-stained cell nuclei from figure (**B**). (**D**) Type I afferent nerve fibers and synapses were marked in green with anti-Tubulin antibody in the same region of the macula of the utricle. (**E**) The nuclei of vestibular hair cells in the same region were stained blue with ToPro-3. (**F**) Merged image of type I afferent nerve fibers and their terminals labeled with anti-Tubulin antibody from image D and ToPro-3-stained cell nuclei from figure (**E**). Apparently, double immunohistochemical staining of anti-Peripherin antibody and anti-Tubulin antibody could effectively distinguish the type I afferent nerve fibers and their synapses, and the type II afferent nerve fibers and their terminals

12.6.3 Immunohistochemical Staining to Reveal the Nerve Terminal Synapses in the Inner Ear

Complementary presynaptic and postsynaptic markers allow precise mapping of the synaptic architecture of inner ear hair cells: Rabbit anti-C-terminal binding protein 2 (anti-CtBP2 antibodies) selectively label the presynaptic membrane of the inner ribbon of hair cells, while antibodies such as anti-PSD95, anti-GluA2, and anti-Shank1 specifically recognize postsynaptic membranes at synapses [29, 49, 50]. Because these antibodies accurately label and differentiate between presynaptic and postsynaptic membranes in cochlear and vestibular nerve terminals, they provide a key tool for studying synaptic pathology in inner ear nerve terminals.

Immunohistochemistry detection of CtBP2 protein was performed by immersing the fixed cochlear and vestibular end-organs in a blocking solution containing 3% Triton X-100 and 10% goat serum in phosphate buffer for 2 h, and then immersing the cochlear and vestibular tissue in the solution containing rabbit anti-presynaptic C-terminal binding protein 2 antibody, which was diluted 100-fold in 0.2% Triton X-100 and 3% goat serum in 0.01 M phosphate buffer at 4°C overnight. After rinsing with the phosphate buffer, specimens were incubated in a solution of fluorescently labeled goat anti-rabbit secondary antibody in a dilution of 200-fold with 0.2% Triton X-100 and 3% goat serum in 0.01 M phosphate buffer for 2 h at room temperature. Immunohistochemistry to reveal PSD-95 protein was performed by immersing samples in mouse anti-post-synaptic density protein 95 (PSD P95) antibody diluted 100-fold with 1% Triton X-100 and 3% donkey serum in 0.01 M phosphate buffer at 4°C in the refrigerator overnight. After rinsing, the specimens were immersed in a solution of fluorescently labeled donkey anti-mouse IgG secondary antibody diluted 200-fold with 1% Triton X-100 and 3% donkey serum in phosphate-buffered saline for 2 h. The above immunohistochemical double labeling can be accomplished in two steps, complete the labeling of one protein, and then perform

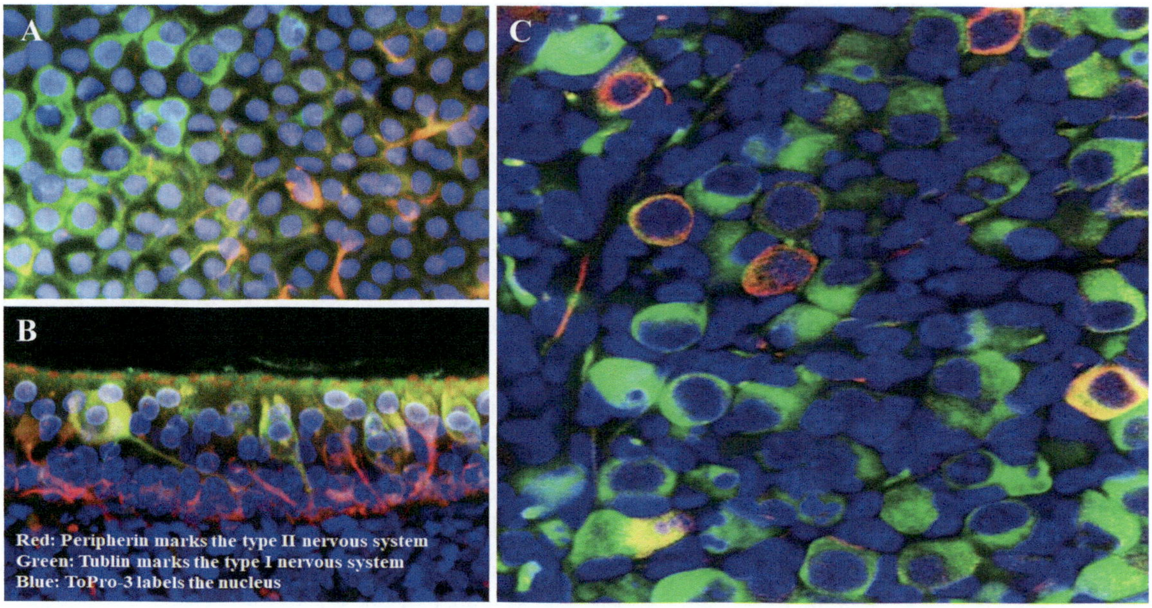

Fig. 12.19 Vestibular afferent nerve terminals and vestibular ganglion neurons with triple staining of anti-Peripherin antibody, anti-Tubulin antibody, and ToPro-3. (**A**) On the surface preparation of the macula of utricle, anti-Tubulin antibody was used to label the type I afferent nerve fibers and their synapse in green, anti-Peripherin antibody was used to label the type II afferent nerve fibers and their synapse in red, and ToPro-3 was used to stain the nuclei in blue. (**B**) In a cross-section of the macula of the utricle, type I afferent nerve fibers and their terminals were stained green with anti-Tubulin antibodies, and type II afferent nerve fibers and their synapses were stained red with anti-Peripherin antibodies. (**C**) From the perspective of the superior vestibular nerve bundle section, type I afferent neurons were immunolabeled with anti-Tubulin antibody and labeled in green, and type II afferent neurons were immunolabeled with anti-Peripherin antibody and labeled in red. This multiscale approach enables correlative analysis of afferent morphology across synaptic, epithelial, and ganglionic levels

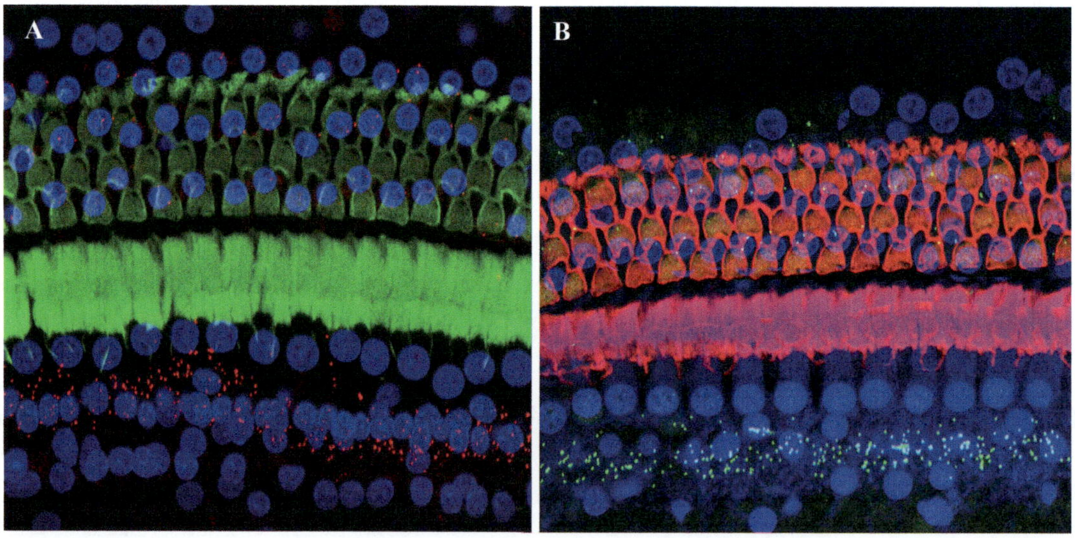

Fig. 12.20 Synaptic organization beneath the inner hair cells of the rat using dual immunofluorescence. (**A**) anti-CtBP2 antibody immunoreactivity (red) is precisely localized to presynaptic ribbons within inner hair cells, marking the original site of neurotransmitter formation and the active zones for neurotransmitter release. (**B**) anti-PSD-95 antibody labeling (green) reveals postsynaptic membrane in type I afferent terminals, showing their precise opposition to presynaptic elements. This paired staining visualizes the complete synaptic complex between sensory hair cells and afferent neurons, enabling functional assessment of auditory neurotransmission machinery. The complementary distribution patterns confirm the corresponding positional relationship between the presynaptic membrane and the postsynaptic membrane beneath the inner hair cells

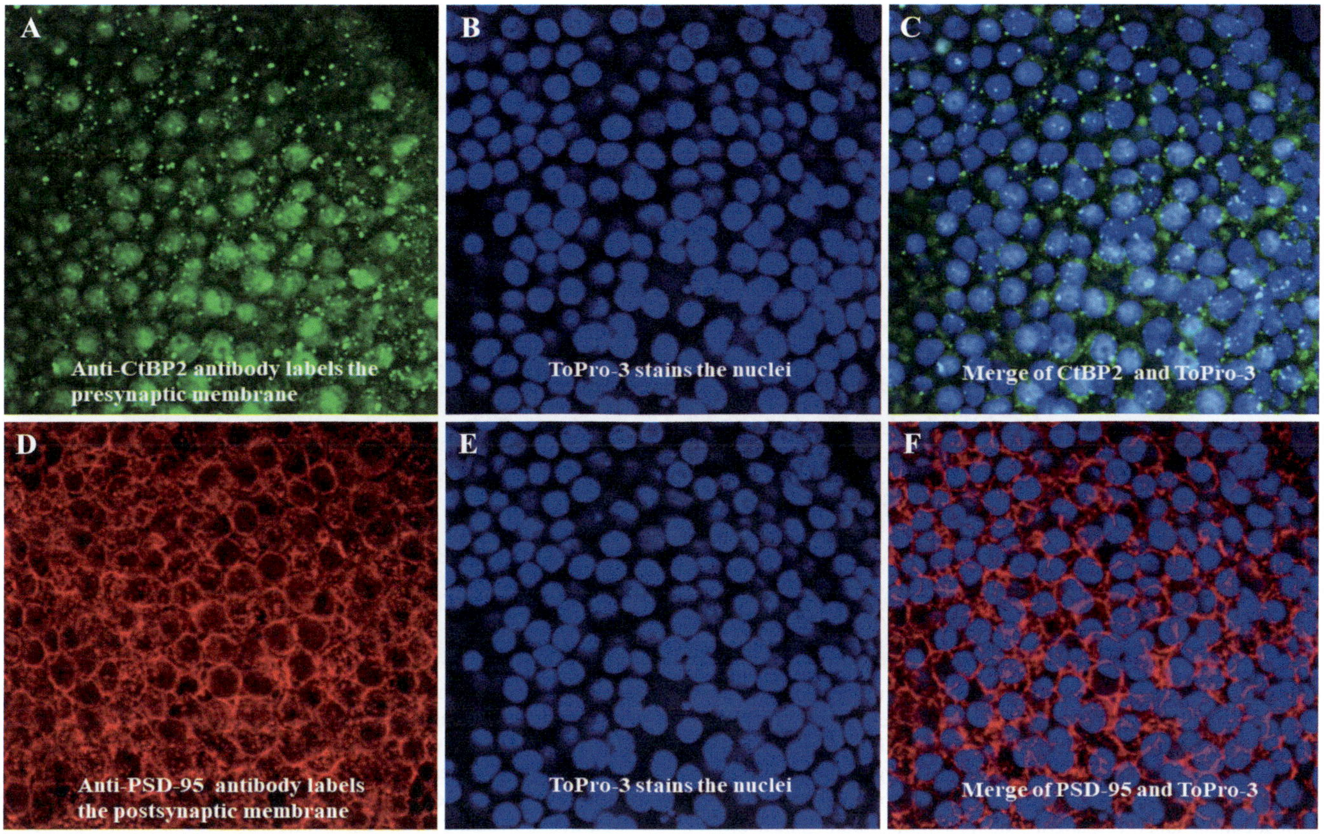

Fig. 12.21 Synaptic organization in the macula of the utricle of the rat using complementary immunofluorescence labeling. (**A**) Anti-CtBP2 antibody immunostaining reveals presynaptic membrane at ribbons (green) within vestibular hair cells. (**B**) ToPro-3 counterstain (blue) identifies cellular nuclei in the same region of figure (**A**). (**C**) Merged image of anti-CtBP2 antibody labeled presynaptic membrane in figure (**A**) and ToPro-3 staining in the same region in figure (**B**). (**D**) Anti-PSD-95 antibody labeling (red) marks the postsynaptic membrane in afferent nerve terminals opposite the base of hair cells. The circular postsynaptic membrane marks type I afferent nerve terminals connecting type I hair cells, and the punctate postsynaptic membrane marks type II afferent nerve terminals connecting type II hair cells. (**E**) The nuclei of vestibular hair cells in the same region of figure (**D**) were visualized by ToPro-3 staining. (**F**) Merged image of anti-PAD-95 antibody labeled postsynaptic membrane in figure (**D**) and ToPro-3 staining in the same region in figure (**E**). These paired labelings illustrate the precise molecular specialization of vestibular synapses, with presynaptic CtBP2 clusters in hair cells precisely aligned with postsynaptic PSD-95 domains in nerve terminals, separated by the synaptic cleft yet functionally coupled for neurotransmission. The nuclear counterstain provides essential cellular context for synaptic localization analysis

the staining of another protein, or the labeling of the two proteins can be mixed together and performed simultaneously. In the immunohistochemical staining process of simultaneously labeling two proteins, the two primary antibodies from different hosts will bind to their specific target proteins, respectively, and the two different fluorescently labeled secondary antibodies will specifically bind to the corresponding immunoreaction products of their primary antibodies in their original locations, respectively. Under a confocal microscope, the image data of the presynaptic membrane and the postsynaptic membranes will be acquired using different excitation fluorophores [29, 49, 50] (Figs. 11.2 and 11.3; Figs. 12.20 and 12.21). The dual-labeling approach enables precise analysis of synaptic pairs, simultaneously detecting distinct protein specificities in the presynaptic and postsynaptic membranes through differential fluorescence in confocal imaging. This allows for specific and reproducible labeling of synaptic specializations at the base of inner ear hair cells.

12.6.4 Immunohistochemical Staining of Efferent Nervous System of the Inner Ear

While inner ear hair cells are known to function as both sensory receptors for afferent pathways and targets for efferent modulation, the precise mechanisms underlying efferent synaptic regulation of hair cell activity remain incompletely characterized. This knowledge gap persists despite established anatomical understanding of efferent innervation patterns, highlighting the need for further investigation into the functional dynamics of these synaptic interactions. Current research continues to elucidate the complex interplay between efferent neurotransmitter

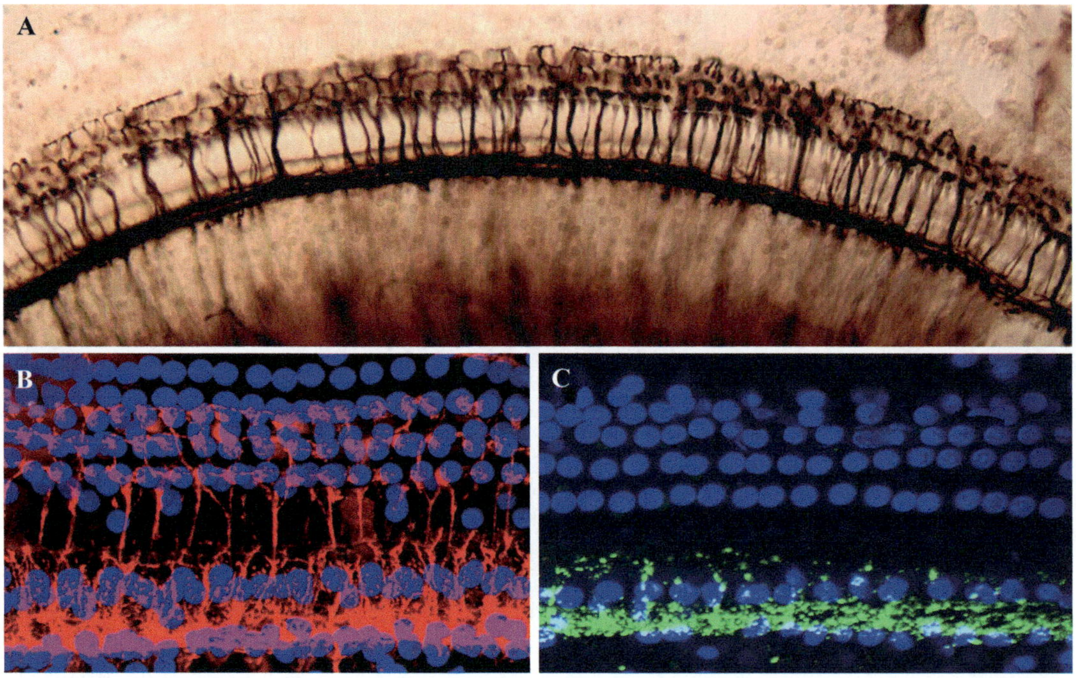

Fig. 12.22 The efferent innervation patterns in the rat cochlea using complementary labeling techniques. (**A**) Copper sulfide histochemistry reveals complete acetylcholinesterase-positive efferent pathways, including fibers and synapses throughout the organ of Corti. (**B**) Anti-acetylcholinesterase immunohistochemistry confirms these findings with identical labeling patterns, demonstrating tulip-shaped efferent terminals. (**C**) Anti-CGRP antibody immunostaining selectively labels granular efferent synapses at internal spiral bundle terminals beneath inner hair cells, while failing to stain efferent fibers or tunnel crossing bundles (Reproduced with permission from Ding et al. [13]). These differential staining patterns demonstrate the utility of acetylcholinesterase for comprehensive efferent pathway mapping versus CGRP's specificity for particular synaptic terminals, highlighting the importance of method selection based on experimental objectives

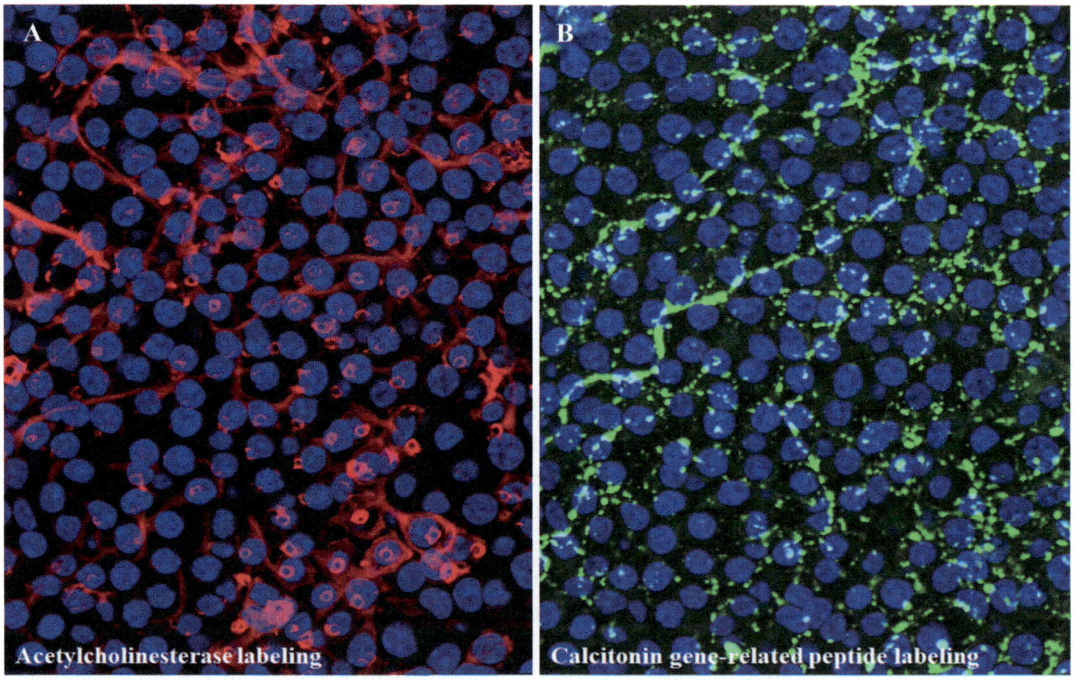

Fig. 12.23 Differential localization of efferent synaptic markers in rat utricular macula. (**A**) Acetylcholinesterase immunoreactivity reveals a small ring of efferent nerve endings surrounding the base of type I vestibular hair cells, but only granular efferent nerve endings are present below the base of type II hair cells. This confirms the distinct structural patterns of cholinergic innervation of type I and type II hair cells. (**B**) CGRP labeling shows distinct granular efferent endings in adjacent but non-overlapping regions, suggesting functional specialization of efferent synaptic subtypes. These complementary staining patterns reveal spatial and molecular heterogeneity in vestibular efferent innervation, with acetylcholinesterase-positive terminals likely mediating cholinergic modulation while CGRP-containing endings may represent peptidergic signaling pathways. The non-overlapping distributions imply separate regulatory mechanisms operating through distinct efferent synaptic populations

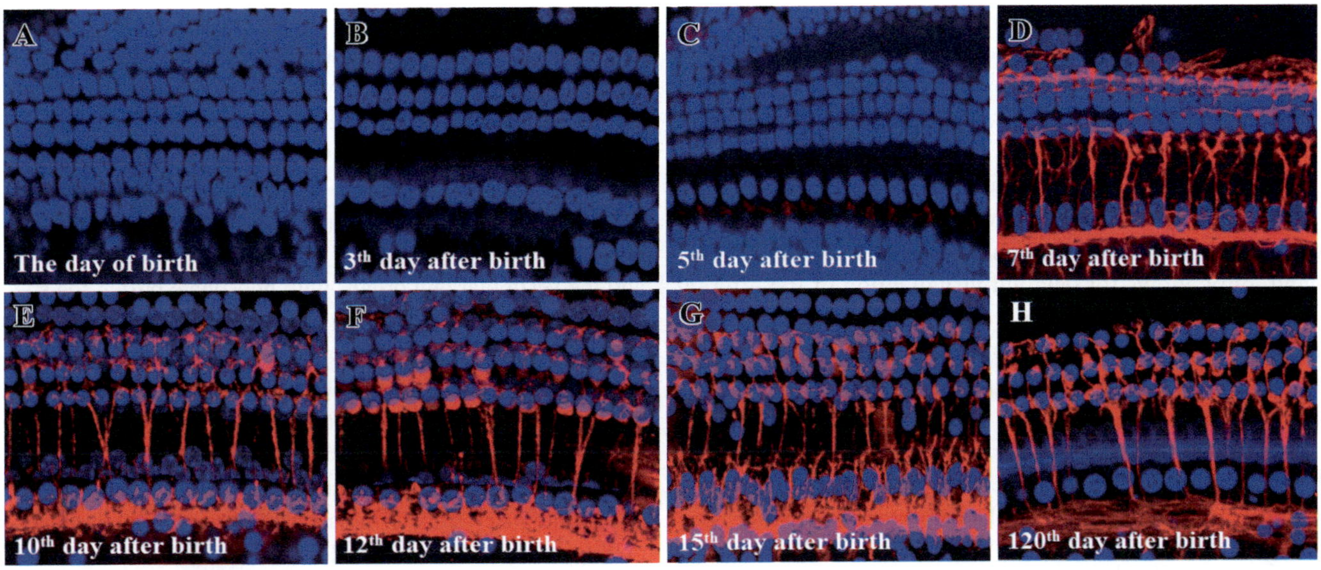

Fig. 12.24 The postnatal development of cochlear efferent innervation in rats using acetylcholinesterase immunohistochemistry. (**A–C**) The complete absence of acetylcholinesterase-positive fibers during the first five postnatal days indicates delayed efferent pathway maturation relative to afferent system development. (**D–H**) From postnatal day 7 onward, distinct efferent projections emerge, with acetylcholinesterase labeling revealing both the internal spiral bundle (innervating inner hair cell afferents) and tunnel-crossing fibers (targeting outer hair cells), confirming parallel development of medial and lateral olivocochlear systems (Reproduced with permission Ding et al. [13]). These temporal patterns suggest critical periods for efferent synapse formation that may influence auditory circuit refinement during early development

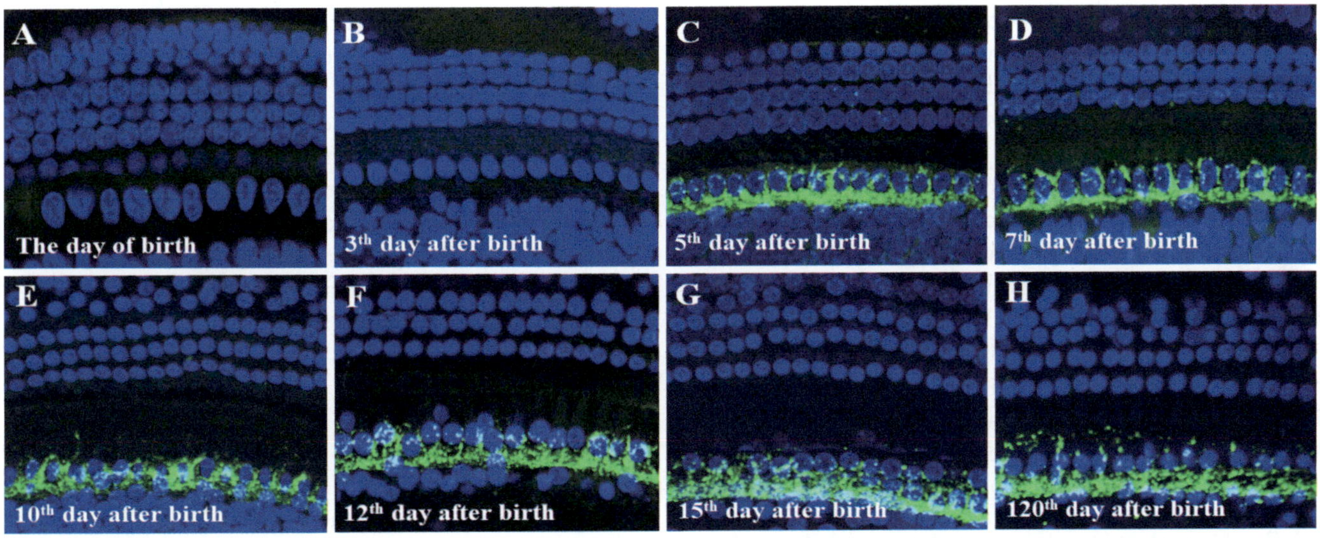

Fig. 12.25 The selective postnatal development of peptidergic efferent innervation in the rat using CGRP immunohistochemistry. (**A** and **B**) The absence of CGRP-positive terminal neurons during the first three days after birth indicates that peptidergic efferent synapses are not mature by postnatal day 3. (**C–H**) From postnatal day 5 to postnatal day 120, CGRP labeling was only present in the inner spiral bundle below the inner hair cells, but no CGRP expression was detected in the tunnel fibers leading to the outer hair cells. This suggests that CGRP is only expressed in the cochlear efferent nerve terminals of the lateral olive bundle but not in the efferent nerve system of the medial olive bundle (Reproduced with permission Ding et al. [13]). These findings confirm CGRP as a specific marker for the lateral olivocochlear system targeting inner hair cell afferents, while being absent from the medial olivocochlear pathway to outer hair cells, highlighting the neurochemical heterogeneity of efferent subsystems during cochlear development

release, postsynaptic receptor activation, and subsequent modulation of hair cell mechanoelectrical transduction.

Acetylcholinesterase immunohistochemistry provides comprehensive labeling of the efferent nervous system by targeting the enzyme's ubiquitous expression in efferent neuronal soma, axons, and synaptic terminals (Figs. 6.23, 8.23E, 11.5, and 11.6; Figs. 12.22A, B and 12.23A). In contrast, Calcitonin gene-related peptide (CGRP) immunostaining selectively identifies efferent synaptic terminals of lateral olivocochlear efferent terminals contacting type I afferent fibers beneath inner hair cells; however, the medial olivocochlear efferent nerve fibers and their synapses leading to the outer hair cells could not be labeled (Fig. 1.30; Figs. 12.22C and 12.23B). It can be seen that acetylcholinesterase staining enables complete efferent pathway tracing from cell bodies to nerve endings, CGRP immunohistochemistry, on the other hand, only allows for detailed visualization of the efferent synaptic regions of type I afferent nerve fibers at the base of inner hair cells [12, 51–53] (Fig. 12.22C). These complementary techniques thus serve different experimental purposes in efferent system analysis.

Acetylcholinesterase in the cochlear basilar membrane can be specifically labeled using cuprous sulfide histochemical staining. The fixed cochlear basilar membrane was immersed in 0.1 M acetate buffer for 30 min, and the cochlear basilar membrane was then immersed in freshly prepared acetylcholinesterase histochemical reaction solution (the acetylcholinesterase histochemical reaction solution contains 6.5 mL of 0.1 M acetate buffer (pH6.5), 5 mg of acetylthiocholine iodide, 0.5 mL of 0.1 M sodium citrate solution, 1 mL 30 mM copper sulfate, 1 mL of double distilled water, 1 mL 5 mM potassium ferricyanide solution) for 30 min. The cochlear basilar membrane was rinsed with 0.1 M acetate buffer and then immersed in 1% ammonium sulfide solution for 1 min to develop color. The specimen was fully rinsed with 0.1 M sodium nitrate solution, and then immersed in 0.1% silver nitrate solution for staining for 1 min. Finally, the sample was rinsed sed with sodium nitrate solution again, and the cochlear basilar membrane was routinely placed in a drop of glycerin on a glass slide as surface preparations. Under the light microscope, the cochlear efferent nerve fibers and their terminals were brownish-black deposits [5, 12, 52] (Figs. 6.23A, 8.22E, and 11.5; Fig. 12.22A). This multistep enzymatic method provides high-contrast labeling of cholinergic efferent innervation patterns throughout the organ of Corti, while staining labels are permanently preserved for subsequent light microscopy analysis.

Immunohistochemistry to label the acetylcholinesterase was performed by immersing the fixed cochlear basilar membrane and vestibular end-organs in a mouse anti- acetylcholinesterase antibody diluted 100-fold in a solution of 1% Triton X-100 and 0.3% goat serum in phosphate-buffered saline solution for 12 h in 4°C. After rinsing with PBS, the specimen was immersed in the secondary antibody solution of Alexa Fluor 555-conjugated goat anti-mouse IgG with 200 times dilution with 1% Triton X-100 and 0.3% goat serum solution prepared in phosphate buffer for 2 h. Observation and photography of the cochlear basilar membrane and vestibular end-organs were performed under a confocal microscope [5] (Figs. 12.22B, 12.23A, and 12.24). This method provides specific fluorescence labeling of efferent pathways while maintaining tissue integrity for high-resolution imaging of cholinergic innervation patterns in both auditory and vestibular systems.

Immunohistochemistry to visualize CGRP protein was performed by immersing the fixed cochlear basilar membrane or vestibular end-organs in the solution containing rabbit anti-CGRP primary antibody at a 1:100 dilution in a solution of 1% Triton X-100 and 5% donkey serum in phosphate buffer at 4°C for 12 h. After rinsing the cochlear basilar membrane and the vestibular end organs with phosphate buffer, the specimens were immersed in the solution containing secondary antibody of Alexa Fluor 488-conjugated donkey anti-rabbit IgG in a dilution of 400-fold for 2 h. The specimens were mounted on a glass slide and imaged under a confocal microscope [5] (Fig. 1.30; Fig. 12.22C, 12.23B, and 12.25). This optimized method provides sensitive and specific fluorescence labeling of peptidergic efferent terminals while maintaining tissue morphology for precise synaptic localization analysis in inner ear sensory epithelia. This also allows for precise comparison and analysis of acetylcholinergic and calcitonin gene-related peptide synapses in the cochlear efferent terminals (Figs. 12.24 and 12.25). Immunohistochemistry reveals distinct morphological representations of efferent innervation despite both targeting efferent pathways. While CGRP selectively labels specific synaptic terminals, acetylcholinesterase staining provides more comprehensive visualization of the entire efferent system, including neuronal soma, axonal projections, and synaptic endings. This broader coverage makes acetylcholinesterase histochemistry the preferred method for complete efferent pathway mapping, particularly when studying developmental or degenerative changes affecting multiple components of the efferent circuitry. The choice between these markers should therefore be guided by whether the research requires focused synaptic analysis (CGRP) or system-wide efferent evaluation (acetylcholinesterase).

References

1. Ding D, McFadden SL, Salvi R. Cochlear hair cell densities and inner-ear staining techniques. In: Willott JF, editor. Handbook of mouse auditory research from behavior to molecular biology. Boca Raton: CRC Press; 2001. p. 189–204.
2. Ding D, He J, Allman BL, et al. Cisplatin ototoxicity in rat cochlear organotypic cultures. Hear Res. 2011;282(1–2):196–203. https://doi.org/10.1016/j.heares.2011.08.002.
3. Ding D, Jiang H, Zhang J, et al. Cisplatin-induced vestibular hair cell lesion-less damage at high doses. J Otol. 2018;13(4):115–21. https://doi.org/10.1016/j.joto.2018.08.002.
4. Zhang J, Sun H, Salvi R, Ding D. Paraquat initially damages cochlear support cells leading to anoikis-like hair cell death. Hear Res. 2018;364:129–41. https://doi.org/10.1016/j.heares.2018.03.014.
5. Ding D, Zhang J, Jiang H, et al. Some ototoxic drugs destroy cochlear support cells before damaging sensory hair cells. Neurotox Res. 2020;37(3):743–52. https://doi.org/10.1007/s12640-020-00170-8.
6. Ding D, Chen GD, Zhang C, et al. Supporting cell involvement in cochlear damage and repair: novel insights from a quantitative

analysis of cyclodextrin-induced ototoxicity in mice. Hear Res. 2025;459:109201 https://doi.org/10.1016/j.heares.2025.109201.
7. Ye M, Zhang C, Ding D, et al. Organ of Corti macrophages: a distinct group of cochlear macrophages with potential roles in supporting cell degeneration and survival. Front Immunol. 2025;16:1617146 https://doi.org/10.3389/fimmu.2025.1617146.
8. Ding D, Zhao J, Huangfu M. Modified cochlear surface preparations. Zhonghua Er Bi Yan Hou Ke Za Zhi. 1981;16(4):207–9.
9. Ding D, Jiang H, Wang P, Salvi R. Cell death after co-administration of cisplatin and ethacrynic acid. Hear Res. 2007;226(1–2):129–39. https://doi.org/10.1016/j.heares.2006.07.015.
10. Ding D, Jiang H, Salvi RJ. Mechanisms of rapid sensory hair-cell death following co-administration of gentamicin and ethacrynic acid. Hear Res. 2010;259(1–2):16–23. https://doi.org/10.1016/j.heares.2009.08.008.
11. Ding D, Manohar S, Jiang H, Salvi R. Hydroxypropyl-beta-cyclodextrin causes massive damage to the developing auditory and vestibular system. Hear Res. 2020;396:108073. https://doi.org/10.1016/j.heares.2020.108073.
12. Ding D, Zhang J, Liu F, et al. Antioxidative stress-induced damage in cochlear explants. J Otol.. 2020;15(1):36–40. https://doi.org/10.1016/j.joto.2019.11.005.
13. Ding D, Zhang J, Yang K, et al. Growth and development process of Calcitonin Gene-Related Peptide and Acetylcholinesterase in rat cochlear efferent nervous system. Chin J Otorhinolaryngol Skull Base Surg. 2020;28(6):662–8. https://doi.org/10.3969/i.issn.1006-7299.2020.06.012.
14. Ding D, Li P, Qi W, Zhang J. Different patterns of age-related damage to cochlear hair cells in different species of experimental animals. Chin J Otorhinolaryngol Skull Base Surg. 2023;29(4):7–13. https://doi.org/10.11798/j.issn.1007-1520.202323084.
15. Ding D, Manohar S, Kador PF, Salvi R. Multifunctional redox modulator prevents blast-induced loss of cochlear and vestibular hair cells and auditory spiral ganglion neurons. Sci Rep. 2024;14(1):15296. https://doi.org/10.1038/s41598-024-66406-1.
16. Ding D, Shi L, Xing Y, et al. Secondary neural damage in the inner ear induced by intratympanic gentamicin injection. Chin J Otorhinolaryngol Skull Base Surg. 2024;30(6):11–19. https://doi.org/10.11798/j.issn.1007-1520.202424356.
17. Ding D, Jiang H, Chen GD, et al. N-acetyl-cysteine prevents age-related hearing loss and the progressive loss of inner hair cells in gamma-glutamyl transferase 1 deficient mice. Aging (Albany NY). 2016;8(4):730–50. https://doi.org/10.18632/aging.100927.
18. Ding D, Jiang H, Manohar S, et al. Spatiotemporal developmental upregulation of prestin correlates with the severity and location of cyclodextrin-induced outer hair cell loss and hearing loss. Front Cell Dev Biol. 2021;9:643709. https://doi.org/10.3389/fcell.2021.643709.
19. Ding D, Jiang H, Fu Y, et al. Ototoxic effects of carboplatin in organotypic cultures in chinchillas and rats. J Otol. 2012;7(2):92–101. https://doi.org/10.1016/S1672-2930(12)50023-1.
20. Wu X, Ding D, Jiang H, et al. Transfection using hydroxyapatite nanoparticles in the inner ear via an intact round window membrane in chinchilla. J Nanopart Res. 2012;14(6):708. https://doi.org/10.1007/s11051-011-0708-1.
21. Deng L, Ding D, Su J, Manohar S, Salvi R. Salicylate selectively kills cochlear spiral ganglion neurons by paradoxically up-regulating superoxide. Neurotox Res. 2013;24(3):307–19. https://doi.org/10.1007/s12640-013-9384-5.
22. Ding D, Qi W, Yu D, et al. Addition of exogenous NAD+ prevents mefloquine-induced neuroaxonal and hair cell degeneration through reduction of caspase-3-mediated apoptosis in cochlear organotypic cultures. PLoS One. 2013;8(11):e79817. https://doi.org/10.1371/journal.pone.0079817.
23. Ding D, Salvi R, Roth JA. Cellular localization and developmental changes of the different isoforms of divalent metal transporter 1 (DMT1) in the inner ear of rats. Biometals. 2014;27(1):125–34. https://doi.org/10.1007/s10534-013-9692-5.
24. Ding D, Salvi R, Roth JA. Cellular localization and developmental changes of Zip8, Zip14 and transferrin receptor 1 in the inner ear of rats. Biometals. 2014;27(4):731–44. https://doi.org/10.1007/s10534-014-9765-0.
25. Qi W, Ding D, Zhu H, et al. Efficient siRNA transfection to the inner ear through the intact round window by a novel proteidic delivery technology in the chinchilla. Gene Ther. 2014;21(1):10–18. https://doi.org/10.1038/gt.2013.49.
26. Li P, Ding D, Salvi R, Roth JA. Cobalt-induced ototoxicity in rat postnatal cochlear organotypic cultures. Neurotox Res. 2015;28(3):209–21. https://doi.org/10.1007/s12640-015-9538-8.
27. Gao K, Ding D, Sun H, Roth J, Salvi R. Kanamycin damages early postnatal, but not adult spiral ganglion neurons. Neurotox Res. 2017;32(4):603–13. https://doi.org/10.1007/s12640-017-9773-2.
28. Ding D, Prolla T, Someya S, Manohar S, Salvi R. Roles of Bak and Sirt3 in paraquat-induced cochlear hair cell damage. Neurotox Res. 2021;39(4):1227–37. https://doi.org/10.1007/s12640-021-00366-6.
29. Ding D, Qi W, Jiang H, Salvi R. Excitotoxic damage to auditory nerve afferents and spiral ganglion neurons is correlated with developmental upregulation of AMPA and KA receptors. Hear Res. 2021;411:108358. https://doi.org/10.1016/j.heares.2021.108358.
30. Li L, Chen D, Lin X, et al. Antioxidative stress-induced destruction to cochlear cells caused by blind antioxidant therapy. Otolaryngol Head Neck Surg. 2024;170(5):1421–29. https://doi.org/10.1002/ohn.659.
31. Ding D, Stracher A, Salvi RJ. Leupeptin protects cochlear and vestibular hair cells from gentamicin ototoxicity. Hear Res. 2002;164(1–2):115–26. https://doi.org/10.1016/s0378-5955(01)00417-8.
32. Ding D, Seigel GM, Salvi RJ. Migration of R28 retinal precursor cells into cochlear and vestibular organs. J Otol. 2006;1(1):51–56. https://doi.org/10.13489/j.cnki.11-4883/r.2006.01.009.
33. Qi W, Ding D, Salvi RJ. Cytotoxic effects of dimethyl sulphoxide (DMSO) on cochlear organotypic cultures. Hear Res. 2008;236(1–2):52–60. https://doi.org/10.1016/j.heares.2007.12.002.
34. Ding D, Qi W, Yu D, Jiang H, Salvi R. Ototoxic effects of mefloquine in cochlear organotypic cultures. J Otol. 2009;4(2):76–85. https://doi.org/10.13489/j.cnki.11-4883/r.2009.02.008.
35. Ding D, Roth J, Salvi R. Manganese is toxic to spiral ganglion neurons and hair cells in vitro. Neurotoxicology. 2011;32(2):233–41. https://doi.org/10.1016/j.neuro.2010.12.003.
36. Wu X, Ding D, Sun H, et al. Lead neurotoxicity in rat cochlear organotypic cultures. J Otol. 2011;6(2):45–52. https://doi.org/10.13489/j.cnki.11-4883/r.2011.02.002.
37. Watanuki K, Kawamoto K, Katagiri S. Surface structure of the cochlea. Tohoku J Exp Med. 1970;100(4):359–68. https://doi.org/10.1620/tjem.100.359.
38. Guo Y, Ding D, Wang Q, Zhu H. Experimental observation on gentamicin vestibular damage alarming deafness. Chin J Integr Trad West Med Otorhinolaryngol. 2000;8(3):108–110. https://doi.org/10.16542/j.cnki.issn.1007-4856.2000.03.002.
39. McFadden SL, Ding D, Jiang H, Woo JM, Salvi RJ. Chinchilla models of selective cochlear hair cell loss. Hear Res. 2002;174(1–2):230–38. https://doi.org/10.1016/s0378-5955(02)00697-4.
40. Ding D, McFadden SL, Browne RW, Salvi RJ. Late dosing with ethacrynic acid can reduce gentamicin concentration in perilymph and protect cochlear hair cells. Hear Res. 2003;185(1–2):90–96. https://doi.org/10.1016/s0378-5955(03)00258-2.
41. Ding D, Jiang H, Salvi R. Cochlear spiral ganglion neuron degeneration following cyclodextrin-induced hearing loss. Hear Res. 2021;400:108125. https://doi.org/10.1016/j.heares.2020.108125.
42. Ding D, Wang J, Hu BH, Zheng XY, Salvi R. Carboplatin-induced early changes of dehydrogenase activity in chinchilla hair cells. Chin J Integr Trad West Med Otorhinolaryngol. 1998;6(1):20–23.

43. Ding D, Jiang H, Wang J, et al. Inner hair cell missing potentiates noise induced outer hair cell lesion. J Audiol Speech Pathol. 2004;12(6):413–15.
44. Yuan F, Ding DL, Wang J, et al. [Inner hair cells loss by carboplatin and the changes of cochlear compound action potential in chinchillas]. Zhonghua Er Bi Yan Hou Tou Jing Wai Ke Za Zhi. 2020;55(5):506–13. https://doi.org/10.3760/cma.j.cn.115330-20200426-00332.
45. Liu H, Ding D, Sun H, et al. Cadmium-induced ototoxicity in rat cochlear organotypic cultures. Neurotox Res. 2014;26(2):179–89. https://doi.org/10.1007/s12640-014-9461-4.
46. Wang L, Ding D, Salvi R, Roth JA. Nicotinamide adenine dinucleotide prevents neuroaxonal degeneration induced by manganese in cochlear organotypic cultures. Neurotoxicology. 2014;40:65–74. https://doi.org/10.1016/j.neuro.2013.11.007.
47. Yu J, Ding D, Sun H, Salvi R, Roth JA. Neurotoxicity of trimethyltin in rat cochlear organotypic cultures. Neurotox Res. 2015;28(1):43–54. https://doi.org/10.1007/s12640-015-9531-2.
48. Ye H, Xing Y, Zhang L, et al. Bilirubin-induced neurotoxic and ototoxic effects in rat cochlear and vestibular organotypic cultures. Neurotoxicology. 2019;71:75–86. https://doi.org/10.1016/j.neuro.2018.12.004.
49. Martinez-Monedero R, Liu C, Weisz C, et al. GluA2-containing AMPA receptors distinguish ribbon-associated from ribbonless afferent contacts on rat cochlear hair cells. eNeuro. 2016;3(2):1–17. https://doi.org/10.1523/ENEURO.0078-16.2016.
50. Liberman MC, Kujawa SG. Cochlear synaptopathy in acquired sensorineural hearing loss: manifestations and mechanisms. Hear Res. 2017;349:138–47. https://doi.org/10.1016/j.heares.2017.01.003.
51. Ding D, Zheng XY, Hu BH, Henderson D, Richard S. Quantitative analysis of cochlear efferent fibers in the tunnel of Corti. Acta Otorhinolaryngol. 1998;12(2):65–68.
52. Zheng XY, Henderson D, McFadden SL, Ding DL, Salvi RJ. Auditory nerve fiber responses following chronic cochlear deefferentation. J Comp Neurol. 1999;406(1):72–86. https://doi.org/10.1002/(sici)1096-9861(19990329)406:1<72::aid-cne5>3.3.co;2-1.
53. Dickerson IM, Bussey-Gaborski R, Holt JC, Jordan PM, Luebke AE. Maturation of suprathreshold auditory nerve activity involves cochlear CGRP-receptor complex formation. Physiol Rep. 2016;4(14):e12869. https://doi.org/10.14814/phy2.12869.

GPSR Compliance

The European Union's (EU) General Product Safety Regulation (GPSR) is a set of rules that requires consumer products to be safe and our obligations to ensure this.

If you have any concerns about our products, you can contact us on ProductSafety@springernature.com

In case Publisher is established outside the EU, the EU authorized representative is:

Springer Nature Customer Service Center GmbH
Europaplatz 3
69115 Heidelberg, Germany

Batch number: 10731528

Printed by Printforce, the Netherlands